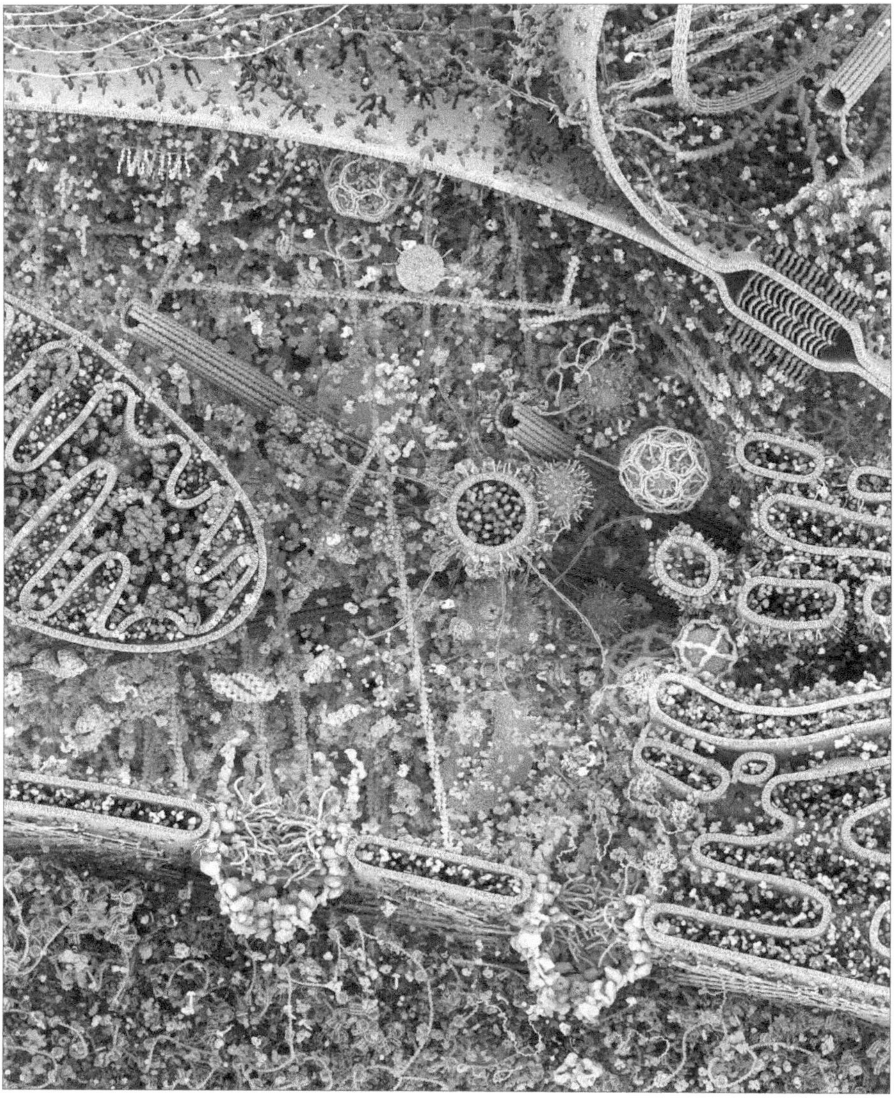

Interior of a Eukaryotic Cell

"Transformation of the Cellular Landscape through a Eukaryotic Cell" by Evan Ingersoll, Ingersoll Gael McGill – Digizyme's Custom Maya Molecular Software, Biologia Al Instante

The human body consists of 37.2 trillion cells.

Thanks to Clifford Gomes: "This image shows the complex landscape of a single cell in your biological body, and no one has a right to do anything to it without your consent . . . Physical sovereignty is the most important political battlefield in your life."

Geoengineered Transhumanism

How the Environment Has Been Weaponized by Chemicals, Electromagnetism & Nanotechnology for Synthetic Biology

Elana Freeland

Sequel to

Under An Ionized Sky: From Chemtrails to Space Fence Lockdown (2018)

Chemtrails, HAARP, and the Full Spectrum Dominance of Planet Earth (2014)

Geoengineered Transhumanism: How the Environment Has Been Weaponized by Chemicals, Electromagnetics, & Nanotechnology for Synthetic Biology

Paperback ISBN 9780578927053
Ebook ISBN 9780578927060

Front cover art by Ethan Clark (*www.BroadastTheory.com*)
Back cover art: Rudolf Steiner's drawing of the *Doppelgänger* or Double, *Studie_Grünes Fenster_Norden.tif.*

Cover design: Robert Ross, Last Word Books & Press, Olympia, WA

The terrain is everything; the germ is nothing.

— Claude Bernard (1813-1879), physician / physiologist

Dedication

To early anti-geoengineering pioneers,
several of whom have died for speaking out:

Carolyn Williams Palit ("I am being disappeared"); naturopath Gwen Scott; Santa Fe radio personality Alan Hutner; industrial polymer chemist R. Michael Castle; Keynote Speaker at the 60th UN DPI/NGO Conference on Climate Change in New York (September 5-7, 2007) Rosalind Peterson; activist Harriett Fels; A.C. Griffith, NSA; futurist-scientist Fred Bell, PhD; former LAPD journalist Mike Ruppert; former FBI Special Agent Ted Gunderson; DARPA RF engineer "Gnarly" Carly Lebrun; aerospace illustrator Mark McCandlish; filmmaker Michael J. Murphy; Behind the Green Mask author Rosa Koire; Canadian activist Suzanne Maher of Bye Bye Blue Sky. . .

. . . and more.

Acknowledgements

CLIFFORD AND CAROL CARNICOM FOR the years of expertise-sharing and team work, webmistress Frankie Styles for my outrageously creative website, Diana Thatcher for proofreading beyond the call of duty, Kate Magdalena Willens for her generous support of this book, David Luxton for photo dpi enhancement, Chase Patton for photo attributions, Tony Pantalleresco for nanotech email clarification, Frank Dauenhauer at https://rudolfsteinerbookstore.com and *MysTech* magazine, farmer Galilee Carlisle for organic produce, activist Rebecca Campbell for neighborly backup; local and far-flung friends who know what I'm looking for and share their ongoing research, reading and thinking; and the far-seeing who put on conferences and host visionary radio shows.

My greatest thanks go to the spiritual world that keeps me safe and dedicated, Rudolf Steiner and the Michaelic School, Christ and the Holy Spirit; family and close friends over the years who continue to carry me in their hearts, despite my imperfections; the astounding ideas that continue to live and breathe even in this difficult era, replenishing my deep energy so I can continue to serve our precious evolving humanity.

I invite those who follow my work to find updates at https://www.elanafreeland.com where my email and PayPal button are available.

Keeping faith for the future . . .

Table of Contents

Index, Remedies and Resources are available at elanafreeland.com

Preface

The Wuhan Showcase

Chinese New Year 2020

> *. . . the cruelty of the heavens—and perhaps, in some measure, that of men, too—was so great and so malevolent that from March to the following July, between the fury of the pestilence [the Black Plague of 1348] and the fact that many of the sick were poorly cared for or abandoned in their need because of the fears of those who were healthy, it has been reliably calculated that more than one hundred thousand human beings were deprived of their lives within the walls of the city of Florence, although before the outbreak of the plague perhaps no one would have thought it contained so many.*
>
> – Giovanni Boccaccio, *The Decameron*, 1353

So off went the Emperor in procession under his splendid canopy. Everyone in the streets and the windows said, "Oh, how fine are the Emperor's new clothes! Don't they fit him to perfection? And see his long train!"

> *Nobody would confess that he couldn't see anything, for that would prove him either unfit for his position, or a fool. No costume the Emperor had worn before was ever such a complete success.*
>
> *"But he hasn't got anything on," a little child said.*
>
> *"Did you ever hear such innocent prattle?" said its father.*
>
> *And one person whispered to another what the child had said, "He hasn't anything on. A child says he hasn't anything on."*
>
> *"But he hasn't got anything on!" the whole town cried out at last.*
>
> *The Emperor shivered, for he suspected they were right. But he thought, "This procession has got to go on." So he walked more proudly than ever, as his noblemen held high the train that wasn't there at all.*
>
> – Hans Christian Andersen, "The Emperor's New Clothes," 1837

NINETEEN YEARS AFTER 9/11—A METONIC cycle in astronomical parlance—a most extraordinary world psyop of fear and economic destruction was loosed. Novelist Dean Koontz foretold it in his 1981 book *The Eyes of Darkness*[1]:

---

1 The CIA "culture wars" have entailed control over various writers, cartoonists, artists, musicians, etc.

[Carl Dombey, PhD:] ". . . It was around then that a Chinese scientist named Li Chen defected to the United States, carrying a diskette record of China's most important and dangerous new biological weapon in a decade. They call the stuff 'Wuhan-400' because it was developed at their RDNA labs outside of the city of Wuhan, and it was the four-hundredth viable strain of manmade microorganisms created at that research center.

"Wuhan-400 is a perfect weapon. It afflicts only human beings. No other living creature can carry it. And like syphilis, Wuhan-400 can't survive outside a living human body for longer than a minute, which means it can't permanently contaminate objects or entire places the way anthrax and other virulent microorganisms can. And when the host expires, Wuhan-400 within him perishes a short while later, as soon as the temperature of the corpse drops below eighty-six degrees Fahrenheit. Do you see the advantage of all this?"

. . . Elliot knew what the scientist meant. "If I understand you, the Chinese could use Wuhan-400 to wipe out a city or a country, and then there wouldn't be any need for them to conduct a tricky and expensive decontamination before they moved in and took over the conquered territory."

The fact that the Wuhan event that occurred exactly on the Chinese Lunar New Year of the Rat had been forecast in a work of Western fiction two Metonic cycles before points to how well planned it all was. Rather like the Spanish flu (1918-1920) that began in America and not in Spain 99 years before, lies and obscuration have been present from the very beginning so as to churn out public confusion and fear, as is proper to carefully manufactured psychological operations (psyops).

Ordo ab chao. Subvert order to produce chaos so the solution can be manipulated.

What actually arose in Wuhan? From Italy in September 2019 to China and South Korea by early March 2020, was there a virus at all, other than a normal coronavirus flu blown out of proportion by a 5G flick of the switch quickly picked up by globalist-controlled media? From thousands of coronavirus, only six have supposedly infected humans, four of which cause the common cold. The final two are deadlier because they were weaponized years ago: SARS (severe acute respiratory syndrome) and MERS (Middle East respiratory syndrome). Had a weaponized SARS-Cov-2 gain-of-function version been loosed[2]?

---

2 See "Unexpected detection of SARS-Cov-2 antibodies in the pre-pandemic period in Italy," National Tumors Institute, Italian Ministry of Health, November 11, 2020.

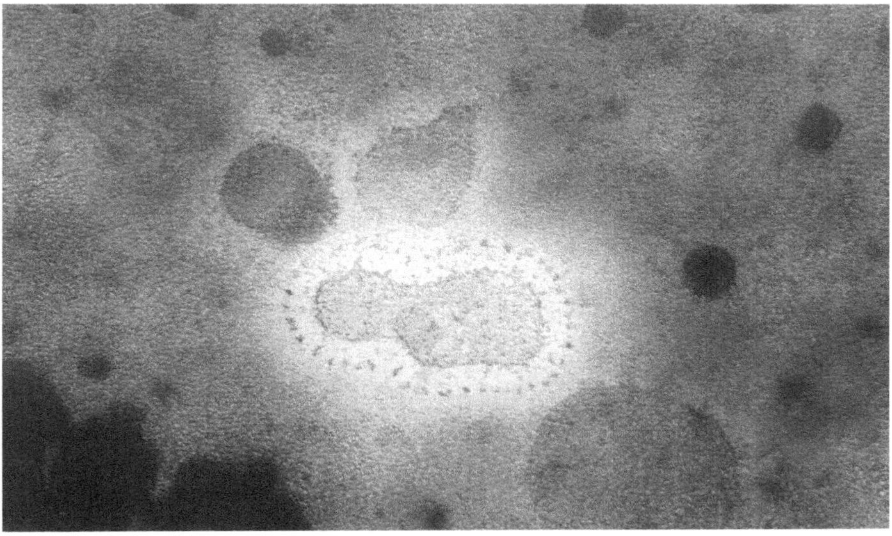

Coronavirus.
http://www.gettyimages.com/detail/news-photo/the-crown-shape-of-the-virus-gives-its-name-coronavirus-news-photo/151036463

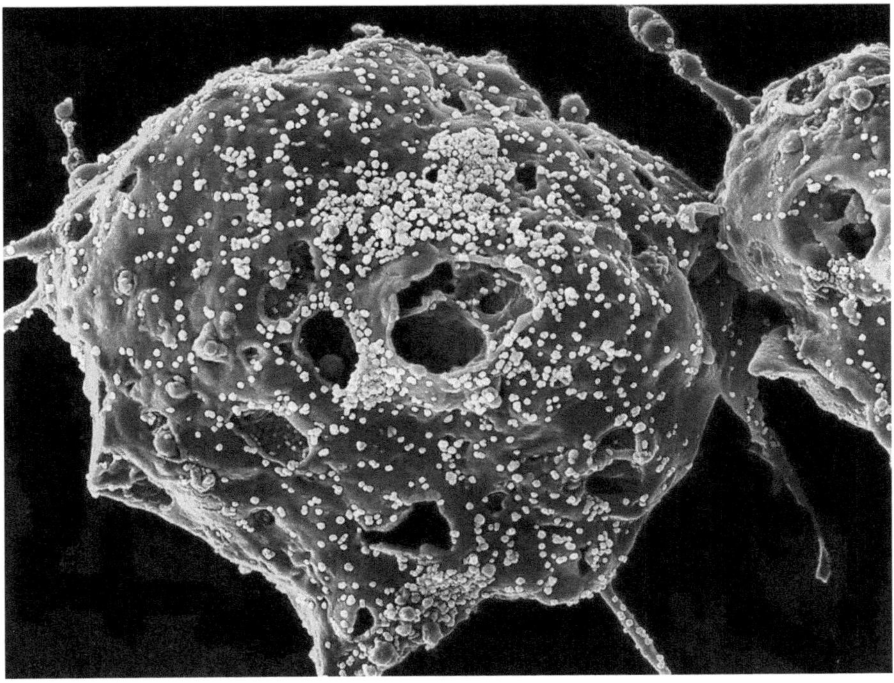

MERS (Middle East Respiratory Syndrome) virus particles (yellow) attached to the surface of an infected VERO E6 cell (blue). Captured and color-enhanced at the NIAID Integrated Research Facility, Fort Detrick, Maryland.

As the Spanish flu announced electricity and 9/11 announced scalar weapons, the Wuhan event announced digital synthetic biology (*synbio*) transmission. Genetics, geoengineering, and artificial intelligence for a world pandemic psyop based not on a virus but on a *nano-synthetic*, the fusing of biological and robotic for "a construct, a new life form," according to Celeste Solum.[3]

A healthy blood cell wall is comprised of plasma which responds to frequency to uptake and discharge gases, nutrients and waste. Natural charges are miniscule compared to mm wave (5G) frequency which is raw kinetic energy that does catastrophic damage. It blasts these ion gates (gates of the gods) wide open to allow pathogenic sRNA[4] *to pass, and also fractures healthy DNA. What you end up with is sRNA exposed to fractured DNA recombined into the biological information.*

– Sine Nomine, Facebook

The media lead-up to what happened in Wuhan—not exactly the same as what happened in Italy, Seattle, New York City, etc.—began with warnings in the West about China's giant telecom Huawei and how China was taking the lead in 5G infrastructure. It wasn't just about the threaten to the global market; it was about technology and the future. Huawei had its own 5G plans, software backdoors, and Space Fence objectives—all, of course, subject to Chinese Communist Party (CCP) while Western telecoms were subject to their own military intelligence tech specifications regarding sensors, high data rate communications, security industries, aerospace robotics, and machine learning AI.

XinhuaNet (May 27, 2019) announced 300+ 5G base stations in Hubei Province—full 5G signal coverage in prefecture-level cities like the capital city of Wuhan: smart education, smart medicine, smart everything up and running. Five months later:

> Wuhan City, the capital of Hubei, is expected to have 10,000 5G base stations by the end of 2019, said Song Qizhu, head of Hubei Provincial Communication Administration . . . China Mobile Hubei Branch has activated 1,580 5G base stations in the city, as of mid-October . . .[5]

---

3 "Former FEMA operative Celeste Solum talks with David Icke," 20 November 2020.

4 sRNA: originally soluble RNA, now transfer RNA (tRNA).

5 "Central China province launches commercial 5G applications." XinhuaNet, October 31,

The next day, CNN didn't even mention Wuhan. (Was it because of American involvement in the labs there?)

> 5G commercial services are now available in 50 cities, including Beijing, Shanghai, Guangzhou and Shenzhen . . . In Shanghai, nearly 12,000 5G base stations have been activated . . . China's commercial network is the biggest, according to Bernstein Research, giving the county [sic] more influence over the technology's global evolution.[6]

In the fall of 2019, all Chinese citizens underwent inoculation with Sinovac (private) and Sinopharm (state) vaccines containing replicating, digitized *synbio* RNA but not mRNA; after studying Pfizer and Moderna vaccine outcomes, mRNA "entered the clinical trial stage" in April 2021.[7] On December 30, 2019, it went public that ophthalmologist Li Wenliang had seven cases of severe acute respiratory syndrome (SARS) quarantined in Wuhan. Panic ensued. Ten days later, Wenliang and his parents became ill. Tests for SARS-CoV-1 were negative, perhaps because it was atypical pneumonia, *SARS symptoms being the same as those of atypical pneumonia.* On January 30, things were kicked into high gear: thanks to German virologist Christian Drosten's scientifically untested fast-track PCR test, Wenliang's SARS test came back positive, and Wenliang died not long after.

Back in 2003, it had been similar: 800 people came down with atypical pneumonia labeled SARS CoV-1. The multitude of causes for atypical pneumonia—*none of which are viral*—was laid at the door of the usual "germ warfare" paranoia regarding viruses and bacteria instead of out of balance, EM-weakened cells. According to German molecular biologist Stefan Lanka, MD, it is "serious medical malpractice" not to consider the possibility of atypical pneumonia in the pell-mell quest of a "new virus" (and lucrative vaccines and patents) in that the wrong diagnosis often ends in wrong treatment and death. Dr. Lanka also points out that scotch-taping together short SARS CoV-1 gene sequences does not take the place of isolating a single SARS virus or the discovery of a complete genome.[8]

2019.

6 Sherisse Pham, "China just launched the world's largest 5G network." CNN, November 1, 2019.

7 Joe McDonald and Huizhong Wu, "Top Chinese official admits vaccines have low effectiveness." AP, April 10, 2021.

8 Stefan Lanka, MD, "The Virus Misconception, Part II: The beginning and the end of the corona crisis." WISSENSCHAFFTPLUS magazin, February 2020.

The Thousand Talents nano connection

Most of the patents and papers connected with synthetic biology, bioengineering, neuroengineering, and artificial intelligence feature Chinese names, American universities, and U.S. government "public-private partnerships." China's Thousand Talents Plan has paid thousands of international scientists working in sensitive U.S.-funded research programs to send their research to Chinese "shadow labs." Thus far, 54 scientists who received $165 million in grants from the National Institutes of Health (NIH) have been fired for failing to disclose ties to China, leaving 245 Chinese and American "scientists of concern").[9] By December 2020, after a year of lockdowns and growing public suspicion regarding the "pandemic" and Chinese involvement, more than 1,000 Chinese military-linked researchers had left the U.S.,

> . . . a "vast network of suspected undercover People's Liberation Army researchers across the country" . . . The arrests formed part of a spate of prosecutions brought by the Justice Department targeting the Chinese regime's broad efforts to steal U.S. technology and research. The Trump administration also forced the Chinese consulate in Houston to close in July, saying it was a center for espionage and malign influence operations. William Evanina, director of the National Counterintelligence and Security Center, said that of the 1,000 PLA-linked researchers, he's most concerned about the risks associated with graduate-level students.[10]

Harvard University chemistry chair Charles Lieber was such a Thousand Talents scientist. Lieber and a Chinese researcher at Boston University—previously a lieutenant in the Chinese military—would eventually be arrested for supplying a foreign government with American innovations in chemistry, nanotechnology, polymer studies, robotics, computer science, biomedical research, etc. Lieber's work pivoted around nanotechnology—nanowires for a transistor able to enter and probe cells, semiconductor switches to enable two-way cell communication (cell signaling), ultra-flexible 3D mesh scaffolding with hundreds of remote-controlled nanobots fused with living tissue. Lieber's Harvard team—Jia Liu, Tian-Ming Fu, Zengguang Cheng, Guosong Hong, Tao Zhou, Lihua Jin, Madhavi Duvvuri, Zhe Jiang, Peter Kruskal, Chong Xie, Zhigang Suo, and Ying Fang—concentrated on electronic neural mesh that fully integrates with the biological web of neurons in the brain. Lieber was obviously heading for the same "cyborg" Transhumanism that Elon Musk's "neural lace" was in service to "cyborg" Transhumanism:

---

9 Adam Kredo, "54 Scientists Given NIH Grants Fired for Failure to Disclose Foreign Ties." FreeBeacon.com, June 14, 2020.

10 Cathy He, "Over 1,000 Military-Linked Researchers Have Left the US Since Federal Crackdown: DOJ Official." Epoch Times, December 2, 2020.

It's hard to say where this work will take us, but in the end I believe our unique approach will take us on a path to do something really revolutionary . . . By focusing on the nanoelectronic connections between cells, we can do things no one has done before. We're really going into a new size regime for not only the device that records or stimulates cellular activity, but also for the whole circuit. We can make it really look and behave like smart, soft biological material, and integrate it with cells and cellular networks at the whole-tissue level . . . But if you want to study the brain or develop the tools to explore the brain-machine interface, you need to stick something into the body . . .[11]

In 2015, the *Harvard Gazette* did a glowing feature entitled "Injectable device delivers nano-view of the brain" (Peter Reuell, June 8, 2015). Lieber was praised for his work on the mesh electronic scaffolding "almost invisible and very flexible, like polymer . . . connected to devices and used to monitor neural activity, stimulate tissues, or even promote regeneration of neurons." Lieber used heart and nerve cells to create "cyborg" tissue and record the electrical signals generated by the tissue.

To create the scaffold, researchers lay out a mesh of nanowires sandwiched in layers of organic polymer. The first layer is then dissolved ["the fabrication substrate"], leaving the flexible mesh, which can be drawn into a needle and administered like any other injection.

Harvard and China had worked out the patent arrangements for Lieber's scaffolding technology, and yet we are expected to believe that Harvard University, the NIH, Department of Defense (DoD), and U.S. Air Force, knew nothing of Lieber's 2012 Thousand Talents contract with Wuhan University in 2012 or his formal relationship with Wuhan University through 2017 to the tune of $50,000 per month, plus $150,000 living expenses and $1.5 million for his Wuhan research lab.[12] How could anyone believe that a Communist nation would allow their best and brightest to attend U.S. universities and work in U.S. labs without political strings? It was similar to the 1940s and 1950s when Chinese grad students at California Institute of Technology were involved in the GALCIT Rocket Project, along with Paperclip Nazis. Was it just coincidental that the world-renowned German scientific publishing house Springer-Verlag relocated to Wuhan? In August

11 American Chemical Society, "On the Frontiers of Cyborg Science." Newswise.com, 29 July 2014.

12 Aruna Viswanatha and Kate O'Keeffe, "Harvard Chemistry Chairman Charged on Alleged Undisclosed Ties to China," Wall Street Journal, January 28, 2020.

2018, Wuhan hosted the International Conference on Control Science and Systems Engineering, joined at the hip with the China Aerospace Laboratory of Social System Engineering (CALSSE) and China Academy of Aerospace Systems Science and Engineering in Beijing.[13]

Wuhan appears to have been chosen to lead the way to a 5G "global reset."

In 2017, via immunologist Anthony Fauci, director of the National Institute of Allergy and Infectious Diseases since 1984, the shady NIH lifted the "unusual three-year moratorium on federal funding" for research into influenza, SARS, and MERS.[14] Was lifting the ban about moving research into new "gain of function" pandemic strains ($3.7 million taxpayer money) from the U.S. Army Medical Research Institute of Infectious Diseases (USAMRIID) at Fort Detrick to the University of North Carolina at Chapel Hill biowarfare lab, and finally to the Wuhan Lab built by Charles Lieber[15]?

The creation of mass electronic scaffolding sounds like Morgellons-hydrogel scaffolding. The presence of the U.S. Air Force and the word "implant" suggest that Lieber's "flexible mesh . . . drawn into a needle and administered like any other injection" (such as Elon Musk's "minor surgery" for his "neural lace") is actually referencing "cyborg tissue" or "fabrication substrate" materials aerially delivered by geoengineers for more than two decades. Needles and minor surgeries may be called for in regenerative medicine, but for the billions on planet Earth, fabrication substrate must be remotely manipulated by means of 5G / 6G armed environments. This was what spoke loud and clear in the early Wuhan footage of people dropping like flies once the 5G switch was flipped.

5G-IoT / 60 GHz / O2

> *Breathing pure oxygen lowers the oxygen content of tissues; breathing rarefied air or air with carbon dioxide oxygenates and energizes the tissues. If this seems upside-down, it's because medical physiology has been taught upside-down, and respiratory physiology holds the key to the special functions of all the organs and too many of their basic pathological changes.*
>
> – Ray Peat, PhD, biologist (*http://raypeat.com*)

13 See Amazing Polly's YouTube "Maxwell, Epstein, and the Control of Science since WW2," July 11, 2020. For Wuhan, begin at ~24:00.

14 "NIH Lifts Ban On Research That Could Make Deadly Viruses Even Worse." NPR.org, December 19, 2017.

15 See the transcript of the interview with biological warfare expert Francis Boyle, PhD: Mike Adams, "Full transcript of 'smoking gun' bombshell interview: Prof. Francis Boyle exposes the bioweapons origins of the CoVid-19 coronavirus," Natural News, February 20, 2020.

At the very beginning of 2019, the *South China Morning Post* announced the completion of the 3,700 square kilometer (1,400 square mile) Wireless Electromagnetic Method (WEM) phased array antenna (ELF waves 0.1-300 Hz). The exact site was not disclosed, but it was in the part of central China that includes Wuhan's Hubei province.[16]

Throughout 2019, state-of-the-art 5G, its Internet of Things (IoT), and thousands of base stations were installed in and around Wuhan. *In the fall of 2019, the Chinese people underwent mandatory vaccines containing synthetic DNA ("synbio").*[17] By the end of 2019, the stage was set. On December 31, 2019, China announced a pneumonia cluster of *novel infectious coronavirus* in Wuhan. The first American case was reported January 20, 2020, then two Chinese tourists in Rome tested positive—and the U.S. and Italy were off to the races. By March, 110 nations were reporting infections. The TikTok footage of men in HazMat suits picking up people dropping to the pavement in Wuhan went out on January 24, 2020. The sudden collapse pattern did not really fit with fever, dry cough, shortness of breath and breathing difficulties, but *novel infectious coronavirus* was blamed, anyway.

On February 22, 2020, Dana Ashlie's one-hour video calling attention to the 5G / 60 GHz oxygen factor behind the early Wuhan scenes went viral. Were we watching the very moment that the new massive 5G system was switched on in the Wuhan 5G Demonstration Zone? Reports of large numbers of crows circling and fish jumping out of lakes and waterways were everywhere in Hubei province. Half a world away, we watched as Chinese people in extreme respiratory distress flooded hospital emergency centers, experiencing loss of smell and taste, fever, aches, fatigue, dry cough, diarrhea, stroke, seizure, "fizzing,"[18] an electric or burning sensation on the skin), and the breathlessness of oxygen distress.

In early April 2020, emergency medical physician Cameron Kyle-Sidell at Maimonides Medical Center in Brooklyn, New York noticed that lungs of COVID-19 victims were damaged, and their blood registered very low in oxygen. In fact, they seemed to be suffering oxygen starvation (hypoxia), as if they were in a jet at 35,000 feet with the cabin pressure dropping. Patients were breathing, but their oxygen was low, and ventilators made them *over*-breathe. Inadequate oxygen delivery to cells is neither acute respiratory dis-

16 Stephen Chen, "China has built an antenna five times the size of New York – but at what risk?" South China Morning Post, 11 January 2019. In Chemtrails, HAARP (2014), see the Google Earth photo of China's "HAARP" (possibly the Super Low Frequency transmission station of 2009).

17 Synthetic biology (synbio) aims to engineer cells with "novel biological functions." Biotechnology and synthetic biology (synbio) are not the same thing. See Chapter 14 for more.

18 Lauren Steussy, "Coronavirus patients report strange new symptom: 'Fizzing.'" New York Post, April 10, 2020.

tress syndrome (ARDS) nor pneumonia. In fact, losing oxygen (*desaturation*) is the fast track to organ failure.

5G is a millimeter wave weapon system destined to rule from space over the entire planet. To elite Chinese and Western secret societies with their eyes on the ancient past and distant future, and access to far more knowledge and technology than the public has access to, it has been essential to convince the planetary public that the drop-dead physiological reaction to switching on what was carefully prepared in Wuhan was not due to "millimeter wave contagion" but to viral contagion.

The situation is similar to the Spanish flu epidemic of 1918 set forth by Arthur Firstenberg in his 2017 book *The Invisible Rainbow*. When the U.S. entered World War One in 1917, its ships were powered by transmitters more powerful than ever, with 30-kilowatt Poulson arcs spraying the air with "unwanted harmonics," then an even more powerful 500-kilowatt arc and 200-kilowatt alternator that together availed command-and-control (C2) transmissions to cross the Atlantic Ocean "clearly, continuously, and reliably," whose *"signal was heard over a large part of the earth."*

> . . . there is no evidence that the disease of 1918 was contagious. The Spanish influenza apparently originated in the United States in early 1918, seemed to spread around the world on Navy ships, and first appeared on board those ships and in seaports and Naval stations. The largest early outbreak, laying low about 400 people. Occurred in February in the Naval Radio School at Cambridge, Massachusetts. In March, influenza spread to Army camps where the Signal Corps was being trained *in the use of the wireless:* 1,127 men contracted influenza in Camp Funston in Kansas, and 2,900 men in the Oglethorpe camps in Georgia. In late March and April, the disease spread to the civilian population and around the world.
>
> Mild at first, the epidemic exploded with death in September, everywhere in the world at once. Waves of mortality traveled with astonishing speed over the global ocean of humanity, again and again until their force was finally spent three years later.[19] (Emphasis added.)

When 5G was switched on in Wuhan, it too was "a signal heard over a large part of the Earth," pulsing throughout the nanoparticulate-saturated atmosphere from which we all draw our breath and ringing the Schumann Well like a dissonant bell. The human population of 1918 underwent a mas-

---

19 Arthur Firstenberg, The Invisible Rainbow: A History of Electricity and Life. Santa Fe: AGB Press, 2017.

sive electric atmospheric “injection” (or *initiation*?), and a third of the world’s population was devastated by “radio wave influenza” from extremely high RF signal ranges and ultra-strong microwave transmissions.[20] Now, 100 years later, the Earth population is undergoing an even more invasive injection / initiation of which Wuhan was the chosen nuncio.

In the summer of 2020, floods plagued 27 provinces along the Yangtze River, Huai River, and Yellow River, as well as southern China. Had the Three Gorges Dam burst, Wuhan would have borne the brunt ten hours later. Geoengineered warning?

Do the elite really call the 60 GHz 5G wave “the V wave” (virus)?

20 Were the insiders of WHO and the CDC who spouted inflated death figures early on aware of what really happened in 1918 and thus projecting what might happen with a 5G switch-on?

Introduction

All life on earth can be considered a unit, a glaze of sentience spread thinly over the crust. In toto, its field would be a hollow, invisible sphere inscribed with a tracery of all the thoughts and emotions of all creatures.

– Robert O. Becker, MD, *The Body Electric*, 1985

The original conception of synthetic biology was to build the infrastructure to make the engineering of new biological function vastly more efficient, predictable, transparent and safe.

– Adam Arkin, synthetic biologist, UC Berkeley

If there is a physical body, there is also a spiritual body.

– St. Paul, I Corinthians 15:44

How far does the military doctrine of full spectrum dominance extend? All the way from the atmosphere into the living cell and its DNA, all the way into your thoughts.

From the PFN/TRAC patent that brings down jets and stops cars and controls the Internet of Things (IoT), to vaccines that install *kernels*[1] so dead man switches can be flipped and pilots die in flight, a death cult is running the "dual use" technology that Smart Cities embody.

Across and above America, pulsed signals streak to and fro, power lines glow, toaster ovens and electric lights and hair and clothes dryers emanate, exude, lead. Cell phone, laptop, and wireless frequencies pulse billions of times per second at low power. Human and animal bodies and brains attempt to pulse at their ancient natural frequencies, but radiation drowns out the Schumann life signal of 7.83 Hz. Neural conditions like amyotrophic lateral sclerosis (ALS or Lou Gehrig's disease) are on the increase, along with breast and testicular cancer, childhood leukemia, immune system dysfunction, Alzheimer's, brain tumors, thyroid imbalances, headaches, difficulty concentrating, chronic fatigue, miscarriages, low sperm counts, assaults on DNA. Blood flow fluctuates with pulsing electromagnetic waves. Eyeballs have trouble moving, pupils can no longer take in much light.

It is obvious to those who know what they're looking at that the secret

1 Kernal: a computer program at the core of a computer's operating system with complete control over everything in the system; the portion of the operating system code that is "resident in memory" and facilitates interactions between hardware and software components.

space program of the "breakaway civilization"[2] is going great guns to dominate all aspects of planet Earth, including control over our Sun and its systems. It all goes back to the Cold War and when the criminal intelligence-military-industrial phalanx of power in league with the nuclear industry was hijacked by the Jet Propulsion Lab Oversight Committee whose Cal Tech chair was intelligence community superstar (according to *Newsweek*) U.S. Navy Admiral Bobby Ray Inman, long-time insider of the George H.W. Bush crime syndicate in alliance with Texas Big Oil and the Carlyle Group.

Still, every era has its challenges. Ours just happens to be planetary powers running world-class technologies to subvert nations and Nature and the very *genetics* of what it is to be human. Still, the desire for technological planetary domination is hardly new; what is new is the technology, particularly nanotechnology. In the 17th century, alchemist John Rudolf Glauber (1604-1670) envisioned:

> . . . the existence of a group of scholars—"men endowed with a quick and penetrating mind"—whose only task must be to develop and perfect more and more sophisticated armaments . . . war will no longer be won by brute force but by the intelligence of scholars and engineers: "Force will yield to skill, for skill often succeeds in overcoming force."[3]

British Empire movers and shakers spent the next few centuries making sure that the masses lived by "faith alone" while the intelligentsia were indoctrinated with materialism and the maxim to live by "power alone." Hardly anyone now can imagine (much less perceive) that human thought is not produced by the brain like sausage but is scalar and originates in holographic dimensions beyond the four (3-space and Time) we are limited by the electromagnetic spectrum to perceiving.

Plato spelled out our existential dilemma long ago in his "Allegory of the Cave," which I chanced to read when I was nine years old. That subtle bodies interpenetrate all living physical bodies to create *biofields*, and that less perceptible entities share our planet's quantum in-folded dimensions (*inorganic life*[4]*?*) are truths that were consigned to mysticism and science fiction until sophisticated instruments and sense-free thinking were allowed in universities.

Heisenberg's uncertainty principle further loosened the bands constricting free thinking by postulating the existence of multiple dimensions that

2 A term I learned from Oxford scholar Joseph P. Farrell and investment analyst Catherine Austin Fitts.

3 Ioan P. Culianu, *Eros and magic in the Renaissance*. University of Chicago Press, 1987.

4 University of Glasgow, "Scientists take first step toward creating 'inorganic life,'" *Phys.org*, September 12, 2011.

obeyed their own laws of consciousness. Even the microcosm of atoms, whether as particle or wave, defied exact measurement *in the presence of a human consciousness.* Obviously, old terms like forces, æther, angels, demons, and death needed revisiting.

Today, techno-magicians control machines that detect and read the radio frequency to gamma waves spectrum and beyond as they extend human perception and thinking into quantum dimensions. As the Earth environment was prepared for full spectrum dominance, biotechnology talents were turned to the epigenetics of creating a new species of human being, the famed free will creation that scientist Rudolf Steiner said comprised the religion of the gods.

. . . if you penetrate through and look at the universe with a holographic system, you arrive at a different view, a different reality. And that reality can explain things that have hitherto remained unexplainable scientifically – paranormal phenomena, synchronicities, the apparently meaningful coincidence of events.

– Karl H. Pribram, MD (1919-2015); quoted in
The Technology of Success, ed. Susan Ford Collins, 2003

My previous two books on geoengineering studied weather engineering, chemical and electromagnetic atmospheric operations, planetary / geophysical operations, directed energy warfare operations (C4ISR), and detection / obscuration of exotic propulsion craft, along with some of the politics of control the operations serve.

Geoengineered Transhumanism: How the Environment Has Been Weaponized by Chemicals, Electromagnetics, & Nanotechnology for Synthetic Biology, the third and final book in my geoengineering trilogy, is not simply more of the same but takes a radical turn into synthetic biology. Part 1 ("As Above, So Below") brings readers up to speed on what is still going on in the heavens under the chemistry and electromagnetics of geoengineering, much of whose carefully devised flotsam and jetsam fall earthward to assault all that is living through the environment they must breathe and eat from.

In Part 2 ("Surviving the Smart City"), we turn our attention to the "dual-use" technologies of surveillance, neural weapons and biowarfare operations embedded in the UN "sustainable development" Smart City restructuring of society for the impending Transhumanist transformation of Human 1.0 into the "enhanced" Human 2.0 being genetically altered from the inside out.

With Part 3 ("The Transhumanist Trojan Horse"), we enter the decidedly *occult* precincts of eugenics-minded global elite bloodlines and secret societies that have sought for millennia the technology by which to turn the human masses into *synbio* (synthetic biology) *golems* or *homunculi.*[5] From "The Magical Human Head, Brain, & 'Second Brain'" to the genetics of the recent bold COVID-19 occult assault on the human genome, the intent being to replace the natural human body and brain (protein, carbon) with a nanoparticle silicon / polymer / graphene-based hydrogel brain-computer interface (BCI) for total artificial intelligence (AI) Cloud domination over any and all future attempts to individually develop or fine-tune free will.

Planetarily, *Geoengineered Transhumanism* configures a *unified digitized AI exotic weapons system* conjunct with the doctrine of full spectrum dominance that serves the secret space program whose sights are set on Earth and space domination. While the slow-to-awaken Child of Man is the embattled protagonist of this book, the central Faustian antagonist is actually the quantum subatomic world of nanotechnology, populated at this point by natural and synthetic smart dust, bacteria, viruses, nano-sensors, microprocessors, all being inhaled and ingested and implanted in weaponized and genetically engineered forms—like the earlier Morgellons "intelligence agents" now being supplanted by gene therapies loaded with graphene-based hydrogel (GBH) and quantum dots—all working in concert with chemical synergies triggered by 5G / 6G transmitters. From the heat pyrolysis of jets to our ionized plasma atmosphere, nanobots are in sync with RF and microwave pulses calibrated and recalibrated for exact pulsing between sky-based satellites, ISS, and geostationary battlespaces, all the way down to ground-based towers, OTH radar units, NexRads, wind farms, fracking liners, utilities, smart meters, 5G / IoT, radio telescopes, particle accelerators like CERN, and inevitably into our bodies and brains.

Is this simply the latest bid for world power by cunning, wealthy technocrats bent on milking human societies for profits and subjecting them to a genetic "shortcut" for space travel and an irradiated AI-run civilization? No, this bid is far more nefarious, as these genetic shortcuts change entire lineages forever and impact individual subtle bodies and souls / psyches. The COVID-19 power play is about supplanting the natural *soma* and *psyche* with synthetic genomes *already machine.*

At this point, we must admit that world events have spun into the precincts of evil disguised as technological achievement. It is difficult for the

5 *Golem:* animated anthropomorphic being created from inanimate matter; *homunculus:* in neurology, the alchemically created "little man inside the brain."

majority of humanity to imagine both the mindset and the means that seek to control all of life for eugenic and planetary goals. The sheer *scale* of massive corporate entities (*Egregores*) at every level of governance, media, and society colluding with controlled government bureaucrats to dominate every level of society and individual free will by means of technology and fear, is simply too great to fathom, much less fathoming the prospect of *organized evil.* In Appendices 1 and 13, "Invisible Mindsets" and "Movers and Shakers" respectively, this problem is examined.

In the 19th century, the poet William Wordsworth (1770-1850) sagely wrote, *The Child is Father of the Man.* Destroy the child, and you destroy the human being. Destroy enough children's souls, and the future of human consciousness is doomed. Define evil simply as deep hatred for the human being and all of life, and it is not difficult to see how the struggle between *biophilia* and *necrophilia* (psychoanalyst Erich Fromm's paradigm) is *right now* at a fever pitch as we face what may be the ultimate challenge for all of humanity.

Millions have now been inoculated with a "gene therapy" that implants into the natural human genome both software and a weaponized Spike protein while "5G flu" is sold to the public as a pandemic. In the Smart City environment that has been epigenetically prepared by chemicals, electromagnetics, and nanotechnology for AI control, natural human health, physical and mental, is at an all-time low, as the ancient immune system struggles with what has been intentionally bioengineered to weaken and sneak around it for Transhumanist *synbio* transformation.

Once you have read and grasped how this has been done, you will be ready to consider what it takes to remain human in an Earth period populated by artificial life, intelligent machines, hybrids, synths, clones, and nano robots everywhere outside in society and inside our bodies and brains. Yes, programmed tiny machines with a swarm hive mind consciousness have been implanted in us.

We cannot solve such problems with
the same thinking that created them.

Ruminate on this sage insight as you read and finally arrive at the Conclusion, "Remaining Human."

Finally, apologies for the forest of acronyms I lead you through. Acronyms now constitute a whole new cipher we must study. Also, no index: too many terms. Please make notes as you go and make use of the Glossary. The wise will read the Appendix 1 before beginning the book.

PART 1: As Above, So Below

In the shade, Thomas was studying the glowing brochure *ECCO Earth Coincidence Control Office Planetary Council of Elders* that Mannie had liberated. ECCO was a low-orbiting satellite system that relayed voice, data, global position location (GPS), and other mobile satellite services. Thomas thought the System Overview specs, Beam Pattern specs, Gateway Segment specs, Subscriber Services and Equipment specs, Phased Implementation, Service Provision, etc. would be useful to him. *20-35 kHz, 2.56 GHz.* The NSA was bent on "electronic incarceration" and "persuasive coercion" in the privacy of people's own brains. Decoding spontaneous thought from infrared brain imaging on headbands fitted with fiber optics zapping the pre-frontal cortex. Embedded interlinked *arphids*, whatever those were.

Thanks to the Global Information Grid (GIG) on the U.S. Navy Space and Naval Warfare Systems Command "dual use" Mobile User Objective System (MUOS), wireless handheld receivers picked voices and data from brains like cherries. Built by Lockheed Martin, Boeing, and General Dynamics, MUOS was 4,000 networks and 6,000 users at once on geosynchronous satellites, including TSATs and AEHFs. Cross-country "observatories" every 250 miles in urban, suburban, agricultural, managed and wild lands, plus 3,000 stations of EarthScope tracking tremors and crustal deformation. The cover story was about tracking birds and weather, drones and sensors, but it was really about discovering, accessing, collecting, managing, archiving, processing, and modeling human "integrated processes." *Unbelievable.*

Thomas read the small print on the back panel: Even the National Ecological Observatory Network (NEON) under the National Science & Technology Council and its *Strategic Plan for the US Integrated Earth Observation System* was in on it. Cybernetic voices. Primary frequency allocations via mental channels. E-mind control (EMC) would be "the ultimate in information protection," according to Raytheon's eCenter Technologies in Aurora, Colorado. From multiple 3,000-square-foot pods protected by security forces and reinforced cement walls impervious to infrasound attack or eavesdropping, Raytheon had formed a cross-discipline ISRnet (Intelligence / Surveillance / Reconnaissance) with encased conduits for multiple customers on multiple server platforms under Electronic Warfare, Computer Network Operations, Psychological Operations, Military Deception, and Operations Security—all to influence, disrupt, corrupt, or usurp human and automated decision-making (DoD, 2003: *Information Operations Roadmap,* 22). Total control of the electromagnetic spectrum meant the ability to deny, degrade, disrupt, and destroy all systems—the D words Strangeloves loved.

Elana Freeland, Book IV, "From Trinity to Trinity,"
Sub Rosa America: A Deep State History

1

Still *Under An Ionized Sky*

The Ionosphere
Jets and "Contrails"
Geoengineered Fires

Biodistribution to organs & tissues: Inhalation is probably the most significant human exposure . . . Part of inhaled particles will deposit within the lung alveoli, while a fraction will be absorbed within the epithelial cells of alveoli, and some of the nanoparticles will cross the air-blood barrier of the lungs. These nanoparticles will enter the circulatory system and travel further to the organs, becoming systemic . . . organs and tissues such as blood, heart, lymph nodes, tonsils, spleen, bones, brain, thyroid, liver, colon, and kidney.

– From *Nanotechnology in Eco-efficient Construction, Materials, Processes & Applications*, Woodhead Publishing, 2019

Ask yourself this: when was the last time you encountered a climate change apocalypse-predicting paper full of computer models that took into account and incorporated the geoengineering technologies—cloud seeding, chemical spraying, ionospheric heaters, and so on—as a component of the computer modeling?

– Joseph P. Farrell, PhD, "Oh, by the way, it's no longer to be called...," *gizadeathstar.com*, June 2019

Thanks to sophisticated planetary warfare technology, we are now ensnared in electromagnetic fields outside and inside our bodies and brains. Delivery via chemical trails, GMO foods, and vaccinations of biowarfare nano-scale components such as Morgellons and fungi, polymers, desiccated red blood cells, microprocessors, sensors, nanobots, and disease tell the tale of the weaponization of our Earth environment.

For millions of years, a natural infusion of galactic rays, meteor debris, corona mass ejections (CMEs), and solar flares merged with atmospheric elements like lightning and volcanic ash to create nanoparticles in the atmosphere by a factor of more than ten.[1] Then came the manmade infusion of the industrial and post-industrial revolutions with their multiplying pollutants in the name of "progress." Now, we are 20+ years into an intentionally

1 Geoff Brumfiel, "Cloud formation may be linked to cosmic rays." Nature, 24 August 2011.

geoengineered global atmosphere awash in chemicals and nanoparticles of conductive metals, sensors, microprocessors, and pathogens delivered along with the effluvium of jets, sounding rockets, and drones. Clouds and rain are no longer natural, snow is chemically nucleated, wind and pressure zones are unnaturally manipulated, and even the jet stream[2] is utterly controlled via manipulation of the Rossby waves, which, according to Electric Universe advocate Christopher Fontenot, are actually Alfvén waves—

> These "planetary" waves [see "Planetary waves, first found on Earth, are discovered on Sun," *Phys.org*, March 27, 2017] aren't new to science. Hannes Alfvén discovered magnetohydrodynamic waves (Alfvén waves) years ago. Yet scientists continue to under-inform the public on the electrical dynamics associated with weather phenomena and Earth-Sun interconnectivity. This mechanism goes by many names, including sympathetic resonance, quantum entanglement or Einstein's "spooky action at a distance" . . .

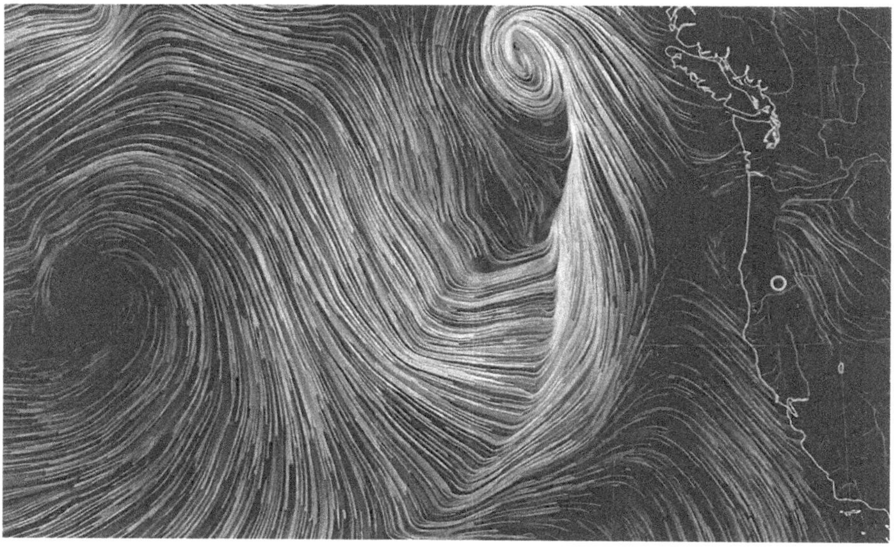

Control over the jet stream. From *www.earth.nullschool.net*, thanks to Lucretia Smith in Oregon.

Besides the endless disinformation and shell games of shifting names and acronyms we have to put up with, this era—unlike the previous era of industrial pollution—has been coerced into an unprecedented inundation of

2 Actually, there are two jet streams: one about 80 miles (128 km) above the Earth's surface with 300 mph (482 kph) winds; the other lower where strong electrical currents occur in the ionosphere (begins 50 miles / 80 km up). The lower altitude jet stream is now fragmented. It is well known that solar minimum effects can be cloned by manipulating the jet stream and polar vortices.

manmade nanoparticle infusions triggered by radio waves and microwaves to quicken synergies and compounds that impact what for millions of years constituted *life* in the biosphere at the bottom of our Schumann Well.

The secretive silence surrounding this illegal and antihuman anthropogenic assault is deafening. Corporate mainstream media and complicit "science" gatekeepers like NASA and the National Sciences Foundation (NSF) bewail "climate change" and "global warming," blaming carbons[3] and the grand solar minimum despite more honest scientists' insistence in the Royal Society's *Proceedings A* that the Sun's output and galactic cosmic rays have nothing to do with "climate change"[4] and carbons are at an all-time low of 400 ppm.[5] Blaming carbon emissions and greenhouse gases is nothing more than the political maneuvering of globalists seeking control over nation states.[6]

Ever since the 2015 UN Climate Chance Conference in Paris, carbon has been under assault as the secret space program grants it a high priority regarding life in space and retracing "the chemical steps leading to the formation of complex carbon-containing molecules in deep space."[7] Carbon-containing ringed molecules called PAHs (polycyclic aromatic hydrocarbons) in emissions and soot from fossil fuel combustion are collected and studied "as precursors to the interstellar nanoparticles" that account for 20 percent of all carbon in our galaxy (in "the vicinity of carbon-rich stars") via free radicals (which contain unpaired electrons).

In the YouTube "Polar Vortex Secret disclosure, BEST SCIENCE, DBAS Aerosol Spray" (November 12, 2019), The HAARP Report explains how for six winters, North America has been forced into a polar vortex[8] deep freeze (in winter 2020-2021, as far south as Texas) while mainstream media spew threats of a mini-Ice Age. Beginning with designer chemicals in dry powder aerosols that produce a *differential buoyancy aerosol spraying (DBAS)* to melt the Arctic, two tanker jets with separate chemicals attack the moisture system rolling in from the South Pacific, one heating with aluminum sulfate, the

---

3 See Kenneth Richard, "Physicist: CO2 Retains Heat For Only 0.0001 Seconds, Warming 'Not Possible.'" Climate Change Dispatch, October 18, 2019.

4 Richard Black, "No Sun link to climate change." BBC News, July 10 or October 7, 2007.

5 P. Gosselin, "Atmospheric CO2 Concentrations At 400PPM Are Still Dangerously Low For Life On Earth." NoTricksZone, May 17, 2013. Plants suffer below 500 ppm, and all of life on Earth depends upon plants.

6 For example, Syria's debilitating drought between 2007 and 2010: crop failure and livestock mortality in 60 percent of the nation with displacement of 1.5 million people. The year after the drought ended, Syria was wracked with political chaos.

7 DOE / Lawrence Berkeley National Laboratory, "Scientists Discover New Pathway to Forming Complex Carbon Molecules in Space." SciTechDaily.com, September 8, 2019.

8 Vortex, vortices: a mass of fluid or air (or plasma) with a whirling or circular motion that forms a cavity or vacuum by means of its angular velocity.

other cooling with aluminum fluoride. While maintaining stationary high pressure west of California, warm humid air is then driven north into the Arctic, producing global heating and fires for profits from Arctic oil and an open Northern Passage.

Meanwhile, supposedly green renewable systems like solar panels and wind farms, in tandem with carbon capture and nuclear energy,[9] are encouraged as UN "sustainable development" mandates and a global "affordable decarbonized energy system" when the truth is that they are calibrated to serve regional weather engineering and the Space Fence smart grid.

Canadian herbalist Tony Pantalleresco studies the carbon nanotubes (CNTs) we're breathing in because many who turn to him for their health issues are among the North Americans whose body composition is carbon, despite the fact that *we are not carbon-based but protein-based.* Are we undergoing genetic modification via the CNTs we're breathing in? This from Tony:

> Here is your space fence composition: carbon (more than likely C60 or C70). The fence just got denser and amplifies more frequencies. Carbon is super-conductive, zero resistance; 3X harder than diamond, 100X stronger than steel. If they are using carbomers (polymers functioning as thickening, dispersing, suspending, and emulsifying agents in cosmetics and personal care products) or diamines (binds monomers or molecules that can be bonded to other identical molecules to form a polymer), then it is even more than C60 / C70. Carbomer or diamine body armor would resist a .50-caliber and could be programmed to assemble into any form or pattern. Fire it in terahertz, 5G, or a multiple-band frequency and it will distribute with zero resistance. It also increases visibility and amplifies whatever you're looking at. They're now making lenses out of it.[10]

Experimenting on populations via aerosols comes under the secret space program pursuing Soviet astronomer Nikolai Kardashev's 3-fold model of a true Space Age:

I. Full spectrum dominance over planet Earth
II. Control over the Sun and its systems
III. Control over the galaxy and its systems

9 Matthew J. Lauridsen and Brian C. Ancell, "Nonlocal Inadvertent Weather Modification Associated with Wind Farms in the Central United States." Advances in Meteorology, August 6, 2018; also, John Reilly, "Too much wind and solar raises power system costs. Deep decarbonization requires nuclear," UtilityDive.com, December 2, 2019.

10 Email, Tony Pantalleresco, September 8, 2019.

Just as natural forests that convert carbon to oxygen are slated for replacement by GMO virtual forests, human beings are slated to become GMO / BCI (brain-computer interface) cyborg Transhumans. Meanwhile, billions of the biologically ignorant accept the lie that carbons are causing "climate change."

Geoengineering Operations in the Ionosphere

- *Weather engineering*
- *Chemical / Electromagnetic*
- *Planetary / Geophysical*
- *Directed energy warfare (C4 / C5ISR[11])*
- *AI Surveillance / neural operations*
- *Biological / Transhumanist operations*
- *Detection / obscuration of exotic propulsion technologies[12]*

The weapon potential of weather control has been coveted by militaries for centuries. A single natural tornado funnel is equal to 50 kilotons of explosives; a thunderstorm tower has the power of 500 kilotons; an Atlantic hurricane draws 1,000 megatons of energy from the sea. Perhaps this is why people are willing to believe in a climate change gone rogue without considering the possibility of technological control over the weather.

In the 1960s, Gordon J.F. MacDonald, science adviser to unelected President Lyndon B. Johnson, cautioned the military not to introduce "chaff" into the stratosphere to absorb incoming light or outgoing heat—exactly what geoengineer David Keith and his handler Bill Gates have been doing for 20+ years.[13] "The temptation to release materials from high-altitude rockets might exist . . . might be carried out covertly since nature's great irregularity permits storms, floods, droughts, earthquakes, and tidal waves [tsunamis] to be viewed as unusual but not unexpected. Such a 'secret war' need never be declared or even known by the affected populations."[14]

MacDonald lived during the CIA's early MK-ULTRA era, which may have awakened him to what weather control over the Earth-ionosphere cavity

11 Full spectrum dominance: Command, Control, Communications, Computers, Combat, Intelligence, Surveillance, and Reconnaissance.

12 The framework of these seven overarching, intertwined operations was proposed by Clifford Carnicom in 2005 in his film Aerosol Crimes, later edited as Cloud Cover.

13 Katie Schoolov, "This Bill Gates-funded chemical cloud could help stop global warming" (CNBC, September 7, 2019): Solar engineering could "mimic the effects of a giant volcanic eruption. Thousands of planes would fly at high altitudes, spraying millions of tons of particles around the planet to create a massive chemical cloud that would cool the surface."

14 Gordon J.F. MacDonald, "How to Wreck the Environment"; in Until Peace Comes: A Scientific Forecast of New Weapons, ed. Nigel Calder. New York: Viking Press, 1968.

might mean *beyond* weather, given how weak oscillating [pulsed] fields can influence human behavior.

> Perturbation of the environment can produce changes in behavior patterns . . . No matter how deeply disturbing the thought of using the environment to manipulate behavior for national advantage is to some, the technology permitting such use will very probably develop within the next few decades.[15]

Manipulate tropical thunderstorms with exactly timed artificially excited strobes (laser) and a pattern of oscillations (pulses) can be produced according to exact latitude and longitude that can "seriously impair brain performance in very large populations in selected regions over an extended period."[16] In 2014, British particle physicist Jasper Kirby admitted during the CERN CLOUD experiment[17] that clouds were being seeded by jets dumping aerosols into the upper atmosphere.

Geoengineering is used for weather engineering and to keep the atmosphere ionized and antenna-primed for six other operations (as listed above). But technology attributed to Nikolai Tesla has been undergoing weapons experimentation dedicated to full spectrum dominance since before his death in 1943,[18] with radio waves being bounced off the ionosphere since 1924.[19] By the mid-1970s, ionospheric heating experiments were being conducted out of Platteville, Colorado, Armidale, South Wales, Australia, and Arecibo, Puerto Rico. By the late 1970s, the Max Planck Institute had built EISCAT (European Incoherent Scatter Radar), a 100-megawatt heater in Tromsø, Norway now run by a 5-nation consortium.

Radio waves forced into a narrow beam that vibrate the ionosphere produces a repetitive excitation that heats our troposphere ("global warming"). In July 2010, the thermosphere (50 miles / 80 km above the Earth) collapsed, then rebounded; NASA and the Naval Research Lab called it a "Space Age record."[20] That it was caused by tampering with the upper atmosphere was

---

15 Ibid.

16 Ibid.

17 CERN explored solar / cosmic ray forcing that would lead to making cloud condensation nuclei (CCNs) form from aerosols. (Were cosmic rays enhancing production of nanoparticles in the aerosols, or were they radio waves?)

18 Under An Ionized Sky has been translated into Serbian, Tesla's language and nationality, and is recommended at the Technical College of Applied Studies.

19 The Sun's radiation creates and maintains the ionosphere as well as plasma in the magnetosphere.

20 John Emmert, Naval Research Lab, "Collapse in Earth's Upper Atmosphere Stumps Researchers." Tech Talk, CBS News, July 16, 2010.

perhaps a little too obvious, so Harvard University geoengineer David W. Keith was trotted out to blame carbons and greenhouse gases for the warming being caused by ionospheric tampering. In his 2010 paper, Keith blames greenhouse gases and references dangerous "side effects," but doesn't name them. Could some of those dangerous side effects be our health?

> Abstract: Aerosols could be injected into the upper atmosphere to engineer the climate by scattering incident sunlight so as to produce a cooling tendency that may mitigate the risks posed by the accumulation of greenhouse gases. Analysis of climate engineering has focused on sulfate aerosols . . . [but] engineered nanoparticles could exploit photophoretic forces, enabling more control over particle distribution and lifetime than is possible with sulfates, *perhaps allowing climate engineering to be accomplished with fewer side effects.* The use of electrostatic or magnetic materials enables a class of photophoretic forces not found in nature. Photophoretic levitation could loft particles above the stratosphere, reducing their capacity to interfere with ozone chemistry; and, by increasing particle lifetimes, it would reduce the need for continual replenishment of the aerosol. Moreover, particles might be engineered to drift poleward enabling albedo modification to be tailored to counter polar warming while minimizing the impact on equatorial climates.[21] (Emphasis added.)

With carbon pollution taking the rap for weather engineering experiments far beyond cloud-seeding, military and commercial jets and sounding rockets continue to load chemical trails with particulate matter and conductive metals like aluminum, titanium, boron, barium, strontium, lithium, europium, even calcium, in large part to keep the atmosphere battery-ready while feeding conductive nanometals into the Space Fence ring around the equator—the "Star Wars" Strategic Defense Initiative (SDI) "shield" back online.

Physicist Bernard J. Eastlund's 1987 High-frequency Active Auroral Project (HAARP) patent clarifies how "global warming" heat is generated not by carbons but by *electron cyclotron resonance* that increases ion density along with, one assumes, the daily deliveries of endless manmade nanoparticles:

> Abstract: A method and apparatus for altering at least one selected region which normally exists above the earth's surface. The region is excited by electron cyclotron resonance heating to thereby increase its charged particle density. In one embodiment, circularly polarized electromagnetic

---

21 David W. Keith, "Photophoretic levitation of engineered aerosols for geoengineering." PNAS, September 21, 2010. Also note his reference to "magnetic materials" that we are breathing in.

radiation is transmitted upward in a direction substantially parallel to and along a field line which extends through the region of plasma to be altered. The radiation is transmitted at a frequency which excites electron cyclotron resonance to heat and accelerate the charged particles. This increase in energy can cause ionization of neutral particles which are then absorbed as part of the region, thereby increasing the charged particle density in the region.[22]

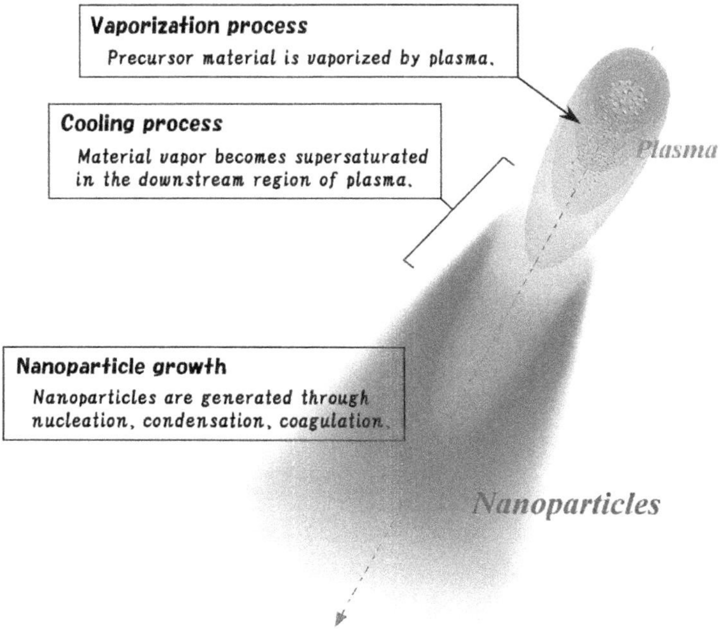
Vaporization process
Precursor material is vaporized by plasma.
Cooling process
Material vapor becomes supersaturated in the downstream region of plasma.
Plasma
Nanoparticle growth
Nanoparticles are generated through nucleation, condensation, coagulation.
Nanoparticles

Plasma and nanoparticle growth. The plasma process of growing nanoparticles requires heat and matter (nanoparticles). Review what Harald Kautz-Vella says about air pharmacology and pyrolysis in Chapter 1, "Project Cloverleaf," of *Under An Ionized Sky*, and in his paper "The Chemistry in Contrails: Assessing the Impact of Aerosols From Jet Fuel Impurities, Additives and Classified Military Operations on Nature" regarding the alchemy that occurs in the combustion chamber; includes a deep consideration of the biological operations of chemical trails. As this graphic says, nanoparticles are heat-generated via nucleation, condensation, and coagulation (blood?). https://iopscience.iop.org/article/10.1088/0022-3727/44/17/174025

By means of cyclotron resonance, heat, and nanoparticles, conductivity between the lower and upper atmospheres basically becomes contiguous,

22 Bernard J. Eastlund (1938-2007), Patent #US4686605 A, "Method and apparatus for altering a region in the earth's atmosphere, ionosphere, and/or magnetosphere," 1987.

making of our atmosphere a charged sky antenna of fully ionized plasma. In 2003, independent scientist Clifford Carnicom in Santa Fe, New Mexico measured the conductivity of the lower atmosphere with a 200,000-volt Van de Graaf generator. After determining the spark length, he realized that *the fundamental electrical nature of the atmosphere had been altered* as a result of the aerosol operations that continue to this day.[23] Planet Earth is now trapped under a conductive CD-ROM-like ring and ionized plasma cloud cover, which runs interference with our God-given cosmic frequencies.

HAARP—the phased array ionospheric heater in the Arctic Circle—is still very much alive, revamped, and calibrated. As Billy Hayes "The HAARP Man" put it in March 2017:

> TAKE CLOSE NOTE of new high-frequency riggings and elevated grounding grids. New multi-band antenna systems installed to initialize lower atmosphere plasmatic triggering . . . the new "CURTAIN OF DEATH." A 5.5 EQ [earthquake] — 42 km WSW of Anchor Point, Alaska, 2017-03-02 02:11:30 (UTC) 76.9 km —12 miles from HAARPoon Gakona while standby crew awaits tomorrow's Poker Flats NASA campaign on March 3.

People in Riga, Latvia and Gomel, Belarus, are waking at 4 a.m. robbed of their Schumann resonance communion with the planet and are thus forced into another brain entrainment entirely.

High gain sources of EM radiation from directed energy weapons like HAARP increase power density without the attenuation the inverse square law says antennas should have.[24] Again and again, it becomes apparent that the technology and science we are confronting is neither Newton's nor Einstein's but Tesla's, and not at all in the way he envisioned.

Jets and "Contrails"

> *Unlike low-level clouds that have a net cooling effect, these contrail-formed clouds warm the climate . . . The effect of these contrail clouds contributes more to atmospheric warming than all the carbon dioxide (CO2) produced by planes since the dawn of aviation . . .*[25]

---

23 Clifford E. Carnicom, "Atmospheric conductivity II," carnicominstitute.org, May 7, 2003. Also see "Atmospheric conductivity I," July 2001. The increase in conductivity in 2003 was by a factor of 3 to 20.

24 Christopher Fontenot, "Phased Array Antenna (HAARP) Breaks the Rules." A Microwaved Planet, May 18, 2016.

25 Katie Camero, "Aviation's dirty secret: Airplane contrails are a surprisingly potent cause of global warming." Science, June 28, 2019.

From the beginning, the classified HAARP / chemical trail "research projects" smacked of intelligence operations[26] beginning with turning the U.S. Air Force Academy's Chemistry 101 manual term "chemtrails" into a "tinfoil hat" pejorative and the August 23, 2000 "chemtrails are contrails" letter that scientist Carnicom received from USAF Lt. Col. Michael K. Gibson, master intelligence officer who the following year assumed command of the 451st Information Operations Squadron at RAF Menwith Hill.[27]

In 2008, the German government admitted to spraying chemical trails to disrupt radar signals[28] but not to plasma experiments regarding earthquake generation and psychotronic weapons, nor to increasing high frequency skip-enhancement for deliveries of energy to target sites exposed by "HAARP rings" generated by pulses of radio frequency seen in weather radar maps. Dual HAARP-like beams crossed like swords can open up a scalar zone, one beam stripping the electrons and forming superheated *plasma rings*, the other beam pumping and sustaining it. NEXRAD radar stations are also used to make similar *ping* rings—including cloud condensation nuclei (CCN) quickened by lasers and high-powered microwaves (HPM) or amped-up wind rotation—above the transmitters two days in advance of incoming manmade stormfronts.[29] Christopher Fontenot:

> As dipole phased array radar ionizes the sky, a Townsend cascade occurs where electrons collide and increase attenuation of the atmosphere. These rings are a product of that phenomenon.

From the nanoscale alumina particles added to liquid fuels for combustion performance, to "aerosol dispensing aircraft" described by Evergreen International Aviation's patent #US7413145, "Enhanced Aerial Delivery System," August 24, 2010, both military and commercial jets are complicit in the deliveries of nanoscale chemicals and conductive metals, many of which are experimental:

> An enhanced aerial delivery system addresses issues raised when large quantities of fluids, powders, and other agent materials are to be trans-

26 For example, Steve Watson, "CIA Is Funding Government-Led Chemtrail Project: Spy Agency to Help 'Security Impacts' of Geo-engineering." Global Research, July 20, 2013.

27 "Air Force Lies to America," September 11, 2000, www.carnicominstitute.crg/articles/af1.htm.

28 Dave Lambert, "Germany becomes First country to admit Clandestine Chemtrails Operations." gatherinespot.net, February 13, 2008. Immediately, the veracity of this revelation was called into question as a misunderstanding and "conspiracy theory."

29 Michael Janitch (aka Dutchsinse), "3/08/2016 – US Military confirms HAARP 'ring' formed by Radio Waves hitting Atmosphere / Ionosphere." Dutchsinse.com, March 8, 2016.

ported in and aerially dispersed by aircraft. Some aspects include positioning and securing of tanks aboard the aircraft . . . Other aspects address *coupling of the tanks and associated piping* to lessen structural effects upon the aircraft. Further aspects deal with *channeling, containing, and dumping stray agent materials* that have escaped from the agent tanks on board the aircraft. (Emphases added.)

Atmospheric physics professor Ulrike Lohmann studies cloud formation. In the 2016 film *Overcast*, Prof. Lohmann discusses her team's study of aircraft engine exhaust and jet fuel (mobile Jet A-1) from various turbines at Zurich Airport—not just the soot and particulate matter but the "very rare" chemical composition measurements. The team confirmed 16 different metals, especially aluminum and barium.[30] Twelve mixtures are electrically different; the other four are time tags that log how mixtures work from all layers, a vertical wall of connectivity between them. They want 24 to extend to the higher frequencies in outer space. *Terahertz wavelengths*—so small that they can manipulate individual atoms—will be the cloak of invisibility. Things will disappear before your eyes.

Sixty billion gallons of kerosene-based jet fuel are annually burned worldwide—jet propulsion JP-8 and JP-5, civil aviation Jet A and Jet A-1, and now biofuels (which are not all that bio). JP-8 is

> . . . the largest single chemical exposure in the U.S. military (2.53 billion gallons in 2000) . . . raw fuel, vapor phase, aerosol phase, or fuel combustion exhaust by dermal absorption, pulmonary inhalation, or oral ingestion routes. Additionally, the public may be repeatedly exposed to lower levels of jet fuel vapor / aerosol or to fuel combustion products through atmospheric contamination, or to raw fuel constituents by contact with contaminated groundwater or soil."[31]

Thus far, *regulation of aircraft exhaust is nonexistent.* (Major NATO and NASA fuel formulae remain classified.)

As the above patent Abstract's references to "tanks" and "piping" suggest, various ducts and bleed-air valves probably serve as "dual use"[32] nozzles in line

---

30 "Overcast Prof Ulrike Lohmann (English) – aluminum and barium in the jet fuel." Chemtrails Nederland, February 18, 2018.

31 G. Ritchie et al., "Biological and health effects of exposure to kerosene-based jet fuels and performance additives." Journal of Toxicology Environmental Health, Jul-Aug 2003. Also see Jim Lee's "Geoengineering and Weather Modification Exposed," https://climateviewer.com/geoengineering/.

32 For one example among many, at 00:28 in the YouTube "What have I found here? Have the BBC messed up releasing this video." Alex Alexander, March 25, 2015.

with the exhaust output and fuel "evac" nozzles off the wings exuding pyrolytic compounds of carbon, chlorine, calcium, copper, aluminum, silicon, sulfur, phosphorus, iron, potassium, titanium, chromium, and magnesium[33] from the combustion chamber that contribute to the Aerotoxic Syndrome suffered by aircraft personnel. Cabin air quality includes lubricants, "stray agent materials" in the dual-use duct system, and now 5G throughout for downloading movies during the flight. (Are they aerosoling "5G Fixer in a Can"?[34])

Jet engines sit forward of the wings on pylons so as to create magnetic fields for vortex lift. Once the jet goes into cruise mode, you can hear the engine change pitch. In the video "A380 Jet Fuel Deception," the assumption that 255 tons of fuel are loaded into the wings of the Airbus A380 is shown to be ridiculous. Once lofted, such a load along with 853 passengers is feasible, but not while on the ground and during liftoff. The airline industry uses less fuel than you think. Consider the bumblebee's tiny wings resonating the hollow cavity next to its larynx while lifting its massive weight. Once its resonance equals that of the magnetic field around its body, a magnetic bubble forms and the bee is levitated above the Earth and into the air æther[35] where it will fly at 30 miles per hour, *the wings steering* but not adding to the thrust.

Ninety percent of a jet's thrust comes from compressed bypass air, not from the combustion chamber. In the video "Important info for all air travelers / jet fuel hoax" (Spacebusters, March 19, 2018),[36] we learn of naturalist and inventor Viktor Schauberger,[37] then of entomologist Viktor Grebennikov, who studied levitation and propulsion through the æther, implosion, and vortices. We learn that aircraft engineering actually uses the vortex to "suck" the jet through the æther. (Vortices exist between scalar waves and the heat from decaying vortices, as well.) Conversion of matter (air, particulates, gases) and "synthesis electricity" (Schauberger) are emitted while a "biological axis" is created along the axis in front of the turbofan into which the airplane is sucked. The *strake effect* kicks in when the engine strake vortex between the jet engine intake and the wet runway spins *over the wings* and sucks the jet

33 "Analysis supports proposition that chemically induced contrails a factor in bleed-air valve, cabin-air contamination (Aerotoxic Syndrome)." Compagnie Africaine d'Aviation, April 2004.

34 Bill Schweber, "Aerosol Delivers 5G as Mist, Solves Countless Technical Problems." ElectronicDesign.com, April 1, 2020: "easy-to-manufacture nanoparticles in the shape of the 5G designation, internally code-named 5G-hype nanoparticles . . ."

35 Review æther in Chapter 3 of Under An Ionized Sky.

36 Followed by "Part 2 important info for all air travelers: Jet Fuel Hoax Nobody owns the air." Spacebusters, January 27, 2019. At 1:25, the æther.

37 Much is said about Schauberger in Nick Cook's The Hunt For Zero Point: Inside the Classified World of Antigravity Technology (New York: Broadway Books, 2001). Cook was aviation editor at Jayne's Defence Weekly.

up—the sudden levitation you feel while sitting inside the jet.[38] Some videos show heavy jets *hovering* ("stalling"); small vortex generators from Micro Aerodynamics can be installed to increase stall ability.

> Powering virtually all commercial aircraft today, *turbofans generate thrust by drawing in air at the front with a fan.* While most of the air goes around the engine, some passes through it, drawn in by a compressor comprising many blades attached to a shaft. The compressor pressurizes the air, greatly increasing its temperature. The hot air is then forced into a combustion chamber where it's sprayed with fuel and ignited, resulting in hot, high-pressure gas that, as it expands, spins a turbine before blasting out of the nozzle at the rear of the engine, thrusting the aircraft forward. Because all the engine's components are connected through a central shaft, a rotating turbine not only drives the low-pressure compressor but also spins the fan, providing additional thrust.[39] (Emphasis added.)
>
> *A turbofan is not a turbine.*[40]

If this is in actuality how jets achieve thrust, then the chemical effluvium from the combustion chamber only occurs in quantity at takeoff and landing. The "contrail clouds" that form from what is spewing out of jets (often along the wings, not from beneath the tail) must be from chemicals ejected from a supplementary duct system. In a 2004 video interview entitled "Airport Employee Interview," Enrico Gianini, an aircraft loading operator at Malpensa Airport in Milan, Italy, offers thought-provoking testimony. As a loading operator, he observed the underbellies of commercial jets, the ducts along the wings for condensation drainage, special ducts said to be "sensors"[41] along the blades of the turbine, and pre-drilled holes under the fuselage. Clearing the ducts of water and oil often included having to *push out* materials that nebulized (converted to a fine spray) as they were discharged. Gianini concluded that the core components of geoengineering might be in the fuel, but other elements, including catalysts, are ducted from tanks and canisters in the extreme aft of the jet.

---

38 "Plane strake lift – Cerebral Vortex / UAP." UAP, March 10, 2018.

39 "Aircraft Geared Architecture Reduces Fuel Cost and Noise," Spinoff 2015 Technology Transfer Program, NASA, n.d. A compelling theory is that compressed air moves the jet forward, with fuel being used only for takeoff, landing, and taxiing.

40 A turbofan (fanjet) is an airbreathing jet engine widely used in aircraft propulsion; a turbine is a steam-powered machine whose shaft produces electricity through movement.

41 The wireless sensor network (WSN) monitors engines, airframes, structures, gearboxes, etc.

...sensor networks are spatially aware and are most closely linked to geographic location and the physical environment than centralized systems. A sensor node in a typical sensor network has a battery, a microprocessor, and a small amount of memory for signal processing and task scheduling. Each node is equipped with one or more sensing devices such as sensors for visible or infrared light, changing magnetic field, electrical resistance, acceleration or vibration, pH, humidity, or temperature; acoustic microphone arrays, and/or video or still cameras. Each sensor node communicates wirelessly with a few other neighboring nodes within its radio communication range. A wireless sensor network may also be augmented with a higher tier of more powerful, wired nodes with greater network capacity and computation power, as in the Tenet architecture. Nodes in this higher tier are sometimes called masters *or* microservers. - Elaine Cheong, "Actor-Oriented Programming for Wireless Sensor Networks," dissertation for Doctor of Philosophy in Electrical Engineering and Computer Sciences, UC Berkeley, 2007

"Aerosol dispensing aircraft" fly under a cloak of secrecy. Air traffic control (ATC) uses passive radar, not active, which means that aircraft transmit their call numbers with a transponder that can be turned off, or they can use fake identifiers. Ships and jets can be made to "go dark," meaning they no longer register on automatic identification systems (AIS) and go "off grid," i.e. vanish from radar.[42] "Phantom" jets lay long aerosol trails, then *disappear*, "phantom" referring to the radar absorbent material (RAM) that turns on and off. [RAM is a coating containing carbonyl iron ferrite ("iron ball" paint or tiles). When radar encounters RAM, a magnetic field forms inside the metallic elements and an alternating polarity dissipates the signal.[43]]

Whether under space surveillance or air traffic control, aerosol dispensing aircraft have a perennial green light. The Proba-V satellite (less than a cubic meter in size) picks up 25 million positions of more than 15,000 jets from space with its Automatic Dependent Surveillance Broadcast (ADS-B).[44]

42 Michael Forsythe and Ronen Bergman, "To Evade Sanctions on Iran, Ships Vanish in Plain Sight." New York Times, July 2, 2019.

43 See these patents: https://www.google.com/patents/US3630594; https://www.google.com/patents/US3810687; https://www.google.com/patents/US3782804; https://www.google.com/patents/US3653736. Thanks to RichieFromBoston.

44 "15,000 planes, 1 image: Stunning satellite map shows jet signals worldwide." RT, 8 May 2015.

Thanks to remote telemetry, computers run all aspects of jets in flight, even to filing the flight plans. As Judson Singer wrote on Facebook in response to one of 1PacificRedwood's excellent Pacific weather reports[45]:

> Spraying patterns by individual aircraft and clusters of aircraft are reported by whistleblowers to be satellite-controlled & coordinated through transponders on each aircraft. Think how complex flight instructions would have to be when manually delivered, given the scope and scale of worldwide spraying. Applied artificial intelligence would make the task easier.

If the jet is using a Rolls Royce engine, then Rolls Royce supercomputers monitor the engine and receive telemetry reports. Dissemination of chemicals is run by on-the-ground (Big Pharma) supercomputers that instruct the flight guidance system as to where and when to release them per their frequency signatures. Finally, the flight termination system (FTS) can take full control over drones, military or passenger jets, as per their frequency signatures.[46]

Getting the picture? Pilot brainwaves may be able to control their instruments, but who's directing those brainwaves from the ground?

> . . . the system monitors and interprets signals in brain electrical activity that translate to movement commands. Once a pilot is connected to the system using a set of 32 electrodes, he can monitor his brain activity using a brain-computer interface [BCI]. The pilot focuses on arrows on the interface that will tell the computer what he wants the plane to do.[47]

Geoengineered Fires

Just as I have been saying now for nearly two decades, Super Nano Thermite Extension is just a part of the atmospheric aerosol chemming.

– Billy Hayes "The HAARP Man"

What we can do is focus this very high energy into a very small spot for a very short time, and when that happens, we get the conditions that are very much like inside our Sun.

– Edward Moses, National Ignition Facility

---

45 See 1PacificRedwood YouTube channel at https://www.youtube.com/channel/UCX-cnHuosOLaKOGU0qQoYzfA.

46 See Chapter 5, "5G Wi-Gig & the Internet of Things (IoT)" regarding the PFN-TRAC patent.

47 Dom Galeon, "Mind Control: New System Allows Pilots to Fly Planes Using Their Brainwaves." Futurism.com, November 22, 2016.

I left my home shortly before it burned as a 5G tower was erected nearby and then tested. I inferred this was a weapon from my observation of readings of ~1 million times or so over background with my meter pegged, indicating illegal levels of radiation. 6 decimal places. 0.0005 mW/m² background. 0.0012 when presumably acting as a cell tower, or some other modern active source of radiation. 150.0000 and change when tested on "bake cycle." Geoengineering is part of a plasma weapon, a military system now surrounding Earth. The effects of the plasma overhead are the certain thing in the burn; the tower is only a presumed part of the system.

– Richard Lawrence Norman, email, 2020

1100°F (593°C)	Normal fire burning point
1220°F (600°C)	Aluminum
2600°F (1426°C)	Tempered glass
2700°F (1482°C)	Stainless steel

What if the "wildfires" along the U.S. West Coast are actually *prescribed burns* prepared by geoengineering with years of drought and tons of aluminum nanoparticles dropped from the upper atmosphere and pounded by scheduled, short-lived floods? As nano-researcher Pete Ramon put it:

> Wildfires destroy Earth's ability to propagate cloud formation through New Particle Formation events (fancy for cloud nucleation) by removing isoprene, Earth's own dual-use bioaerosol that can inhibit and promote. While large biomass burning does put vast amounts of CO and particulates in the air, it's ultimately vanquishing Earth's ability to generate her own weather patterns. If you're trying to control global weather patterns, you do indeed have to cut out the middle-men: the Earth and Sun.

In 2014, mainstream news had it that trees were dying in the Rocky Mountains "for no apparent reason" other than the usual "climate change" cover story. In 2015, the U.S. Forest Service estimated that 12.5 million trees in southern and central California forests were dead, with another 120 million trees stressed from years of drought and soon to be dead, as well—20 percent of the state's forests, not including the fires.

Geoengineered drought, geoengineered fires.

Something very VERY TOXIC was clearly sprayed on the trees on Mt. Ashland this winter. I drove up there today and was blown away by the death. To have the trees going from looking very healthy this last fall (DESPITE the drought) to now looking very very sick—and with many already dead that were healthy and well last fall is mind-blowing. The tree bark is no longer the healthy brown-red color as last fall; instead, it looks totally grayish white with white or black mold or moss growing in them (an absolute indication of the trees dying, especially when so thick and all up and down the trees). Branches are strangely bending down like they are made of rubber (like NOTHING I HAVE EVER SEEN BEFORE, even with trees under 10 feet of snow), and branches just snapping off. Unbelievable and beyond sad and sick. Absolutely our forests have been sprayed. No way is this quick die-off normal.

– Lucretia Smith, Ashland, Oregon, February 29, 2016

In 2012, the first of its kind U.S. Forest Service Forest Products Laboratory began producing forest-based nanomaterials known as *nanocellulose*—organic matter stronger than Kevlar fiber, low weight. All of the industries wanted it, including the military. Did the 12.5 million dead trees contribute to this industry? Killing off the natural forests so GMO forests ("growth platforms") can be planted to provide genetically modified pulpwood fiber for the production of nanocellulose substrate, "a crystalline cellulose rich waste"[48] similar to the "cell growth substrate" for growing human body spare parts?

In the next chapter, nanotechnology is discussed in detail. *Neural* and *smart dust* is nanotechnology. Nano-drones are nanotechnology. Aerosols deliver smart dust as sensor networks to the environment and bodies (e.g. "Internet of Bodies"), GMO foods and vaccines deliver neural dust to monitor the brain from the inside. Even natural nanoparticles have a *swarm consciousness* that in manmade microprocessor-armed nanobots becomes a nano-drone army.[49]

In an obscure trade magazine, Finnish observer Arto Lauri read a feature story about a Rauma biopharmaceutical professor busy growing human cells on nanocellulose and how three factories in Finland are producing nanocel-

48 Roi Paretz et al., "Nanocellulose production from recycled paper mill sludge using ozonation pretreatment followed by recyclable maleic acid hydrolysis." Carbohydrate Polymers, 15 July 2019.

49 "SWARM – Exposing the Swarm at the Edge of the Cloud & the Integrating Man / Machine Transhumanism." A Call to Actions, June 1, 2016.

lulose substrate.[50] In Chapter 6 under "The Nuclear Behemoth," Finland's nuclear industry is discussed, especially Rauma being rife with Pu-239 ion gas leaks and how deeply invested in the chemical trails and polymerization industries (including nanocellulose / hydrogel production[51]) and plutonium ion experiments Finland is. The phlegm-like cellulose substance Lauri collected from rainwater in mid-January 2016 reminded me of the Oakville, Washington (pop. 665) "gelatinous goo" of human white blood cells, two species of bacteria, and live eukaryotic cells that fell from the sky six times in three weeks in 1994.[52]

What *is* going on with the forests? Fire is habitually considered to be a natural phenomenon or individual arson, but it can also be ignited and accelerated with directed energy technologies like lasers and nano-chemicals for purposes of warfare and experimentation.[53] Under the cover story of weather management, the space-based Planetary / Geophysical operations like the California "wildfires" of 2017 and 2018 (Santa Rosa, the Carr fires near Woolsey, Redding, Noland, Delta, Boots, Hill, Malibu, Paradise, etc.[54]) were geoengineered to clear a 300-mile right-of-way for the Great Redwood Trail alongside the North Coast Railroad Authority's Northwestern Pacific Railroad just as the "wildfires" for the TransMountain pipeline in British Columbia.[55] As ionospheric heaters melt the Arctic glaciers to clear the way for ship lanes, the Redwoods were torched to serve disaster capitalist acquisition of more and more mineral resources.

October 2017	Napa / Sonoma	154,654 acres
December 2017	Santa Barbara / Thomas	281,893
July 2018	Yosemite	97,000
	Redding / Carr	229,651
	Mendocino Complex	459,123

50 "ArtoLauri169," February 24, 2016, https://www.youtube.com/watch?v=ivaBxBUk0uI&t=0s.

51 Nanocellulose preprogramming is used in plant cells. From a mechanical perspective, wood hydrogels outperform manmade 3D-printed nanocellulose hydrogels. Hydrogel is taken up in Chapter 14, "The COVID-19 'Vaccine' Event."

52 From the mid-1970s, the 5 kingdoms of Nature have been reclassified by cell structure into 3 domains: Archae, Bacteria, and Eukaryota.

53 See DEW capability to bend steel in "DEW – Steel Bridge wiped out. My most weird year and most serious as an activist," chemtrail chemtrail, November 12, 2018.

54 The Kincade fire in Sonoma County (77,758 acres) burned from October 23 to November 6, 2019. Regarding the July 2018 fire in Redding, Cat Brown at The Con Trail pointed out the blood moon (lunar eclipse) and redding. Further Onomancy in news accounts: Andrew Moon, Sherry Bledso, Jeremy Stoke the fire inspector . . .

55 P.J. Taylor, "Federal government thank wildfires for clearing path for Trans Mountain pipeline," The Beaverton, August 20, 2018.

2015-2018	Lake County, Rocky River	171,539
November 2018	Woolsey / Malibu	96,949
	Paradise / Camp	153,000[56]

The Woolsey fire began at the defunct Santa Susana Field Laboratory in Simi Valley (ceased operation in 2006), home of Rocketdyne's research reactor and ten other reactors—four cores dissipated radioactivity, with iodine-131 radionuclides, trichloroethylene, perchlorate, dioxins, heavy metals multiplying the contamination. During the Paradise fire, the local hospital's radionics wing had all the markings of having been intentionally torched to release maximum radiation.

In December 2018, videographer Jamie Lee interviewed a microwave specialist whose home was torched. His expert opinion was that smart meters had been involved in prepping homes slated for immolation. Blue flames playing among the unburned trees pointing to the white powder (the incendiary phosphorus?) dropping from helicopters and mixing with natural gas to create a vacuum for combustion in turn pointed to the smart meters that appear to have opened propane tank gas lines to flood houses with natural gas. Interestingly, California is banning natural gas from all new buildings so that electric is the only option.[57]

Citizen eyewitness accounts from drone footage and cell phone cameras[58] have been invaluable to interpreting the "wildfires" along the West Coast, given that mainstream media bend the facts to obey their corporate masters. First, jets and drones strafed the sky over target zones with nanometals / -chemicals for the indices of refraction required. Then, as sharp observer Krispy Verbakel noted during the 2017 Santa Rosa fires,[59] blue laser light—*Teramobile infrared femtosecond laser? LiFi LED satellite optics on-off energy transfer switch?*—descended in a column of ionized air for ignition of the nano-swarm brigades resurrected from the drought-compacted soil or summoned from the air.[60]

Think of the chemicals laid by jets and drones over fire target areas—the

---

56 James W. Lee (Jamie Lee), Paradise Lost: The Great California Fire Chronicles, 2019, https://planetruthblog.files.wordpress.com/2020/08/ccthe-california-fire-chronicles-first-edition.pdf.

57 Mallory Moench, "California regulators clear way for natural gas bans to take effect." San Francisco Chronicle, December 11, 2019.

58 Not everything is picked up by iPhone cameras, due to their filters.

59 The official account is 14 fires, but it is more like 170, most of which have not been made public. Multiple experimental deployments of various elements.

60 Laser visibility or invisibility is determined by (1) frequency of the laser, (2) strength of the laser, and / or (3) dust or mist in the air.

U.S. Naval Research Laboratory and SuperDARN[61] network are engaged in thermosphere (56 miles / 90 km above the Earth) and low-orbit satellites research—as "chempiles" of nano-super-thermite components, with "burn" meaning combustion. Space launches use aluminum oxide as the propellant for a thermite burn of lithium with aluminum and barium, thermite being a pyrotechnic composition of nanometal powder fuel and nanometal oxide. When ignition occurs, firefighters experience it as a *vaporific effect*, a sudden flashfire due to the impact of a high-velocity projectile (laser? maser?) with metallic objects. Nanoparticles of magnesium (Mg) could burn at 3600°F (2000°C), splitting water into hydrogen (H) and oxygen (O), after which each element undergoes combustion. Magnesium nanoparticles can burn a hole through an engine block, just as the exothermic redox of thermite (metal powder fuel and metal oxide) melts iron fences and bolts in creosoted guard rails. The range of thermite in jet fuel spans aluminum (Al), magnesium (Mg), titanium (Ti), zinc (Zn), silicon (Si), and boron (B), coupled with oxidizers boron(III) oxide, silicon(IV) oxide, chromium(III) oxide, manganese(IV) oxide, iron(III) oxide, iron(II,III) oxide, copper(II) oxide, and lead oxide.

Metal fires burn hotter and longer with less oxygen—Agent Orange for Vietnam chemical warfare experiments, nano-metal particles for California combustion. USAF aerospace illustrator Mark McCandlish (recent suspicious death) adds to the picture:

> Imagine then how this affects the conflagration that is a forest fire with these materials present in the environment. I have personally spoken to a number of career CDF personnel who have told me unequivocally that fires over the last ten years have become significantly more difficult and costly to suppress. They burned unusually hot, but officials were at a loss to explain why . . .
>
> Now as if that weren't bad enough, with aluminum being a conductor of electricity, spraying countless microscopic-sized particles into the sky does something else you might not have considered: It dramatically increases the electrostatic potential of the air. That is, its ability to conduct electricity. So those storm clouds that always seem to follow heavy chemtrailing are primed to produce many more lightning strikes. In late July of 2010 (if memory serves), one such storm produced over 8,000 lightning strikes in our region, many of which created fires. When it was all over a month later, California had totaled over $23M in suppression costs. And since the chemtrailing started around 1999-2000, the amount of acreage burned

61 The Super Dual Auroral Radar Network is an international scientific radar network of 35 high-frequency (HF) radars in the Northern and Southern Hemispheres.

and suppression costs have doubled, according to NOAA figures.[62]

As for the money angle, investment analyst Catherine Austin Fitts called the California fires "9/11 West," surmising that the fires were set in areas of mortgage fraud so as to clear properties for wealthy Asians. During a disaster, laws are more "flexible" and skimming out the back door is common—for example, writing off mortgage fraud (see "Inflated Home Appraisals Drain Billions From Government Insurance Fund," *Wall Street Journal*, November 16, 2018) and pilfering from disaster recovery funds. Citizen deaths lower life expectancy when it comes to social security outflow. The Red Cross took in $425 million from people wanting to help fire victims but only provided water bottles. Where did the rest go? Insurance and reinsurance money; catastrophe (cat) bonds[63] for money laundering; lucrative real estate deals while the devastated and desperate are crammed into pack-and-stack lockstep Smart Cities; burned and scorched Douglas firs and Ponderosa pines clear-cut for high-priced lumber and polymerization factories (mentioned above); and on and on.

The "Paradise Lost" fires appear to have been carefully scheduled to follow midterm elections on November 6, 2018, followed on November 7 by remote-controlled U.S. Marine Ian David Long, 28, shooting and killing a dozen people at the *Borderline Club* in *Thousand Oaks*, then killing himself for the favored number 13. *Fire walk with me.*[64] "Camp Fire" was immersed in symbolic language and burned like a microwave oven through November 8 and 9. Paradise (pop. 27,000) lost 6,700 structures, at least 88 citizens (many immolated in metal vehicles) with 1,276 missing and 52,000 displaced and / or unaccounted for. PG&E trucks, MRAPs (mine-resistant ambush protected) filled with militarized police, tactical vehicles, sabotage teams and private security forces[65] were everywhere.

Overhead, TR-3Bs—hovering triangular ships with three lights on their hulls—were cloaked in chemical clouds and now and then captured by cell phone cameras. One acute observer noted a *3-holed pattern* on the burned hoods of cars (and even inside on the ceilings), in the soil, in stainless steel sinks in burned-out houses, concrete, glass, even plastic containers—"damning evidence against the United States government" (Heath, "The Most Important News of 2018 / Please Share," February 6, 2018). The energy

62 Most of Mark's clients were top military contractors like General Dynamics, Lockheed, Northrop, McDonald-Douglas, Boeing, Rockwell International, Honeywell, and Allied Signet Corporation. Mark spoke these words at the Shasta County Board of Supervisors Hearing on Chemtrails, July 15, 2014.

63 Catastrophe bonds are collateralized debt obligations between sponsors and investors.

64 From the David Lynch series Twin Peaks.

65 High-value murders are often hidden amidst chaos and mass casualties.

of the Sun can be focused with a magnifying glass to melt rock in 15 seconds, dirt in 45 seconds, wood in 2 seconds, and steel nails in 30 seconds, so what directed energy weapon (DEW) did this? "Heath" mentions microwaves, namely MASERS. (Lasers to ignite, masers to melt?) Alleging that the National Guard "tampered with the crime scene" by attempting to cover the larger 3-holed patterns, he appealed to U.S. Army General Martin Dempsey regarding one final crucial observation: two antennas, one on each side of the rear of a burned-out car seemingly stopped the fire raging over the car roof in its tracks. Indeed, the trunk is unblemished. Bingo: the "wildfire" was conducted via frequency with a high-powered microwave pulsing weapon.[66]

It just so happens that off the coast of California running north and south is a string of *underwater microwave transmitters*[67] that have played a big role in evaporating moisture since the Great California Drought began in January 2011 just after Governor Jerry Brown took office.

Temperatures and summer "wildfires" temperatures are geoengineered, thanks to an entire industry of complicit corporations.

- Since 2018, the Department of Energy's Argonne National Laboratory (ANL) Combustion Synthesis Research Facility in Illinois has utilized Flame Spray Pyrolysis (FSP) to manufacture the masses of nanomaterials in silica, metallic, oxide and alloy powders or particulate films—much as the spray pyrolysis going on in aircraft engines produces artificially nucleated condensation trails.[68]
- Nanowave Technologies Inc. calibrates high-powered transmitters (including those offshore) so they work in tandem for and with *film combustion synthesis*—in other words, preparing the immediate environment for combustion. Chemical trails load nanoscale oxides, metals, alloys, and sulfides necessary for *combustion synthesis (CS)* of reactive agents guaranteed to produce the thermodynamic-kinetic "rapid self-sustained combustion reactions" like fires and explosions.[69] All in all,

---

66 U.S. Navy-trained radar expert Christopher Fontenot: "The use of MASER (DEW) technology to heat the atmosphere for weather modification, increase evaporation, or even conduct microwave-induced combustion operations in which temperatures reach 950 degrees Centigrade (1742 degrees Fahrenheit) is relatively recent."

67 See the infrared satellite map in the YouTube "7-29-2018; Moisture Superheated As It Approaches CA" by 1PacificRedwood. US West Coast weather reports by 1PacificRedwood are excellent, plus the underwater transmitters may still be visible on Google Earth. Thanks to scientist Harald Kautz-Vella for pointing this "microwave farm" out to me.

68 Review Chapter 1 in Under An Ionized Sky.

69 Arvind Varma et al., "Solution Combustion Synthesis of Nanoscale Materials," Chemical Reviews 2016. Also, Fa-tang Li et al., "Solution Combustion Synthesis of metal oxide nanomaterials for energy storage and conversion." Nanoscale, Issue 42, 2015.

metal oxide nanomaterials are a large part of how the chemical trail delivery system serves operations from communications to for "highly efficient energy conversion and storage" and mind control.

The YouTube "Solution combustion synthesis" (Velaga Srihari, July 19, 2008) and footage of the California fires, coupled with the following from Richard Lawrence Norman[70] about how combustion synthesis might be conducted in a target area will help you learn to recognize what is obviously not a "wildfire":

1. Metals in the system are preloaded with microwave, millimeter wave, or infrared—all present in satellite systems currently deployed. However, massive spontaneous combustions indicate *a ground source of preloaded energy.*[71]
2. Once the system is PRELOADED WITH ENERGY, it is ready to burn in complete efficiency.
3. As film combustion synthesis (CS) and ignition pulse are added, the metals and proximately associated materials (which also absorb energy) suddenly burst into flame, the laser being the match.

Regarding the preloaded environment, retired USDA biologist Francis Mangels[72] in the Mt. Shasta region measured 4,610 ppm aluminum in water and soil samples—25,000X World Health Organization (WHO) safety levels.

Explosions are combustion synthesis technology as well, thus I can only surmise that the six explosions between August 3 and August 5, 2020 were preplanned as well:

August 3	Hyesan, North Korea
August 3	Xiantao (outside Wuhan), China
August 4	Beirut, Lebanon[73]
August 4	St. Paul, Minnesota, U.S.
August 5	Ajman, United Arab Emirate
August 5	Naiaf, Iraq

---

70 Editor of The Journal of Unconscious Psychology and www.mindmagazine.net.

71 For me, preloading is not just the nanochemical deliveries three days in advance of geoengineered events (fires, earthquakes, storms, etc.) but the impacted nanometals and nanobots already in the soil, walls, bark of trees, etc., from years of geoengineering.

72 See "Retired USDA Biologist Francis Mangels on Geoengineering - FULL HD (Interview by John Whyte)," ChemtrailsConference, September 1, 2012 (41:53) https://www.youtube.com/watch?v=9jf_nVLGDTo.

73 A TR-3B was filmed during this "multiplex" explosion. See "TR3B's Caught Bombing Beirut," aplanetruth5, August 5, 2020. Also see Sean Gautreaux, "What is in Our Skies, Part 1 – Introduction," June 2, 2012, to better understand Geoengineering Operation #7.

A few suspects from a very long list include:

- Solaren Space contracted to transfer space-based satellite solar power via MASER technology to ground stations (which may in part explain the PG&E power surges and outages prior to the fires); it has space solar power (SSP) patents in the U.S., Canada, European Union, Russia, Japan, India, and China. Its patent for modifying weather via satellite is Patent No. US20100224696:

Space-based power system and method of altering weather using space-born energy. The space-based power system maintains proper positioning and alignment of system components without using connecting structures. Power system elements are launched into orbit, and the free-floating power system elements are maintained in proper relative alignment, e.g. position, orientation, and shape, using a control system. Energy from the space-based power system is applied to a weather element, such as a hurricane, and alters the weather element to weaken or dissipate the weather element.[74] The weather element can be altered by changing a temperature of a section of a weather element, such as the eye of a hurricane, changing airflows, or changing a path of the weather element.

- The Canadian corporation Maxar Technologies ("We are the nexus of the new space economy") has drag-and-drop interface technology able to target specific targets pre-mapped by the National Geospatial-Intelligence Agency (NGA) (previously the National Imaging & Mapping Agency or NIMA) while the British corporation Serco (discussed in Appendix 15, "Movers and Shakers")—the world's largest non-state air traffic controller (ATC)—oversees and controls satellite computer algorithms as well as jet / drone chemical deliveries.[75]
- Based in Utah, ChamTech Operations produces a nanoparticle spray that acts as a nanocapacitor to turn trees into antennas and extend existing antennas by a factor of 100X. Sprayed along the median of roads, it produces high bandwidth connectivity with vehicles. It is no surprise that spray-on nano was originally intended for military use.[76] (See barium-strontium-titanate in Chapter 2.)

---

74 Or build and intensify.

75 "Did Serco ConAir Patents Cause California Wildfires via CIA Nanowaves? Special Guest David Hawkins." Jason Goodman, November 28, 2018. Hawkins is a forensic economist with a Cambridge University background in the Science of Waste and Chaos.

76 Dexter Johnson, "Spray-on Nanoparticle Mix Turns Trees Into Antennas." IEEE Spectrum, 16 February 2012. Also see Michael Irving, "Sprayable antennas turn surfaces into ultra-thin, transparent transmitters," NewAtlas.com, September 24, 2018.

We used similar technologies in Operation Igloo White (1968-1973) in Vietnam and Laos but on VHF [very high frequency], trimming back long-leafed plants and tree leaves for low SWR [standing wave ratio], then adding sensors and transmitters to same plants. SWR meters measure how well the transmit power signal emitted from a transceiver (radio) is traveling through the antenna system into the atmosphere.

– Billy Hayes "The HAARP Man"

Fires almost identical in every way to the Santa Rosa fires, including the date (October 15, 2017), burned for six intense hours in Oliveira do Hospital, Portugal: 93 percent of the surrounding forest destroyed, 20,855 houses and buildings, 54 dead. Drones were spotted when it started, the laser trigger from out of the plasma cloud cover. Eyewitness Conny Kadia wrote in an email:

At the northern border an airplane [or drone] over our forest, everything went dark, five minutes later a fire tsunami, a 20-meter wall of fire arose. Wooden factory in village 3 kilometers away – I saw a beam, heard sounds like glass falling on metal, the sound of electricity, almost like iron in a microwave. We found thousands of empty bottles at the northern border in the deep forest, beside roads, in villages . . .

In July 2018—while "wildfires" raged in Yosemite, Redding / Carr, and the Mendocino Complex—"wildfires" beset Greece, killing 102 people and said to be "the second-deadliest wildfire event in the 21st century, after the 2009 Black Saturday bushfires in Australia that killed 173" (Wikipedia). As both Portugal and Greece are NATO members, it is suspicious that their "wildfires" erupted *simultaneous* with the California "wildfires"—Portugal in October 2017, Greece in July 2018.

A primary difference between the Santa Rosa fire and the Portuguese fire was the *acceleration* of the Portuguese fires by the category-3 Hurricane Ophelia, the 10th and final hurricane of a very active 2017 hurricane season. Sweeping up from the southeast Atlantic Ocean, Ophelia arced past Portugal and Spain all the way to Ireland. Though hurricane wind fanned the flames of the fires, this fact was not mentioned in the report by the National Hurricane Center. From Wikipedia:

Starting on 15 October 2017, winds from Ophelia fanned wildfires in both Portugal and Spain. The wildfires have claimed the lives of at least 49 individuals, including 45 in Portugal and four in Spain, and dozens more were injured. In Portugal, more than 4,000 firefighters battled around 150 fires.

Ophelia's presence reminded me of Hurricane Erin (also a class 3) that on September 11, 2001 was parked 200 miles east of New York City before and during the destruction of the World Trade Towers. Major airports recorded "distant thunder" as U.S. Navy planes flew into Erin's eye to assess her strength. It was obvious that Erin had been created and placed to generate the high-voltage potential gradient needed for molecular dissociation via the Hutchison Effect (wilting steel, evaporation of metal, cold "heat," dustification, binding of metal and non-metal, etc.) discussed by Judy Wood, PhD, in her excellent book *Where Did the Towers Go? The Evidence of Directed Free-Energy Technology on 9/11.* Michael Brenden at *Toxi.com* wrote:

> This topic involves deeply occulted dark military advanced weaponry science, so open your mind to the incredible possibilities of the best minds limitlessly funded with results bent not for 'free energy' or any good but primarily for cultish mass murder (Purim sacrifice?) and geopolitical leverage. It was Trump's uncle who is bragged to have been involved in the infamous gov-grab of Tesla's papers, particularly regarding his Death Ray—an almost inconceivable energy and particle beam weapon that required high-voltage gradient established over target (by Hurricane Erin), into which particles are injected at high velocity (from Brookhaven National Lab's RHIC and ASYNCH LASER to clear the path in the atmosphere between BNL and WTC) and excited into microwave resonance such that aluminum, steel, and hard brittle materials are vaporized into nanoparticulate dust . . .[77]

Was Ophelia used to ramp up the uncanny wind whose peak intensity of 115 mph occurred just south of the Azores on October 14, seemingly like it was coming from a crack between non-scalar and scalar worlds?

And let's not forget the 130 fires in Australia—72,000 square miles, 3,500 homes and other buildings, 34 people dead, countless wildlife—between June 2019 and March 2020; in August and September, fires raged in California and Oregon.

---

77 File name: "HAARP Weather Mod Disrupts Earth Magnetosphere": "[ionospheric heating experiments at Arecibo] showed that HF heating can excite instabilities that generate large-scale irregularities and striations along the [Earth's] magnetic field." Toxi.com, 18 August 2020. From the work of William Edwin Gordon (1918-2010), Arecibo Ionospheric Modification HF Facility, Puerto Rico. See the National Academy of Sciences (NAS) biography on Gordon.

> *The Great Plume in Paradise: At 6:33 am on November 8, 2018, fire was ignited and immediately traveled WEST from Concow to Paradise with a tight plume that exploded over us within an hour. I was outside until 10 am, and it was bluebird. An hour later, complete [chemical cloud] coverage . . . Paradise got hit last year as well; they keep coming back to the same areas. I've been the only one until recently who has chronicled the worldwide DEW attacks the past 3 years, but it really goes all the way back to the Oakland '91 fires at the same time we were using laser in Iraq 1.*
>
> – Jamie Lee, author of *Paradise Lost: The Great California Fire Chronicles,* 2019

The 2016 film *Geostorm* preprogrammed the public for "new normal" fires ignited in carefully prepared electrostatic, ionized environments. The mainstream media outdo themselves to invent new "wildfire" terms: *firenado, firestorm, pyrocumulus clouds* (that collapse at night and create strong downdrafts), *plume-dominating fires,* etc., all the while blaming "poor forest management" and "strong Santa Ana winds."

Take the fire in Walker, California in 2020 that generated enormous pyrocumulus and pyrocumulonimbus clouds visible from space—NASA's "fire-breathing dragon of clouds" injecting masses of nanoparticles into the lower stratosphere ten miles above Earth. *Plume-dominated* means high pressure vertical updraft resulting in strong erratic winds and extreme fires (fire tornadoes) that sustain and grow themselves, thanks to all the nanoparticles.[78]

The truth is that there was virtually no natural wind, only *blast waves* from pressure expanding *supersonically* (meaning in a *scalar* dimension) due to explosive cores of compressed gases followed by blast waves of negative pressure.[79] The fires moved at an uncanny 80 football fields a minute. Firemen stood in bewilderment.

The "new space economy" obliquely references *full spectrum dominance* over everything and everyone on the planet in the name of decreasing carbons / increasing carbon credits, global warming, climate change, and all the rest, but actually including 3D battlefield monitoring, reading DNA signatures and brain evoked potentials, with cavity magnetrons reading the metal in our brains and bloodstream, in soil, buildings, and cars—all from space. Interference patterns can be used to direct phase conjugation so as to heat

---

78 Paul Duginski, "The fire that devastated a Sierra town created a pyrocumulus cloud. What does that mean?" Los Angeles Times, November 19, 2020.

79 See Mike Morales's YouTube "More Proof West Coast Was Attacked By Fire Storms!!!" November 10, 2018.

nanometal components and ignite prechosen buildings without igniting trees via the nanotech in the air and soil.

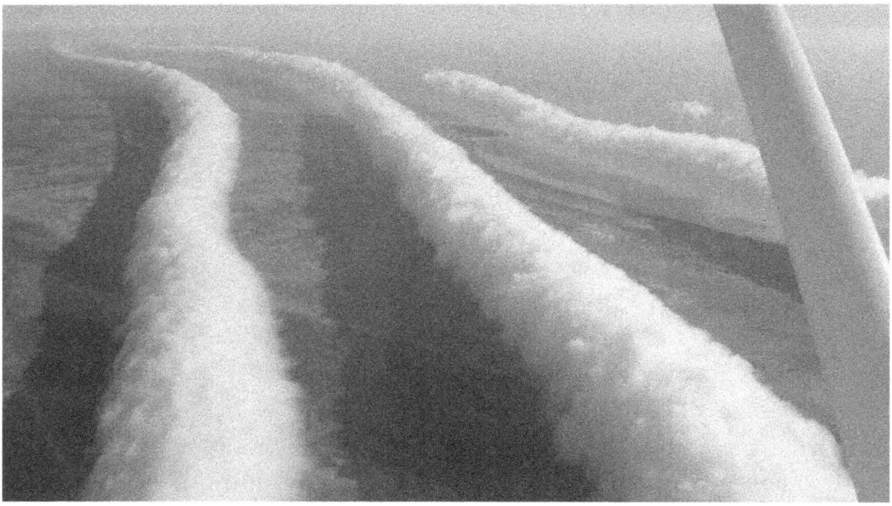

Soliton clouds (Morning Glory). Soliton clouds can reach 1,000 km long while maintaining their shape and moving.

https://en.wikipedia.org/wiki/Morning_Glory_cloud

The metal nanotechnology that came from the sky and is now wedged into the soil 6-8" down[80] is a byproduct of *utility fog (foglets)*—the flying, intercommunicating nanomachines that shapeshift for whatever programmed task they have been given[81]—nano-swarmtroopers whose hive intelligence is yoked to computers armed with AI algorithms that track and correct their itinerary as they travel in ember-like phalanxes to buildings, cars, and parts of forests slated for immolation. (Wildfires don't selectively burn and not burn.) These swarms of "programmable matter" self-assemble, self-replicate, destroy or build. They and their kin—wherever they are, and they are everywhere, even inside our bodies and brains—are the foglets being used to replace yesterday's world with a brave new world run by nano and the human hive mind of Transhumanism.[82]

80 Nubia Zuverza-Mena et al., "Exposure of engineered nanomaterials to plants: Insights into the physiological and biochemical responses – A review." Plant Physiology and Biochemistry, January 2017: "Carbon-based and metal-based engineered nanomaterials (ENMs) . . . have the potential to build up sediments and biosolid-amended agricultural soils . . ."

81 See Wil McCarthy's article "Ultimate Alchemy," Wired, October 1, 2001, plus Tim Ventura's article "Smart Dust, Utility Fog & virtual People: The Future of Programmable Matter," Medium.com, December 6, 2019.

82 Thanks to Michelle Ewens, "Future Foglets of the Hive Mind," March 24, 2011. Also see

The fact that trees near thoroughly torched vehicles and buildings didn't burn was the first obvious clue that the "wildfires" were not wildfires at all, while other trees burned *from the inside out*. Laser strafe marks were everywhere around Paradise.

The Earth being a capacitor storing electrical charge in electrical fields means that lightning discharges can occur underground naturally, as Stephen Smith of *The Thunderbolts Project* explains in his essay "Lightning discharges in the atmosphere are familiar, but what about the ones underground?"[83] But natural subterranean conductivity can be amped up considerably by scalar waves traveling through the Earth. The ULF "lightning" erupting from inside trees and underground pointed to this, as did the fact that the "wildfire" was moving at 273 mph until arriving at what seemed to be its destination: Paradise, the town whose gold and silver deposits added to the conductivity factor. Now, a real "kill charge" could be triggered from above by laser or maser, along with the tomography that gave the technology far above the Earth the eyes it needed to peer deep underground.

Months ago, while examining some drone and dashboard footage that came my way, I suddenly realized that I was not looking at blowing embers blowing but phalanxes of nano-swarmtroopers flying *against* the blast surges, marching into housing developments and along the edges of buildings, even along highways, intent on getting to where they were programmed to go so as to burn what they were programmed to burn.[84] *I was looking at an intelligent operation, not random in any way*—the swarm intelligence of the technology, the intelligence of a distant ion-driven satellite, and the intelligence of those manipulating and following the operation on their monitors.

It was a moment of revelation: the ability to destroy from space was here, and thanks to nanotechnology, it could be highly specific.

G.O. Mouteva et al., "Black carbon aerosol dynamics and isotopic composition in Alaska linked with boreal fire emissions and depth of burn in organic soils." Global Biogeochemical Cycles, November 2015.

83 Posted by Teo Blaskovic at The Watchers, September 12, 2011. See "Oregon fires burning underground post new threat," KGW News, September 21, 2020.

84 See "Paradise Lost #91 – The Malibu Ember Chronicles," aplanetruth3, June 28, 2019.

More on the fires

"Santa Rosa & Northern CA Fires THE LAWS OF PHYSICS (where'd the houses go??)" InTruthbyGrace, October 10, 2017
"Exactly like September 11 . . . twigs didn't burn but buildings 'ignited to desolation' . . ."

"EMF signatures in California Fires: plant / tree electro-physiological responses to high EMF fields," InTruthbyGrace, August 8, 2018
How trees react to EMF. Trees catching fire from the inside out; cedar branches splaying out.

"Fires Burn Hotter with Nano Metals in Chemtrails," *TheTruthDenied.com*, July 30, 2014

"California Gets Cooked / Fires Created by Microwave Directed Energy Weapon," ODD TV, October 18, 2017
Fires 500 Terawatts of power in 2 billionths of a second.

"California Drought and Fires Caused by USAF Pillar Point Radar? 2018 09 27," The HAARP Report
Breakdown of drought factor behind the 2018 fires. How ionospheric heaters are used.

"Were Black Triangle Craft Used in Calfires?" James Munder, November 17, 2018
Mike Morales clip. Explosion just before fires. Beams shooting out of NexRads.

"DEW Weapons Shock Wave Rocket?? Camp Fire Paradise lost via Mike Morales," November 12, 2018
Mike has more videos about the fires.

Jamie Lee, "Paradise Lost #25[85] ~ How the Houses Were Torched Interview with 30 yr Microwave Engineer," December 9, 2018
How the environment was "loaded" for the fires.

Jamie Lee, "Proof ~ Some CA Fires Caused by

---

85 Jamie Lee aplanetruth3 has an entire series on the fires, particularly on the Paradise, California fires, including his book Paradise Lost: The Great California Fire Chronicles, https://www.youtube.com/channel/UCbM5aiq-du38a05SfseMTPg/search?query=paradise+lost. He lives near Santa Rosa.

Underground Lightning Strikes," aplanetruth5, August 23, 2020

Jamie Lee, "Paradise Lost #56: Did Underground Lightning Create the Burned Trees and Torch the Houses Too?"

Daniel Alexander Cannon's "8888 Trees Struck By Lightning in Paradise, CA," LogicBeforeAuthority, January 5, 2019

J. Marvin Herndon, PhD and Mark Whiteside, "California Wildfires: Role of Undisclosed Atmospheric Manipulation and Geoengineering," *Journal of Geography, Environment and Earth Science International,* October 2018

2

The Three Primary Transhumanist Delivery Systems

The Chemical Aerosol Soup

Water
Ozone
Group 2 Earth Metals:
Calcium (Ca), barium (Ba), magnesium (Mg), strontium (Sr) & fluoride (F)
Barium-strontium-titanate (BST)
Titanium (Ti) / Titanium dioxide (TiO_2 / E171)
Lithium (Li), a "conflict mineral"
(Aluminum & Mercury, see "Vaccinations")
BioAPI (Bio-Application Programming Interface)
Polymers / Filaments / Fibers
Biofilm pseudo-skin
Lyme & Morgellons

GMO Frankenfoods

GMO Meat
GM Marketing
Glyphosate

Vaccines: The Medical Industry's Third Rail

"Herd Immunity"
The strange *pharmakon* of vaccines
Vaccination by aerosol
Aluminum
Mercury

EMR [electromagnetic radiation] is most likely a synergen. The exposures such as pesticides, chemtrails, harvesting of forests and urban sprawl are not causes competing with EMR—they are additive and synergistic [or amplifying] causes. They are insults to the system that requires strong biological compensation to overcome. EMR depletes that ability to compensate, and thus the person or species succumbs to the effects of the environmental insult more severely and more rapidly.

– George Louis Carlo, epidemiologist, January 1, 2008

. . . The dry warm air above San Diego is not conducive to the formation of jet contrails, which are ice condensate. By November 2014 the tanker-jets were busy every day crisscrossing the sky spraying their aerial graffiti. In a matter of minutes, the aerosol trails would start to diffuse, eventually forming cirrus-like clouds that further diffuse to form a white haze that scattered sunlight, often occluding or dimming the sun. Aerosol spraying was occasionally so intense as to make the otherwise cloudless blue sky overcast, some areas of sky turning brownish. Sometimes the navigation lights of the tanker-jets were visible as they worked at night, their trails obscuring the stars overhead; by dawn, the normally clear-blue morning sky already had a milky white haze. Regardless, aerosol spraying often continued throughout the day. The necessity for daily aerosol emplacement stems from the relatively low spraying-altitudes in the troposphere where mixing with air readily occurs, bringing down the aerosolized particulates and exposing humanity and Earth's biota to the fine-grained substance. My concern about the daily exposure to ultra-fine airborne particulate matter of undisclosed composition and its concomitant effect on the health of my family and public health in general prompted my research.

– J. Marvin Herndon, PhD, "maverick geophysicist" (*Washington Post)*

The Chemical Aerosol Soup

The aerosols that have been distributed for 25 years have been loaded with chemicals and conductive nano-sized heavy metals as well as genetically engineered fungi, red blood cells, nanobots, nanosensors, and nano-*synbio* creations piggybacked onto polymer fibers. These flotsam and jetsam and Frankenstein creations permeate the soil, tree bark and roots, aquifers, and foods growing in the open air. We are breathing and ingesting them, and they are challenging our weakened immune systems and making us ill.

The U.S. Navy and enlisted merchant ships produce ship tracks in the South Pacific to feed and direct weather systems (and data "clouds") to carry this detritus across the nation and into the world, supplemented by particles released by industrial plants, proving once again that the "public-private partnership" of military and industry work hand in glove. Floods in Louisiana, West Virginia and Macedonia in the Balkans are not due to any 1,000-year cycle or "inland sheared tropical depression"; such floods are geoengineered with atmospheric rivers and in-place water vapor generation (WSAC). Spray nano-laden aerosols into the atmosphere to capture moisture, then release billions of tons of rainwater with electromagnetic pulsing.

In 2003, a paper from the National Center of Biotechnology Information (NCBI) recommended aerosol "live-attenuated strain" vaccinating of populations, given that "nasal breathing" is more suitable for the old and very young.[1] Corporate media shout from the rooftops about Russia and South America experimenting on their populations, but utter not a word about the thousands of releases by the United States—like the *Bacillus subtilis* (lung damage) released in the Pentagon South Parking Lot in early June 2007, or the open-air "Urban Shield: Crystal City Urban Transport Study" release of perfluorocarbon tracers and sulfur hexafluoride (lung- and neuro-toxicant) in Crystal City, Virginia. Sulfur hexafluoride (SF6) is the *real* greenhouse gas problem, due to the fact that it is used extensively by the electrical industry to prevent short circuits. SF6 is 23,500X more warming than CO2, and being synthetic, cannot be absorbed or eliminated naturally. SF6 *switchgear* is being used more than ever, due to the necessity of coupling "green" power (wind, solar, etc.) to electrical switches and circuit breakers.[2]

Back in 1990—Bernard Eastlund's 1987 HAARP patent was already in the building phase in Gakona, Alaska—CRRES (Combined Release and Radiation Effects Satellite) was placed in an elliptical geosynchronous transfer orbit 22,236 miles up, carrying 24 canisters of chemicals to be released and ionized by the Sun's UV light to create elongated plasma clouds along the magnetic field lines (Birkeland currents) connecting Earth and Sun. These NASA / USAF payload releases into "Earth space"— the magnetosphere and ionosphere space environment, a "dynamic ocean of invisible magnetic and electrical fields and particles" (CRRES press kit)—were augmented by massive chemical releases from ten sounding rockets launched from Arecibo, Puerto Rico and Kwajalein Atoll, home of the Space Fence in the Marshall Islands.

Eighteen years later, CBS-affiliated KSLA investigated the possible source of a substance that fell to Earth in the wake of high-altitude chemtrails. High levels of barium (6.8 ppm), lead (8.2 ppm), and traces of arsenic, chromium, cadmium, selenium, and silver were found, with barium being more than 6X

1 Roth, Y., et al., "Feasibility of aerosol vaccination in humans." NCBI, March 2003.

2 Matt McGrath, "Climate change: Electrical industry's 'dirty secret' boosts warming." RNZ.co, 14 September 2019.

the EPA toxic level. Symptoms of barium poisoning begin with stomach and chest pains and blood pressure problems.[3]

Lies regarding the chemicalizing of the atmosphere and use of electromagnetics for weather engineering skews all other planetary data and leaves PhD and layman researchers in perpetual *cognitive dissonance*.[4] As in the CV-19 "pandemic" for which all causes of death are CV-19, all planetary changes for the worse are filed under "global warming" and "climate change."

Water (H2O)

Water is *the* magic transducer because of its dielectric constant. All the water in our bodies, our oceans and rivers, atmospheric rivers, geoengineered storms of rain and ice, acts as a *sponge* for the electromagnetic radiation that then turns the water acidic—an increase in hydrogen ion concentration (H+) that decreases the pH.[5] We have heard for decades how pollutants acidify our rain, aquifers, oceans, and atmosphere, but we've heard precious little about how this acidity affects our health. For the military-industrial-intelligence phalanx, increased acidity serves the conductivity needed for wireless operations: the lower the pH, the higher the H+ ions, the greater the conductivity.

Private wells, watersheds, and aquifers are now acidic. In the past ten or so years, 85,000 fracking wells[6] from Big Oil's "shale revolution" of horizontal drilling and hydraulic fracturing have gone through 72 trillion gallons of water and 360 billion gallons of chemicals. Human and pet pharmaceuticals end up in public water and watersheds, and so do medicines for pain, infection, high cholesterol, asthma, epilepsy, mental illness, heart problems, anti-anxiety, sex hormones. Corporations that bottle water do not test or treat water for pharmaceuticals,[7] and the same goes for home filtration and sewage treatment systems. Reverse osmosis can do it, but is often cost-prohibitive.

> Cattle are given ear implants that provide a slow release of trenbolone, an anabolic steroid used by some bodybuilders, which causes cattle to bulk up. But not all the trenbolone circulating in a steer is metabolized. Water sampled downstream of a Nebraska feedlot had steroid levels four

---

3 Steve Watson, "CIA Is Funding Government-Led Chemtrail Project: Spy Agency to Help Study 'Security Impacts' of Geo-engineering." Global Research, July 20, 2013.

4 A mental conflict when beliefs are contradicted by new information and in the end affects personal identity and heightens emotional reactions.

5 "How does the concentration of hydrogen ions change with pH," Rehan Muhammed, February 2, 2014, http://www.youtube.com/watch?v=84Y555UfRPg.

6 By 2040, the projected figure for fracking wells is 675,000.

7 Ethan A. Huff, "Bottled water found to contain over 24,000 chemicals, including estrogen disruptors." Naturalnews.com, September 19, 2013.

times as high as the water taken upstream. Male fathead minnows living in that downstream area had low testosterone levels and small heads . . . Our bodies may shrug off a relatively big one-time dose, yet suffer from a smaller amount delivered continuously over a half century . . .[8]

In 2014-15, Flint, Michigan's contaminated water led to Legionnaires' disease (atypical pneumonia), not just the "low chlorine" reported. Dow Chemical's chlorine / chloroform has been added to water treatment since 1908, despite the cancer and premature senility, heart attacks, sexual impotency, strokes, CNS depression, liver and kidney damage, and immune system suppression. Then there is the PVC (polyvinyl chloride), dry cleaning solvents, pesticides like Syngenta's paraquat ($C_{12}H_{14}Cl_2N_2$ usage doubled between 2006 and 2016, according to the National Water-Quality Assessment Project), bleach in the manufacture of paper, chlorine gas, chlorine-based DDT, dioxin, PCBs, etc.[9]

The water molecules in our bodies and brains resonate to frequencies other than our own. The brain (80 percent water) can be entrained at any distance by any bio-phasic waveform that can penetrate the skull—even from satellite. Blood sugar and iron in the blood can be entrained. Target a crystal molecule with a wave resonating at the crystal's own frequency, and it will explode. If it's a sugar crystal, the release charge (*triboluminescence*) can damage the brain or at the very least produce confusion, dizziness, apathy, etc.—similar to what the Lilly Wave does with "the madness frequency" (see Chapter 10, Dual Use II: Pulsed Frequencies").[10]

According to Gerald H. Pollack, PhD, water has a fourth phase beyond solid, liquid, and vapor (gas), namely a *hexagonal geometry* able to draw electric current from sunlight.[11] Tom Bearden addresses the amazing sensitivity of water to everything in its surroundings via its Whittaker[12] substructure inside its bond-structuring, even to the point of its internal bonding structure changing when someone enters the room or an observer blinks an eye. In the Whittaker in-folded EM wave structure, all potentials overlap and water

8 Jeff Donn, Martha Mendoza and Justin Pritchard, "AP probe finds drugs in drinking water." AP, March 9, 2008.

9 Charlie Cray, "Chlorine: The Everywhere Element." ZMagazine, December 1995.

10 HAARP, the GWEN gyrotron system, cell phone towers, and power lines can all carry the Lilly Wave carrier waveform to transmit EM frequencies, including mind control (1-10 MHz).

11 Gerald H. Pollack, The Fourth Phase of Water: Beyond Solid, Liquid, and Vapor. Ebner & Sons, 2013.

12 E.T. Whittaker (1873-1956) was an American physicist whose mathematical work on scalar waves has been shrouded in "national security" for a century. He was the first to prove mathematically that there are far more than four dimensions to spacetime.

transduces the cross currents.[13] Could this be why functional hydrocephalics and people who have lost most of their brain can still think?

> The Whittaker structures ensure intermingling and intercommunication through the internal energy channels of the total bio-potential to all its constituents. Therefore, the water structuring of the fluid in the head of the hydrocephalic serves, bridgewise, as a substitute brain.[14]

That water can serve as a substitute brain bridge means that its infolded structures have multidimensional properties, which is what shamans have indicated for millennia by referring to water as a *road*, a link to the seven worlds below (Toltec), deep lakes and waterholes being in touch with a level of reality just below ours, with rivers and streams acting as transmitters by which human consciousness can travel to places on the Earth's surface and below. Water's reflective nature (think of the Greek tale of Narcissus) can put the shaman in touch with subterranean beings, with the shiny surface at the very bottom of deep waterholes and lakes serving as a window or mirror through which entities can be encountered. I think of the fairy tale "The Nixie of the Pond."[15]

Metaphysics, physics, and myth intermingle at quantum junctures.

Is it, then, just coincidence that our bodies are composed of 70 percent water, and water molecule electrons are made to rotate by the WiFi frequency of 2.4 GHz (2450 MHz), the frequency of microwave ovens and 4G iPhones, to force a dielectric loss of water? WiFi initiated the assault on our bodies via water, and now 5G, "the new Wi-Gig," is initiating the assault on our oxygen.

4G	700 MHz to 5 GHz (wavelengths in centimeters)
5G	5 GHz to 90 GHz (wavelengths 1-10 millimeters)

13 Masaru Emoto (1943-2014) "water messages" books show photographs of water crystals responding to thought forms.

14 Thomas E. Bearden, interview in MegabrainReport, February 4, 1991. Lt. Col. Bearden (ret.) resides in Huntsville, Alabama, home of U.S. Space and Rocket Center, NASA's Marshall Space Flight Center, and U.S. Army Aviation and Missile Command. President and CEO of CTEC, Inc. Consultant on scalar electromagnetics processes. Also see Thomas Bearden, "Scalar Electromagnetics and Weather Control." Esoteric Physics homepage, May 26, 1998.

15 Grimms' Tales for Young and Old, translated by Ralph Manheim (Doubleday & Company, 1977).

Ozone (O3)

Ozone (O3) is an upper atmosphere bluish gas that helps to block UV radiation. Ozone depletion in the stratosphere and increase in the troposphere (if it really is increasing) is supposedly due to burning fossil fuels (cars, jets) that produce nitrogen oxides, etc. Electric Universe proponent Christopher Fontenot has a whole other take on ozone depletion, particularly the relativistic electron acceleration in our ionosphere (60 to 1,000 km above the Earth) due to the high-frequency modulation of Alfvén waves. Ionospheric heaters work with solar radiation management (SRM) geoengineering to ionize the Earth's electrojets by ionizing the endless nanoparticles dumped by jets and rockets.[16]

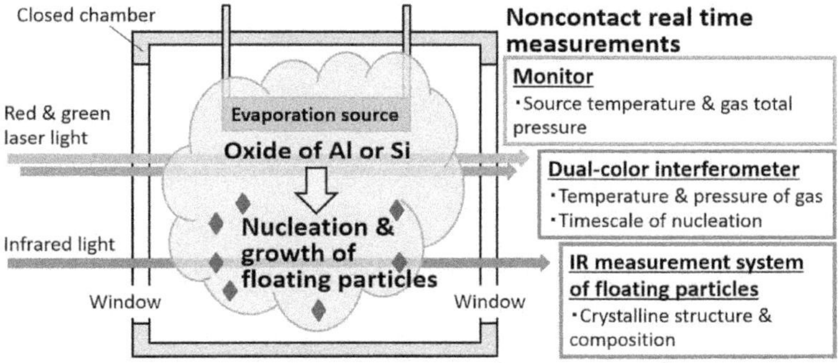

Nucleation & growth of oxide nanoparticles ("**star crumbs**").

Hokkaido University: "We identified the initial conditions required to form nanoparticles, the basic building blocks of earth-like planets. In particular, we searched for conditions where nucleation of oxidized aluminum and silica could easily occur, and we identified the first nanoparticles which govern the evolution of cosmic dust."

https://www.global.hokudai.ac.jp/blog/successful-launch-of-the-sounding-rocket-s-520-30-experiment-using-a-microgravity-environment-to-reproduce-star-crumbs/

SRM's stratospheric aerosol injection (SAI) program is now spraying large quantities of sulfur dioxide into the stratosphere (10-50 km). The "wildfire" biomass burning in the western United States and other places contributes 10-20 percent of the sulfur that then becomes carbonyl sulfide (COS), a long-lived form of sulfur in the troposphere:

> Because it is not easily removed from the troposphere, its distribution is relatively uniform with height and therefore allows COS to migrate to

16 The science-minded might want to read "Study explores wave-particle interaction in atmosphere" (Phys.org, October 27, 2015).

> the stratosphere where it is converted by photolysis to SO2 [sulfur dioxide] and eventually sulfate particles . . .[17]

Besides acid rain, sulfur injections lead to more and more ozone depletion. So it goes when such "save-the-planet" programs are backed by ExxonMobil and Shell Oil.

Group 2 Earth Metals:
Calcium (Ca), barium (Ba), magnesium (Mg), strontium (Sr)

In 2007, the intrepid targeted individual Carolyn Williams Palit explained exactly what the unleashed chemical stew in our skies was all about, especially the barium and aluminum:

> We are dealing with Star Wars. It involves the combination of chemtrails for *creating an atmosphere that will support electromagnetic waves, ground-based electromagnetic field oscillators called gyrotrons, and ionospheric heaters. Particulates make directed energy weapons work better.* It has to do with "steady state" and particle density for plasma beam propagation.
>
> They spray *barium powders* and let it photo-ionize from the ultraviolet light of the sun. Then they make an *aluminum-plasma* generated by "zapping" the metal cations that are in the spray with either electromagnetics from HAARP, the gyrotron system on the ground [Ground Wave Emergency Network or GWEN], or space-based lasers. *The barium makes the aluminum plasma more particulate dense.* This means they can make a denser plasma than they normally could from just ionizing the atmosphere or the air.
>
> More density means that these particles which are colliding into each other will become more charged because there are more of them present to collide. *What they are ultimately trying to do up there is create charged-particle plasma beam weapons.*
>
> Chemtrails are the medium – GWEN pulse radars, the various HAARPs, and space-based lasers are the method, or more simply: *Chemtrails are the medium – directed energy is the method.*
>
> Spray and Zap.[18]

Another targeted individual, Vic Livingston, offers an example:

---

17 Eugene S. Takle, "Biomass Burning Contributes to Stratospheric Sulfate Particles," 2003; from J. Notholt et al., "Enhanced upper tropical tropospheric COS: Impact on the stratospheric aerosol layer," Science, 300, 307-310.

18 Carolyn Williams Palit, "What Chemtrails Really Are," November 9, 2007. Carolyn's emphases.

> Using the microwave weapon system to intensify weather patterns: Manipulate the jet stream to generate high wind gusts, then operatives can precision-target directed MW [microwave] energy to create damaging winds in the immediate vicinity of a target—thus using weather as a weapon and major weather patterns as a camouflage for local precision-targeted attacks, like outbreaks of "thundersnow" or the tornado-strength winds that pushed against my house this morning shortly before 6 a.m. After I took steps intended to ensure that authorities review surveillance of Lockheed Martin CentCom [unified armed forces command] personnel on duty this early a.m. to determine if this highly plausible theory is true, the tornado-strength winds quickly subsided.[19]

On January 30, 2018, MIT-trained scientist Jeffrey Golin, who had worked extensively with gas discharge devices, sent me a chastising email about how dismayed he was that I had neglected to discuss the following in *Chemtrails, HAARP, and the Full Spectrum Dominance of Planet Earth*:

> This particular group of metals together—barium (Ba), strontium (Sr), calcium (Ca), and magnetism (Mg)—are cold cathode emitters used industrially for their unusual special property of having a low electron work function. The important thing to understand is that this special group of unique elements was chosen to aid in *the ionization of gases at low pressures*, just like a neon tube does, just like the air in the ionosphere does. That makes them really useful for HAARP devices.

Two months later, a March 21, 2018 email from Paul Stephen Cox took me a little further down the metal nanoparticle rabbit hole:

> Barium and strontium bind together inside the body. Because they are very similar to calcium and magnesium, the body is fooled into taking them up. They then get into the soft body parts and cause untold medical conditions.

So nanoparticles of Ba, Sr, Ca, and Mg are released in the upper atmosphere to aid in the ionization of gases (plasma) at low pressure, but when they fall earthward and we breathe in their nanoparticles . . .

---

19 Vic Livingston, "'Microburst' winds again hit home of Journo exposing electromagnetic radio weapon crimes," viclivingston.blogspot.com, November 13, 2012. Also consider raising winds to drive fires: Paul Duginski, "This fire that devastated a Sierra town created a pyrocumulus cloud. What does that mean?" Los Angeles Times, November 19, 2020.

Calcium

It is strange to imagine, as Paul Stephen Cox maintains, that barium and strontium can fool the body into thinking they are calcium and magnetism. Microwave phones cause our neurons to release calcium ions, which makes us tired, irritable, and emotional. *Stress* is a key word when it comes to calcium.

> It is child's play to transmit an ELF-modulated signal to be broadcast by the entire mobile phone network—if need be. By this means, all mobile phone users can be behaviourally modified, at the cost of developing cancer from low level microwave exposure from the phones they constantly use, stressing the neural network by constant calcium ion efflux and interference with bioelectric fields.[20]

Martin Pall, PhD, (*bioinitiative.org*), is professor emeritus of biochemistry at Washington State University.[21] He has done extensive research into electromagnetics, 4G and 5G technologies, and points out that now that we live in a constant electrosmog of WiFi fields (2.4 GHz), our stem cells are negatively affected and produce oxidative stress on the *voltage-gated calcium channels (VGCCs)* in the plasma membranes around our cells.[22] The very presence of wireless technologies means no less than a *million ions per second* are being loaded into our cells via the voltage sensors in the plasma membrane surrounding each cell, thus increasing cellular calcium, nitric oxide, and excessive signaling, all of which lead to the physiological stress that undermines and confuses the immune system and produces a host of chronic symptoms: Lupus, rheumatoid arthritis, Crohn's disease, irritable bowel syndrome, Type 1 diabetes, chronic fatigue, fibromyalgia, EHS, etc.[23] Complex calcium signaling overload is the domino effect behind many autoimmune symptoms, from cataracts and breakdown of the blood-brain barrier to lowered nocturnal *melatonin* (and increased nocturnal norepinephrine) and metabolic weakening.

Our amazing neurons have the highest densities of VGCC, due to the cal-

---

20 Tim Rifat, "Electromagnetic Murders & Suicides & How They're Done." The Truth Campaign, Spring 1999.

21 See Dr. Pall's 90-page book, "5G: Great Risk for EU, U.S. and International Health! Compelling Evidence for Eight Distinct Types of Great Harm Caused by Electromagnetic Field (EMF) Exposures and the Mechanism that Causes Them," May 17, 2018, https://peaceinspace.blogs.com/files/5g-emf-hazards--dr-martin-l.-pall--eu-emf2018-6-11us3.pdf.

22 This plasma is not the same plasma of plasma physics. Blood plasma makes up 55 percent of our blood and acts as a gatekeeper between the blood and circulatory system. It is a light yellow liquid that carries water, salts, enzymes, hormones, the proteins albumin and fibrinogen, immunoglobulins (antibodies), and clotting factors to parts of the body that need it, plus removes waste from the body's cells.

23 The trend of misdiagnosing symptoms as diseases is often based on ignorance of electromagnetic radiation.

cium-signaling required for release of neurotransmitters and regulation of synaptic structure and function. Excessive Ca2+ levels in the mitochondria[24] can produce cell death (apoptosis), similar to what follows double-strand breaks in cellular DNA, all of which has to do with chronic electromagnetic radiation exposure that increases hormone levels and releases and thus exhausts the body.

Barium

In 2005, independent scientist Clifford Carnicom used spectral analysis to determine that the combination of the nanometals he was collecting from precipitation and a HEPA filter seemingly had been *designed* to interfere with the cyclotronic resonant frequency of our *potassium (K)* ions when hit by the fifth harmonic of ELF radiation. Barium blocks the passive efflux of intracellular potassium, *the* essential alkali. Potassium depletion can lead to heart fibrillation, arrythmia, and heart attacks. Without potassium, we are vulnerable to gain-of-function virulent diseases: lack of potassium chlorate (lungs); lack of potassium phosphate (cerebrum); lack of potassium sulfate (solar plexus and colon). Possibly, it is the same for the sodium (Na) and chloride (Cl) ions that act as *neuron action potentials.*

It appears that the central nervous system is being intentionally targeted for Transhumanist modification.

> The technical principle of receivers for electromagnetic waves is fully analogous with biological information and communications systems. If several thousand of the hundreds of billions of nerve cells in our brain resonate with manmade centimeter waves, the carrier frequency has to be suppressed when the signal is passed on to the synapses.
>
> To overcome cell membranes, living organisms use electrochemical processes involving sodium and potassium ions. This suppresses the carrier frequency in the high-frequency range just as the demodulation circuit does in manmade receivers. What remains is the signal impressed on the carrier frequency, e.g. in the low-frequency ELF range. This is also the frequency range at which our own nervous system normally works . . . If interference signals are superimposed on the *natural* signals generated by the body, e.g. by using artificially created centimeter waves as a carrier, the brain could be presented with *simulated states that we consciously perceive but which do not exist in reality* . . . In a 'psychotronic war' using microwaves modulated by using ELF waves, it would no longer be necessary to kill whole armies by inducing cardiac or respiratory irregular signals.

---

24 Mitochondria are the powerhouses of our cells, converting nutrients and oxygen into energy. They have their own DNA. Damaged mitochondria = altered DNA.

The enemy can simply be incapacitated by disturbing their states of balance or confusing the ability to think logically . . .[25] (Emphasis added.)

Released into the atmosphere and ionized by light and UV radiation, barium sets up a conductive layer that acts as a filter to short-out the Earth's 800-1,000 volts per meter potential gradient,[26] thus keeping the trillions of nanoparticles discharged by jets suspended. Ionized barium uses the Sun's radiation to form rain (like radiolysis), unlike short-lived isotopes that induce conduction, gather and direct moisture.

Barium is highly refractive (unlike aluminum, which is highly reflective) and absorbs high levels of UV emissions because of its low electron volt work function (barium 2.7 eV, aluminum 4.3 eV), after which it ionizes them and re-emits the energy into our visible spectrum.

Barium has complex synergistic capabilities. For example, barium-strontium-titanate (BST) (BaSr3)TiO3 has the ability to share calcium electrons (valence) that are highly fluoride-reactive. (See below for more on BST.) Barium's synergy with *hydrogen fluoride (HF)* (see Fluoride below) is said to remove fluoride and other acids from atmospheric suspension. Jim Phelps of DOEWatch: "In the mid-1980s . . . massive health problems linked to HF emissions . . . was causing problems ranging from health damage to changing local weather. The study of the Oak Ridge DOE and TVA [Tennessee Valley Administration] system showed this was a national effect. *This is how the major DOE chemtrail operations came into being.*" (My emphasis.) In 1999, Phelps wrote a whistleblower letter about worker illnesses at the Oak Ridge National Laboratory (where he had worked in the 1980s) in which he referenced how burning soluble uranium fluorides releases HF and other toxic fluorides into the air, along with chemical catalysts like methyl cyanide:

The lung damages *and the high blood calcium* are prime indicators of HF exposures. The arthritis, sore joints, thinking impairment, rashes, and fatigue are also prime indicators of increasing amounts of insoluble calcium fluoride rat poison in the body. HF calcium scavenges and will impact nerve myelin and also kill off mitochondria in cells and lead to heart spasms and attacks.[27] (Emphasis added.)

---

25 Wolfgang Volkrodt, PhD, "Can Human beings Be Manipulated by ELF Waves?" Raum & Zeit (June-July 1989). Former Siemens scientist in Germany.

26 The Earth's charge potential is no doubt increasing, due to the increasing power density of EM radiation. It used to be much lower (e.g. 100-300 volts per meter). This artificially induced electromagnetic current impacts solar activity via the connective Birkeland currents.

27 Oak Ridge National Laboratory letter from Jim Phelps, "Concerned about toxic emissions," December 30, 1999. The case is made that Pyrroloquinoline Quinone (PQQ) can grow new mitochondria in "The little-known nutrient that's growing my daughter new mitochondria: PQQ" at recoveringkids.com.

Magnesium

It is odd that the *Introduction to Atmospheric Chemistry* by Peter V. Hobbs (Cambridge University Press, 2000) does not include magnesium or titanium, aluminum, barium, or calcium in its chart of expected components of the atmosphere.[28]

As early as June 2001, while directing his attention to the elements in the periodic table's Groups I and II that kept showing up as crystals in environmental samples, Carnicom noted the presence of substantial amounts of elemental magnesium. Two-thirds the weight of aluminum, magnesium is extremely conductive (like copper and aluminum) and can be ionized by the Sun's UV. Twenty years ago, Carnicom wrote:

> Evidence continues to accumulate that certain metals, i.e. magnesium and barium, as well as certain biologicals and fibrous components, are established as the core elements of the aerosol operations in progress.[29]

If we are thus depleted of real magnesium by the chemical soup raining down on us, we are robbed of the very element that enhances the binding of oxygen to haem proteins for healthy red blood cells (hemoglobin and iron) and therefore oxygen transport and utilization. It is imperative that we attend to magnesium palliatives like Epsom salt baths (MgSO, magnesium sulfate), supplements (with zinc), and liquid magnesium spray that Morgellons sufferers swear by, plus adding magnesium-rich foods in a balanced acid-alkaline diet. Believe it or not, this includes greens, due to the transmutative alchemy of oxidation: $Mg + O \rightarrow Ca$.[30]

---

28 In fact, the publisher formally asked Clifford Carnicom to remove the Hobbs chart from his website. Clifford E. Carnicom, "The Expected Composition," March 28, 2002.

29 Clifford Carnicom, "Atmospheric Magnesium Disclosed," June 10, 2001, carnicominstitute.org.

30 C. Louis Kervran, Biological Transmutations and Their Applications in Chemistry, Physics, Biology, Ecology, Medicine, Nutrition, Agriculture, Geology (Swan House, 1972). «This English edition of the works of Louis Kervran (1901-1983) is intended for everyone: scholar, layman, or college student. In Mr. Kervran's words, as scientists 'have made of science another job,' it would not be ethical to present it to scientists alone. The problems of ecology, medicine, nutrition, and the alarming rise of radioactivity are too acute to be dealt with solely through academic channels. It is within everyone's ability to comprehend the biological transmutations as long as there is a desire for true knowledge. The understanding of the biological transmutations requires nothing more than the casting aside of all rigid thought while studying them. Transmutation is no more and no less than a reality that teaches us about change. In change we find life, and by change we create life. Our only constant is our goal of becoming Man. The principles of biological transmutation affect every phase of our existence..."

Also available is macrobiotics founder George Ohsawa's translation and interpretation of Kervran's work *Biological Transmutations,* 2nd edition, 2011.

Strontium (St) & fluoride (F)

Strontium leads to a deeper consideration of both ionized radiation in the air and fluoride in the public water, and the synergy between the two in the body. The atmospheric nuclear tests between July 16, 1945 and November 4, 1962 poisoned the atmosphere with one billion grams of radium from strontium-90 (Sr90) alone with a half-life of 28.8 years. Add to Sr90 the high-voltage electricity, radar microwaves, nuclear energy, and heat released by reactor spent fuel rods, and it's easy to see how the DOR (deadened orgone) that Wilhelm Reich, MD, talked about has been depleting the life force (orgone / æther) of the living planet and its inhabitants for almost a century. In 1950, Reich conducted the Oranur Experiment that proved orgone (æther) impacted the DOR clouds that cause drought and deserts.[31]

Throughout the Cold War, the synergy between strontium and fluoride was consistently avoided and lied about in the name of national security. An alarm was raised in 1958 by Dr. James G. Kerwin, director of the Passaic Department of Health, in a 1958 *Dental Digest*: "Because of the affinity of strontium and fluoride to form highly insoluble Sr90F2, the consumption of artificially fluoridated water increases the danger of strontium-90 to man and animals." Strontium-90 and fluoride settle in bones and teeth, and the damning synergy of Sr90F2 leads to gene mutation.

Were the environmental releases of radiation intended to prepare the cells of Human 1.0 for Transhumanist modification?

Fluoride (F) rarely occurs naturally in biological molecules,[32] so what has been the reasoning behind accustoming Americans to drinking and bathing in fluoridated water? In 1960, it was 16.6 percent of 180.7 million Americans; now, it's 62.4 percent of 323 million Americans.[33]

Jim Phelps claims that fluoride compounds like HF and fluoride-metals descending from the upper and lower atmospheres are pulled out of the atmosphere and neutralized, just as the fluorides in rocket fuels from 1970 to 1991 were:

> The fuel utilized in fuel tank 11 is either hydrazine (N2H4) or liquid ammonia (NH3) while the oxidizer employed is selected from *the group consisting of liquid fluorine (F2), chlorine trifluoride (ClF3) and oxygen difluoride (OF2).* When using hydrazine as the fuel, barium may be dissolved therein as barium chloride, BaCl2, or barium nitrate, Ba(NO3)2, or a

31 The chemical plasma clouds of today are often darkened by DOR, not withheld rain.

32 The pineal gland sequesters fluoride from the bloodstream, but for how long under duress? Fluoride either lays the groundwork for or produces effects like hearing voices (schizophrenia or V2K?), and if it impairs the left occipital lobe, will power is impaired.

33 https://www.cdc.gov/fluoridation/statistics/FSGrowth.htm.

combination of the two. When using liquid ammonia as the fuel, barium metal may be dissolved therein. The combination found to produce the highest intensity of Ba- and Ba+ resonance radiation in ground-based tests involved a fuel of 16 percent BA(NO3)2, 17 percent BACl2, and 67 percent N2H4; and as the oxidizer, *the cryogenic liquid fluorine F2* in which an oxidizer to fuel-weight ratio was 1.32...[34] (Emphasis added.)

PERTRAS (the perfluorocarbon tracer system) is also tagging air masses with a PFC (perfluorocarbon) compound ("a particle dispersion model") by loading aircraft so they disperse perfluorocarbons (PFCs) as atmospheric tracers (30kg PFCs per flight) through their hot exhaust or, in HALO flights, through the spray nozzles on the fuselage exterior. PFCs then find their way into our lungs, and are in blood plasma processing, blood substitutes, drug deliveries, and liquid ventilation for deep diving and space travel. *PFCs do not metabolize.* Flu-like symptoms may arise, from light fever and myalgia to a 24-hour intense fever, arterial hypertension, tachycardia, high white blood cell count, and thrombocytopenia.

Then there's the decades of SCoPEx (stratospheric controlled perturbation experiment) whose latest balloon launch in Sweden has been refused and tabled.[35] How ironic is it that HALO-type aircraft release *sulfur hexafluoride (SF6)* in order to trace pollutants, like the 45kg of SF6 gases ejected from fuel-oil nozzles and a 1/16" jet in the baggage compartment of jets to produce a plume[36]? Or FACE, DAPPLE—releases of ozone and CO2, SF6 and perfluoromethylcyclohexane (C7F14) "into urban air." As said above, SF6 is the world's most powerful greenhouse gas (22,200X more heat-trapping than CO2). Tracing pollutants with pollutants . . .

Since November 22, 2016, under the 1970 Toxic Substances Control Act (TSCA), the Fluoride Action Network (FAN) has been pursuing a case against the EPA to ban fluoride in public water supplies due to risks to the

34 NASA's US Patent #3813875 A, "Rocket having barium release system to create ion clouds in the upper atmosphere" (June 4, 1974).

35 James Temple, "Geoengineering researchers have halted plans for a balloon launch in Sweden." MIT Technology Review, March 31, 2021.

36 HALO (high altitude and long-range research aircraft) under German Aerospace: aircraft equipped to disperse chemicals into the hot exhaust (dusty plasma). "Liquid-feed flame spray pyrolysis (LF-FSP) is a general aerosol combustion route to unagglomerated and often single crystal mixed-metal oxide nanopowders with exact control of composition." (Jose A. Azurdia et al., "Liquid-feed Flame Spray Pyrolysis as a Method of Producing Mixed-Metal Oxide Nanopowders of Potential Interest as Catalytic Materials," Chemical Materials, January 6, 2006. Also review "Air Pharmacology II: Spray Pyrolysis and Chemi-ionization," pages 65-72, in Under An Ionized Sky. Typically, another HALO acronym exists for the sake of confusion and cover: High Altitude Lidar Observatory.

brain as well as the inhibition of enzyme action, including enzymes necessary for cell oxidation.[37] The TSCA fluoride lawsuit trial began the week of June 8, 2020.[38] Expert witnesses for the plaintiffs confirmed that sodium fluoride is a pesticide and that fluoride parallels lead neurotoxicity with an IQ drop of 3 to 4 points. Not surprisingly, the World Health Organization (WHO) had been infiltrated by a powerful fluoride lobby. Danish environmental epidemiologist Phillip Grandjean, an expert on mercury neurotoxicity, testified that he was threatened at the Harvard Dental School regarding publishing his neurotoxicology studies on fluoride.[39]

As the most electronegative and reactive element of the entire periodic table, fluoride is difficult to work with and yet commonly used in pharmaceuticals (20-30%), possibly because of the tight bonds it forms with carbon, thus making it difficult for enzymes to break down the drugs too quickly. Antibiotics, anti-inflammatories, and anti-depressants all have fluoride in them.

Barium-strontium-titanate (BST)

Barium-strontium-titanate (BST) is "a complex manmade mineral" used in developing "a wide variety of integrated circuits that create, process and receive microwave frequencies on which communication is based" in order to respond to the demand for "higher performance over a wider range of frequencies . . . new materials tested in detail over the entire microwave spectrum (1-50 GHz)."[40]

Thin-film BST capacitors (ferroelectric thin film varactors made from nano-crystals) doped with europium (Eu) are soldered onto circuit boards (such as in LTE smartphones) for tuning miniature antennas—in the case of LTE smartphones, phased array antennas.

As German scientist Harald Kautz-Vella described in a 2017 interview with Susan Ferguson (whose extraordinary cloud photos were featured throughout *Under An Ionized Sky*):

> Microscope resolution (1000-5000x) of raindrops [reveals high-tech]

---

37 Fluoroacetate is used to introduce fluoride into organic molecules, similar to how soil bacteria are made to convert molecules into polyketides, the molecules that incorporate acetate (Lin Edwards, "New method of incorporating fluoride into drugs," Phys.org, September 6, 2013). Sodium fluoroacetate is used to poison rodents and coyotes by impairing their oxidative metabolism. See "Sodium fluoroacetate poisoning," A.T. Proudfoot et al., Toxicology Review, 2006; 25(4):213-219.

38 See http://fluoridealert.org/researchers/government-reports/timeline-the-tsca-law-suit-against-u-s-epa/.

39 Derrick Broze, "Experts Admit Fluoride is a Pesticide." Activistpost.com, June 12, 2020.

40 American Institute of Physics, "For future chips, smaller must also be better." Science Daily, October 18, 2010.

particles in the raindrops, very intelligent, very exotic particle substances and devices and things that work together as one technology. This is what you find under the microscope, and you find it every day. We have thousands of pictures and people who are doing this for years now, every day microscoping rain.

> And to give you an example of how exotic these substances are, you find a type of nano-crystal that converts body heat to visible light. You can switch off the light of your microscope and when you take your finger and start to point in the direction of the raindrop (*probe?*), the moment you reach the distance of 1 cm, the raindrop starts to glow and shine like a neon bulb, just by converting body heat to visible light. And you can check the literature for substances that have the ability to do this, and actually you will find one that is extremely exotic and artificially made and this is barium-strontium-titanate doped with Europium and other rare earth elements . . . This is one of the key components of this technology having these nano-crystals.[41]

Ferguson includes photos of the "white-grey dust" she finds in her home, which she rightly knows to be "crippling our immune system." Identified by a microbiologist as being manmade, the "dust" we are breathing daily is loaded with metal oxides. Ferguson's research led her to the probable provider of BST components (including the rare earth Harald mentions), possibly even THE corporation producing the chemical mixes we inhale: American Elements.

> . . . The company develops and commercializes technology materials in partnership with the U.S. military and 30 percent of the Fortune 50 list of companies. On November 12, 2020, the company announced its expansion into the life sciences industry with a new manufacturing group devoted to life science and organic chemistry products. (Wikipedia)

And the nanoparticle mix that can be sprayed on any vertical object (like a tree) to make it into a high-powered antenna, or extend the range of an already existing antenna by a factor of 100[42]—do these sprays contain the nanocapacitor BST?

---

41 "Harald Kautz-Vella: 7000 tones of nano-crystals raining down per year on just Germany alone / Three generations of Trans-Humanistic technologies!" Susan Ferguson at Metaphysical Musings, September 29, 2017. Harald continues by talking about BST involvement in the pyrolysis he covered in Under An Ionized Sky.

42 Dexter Johnson, "Spray-on Nanoparticles Mix Turns Trees Into Antennas. IEEE Spectrum, 16 February 2012.

Titanium (Ti) / Titanium dioxide (TiO2 / E171)

Above is the compound barium-strontium-titanate. *Titanium*, a Group 2B carcinogen, often accompanies barium and aluminum in aerosol chemical deliveries,[43] in large part because of how highly valued the reactivity of titanium dioxide nanoparticles (TiO2 NPs) to electromagnetics is in jet fuel air pharmacology.[44] Once activated by UV radiation, TiO2 NPs become good UV blockers (as in sunscreen), even as the UV / TiO2 synergy catalyzes reactions that are toxic to fish and other aquatic species. In soaps and detergents, NP TiO2 accounts for the slick film on our skin, the whitening filler in toothpaste, cosmetics, house paint pigment, processed candies, frostings and icings, dairy products, etc.

Layered (50 nm) over pure salt crystal, NP TiO2 is excellent for cloud-seeding and rain enhancement. Once in contact with water vapor, TiO2 initiates and sustains absorption and condensation to make large raindrops. Much research has gone into proving how TiO2 NPs in outdoor environments or close to artificial UV sources produce what is called *reactive oxygen species (ROS)*—namely, a phototoxicant effect, such as what the TiO2 NPs in sunscreen do to the skin.[45] "Airborne ROS could indeed reach the pulmonary system in exposed individuals and generate a potentially harmful oxidative stress."[46] That said, Jim Phelps says that TiO2 pretreats our G-proteins[47] so that fluoride's electronegative nerve-gas blockage of our G-protein switches is neutralized.

Like cerium oxide (CeO), titanium oxide (TiO) is a semiconductor and photo catalyst with excellent ultraviolet (UV) absorption, and yet strangely, titanium is classified as a "food additive." In fact, according to a 2013 Nanotechnology Consumer Products Inventory, besides the NP TiO2 in processed foods and beverages, NP gold (Au), NP zinc oxide (ZnO), and NP silica oxide (SiO) have increased in foods, as well. Are you getting the idea that nanoparticles are a *delivery system* to the cells? For example, gold NPs have an innate ability to bind with biomolecules and possess excellent optical properties (photocatalytic), possibly for LiDAR (light detection and ranging) biotagging. Either through food and air intake or vaccinations, targets can be color-coded by threat level, security clearance, vaccination status, etc.

Titanium is certainly not a nutrient, but Robin D.P. Watson's essay "The

---

43 YouTube "Off Grid Cabin Life Vlog 45 It's Raining Foam and Other Life Updates, Off Grid Homesteading with The Boss of the Swamp," August 4, 2019.

44 Jim Phelps, DOE / DoD Whistleblower, "Air Pharmacology and end time predictions," 2003. Very important insights into Big Pharma's granddaddy I.G. Farben.

45 The endocrine disruptor oxybenzone is also in sunscreen.

46 David Vernez et al., "Airborne nano-TiO2 particles: An innate or environmentally induced toxicity?" Journal of Photochemistry and Photobiology A: Chemistry Volume 343, 15 June 2017.

47 G-proteins: guanine nucleotide-binding proteins that act as molecular switches inside cells, transmitting signals from outside the cell to its interior.

Nano Blenders Thesis" points to the fact that it is a semiconductor that could play into viral epidemics dependent upon a complex interplay between electromagnetic forces (5G?) and the already implanted "food additive" titanium dioxide known as E171. Not only does E171 *shred* the surfaces of vascular systems, but it is insoluble and bioaccumulates in organs, ready to be activated by 5G.

> Recent forensic research has revealed that the genuine victims of COVID-19 have died from a process called *disseminated intravascular coagulation (DIC)* . . . a cascade of micro-thrombi or blood clots . . . Many victims of COVID-19 have been predisposed to having their immunity status critically lowered by prolonged exposure to electromagnetic frequencies (EMF) from photovoltaics (cheap solar panels) which produce adverse electrical fields . . . [T]he co-morbidities in question are the result of prolonged exposure to titanium dioxide, either from food or pharmaceutical products.[48]

Beyond the fact that TiO2 NPs in the air and foods are impacting our lungs and gastrointestinal tracts,[49] the trend toward nanomedicine ("precision medicine") points to TiO2 NPs being used in intravenous injections that end in pathological lesions on the liver, spleen, kidneys, and brain.[50]

In short, TiO2 NPs are dual use. Under UV illumination, the absorption of a photon with a higher energy than the band gap (3.0-3.2 eV) creates an electron-hole pair, which basically means a *moving conductive current*, which no doubt has to do with why TiO2 NPs are used in electronic devices and as a nano-thermite in depleted uranium (DU) munitions. TiO2 adds its share of atmospheric heating.

Europe acknowledges that NP TiO2 is a nanotechnology, but not the U.S. Food and Drug Administration (FDA), which calls it a "nanoscale material"—just a size thing. *Word games.*

Lithium (Li), a "conflict mineral"

"Conflict minerals" refers to minerals gouged out of earth that has been blood-soaked by wars fought over the wealth the minerals promise: gallium (Ga), selenium (Se), gold (Au), mercury (Hg), chromium (Cr), niobium (Nb), tung-

---

48 Robin D. P. Watson, "Disability By Design: Covid-19, Titanium Dioxide and Electromagnetic Radiation." The Light, thelightpaper.co.uk, December 2020. See Chapter 3, "Nanotechnology at the Quantum Threshold," for Watson's explanation of the "Nano-Blender" and how insoluble nanoparticles "excoriate the epithelial lining of vascular systems" and cells.

49 M.C. Botelho et al., "Effects of titanium dioxide nanoparticles in human gastric epithelial cells in vitro." Biomedical Pharmacotherapy, February 2014.

50 Hongbo Shi et al., "Titanium dioxide nanoparticles: a review of current toxicological data." Particle and Fibre Toxicology, 2013.

sten (W), molybdenum (Mo), etc. For example, the coltan[51] providing the niobium and tantalum for cell phones, computers, PlayStations and XBoxes has merited the deaths of *four million* between 2000 and 2004 in the Democratic Republic of the Congo. In 2015, *Tech Times*[52] issued the alarm that electronics-essential "conflict minerals" would get harder and harder to get.

Lithium (Li) is a rare earth mineral and an integral component of laptops, cellphones, and electric car batteries. This makes lithium an economic and political hot potato between the U.S. and the Russian-Chinese Strategic Partnership, thus earning its place among the "conflict minerals" like cobalt (Co) in Congo for rechargeable lithium-ion batteries and coltan in Congo and Venezuela for capacitors. Bolivia, a "plurinational" state of 38 ethnic groups, claims to hold 70 percent of the world's lithium deposits, the Salar de Uyuni salt flat alone holding 21 million tons.[53]

Lithium is a strategic paramagnetic metal with multiple uses. Like aluminum, lithium at the nanoscale in space is light and stays aloft longer than other good conductor metals like silver, gold, and copper. For example, on January 29, 2013, the sounding rocket *Orion* took off from NASA's Wallops Flight Facility with lithium rods embedded in a thermite cake which, once ignited, vaporized the lithium that then left a spectacularly colorful trail of lithium vapor and lithium oxide while the thermite left iron and aluminum oxide, all of which urban centers below breathed in.[54]

Lithium's tranquillizing, short-circuiting role in the brain ("mood stabilization") is known to those diagnosed with bipolar disorder (manic depression) for how it silences dopaminergic neurons[55] and how its paramagnetic character inhibits oxidative damage to cells and glutathione levels in cerebral cortical cells, proteins and lipids.[56] The relationship between lithium-ion batteries and medical implants points to the need for a thorough study of manic

---

51 Coltan is columbite-tantalum whose rare metals tantalum and niobium / columbium are chemically linked.

52 Robin Burks, "The Metals Used To Make Smartphones Could Run Out Soon." Tech Times, 26 March 2015.

53 Andrew Korybko, "Lithium, a Strategic Resource: Here's Why the US Wants To Break Bolivia To Bits With Hybrid War." Global Research, October 26, 2019. Was President Evo Morales forced out of office in November 2019 because he championed a state-run lithium industry, similar to Venezuelan President Hugo Chavez's elimination for nationalizing oil (and possibly coltan)?

54 Joe Rao, "NASA Rocket to Spark Light Show Over US East Coast Tonight." Space.com, January 29, 2013.

55 Anne Trafton, "New clue to how lithium works in the brain." MIT News, July 7, 2016.

56 Rodrigo Machado-Vieira et al., "The role of lithium in the treatment of bipolar disorder: convergent evidence for neurotrophic effects as a unifying hypothesis." Bipolar Disorder, June 2009.

depression in electromagnetic terms, as has been done for electrosensitivity (ES) / electromagnetic hypersensitivity (EHS). Interestingly, when introduced into a magnetic medium, lithium emulates the Lenz effect and makes magnetic devices inoperable.

(See below under "Vaccines" for *aluminum* and *mercury*.)

BioAPI (Bio-Application Programming Interface)

Polymers / Filaments / Fibers
Biofilm pseudo-skin
Lyme & Morgellons

(More in Chapter 14, "The COVID-19 'Vaccine' Event," under "(BioAPI) Hydrogel tissue engineering")

BioAPI is one of those slippery terms (like synthetic biology, *synbio*) that is used for a variety of applications, most of which concern *biometrics*, the measurement and analysis of people's unique physical and behavioral characteristics. What is more difficult to determine (requiring considerable experience in discerning and reading between the lines) is how crucial BioAPIs are to brain-computer interface (BCI).

> "Instead of chemically engineering functions into a composite material, it may be more convenient to take advantage of nanoparticles as carriers of the desired properties [that] can then be used as building blocks for the fabrication of a composite material with the required qualities. Engineered viruses may fulfill the role of the nanoparticles and once a convenient and general strategy to attach them to an interface is found, the setup can be standardized . . . The fabrication of a large variety of functionalized surfaces becomes possible by bringing together the potential of viruses for combinatorial surface display and a general strategy for surface attachment."[57]

Let's begin with polymers / filaments / fibers, then move on to biofilm, both of which qualify as self-replicating BioAPI connectors delivered under geoengineering and Project Cloverleaf. Morgellons was an infrastructure precursor to the BioAPI *hydrogel* covered in Chapter 14, "The COVID-19 'Vaccine' Event," though it is also much more. Other BioAPI connectors have no doubt been essential to the task of replacing the neurons in Human 1.0 with a synthetic neural network that will connect the Human 2.0 to AI systems.

57 Dr. Edwin Donath, professor at the Institute of Medical Physics and Biophysics at the University of Leipzig in Germany, speaking to Nanowerk's Michael Berger, "Viruses as nanotechnology building blocks for materials and devices," March 19, 2007.

> *. . . and [Bernard Eastlund] said that to heat up the atmosphere with HAARP was very difficult, it would go right through the atmosphere, unless you put some element in that airspace that it could heat, and he suggested that polymers would work very well in allowing HAARP to be directed to heat certain sections of the atmosphere. And in fact, we've been seeing . . . cobweb-like material, polymer material all over the United States and other locations, in conjunction with airplanes flying overhead emitting something out of the back end of them. And Eastlund went further and said that heat generation works by adding magnetic iron oxide to the polymer . . .*
>
> – William Thomas on *Coast-To-Coast AM* with George Knapp, December 20, 2009

> *Then there is this [geo]engineering program . . . lots of nanoparticles in the air that we breathe, which has been shown to shrink the volume of the brain, which dumbs us down. It has huge effects on the environment. The oceans are now covered with a layer of nano-beads of plastic spiked with aluminum and titanium. These are meant to be suspended in the sky to shade strong, excessive sunlight, but whatever goes up, goes down. So the oceans are blanketed by that.*
>
> *The media are all looking at plastic bottles and other things that never break down to these nanoparticles. It's manmade stuff covering the oceans and preventing the oceans from evaporating water. The whole atmosphere is drying up dramatically, creating deserts at unprecedented speed . . .*
>
> – Dietrich Klinghardt, MD, "What is The Root of All Diseases?" August 7, 2019

Polymerized viral agents have been dispersed by military jets and ships and commercial airlines since Project Cloverleaf began in the 1990s—nanosized translucent Mylar polymers, high-density polyethylene fiber (HPDE), genetically engineered fungal forms mutated with viruses into polymers—"goo" polymer strands ending up in acidic "chemwebs," the Oakville, Washington event in 1994 being the most infamous. Impact of electromagnetic (not solar) radiation on sprayed high molecular weight (HMW) polymer dumps, biological impact on lungs—much biological analysis has gone into comparing soluble, insoluble, and water-absorbing polymers to determine that water-absorbing polyacrylate polymers present the most "unreasonable risk."[58]

58 "High Molecular Weight Polymers in the New Chemicals Program" EPA, https://www.epa.gov/reviewing-new-chemicals-under-toxic-substances-control-act-tsca/high-molecular-weight-polymers-new.

During the Cloverleaf years, synthetic polymers released into the environment became the favored carriers of all sorts of experimental biologicals. As I explained in *Chemtrails, HAARP* in 2014:

> The fibers exhibited extreme adhesiveness and elasticity with a tendency to form "kinked" wave-like forms that dissipate over time. People became ill after handling the fibers, so [independent scientist Clifford Carnicom] advised caution.[59] Fibers dropping over Sedona, Arizona on July 10, 1999 had a *petrochemical* odor; in Oklahoma, they were chiffon-like; in Sacramento in February 2000, a white powder or granular clumps fell that were 200 microns wide.

Industrial polymer chemist R. Michael "Mike" Castle identified cationic[60] polymers decades ago that form a "dashes" jet-trail pattern in chemical trails:

> . . . separate, individual reaction-injections of a cationic polymer system that has been mixed in a cannister and immediately ejected into the atmosphere using a venture eduction spinneret nozzle . . . cationic polymers have an extremely high capacity for use of heavy metals. They don't coagulate due to catalysis . . . Barium and Aluminum, Cadmium, Selenium and Thorium can be easily sprayed into the atmosphere, are chemically stable and reflect UV and may carry a specific electronic charge. This is the model aerosolized pattern.[61]

Geoengineered droughts and floods, extreme heat and cold, have been crucial to biologicals-encased-in-polymers experimentation, like the outbreaks of valley fever with flu-like symptoms and severe coughs due to breathing in increased numbers of *Coccidiodes* fungus-laced spores. Valley fever increased 850 percent between 1998 and 2011, the years of EM-induced drought in California (from 700 cases in 1998 to 5,500 in 2011) and Arizona (1,400 cases in 1998, 16,400 in 2011).[62]

Polyethylene-silicon-carbon nanofibers and nanowires house combinations of pathogens, red blood cells, and nanosensors loaded with microprocessors made from proteins and powered by cells—tiny cell phones and computers busily recording electrical activity of nerve cells adjacent to blood vessels, then transmitting data to distant supercomputers.[63] From *Chemtrails, HAARP:*

---

59 See Maryna van Wyk, "Strange, sticky, wiry threads similar to spider's web falls in the Karoo." Rapport, South Africa, Cape Edition, 25 June 2000.

60 Cation: a positively charged ion that is attracted to a cathode in electrolysis.

61 Mike Castle, "Chemtrails – Bio-Active Crystalline Cationic Polymers," Rense.com, July 14, 2003.

62 Gosia Wozniacka, "Fever hits thousands in parched West farm season." AP, May 6, 2013.

63 See Aleksandr Noy et al., "Carbon Nanotube Transistor Controlled by a Biological Ion

In 2009, Hildegarde Staninger reported that exposure to aerosols filled with nanocomposites inhibits the cholinesterase that the brain, liver, and red blood cells need. Chronic inhibition of this enzyme causes slow-death poisoning leading to neurological disorders and paralysis.[64] Dementia and anemia have been linked.[65]

The PEDOT polymer poly(3,4-ethylenedioxythrophene) polystyrene sulfonate coating makes it crystal clear that Transhumanism's brain-computer interface (BCI) has been the primary objective since the Cloverleaf days. As David Martin, associate dean at the University of Delaware's College of Engineering, puts it, "Name your favorite biomolecule, and you can in principle make a PEDOT film that has whatever biofunctional group you might be interested in."[66]

Polymerization inside living organisms.

Supposedly an antistatic coating for electronic displays, a layer of PEDOT makes material conductive, thus aiding in linking humans to computers, as in robotics and image processing. Interfacing without scarring and "significantly boosting medical implant performance," PEDOT joins neural lace and other technologies seeking to provide the brain with full-bandwidth data streaming via USB-C.

Commercial jet fuel is dependent upon polymer fibers,[67] the long strands of sticky-to-the-touch polymers ("nanowebs") found on people's windshields, strewn over porches and fields. Sticky to the touch, they are not water soluble. They look like spider webs but are deadly and come from the sky, not spiders.

Kautz-Vella points out that the U.S. Air Force Academy chemistry manual—the manual that coined the term "chemtrail"—discusses the polymerization of nylon and electrolytic coating of thin metal layers. Aluminum-coated nano-nylon fibers in "spoofer sprays" have been found in rain samples. Because nylon cannot endure temperatures higher than 250°C (482°F), spoofer spray operations point to *secondary* delivery systems through nozzles such as Castle mentions—for example, electrospun nanofibers carrying barium salts to cloak aircraft from radar by absorbing moisture, keeping the plasma clouds dry enough for transmissions, all under the auspices of solar geoengineering.

Pump Gate," American Chemical Society Nano Letters, 2010; and "Wiring the Brain at the Nanoscale," Phys.org, 8 July 2005.

64 Hildegarde Staninger, Ph.D., "Exposure to Aerosol Emissions of Nano Composite Materials Resulted in Cholinesterase Inhibition," September 7, 2009. http://1cellonelight.com/pdf/NanoCompositeCholinesteraseInhibition10.2009.pdf

65 "Anemia Linked to Increased Risk of Dementia." ScienceDaily, July 31, 2013.

66 "New 'PEDOT' polymer may allow human brain to merge with AI, cure and detect diseases, scientists say." Tech2Thai, August 17, 2020.

67 Ming-Hsin Wei et al., "Megasupramolecules for safer, cleaner fuel by end association of long telechelic polymers." Science, 2 October 2015.

Polymer-barium salts in the aerosol drops help to shape the atmospheric RF ducts necessary for the U.S. Air Force VTRPE system (variable terrain refractivity parabolic equation) that avails the military of viewing what an enemy radar system is seeing—all part of optics-based communications broadcasting by beams above the Earth instead of fiber optics cable on the ground.

> The mixture of barium salt aerosol when sprayed in a straight line will also provide a ducting path from point A to point B and will enable high frequency communications along that path, even over the curvature of the earth, in both directions. Enemy high frequency communications can be monitored easier with the straight line A to B ducting medium.[68]

Marine cloud brightening (as in ship track[69] cloud releases from ship exhaust or wet surface air cooler technology) creates submicron-sized cloud condensation nuclei (CCN) from seawater via electrospraying from Taylor cone-jets, either micromachined silicon in long capillaries or short capillary polymer substrates.

In London and the French Pyrenees, people breathe in fibrous microplastics and blame it on atmospheric dust, plastic textiles, disposable plastic bags and polystyrene floating and landing everywhere. Nothing is said about the chem-webs from electrospinning electrosprays delivering aluminum and barium. Electrospun nano-webs are also sprayed on GMO crops,[70] much of it remaining airborne with Terminator seed stuck to it and traveling as far as 95 km.[71] It's in the rain and snow as well, from the Pyrenees to the Arctic, Antarctic, and Sierra Nevadas,[72] carried by the wind but primarily issuing from jets, drones, and rockets.

Biofilm pseudo-skin

> *. . . the rise of "smart" materials that can instantly change based on body conditions and integrate into tissues . . . marks a future of computational analysis and restructuring of the body. For successful tissue integration and*

---

68 "Chemtrails Over America: A Special Report," June 2001. For more on VTRPE, see Chapter 11, "The 'Air Loom' Hospital."

69 Lithium is employed for ship tracks because it boils in water and produces steam for clouds.

70 Christoph Hellmann et al., "Design of pheromone releasing nanofibers for plant protection," Polymers for Advanced Technologies, April 2011: "...the release of pheromones from polymer carriers, in particular from nanofibers webs as obtained by electrospinning." Note the 2006 Nanotechnology paper by W. Salalha et al., "Encapsulation of bacteria and viruses in electrospun nanofibers," calling to mind the BioAPI quote above regarding using nanoparticles and viruses for "surface attachment."

71 King's College London, "New study reveals higher microplastics in London air compared to other cities." Phys.org, December 31, 2019; "Otago scientist awarded emerging innovator grant for nano-webs," www.ortago.ac.nz, 1 August 2016.

72 Zoe Schlanger, "Yes, there's microplastic in the snow." Quartz, December 13, 2019.

the prevention of inflammation reactions, special surface coatings were developed by [the Karlsruhe Institute of Technology] under the multidisciplinary program "BioInterfaces."

– Nicholas West, "The Era of Cyborgs Has Begun," *Activist Post,* January 11, 2014

The synthetic creation of invisible sheets of biofilm has been underway since the bacteria genus *Mycoplasma* was patented during World War Two by Shyh-Ching Lo of the Armed Forces Institute of Pathology and the U.S. military. Wikipedia describes Mycoplasma as "a genus of bacteria that lack a cell wall around their cell membranes [which] makes them naturally resistant to antibiotics that target cell wall synthesis. They can be parasitic or saprotrophic [an organism that derives nourishment from decayed organic matter]." *Mycoplasma genitalium* only has 525 genes, making it Nature's smallest genetic organism.

The *Brucella* bacterium has been tested on North American populations since the 1970s, particularly the five genetically armed strains of Mycoplasma made from the crystalline toxin Merck derived (gain of function) in 1946 and thoroughly exploited during the bio-chemical Gulf War of 1990-1991. [See Chapter 9, "Dual Use I: A Smart City Is An Armed City."]

A Mycoplasma infection indirectly causes inhibited production of nitric oxide (NO) that causes endothelial cells to become "sticky" and form the arterial plaque *biofilm.* Making biofilm from viruses and bacteria is simple, as they pretty much make it themselves:

> . . . surface-associated microbial populations in which the individual cells are affixed to surfaces and cohered to each other through an extracellular polymeric matrix [are] often produced by the bacteria themselves . . . [T]he point at which the presence of multiple cells adhered to the surface changes the attributes of the population as a whole can arguably be considered a biofilm.[73]

All bacteria colonize for protection into biofilm, a process that includes Mycoplasmas, archaea, protozoa, fungi and algae. Biofilm colonies attach to host tissues and each other by means of hairlike appendages on a vertical structure so as to take in nutrients and release byproducts more easily. As Mycoplasmas build layers and maintain cell-to-cell communication, they use host cells to replicate, then at a certain point the biofilm ruptures and disperses Mycoplasmas for further colonization. Shapeshifting, rapidly dissolving biofilm being dumped over populations does not require refrigeration. Once inhaled and ingested, it will reconstitute inside the body.

---

73 Tzvi Tzfira and Vitaly Citovsky, editors, Agrobacterium: From Biology to Biotechnology (Springer Science, 2008). This "genetic transformation machine" is liberally used in GMO "precision pharming."

The immune system ignores biofilm because its protein surface has a negative charge. Biofilm is implicated in various infections, dental plaque, gingivitis, contact lens coating, cystic fibrosis, prostheses and heart valves malfunctions. Carpal tunnel surgery entails scraping biofilm from myelin sheaths, and it is found in the brains of Alzheimer's and macular degeneration sufferers.[74] A recent example is the "bacteria, fungi and algae creeping over the once-gleaming dome of the Jefferson Memorial [in Washington, D.C.], leaving black splotches in its wake."[75] The National Park Service historic architect described it in this way: "We've never seen it before. Now it is everywhere"—the Washington Monument, the Lincoln Memorial, Arlington National Cemetery, on our skin, in hospital catheters . . .

The delivery is chemtrails, and the trigger is Agrobacterium.

– Christopher Macklin, PhD

In 2008—while Clifford Carnicom was breaking into the polymer fibers falling to Earth in northern New Mexico—Vitaly Citovsky at Stony Brook University in New York was studying the *Agrobacterium tumafaciens*[76] fibers producing *pseudo-skin* all over the bodies of his ten patients. *Agrobacterium tumafaciens* is the well-known "genetic transformation machine" that forms architecturally complex biofilms on host tissues. Since the 1980s, it has been creating genetically modified plants (GMOs) "because of its ability to transfer a piece of its genetic material, the T-DNA on its tumor-inducing (Ti) plasmid to the plant genome."[77] These "genetic transformation machines" spread over vast acres of GMO soil (and human populations):

> So how could this gram-negative soil bacteria be spread over the population without their knowledge or consent? This constitutes biological terrorism, and is illegal. However, bioprecipitation, the concept of "rain-making bacteria," uses gram-negative soil bacteria to produce rain. And

74 Thanks to lindaemmanuel.com for these insights.

75 Evan Halper, "Uninvited guest leaves behind a mess." Los Angeles times, October 30, 2019.

76 Agro, L., field, soil, crop production; tumere, L., to swell, as in tumescence; facie, L., doing, making. Agrobacterium is a soil bacterium.

77 Mae-Wan Ho and Joe Cummins, PhDs, "Agrobacterium & Morgellons Disease, A GM Connection?" Institute of Science in Society (ISIS) Press Release, 28/04/08. Counter to these findings, Clifford Carnicom never found any Agrobacterium in the specimens he worked with.

> it is used in cloud seeding . . . Leave it to our "friends" at Monsanto. Creating destruction of our environment since 1901.[78]

Since 2012, the genetically altered M13 virus M13 with negatively charged amino acids has been *amping up its piezoelectric effect for more conductivity*:

> Imagine painting a layer of this film onto the casing of your laptop. Every time you tap the keyboard, these [M13] viruses convert the pressure from your fingers into electricity that constantly powers up your battery. Any kind of motion can power up M13 . . .[79]

Think aerosols delivering virus-powered electronics to your lungs and skin. Think pseudo-skin as circuit board *cum* antenna. From Mickael Lallart's 2011 book *Ferroelectrics-Material Aspects,* we learn of how strontium and barium plus niobate (niobium plus oxygen) are used to make similar thin biofilms for dielectric and electro-optic applications. Alter the radio frequency and the oxygen percentage in the plasma, and you alter the film composition.

The cheapest creation of biofilm comes from treating *bio-fungal graphene* with the bacteria *Shewanella oneidensis* to lower the oxygen level so as to increase conductivity—much like 5G 60 GHz does—and turn the skin into a shiny electric generator that reacts with nano-metals in a semiconductor fashion. According to Lookoutfa Charlie, a targeted researcher of Morgellons and other nanotechnology, *Shewanella* coupled with thin, flexible, strong, and conductive bio-fungal graphene is easily remotely programmed and manipulated, even to the degree that its antenna-like nature makes monitoring the host possible.[80] As you will learn in Chapter 14, graphene plays a decisive role in hydrogel. Needless to say, NASA has been extremely interested in *Shewanella.*[81]

Three proteins are involved in the formation and adhesive capabilities of biofilm: *SinR,* the master regulator of biofilm formation (*Bacillus* subtilis); magnesium-dependent *ExoR* that promotes protein-protein interactions while interacting with signal transduction systems; and the fumarate and nitrate reduction (FNR) regulatory protein that controls the expression of a wide range of genes involved in *the switch from aerobic to anaerobic growth.* The human skin being a respiratory organ, a shift from free oxygen to the

78 "Morgellons Disease: The Geoengineering Epidemic," StopChemicalTerrorism.com, n.d.

79 Dan Krotz, "Berkeley Lab Scientists Generate Electricity From Viruses." Berkeley Lab, May 13, 2012.

80 "Electronic Harassment – Delivery Method Explained in Detail . . ." Lookoutfa Charlie, August 21, 2019.

81 "Could Electricity-Producing Bacteria Help Power Future Space Missions?" NASA, June 27, 2018.

lack of free oxygen in a biofilm pseudo-skin covering the human body sounds like a long space voyage experiment with SinR making sure that the biofilm spreads along the body surfaces "in response to the oxygen limitation that occurs as a consequence of oxygen utilization within the biofilm."[82]

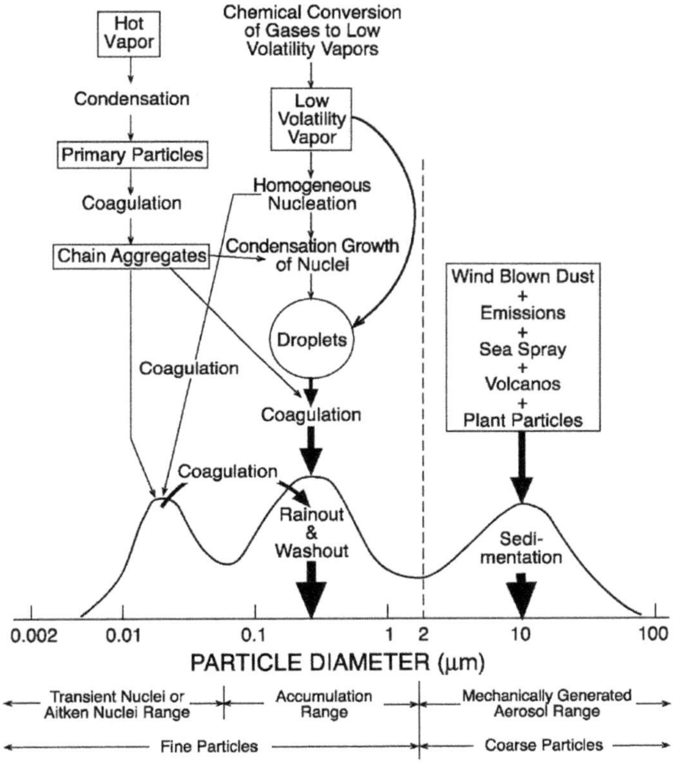

Classical cloud seeding.

http://what-when-how.com/nanoscience-and-nanotechnology/atmospheric-nanoparticles-formation-and-physicochemical-properties-part-1-nanotechnology/

The FNR protein, *Shewanella* coupled with bio-fungal graphene and the 5G 60 GHz frequency are all concerned with oxygen.

Meanwhile on planet Earth, chronic disease is more and more of a concern. At the Heavy Metal Detox Summit in 2019, Dietrich Wittel, MD, PhD, addressed "Unconventional detox protocols and uses of chelating agents," beginning with finding a way to destroy biofilm, given that the toxic metal distribution locked into the biofilm matrix leads to one illness after another.[83]

---

82 Tzvi Tzfira and Vitaly Citovsky.

83 Dr. Wittel has dedicated years to his EDTA magnesium (Mg) chelation biofilm matrix destabilizer approach.

His discovery of calcium crystals forming in bodies of water *and in the bloodstream,* thus clogging arteries, etc., raises the suspicion that the human body is being used like a crystal radio . . .

Lyme & Morgellons

> *And here, below, there is silence. In the air—thin, incomprehensible, almost invisible threads. Every autumn they are carried here from outside, from beyond the Wall. Slowly, they float—and suddenly you feel something alien, invisible on your face; you want to brush it off, but no, you cannot; you cannot rid yourself of it.*
>
> – Yevgeny Zamyatin, *We* (1920-21), translated by Mirra Ginsburg

> *And the first went and poured out his vial upon the earth, and there fell a noisome and grievous sore upon the men which had the mark of the beast, and upon them which worshipped his image.*
>
> – Revelations 16:2

Bioterrorism and its concomitant experimentation on citizens as U.S. policy began long before 9/11, as this book demonstrates. The 2004 Pentagon budget for chemical-biological warfare (CBW) was $10 billion.[84] Mycoplasma pathogens, autoimmune diseases like myalgic encephalomyelitis in Canada and chronic fatigue syndrome in the U.S., recombinant DNA in quest of new organisms, Project Jefferson (vaccine-resistant anthrax), cowpox, the weaponized Lone Star tick—all of it has been of great interest to Cold Warriors and their post-Cold War scientism minions vying for military grants.

As one example among thousands, Paperclip Nazi scientist Erich Traub, PhD—the Third Reich's lab chief under Kurt Blome at Insel Riems, a secret biological warfare lab—first studied at the Rockefeller Institute in Princeton, New Jersey prior to World War Two, then after the War was stationed at the Naval Medical Research Institute in Bethesda, Maryland, often visiting Plum Island while simultaneously directing biological warfare work at the Tübingen lab in West Germany.[85]

Be under no illusion! As Francis Boyle, PhD, reminds Americans—Boyle drafted the law the U.S. Congress enacted in order to comply with the 1972 Biological Weapons Convention—the U.S. has 13,000 "death scientists" in 400 laboratories to enrich the $100bn germ warfare ("biodefense") industry.

---

84 Read Michael Christopher Carroll, Lab 257: The Disturbing Story of the Government's Secret Plum Island Germ Laboratory (HarperCollins, 2004).

85 Scientific American has dismissed these connections. Both Scientific American and Nature magazines are owned by the Holtzbrinck Publishing Group, one of the big five English-language gatekeeper publishing firms.

At University of Wisconsin, Yoshihiro Kawaoka, PhD, resurrected the Spanish Flu and is now increasing flu toxicity; the Galveston National Laboratory in Texas should be shut down, Dr. Boyle stresses, because it is

> . . . an ongoing criminal enterprise along the lines of the SS and the Gestapo—except that Galveston is far more dangerous to humanity than Hitler's death squads ever were. American universities have a long history of willingly permitting their research agenda, researchers, institutes, and laboratories to be co-opted, corrupted, and perverted by the Pentagon and the CIA into death science. These include Wisconsin, North Carolina, Boston U., Harvard, MIT, Tulane, University of Chicago, and my own University of Illinois, as well as many others.[86]

In his 2010 article "National Security Secrecy: Morgellons Victims Across the US and Europe," Hank P. Albarelli Jr. (1947-2019) with Zoe Martell posited that Morgellons research may have begun even before the 1969 Defense Department Appropriations Subcommittee meeting at which high-ranking Pentagon biological warfare expert Donald MacArthur begged for $10 million for Fort Detrick research into

> . . . a new infective microorganism which could differ in certain important aspects from any known disease-causing organisms . . . that might be refractory to the immunological and therapeutic processes upon which we depend to maintain our relative freedom from infectious disease . . . a synthetic biological agent, an agent that does not naturally exist and for which no natural immunity could be acquired.

Immediately after the $10 million was approved, the Frederick Cancer Research Facility of the U.S. Army's Fort Detrick Biological Warfare Laboratory morphed into the National Cancer Institute and the staff and budget tripled.

German scientist Kautz-Vella claims that Morgellons is a hollow-tube quantum dot technology designed to be part of a nanobot BCI network that began with "black goo" in Texas oil fields hit 20,500 years ago by a meteorite. Kautz-Vella says that this "black goo" is also the source of petroleum.[87]

In the early years of Project Cloverleaf's aerosol delivery of Morgellons filaments, the CDC and Kaiser Permanente were in charge of marginalizing and discrediting those experiencing extreme symptoms (rashes, eruptions of

86 Sherwood Ross, "U.S. Biowarfare Programs Have 13,000 Death Scientists Hard At Work." Scoop, 26 February 2020.

87 Interestingly, the term "gray goo" is how nanotechnology discoverer Eric Drexler characterized ecophagy, the global catastrophe of self-replicating nanobots that eventually consume all of the Earth's biomass.

fibers and "glitter"—quantum dots—from skin lesions, subcutaneous sensations of crawling worms and biting insects, etc.) by accusing them of delusional parasitosis, exhibiting the "matchbox sign," and neurotic excoriation. Meanwhile, biotech was hitting its stride: In 2003, the U.S. Army announced the $50 million Institute for Collaborative Biotechnologies (biotech / engineering public-private partnerships); in 2008, the CDC Morgellons "study" was passed to the Armed Forces Institute of Pathology; in 2010, the 21st Century Nanotechnology Research and Development Act authorized $3.7 billion over five years for bio-nanotechnology.

The genesis of Lyme Disease in the United States occurred under the CBW auspices of the CIA's Project MKNAOMI (1950s-1970s) run in concert with the Special Operations Division of the U.S. Army Biological Warfare at Fort Detrick, where "paralysis agents" under K Project (K = kill or knockout) had included the *Dermacentor* tick, then in 1962 focused on creating a "designer disease" that would *incapacitate,* not immobilize, "ticks being a natural breeding and mixing ground for pathogens."[88] The Department of Agriculture facility at Fort Terry on 840-acre Plum Island doubled as a U.S. Army biological warfare research facility where Paperclip Nazi scientists were given carte blanche to pursue their CBW black magic brews.[89]

The first public cases broke out in Lyme, Connecticut in 1975.

> Apparently, the first appearance a mere 13 miles northeast of [Plum Island Animal Disease Research Center] of what we now call Lyme Disease falls under the category of coincidence, as does the mysterious and still unexplained appearance of West Nile virus in Long Island and New York City. Coincidences, it seems, abound at Plum.[90]

The American Lyme Disease (300,000 cases per year)—supposedly a bacteria transmitted through infected deer ticks—differs greatly from the Black Forest German variety, particularly as regards the symptoms that add up to autoimmune conditions and immune suppression. As I have said elsewhere in this book, immune suppression has proven again and again to be a primary objective of CBW experimentation, including the creation of vaccines like the mRNA bioengineered to actually *circumvent the immune system entirely.* Lyme disease expert Ginger Savely, DNP, believes that Lyme sufferers have weaker immune systems and may therefore be more vulnerable to Morgellons. It

88 Hank P. Albarelli, Jr. and Zoe Martell, "National Security Secrecy: Morgellons Victims Across the US and Europe." Voltairenet.org, June 12, 2010.

89 In 2003, Plum Island administration was passed from the USDA to the Department of Homeland Security (DHS).

90 Alan Cabal, New York Press, March 16, 2004.

is obvious—what with all the environmental pollutants, GMOs and junk foods, and wireless electromagnetics—that weakening and deceiving the immune system would have to precede the myriad *synbio* brain-computer interface (BCI) / Transhumanist modifications to Human 1.0.

The chemical nanoparticle is now the favored approach to "modulating" the immune system—for example, silica nanoparticles that penetrate the skin barrier, and titanium dioxide nanoparticles that induce gene expression alterations in the brain. Together, the two induce reproductive and/or liver toxicity.[91]

Dietrich Klinghardt, MD, founder of the Sophia Health Institute, has devoted years to deciphering Lyme Disease, including its autoimmune fallout that parallels the Morgellons fallout, despite the fact that Lyme has been constructed in spirochetes (spirally twisted bacteria) and Morgellons in coccus (spherical bacteria). Dr. Klinghardt agrees that Lyme spirochetes *Borrelia burgdorferi* and *Borrelia mayonii,* both of which shapeshift, have been gain-of-function genetically modified to *aggressively* suppress the immune system, thus leading to chronic fatigue, brain fog, autism, Alzheimer's, MS, ALS, and other nerve conditions by piggybacking Epstein-Barr DNA and other viral components and co-infections (Bartonella, Mycoplasma, etc.) onto spirochete bacteria.[92]

Dr. Klinghardt agrees that Lyme is not caused by microbes so much as a lack of proper immune response. For example, the spirochete's outer surface appears to have been engineered to look like a myelin biofilm nerve sheath so that the immune system attacks the nerve or white blood cells coming to the rescue. *Many Lyme sufferers have no immune response, period.* Dr. Klinghardt maintains that 90 percent of a successful Lyme treatment must be geared to building the immune system, with 10 percent going toward killing microbes. His treatment begins with PCR testing and his own tissue-specific *autonomic response testing (ART)*, then moves on to ultrasound, infrared light, and even urine therapy, plus progesterone for opening the blood-brain barrier to herbal remedies.[93]

The 4-step Klinghardt Protocol (www.klinghardtacademy.com):

1. Decrease toxic body burden
2. Improve disturbed physiology

---

91 Toshiro Hirai et al., "Amorphous silica nanoparticles size-dependently aggravate atopic dermatitis-like skin lesions following an intradermal injection." Particle and Fiber Toxicology, 2012.

92 Morgellons shares much of this, intermingling with intestinal-fungal overgrowth, rash, B12 deficiency, and skin / internal itching and the subdermal sensation of shared of broken glass and lit cigarettes.

93 "Episode 93 Lyme Disease with Dr. Dietrich Klinghardt," Rebecca Risk, October 21, 2017.

3. Decrease microbial count
4. Immune modulation

Morgellons patients tend to test positive for Lyme or Bartonella, but the sores are different: Lyme displays the bull's eye rash (*Erythema migrans* or EM) while Morgellons varies from a red rash to staph-like craters with protruding colored "wires." Treating Lyme often makes Morgellons symptoms disappear.[94] High levels of aluminum nanoparticles are found in both Lyme and Morgellons, and cell phone radiation can block the enzymes necessary to detoxifying the heavy metals in both conditions. Lyme spirochetes do not live in the blood but instead set up sanctuaries in various parts of the body, whereas Morgellons coccus have been engineered to reside primarily in erythrocytes. In a sense, Lyme attacks the immune system so the cross-species technology we call Morgellons can be slipped into place without the immune system noticing.

Between Morgellons filaments dropping from the sky and the nanotechnology that came of age in the 1990s, the tiny subatomic *quantum* world beckons more and more that we examine the synthetic biology (*synbio*) behind the engineering of pathogens, shape-shifting polymers,[95] and cells growing on intricate polymer scaffolds—

> The scaffold is built out of a series of thin layers, stamped with a pattern of channels that are each 50 to 100 micrometres wide. The layers, which resemble computer microchips, are then stacked into a 3D structure of synthetic blood vessels. As each layer is added, UV light is used to cross-link the polymer and bond it to the layer below. When the structure is finished, it is bathed in a liquid containing living cells. The cells quickly attach to the inside and outside of the channels and begin growing just as they would in a human body.[96]

—because it is changing the nature of our human blood and genetics.

In 2014, after nearly two decades of observing chemical-signature trails from jets and analyzing collections of environmental filaments appearing in precipitation and HEPA filters, independent scientist Clifford Carnicom coined

94 Borrelia spirochetes have been found in skin tissue of four "randomly selected" Morgellons patients (Marianne J. Middelveen et al., "Association of spirochetal infection with Morgellons disease," F1000Research, 28 January 2013), but in general the bacteria used for weaponizing Lyme and Morgellons are different, one being spirochete, the other coccus.

95 "Chinese scientists develop shape-shifting material," Xinhua, January 10, 2016.

96 "'Person-on-a-chip': Engineers grow 3-D heart, liver tissues for better drug testing." Phys-org., March 7, 2016.

the term *cross-domain bacteria (CDB)* for the "bacterial-like"[97] sub-micron spherical structure (0.3-0.8 microns) he found inside the tiny filaments he was also finding in the bodily fluids (saliva, blood) of human beings and animals.[98]

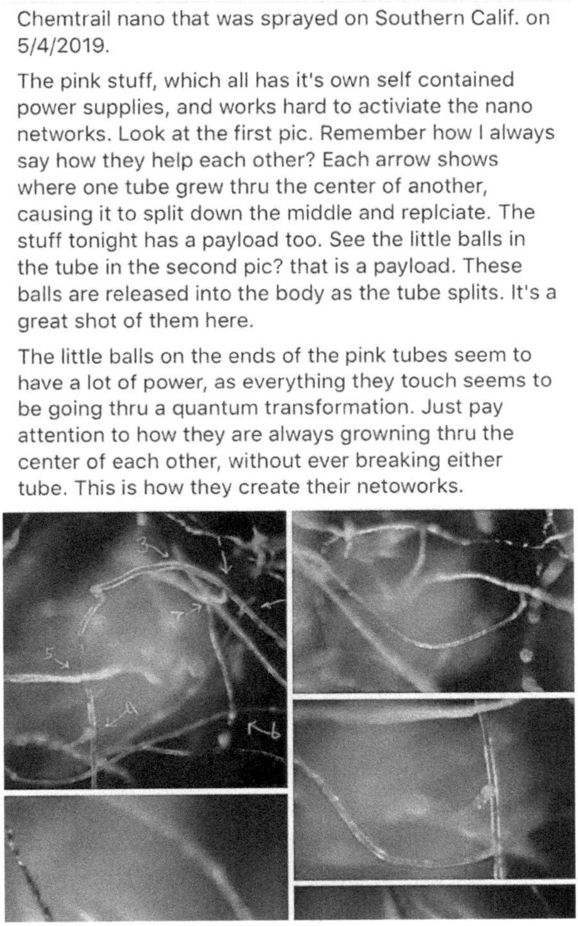

Chemtrail nano that was sprayed on Southern Calif. on 5/4/2019.
The pink stuff, which all has it's own self contained power supplies, and works hard to activiate the nano networks. Look at the first pic. Remember how I always say how they help each other? Each arrow shows where one tube grew thru the center of another, causing it to split down the middle and replciate. The stuff tonight has a payload too. See the little balls in the tube in the second pic? that is a payload. These balls are released into the body as the tube splits. It's a great shot of them here.
The little balls on the ends of the pink tubes seem to have a lot of power, as everything they touch seems to be going thru a quantum transformation. Just pay attention to how they are always growning thru the center of each other, without ever breaking either tube. This is how they create their netoworks.

Cross-domain bacteria (CDB)? Gretchen Ahlers, May 4, 2019, chemtrail nano-sprayed in Southern California.

Relatively early on, he had discovered three components inside the so-called Morgellons filament: an erythrocytic form; a Chlamydia-like structure; and a pleomorphic "ribbon or sausage-like form." Strong parallels piqued his

97 Also "erythrocyte-like" and "Chlamydia-like, with a special interest in Chlamydia Pneumonia" (Clifford E. Carnicom, "Morgellons: A Status Report," October 8, 2009).

98 Review Chapter 8, "Morgellons: The Fibers We Breathe and Eat," in Chemtrails, HAARP, and the Full Spectrum Dominance of Planet Earth (2014).

interest: the Gulf War Syndrome, Lyme Disease, fibromyalgia, and chronic fatigue syndrome. Not only was the CDB part of the "novel and ubiquitous life-form that is known to exist in association with the so-called 'Morgellons' condition," but it also appeared to be the originator of the pathogen's extraordinary growth process and creator of nodes of operation near nerve centers and joints, producing biofilm for self-protection as it moved through the body, quorum sensing (intercellular signaling) and highly adaptable.[99]

On January 18, 2014, Carnicom wrote in "The New Biology" that the Morgellons condition "represents a fundamental change in the state and nature of biology as it is known on this earth. The evidence now indicates and demonstrates that there is, at the heart of the 'condition,' a new growth form that transcends, as a minimum, the plant and animal boundaries."[100] Then in his paper "*Cross-Domain Bacteria* Isolation" (May 17, 2014), Carnicom spelled out the many tests he put the CDB through to determine the original bacterial status (coccus) engineered to enjoin a unique relationship with iron (Fe), even to setting up inside erythrocytes (red blood cells). At his online paper "Morgellons: A Status Report," October 8, 2009, you can see illustrations of erythrocytes infused with "organized, structured and packed" CDB.

In other words, Morgellons is not a "skin condition" (shades of the "climate change" cover story) but an *alteration of the blood* alongside filaments loaded for experimental purposes. The Carnicom paper "The Transformation of A Species?"[101] makes it clear that the bioengineered CDB is altering the fundamental morphology and geometry of human erythrocytes. Carnicom points out that "the blood of every individual does exhibit some degree of variation caused by the presence of the CDB"—some blood cells extremely misshapen, others less so. In some cases, the cell membranes remain surprisingly intact with no material structural damage, despite signs of "gain of function" *synbio* engineering; in other cases, obliteration.

Due to the ubiquity of the chemical aerosol and GMO food delivery systems,[102] it appears that this pathogen is in everyone, not just in those with lesions. Carnicom found normal red blood cells and submicron granular or fibrous anomalous forms in both people suffering lesions and people seemingly healthy, with only the *degree* of presence of these anomalous forms differing, along with more pronounced degradation of cellular integrity in lesions sufferers.[103]

---

99 "Carnicom Institute Disclosure Project – Overview with Clifford Carnicom" (47:00), Transparent Media Truth, November 17, 2020.

100 Also see "Morgellons: A New Classification" (February 2010).

101 https://carnicominstitute.org/research_papers/Carnicom_Institute_Research-2019.pdf.

102 I must include the COVID-19 masks and PCR swabs with filaments in them possibly transporting the CDB into people under the guise of "safety" and "testing."

103 Clifford E. Carnicom, "Blood Testing: Lasers, Morgellons & Fungus (?)" November 21, 2007.

The segregation of only certain individuals as having the "Morgellons" condition is completely and totally false; the general population is involved whether they would like to know of it or not. The pathogens found have now been discovered repeatedly across all major body systems and functions, including skin, blood, hair, saliva, dental (gum), digestive, ear, and urinary samples.[104]

With blood samples and samples of gels falling from the sky in the Pacific Northwest, spider-like web strands in California, discrete filaments in Oregon, and red blood cells (not "juniper pollen") in New Mexico and Colorado, Carnicom established that airborne submicron fibers and the fibrous structures emerging from the Morgellons sufferers were one and the same.[105]

The fibres grow and extend through my body, actively pulsing together, causing uncontrollable muscle spasms. They grow into worms, their eggs 0.8 to 1-2 mm in size placed inside insects with many legs and a T proboscis used to puncture the skin so the beetle-like body with its many rows of eggs can be pulled through the skin opening… The worms go through any tissue and seal the wall behind them. They attach to the back end of blood vessels, go to the edge of the skin, and put eggs wherever you go through the skin… I have no plausible way of getting rid of these things. Sugar or carbohydrate that breaks down into sugar feeds them. While treating myself, the worms encyst in my torso and left leg; when I stop, they disappear and it's business as usual. In a world compendium of worms, there is a DNA connection of 6 different worms, maybe 7, with the beetle.

– Philip Ball, Auckland, New Zealand, July 2019

Graphic photographs of what is extruding from human bodies accompany Carnicom's many papers, from normal vision to 2500X and 5000X magnification of Morgellons microphotographs subjected to laser light (650 nm) in addition to bottom-up light. It is at high magnification that the *artificial nature (nanotechnology)* of the fibers begins to emerge: the single Morgellons fiber is actually composed of innumerable sub-fibers measuring 1 micron or less in thickness—similar to airborne fibers—and the CDB spherical entity

104 Clifford E. Carnicom, "'Morgellons': The Wine-Peroxide Test," March 15, 2008.

105 Clifford E. Carnicom, "Morgellons: First Observations," August 2006; "Morgellons: Morphology Confirmed," November 15, 2007.

inside the fiber measures 1 micron or less, with branching growths of a "budding" structure encapsulating submicron structures of a fungal nature; etc.

Random comments about Morgellons[106]:

- Feeds on fear, sugar, and low pH (Diane Gregory, 2017)
- Because it has its own consciousness, your consciousness matters
- Development of Morgellons doesn't occur in the lungs but in the acids of the digestive tract that produce the crystals for communication and the appendages for motility (Terral@terral03.com)
- A silicon-based lifeform that self-replicates; boron (Borax) is a nanofilament replication inhibitor (Terral@terral03.com)

At 19:25 in his Disclosure Project Overview referenced earlier, Carnicom makes it crystal clear that four agencies—the Environmental Protection Agency (EPA), the U.S. Air Force, the Centers for Disease Control and Prevention (CDC), and the U.S. Patent and Trademark Office—have committed crimes against humanity by burying and obfuscating the issue of Morgellons. A review of Appendix 14, "Visitors to www.Carnicom.com" (August 26, 1999), makes it clear that the so-called "alphabet soup" agencies of Washington, DC followed Carnicom's single-handed, low-budget investigation into their classified delivery of the *synbio* blood infrastructure necessary to their globalist dream of BCI Transhumanism. (Once Carnicom published this list on the Internet, the website visitor identification feature was shut down.)

The saga of Morgellons continues in the Nanotechnology chapter because Morgellons leads us into *digital biology utterly dependent upon nanotechnology*, in keeping with the globalist vision of cyborg Human 2.0.

---

106 For more on Morgellons from sufferers and researchers: carnicominstitute.org, Skizit Gesture, *http://www.dataasylum.com/*, *independz.podbean.com*, *augmentinforce.50webs.com*, *www.Bryan396.com*, *https://lookoutfacharlie.blogspot.com*, Lyme Protocol: *http://www.klinghardtacademy.com/images/stories/Lyme_Disease/klinghardt_biological_treatment_of_lyme_disease_protocol.pdf;* Facebook sites: Finding Hope with Morgellons, Morgellons Coverup, Tommy Target, Morgellons: An Open Forum (closed group), Morgellons Extreme & Emerging Illnesses, Energy Clearing Protocol; etc.

A few recommended papers from carnicominstitute.org

"The Salts of Our Soils," May 11, 2005, Santa Fe, New Mexico
High levels of conductivity (ions) in increasing reactive metals in the soil stressing plant life.

"The New Biology," January 18, 2014

"Preliminary Rainwater Analysis: Aluminum Concentration," November 2, 2015, Wallace, Idaho
Voltammetric testing.

"Preliminary Rainwater Analysis: Organics & Inorganics," November 4, 2015, Wallace, Idaho
Biological red and blue fibers in the rainwater visible under microscope (200x) and infrared spectroscopy (5000x); aluminum level exceeds the US EPA standard for drinking water by a factor of 10.

"The Demise of Rainwater," June 20, 2016, Wallace, Idaho
Ionic consequence in the soil of atmospheric activity.

GMO Frankenfoods

From a genomics standpoint, germline / genome modification was banned in 83 percent of the 30 nations in the Organization for Economic Cooperation and Development (OECD) until the UK broke ranks in 2013 by allowing three-parent babies. That's when Pandora's box tumbled open. Synthetic biology *(synbio)* is the overarching science that engineers cells ("material production") with novel (gain of function[107]) biological functions. GMO foods were the very first inkling I had of the genetic revolution already underway. The corporations making millions from genetically altered seed alter food genetics so as to acquire lucrative proprietary patents over food. *By buying and eating that "food," you are furthering their power.* The same Big Pharma names come up again and again, stretching back centuries: Novartis, Monsanto, DuPont, Dow, Bayer. Big Pharma corporate families are now gobbling up biotech and genomics corporations so as to control the future of GM seed, germplasm, pesticide with *Bacillus thuringiensis* genes, corn (maize), soybeans, wheat, rice, tobacco, cotton, etc.—in other words, humanity's food staples.

Up until the 1990s, the nine-member CGIAR (Consultative Group on International Agricultural Research) review panel was relatively balanced be-

107 Gain of function: activation of genetic mutations to enhance or block; employed not just to alter Nature in order to qualify for a patent but also to weaponize it for unending profits and other agendas.

tween the global North (supply-side science / the head) and global South (end-users growing food / the heart). As biotechnology took over more and more, however, the Northern private sector became dominant. Monsanto spent the late 1990s devouring seed, chemical, and biotech corporations (and buying off politicians). Its *apomictic maize* (US Patent #5,710,367) creates reproducible plant clones that speed up sterile hybrid seed production.[108]

The United States was the first nation to release genetically modified / engineered (GM, GMO, GE) crops and remains the top producer. *The U.S. is not a Party to the UN Convention on Biodiversity.* Only 26 nations currently allow GM foods to be commercially available or grown by *precision farming (site-specific management)* under agrochemical corporations whose access to supercomputers, satellites, nanosensors (smart dust), geospatial intelligence, etc., is dedicated to the ceaseless *ambient intelligence*[109] of smart fields growing GMO foods for Smart Cities filled with BCI cyborgs plugged into the Space Fence lockdown.

Terminator Technology—the RAFI (Rural Advancement Foundation International) term for US Patent #5,723,765, "Control of Plant Gene Expression," controlled by Monsanto—sterilizes farm-saved seed by blocking its reproductive process. The European version is Zeneca's Verminator,[110] a chemically activated seed killer that switches on rodent fat genes bioengineered into crop seed. Plant variety protection is also built into the seed so that crops can be engineered to kill their own seeds in the second generation, thus making it impossible for farmers to save and replant seed.

Monsanto controls the world *transgenic* cotton market:

> . . . the goal is to develop a variety of cotton that will grow normally until the crop is almost mature. Then, and only then, a toxin will be produced in the (seed) embryos, specifically killing the entire next generation of seeds . . . The key to terminator is the ability to make a lot of a toxin that will kill cells, and to confine that toxin to seeds.[111]

---

108 In 1998, the internationally respected British magazine Ecologist announced that its printer Penwell's had destroyed the entire print run of 14,000 copies of the edition devoted to exposing Monsanto and its Terminator seed technology. The Ecologist arranged for another printer to reprint the issue.

109 "Precision Agriculture – Nanotech Methods Used, Such As 'Smart Dust' and Nanosensors." AzoNano, July 25, 2005. Read Steven Druker's Altered Genes, Twisted Truth: How the Venture to Genetically Engineer Our Food Has Subverted Science, Corrupted Government, and Systematically Deceived the Public (Clear River Press, 2015).

110 Zeneca "life industry" is now AstraZeneca of COVID-19 "vaccine" infamy. Bayer / Monsanto, pharmaceuticals and chemicals in the sky, soil, and body—they are all Big Pharma.

111 Martha L. Crouch, PhD, "How the Terminator terminates: an explanation for the non-scientist of a remarkable patent for killing second generation seeds of crop plants." The Edmonds Institute, 1998.

The 1998 Terminator chemical programming bioengineered into the cotton plant DNA is fourfold: (1) a toxin gene controlled by the promoter DNA (responsible for interacting with the cell or environment); (2) a repressor protein coding sequence with a promoter; (3) insertion of a piece of DNA between the promoter and the toxin coding sequence that blocks the manufacture of protein; (4) a recombinase enzyme coding sequence controlled by a promoter but regulated by the repressor protein while the plant grows until it is overridden by the antibiotic tetracycline the seed was treated with before being sold to farmers. (The patent holders, of course, have recourse to an altered version that keeps the promoter active and revives the recombinase just before planting the seed they grow to sell to farmers.)

Transfer methods of getting genes into cells via "gene therapy" have been similar for humans, animals, and plants: injection into the cell nucleus with a tiny needle (microneedle transfection); plant cells soaked in DNA "stews," then electrically forced into the cell (electroporation); DNA attached to tiny metal particles (nanoparticles) and shot into cells (electroporation); viruses or bacteria engineered to infect cells with DNA.

> Once the Terminator seed becomes a mature plant, the Terminator pollen carries the ready-made toxin gene to infect nearby or distant crops wherever the wind or birds carry it. In 1998, the toxin gene ended with a dead plant; today, it is inherited. In 2013, six out of six major rivers in China tested positive for ampicillin antibiotic-resistant bacteria. The *bla gene* was sequenced: it was synthetic, and samples from all six rivers were also resistant to tetracycline.[112]

It is not hyperbole to say that Monsanto and its Terminator patent have been "the neutron bomb of agriculture."[113]

With *molecular pharming*, Monsanto *synbio* turned to genetically modified crops for pharmaceuticals.[114] Ventria Bioscience (CA) began planting rice engineered to produce the synthetic proteins lactoferrin and lysozyme.

> *Lactoferrin* regulates immune functions and controls pathogens by binding iron required for bacterial growth; implicated in fatal asthma

112 "GM Antibiotic Resistance in China's Rivers." Institute of Science in Society (ISIS), February 13, 2013.

113 "Monsanto Takes Terminator," RAFI press release, May 14, 1997. The Rural Advancement Foundation International (RAFI) has been going since 1990. See www.rafiusa.org.

114 Molecular pharming patents date from 1990 ("Protein products for future global good") for production of antibodies, vaccines, proteins, flavorings, biodegradable plastics, seed metabolism, viral systems and vectors, etc.

> *Lysozyme* is normally produced in human milk, saliva, and tears; it breaks down the cell walls of bacteria and may contribute to emphysema

The USDA, another department of Big Pharma,[115] approved Ventria's pharm rice test site right in the middle of Missouri's chief rice-growing region so other fields could be contaminated by cross-pollination and seed spills during transport.

From the beginning, the intention of Big Pharma has been that transgenic proteins enter the human food supply.

> . . . by far, the greater danger is that the transgenic proteins are only approximations of the natural protein both in DNA sequence, Amino-acid sequence and patterns of glycosylation (carbohydrate chains added to the proteins), all of which may make transgenic proteins allergenic, or the transgenic proteins may trigger diseases connected with the inability of human cells to break them down properly.
>
> As these proteins [lactoferrin and lysozyme] both target bacteria, there is a large question mark over the safety of these proteins to beneficial bacteria in our gut . . . [and] horizontal transfer of the transgenes to viral and bacterial pathogens that are everywhere in our environment.[116]

GM fruits, vegetables, and grains (potato, tomato, lettuce, papaya, carrot, rice, quinoa, alfalfa, banana, algae, etc.) are now being genetically modified to produce edible vaccinations.[117] Compounds like resveratrol and genistein[118] are programmed to generate an immune response in the intestinal epithelium, no doubt contributing to the epidemic of gut biome problems in children—inflammatory bowel disease, ulcerative colitis, Crohn's disease, etc.—on the rise since 1990.

The French molecular biologist Gilles-Éric Séralini conducted a two-year study of rats fed on Monsanto GM corn, all of the rats developed dramatic tumors and organ damage, including atrophied kidneys. Séralini's paper was published in the Journal of Food and Chemical Toxicology in September 2012, then retracted due to pressure from Monsanto, then republished (minus crucial data) in the Environmental Sciences Europe journal.

---

115 During the post-World War Two Cold War, the USDA dedicated large plots of land in the U.S. Midwest to "anti-crop germ" (weaponized viral) aerosol tests in concert with Fort Detrick Special Operations Division's "vulnerability tests" on American populations.

116 "Molecular Pharming – the New Battlefront over GM crops." ISIS press release, 19 July 2005. ISIS is the Institute of Science In Society.

117 "Scientists Are Growing Genetically Modified Edible Coronavirus Vaccine," GreatGameIndia, July 30, 2020.

118 Natasha Longo, "GMO Tomatoes May Soon Be Back on Supermarket Shelves." Prevent-Disease.com, November 10, 2015. The question is, like the mouse that must carry a human ear on its back, what does this do to the tomato?

More than a decade ago, cellulose fibers found in the skin of Morgellons sufferers pointed to a possible connection between Morgellons and GMO fields—in other words, the possibility that eating food grown from genetically modified seed in soil treated with chemical aerosols and pesticides and fertilizers can end in Morgellons lesions with protruding fibers produced by the pathogenic soil bacterium Agrobacterium, which is used extensively in agricultural genetic engineering because of its "natural ability to transfer parts of its genetic material to plant cells."[119]

Agribusiness is deeply involved in synbio experimentation. Besides the impact of Agrobacterium transferring its genetics to plant cells that are then consumed by humans and animals—animals that many humans then eat—there is the impact of "microencapsulated insecticidal pathogens" (US Patent #4844896A) loaded with "a virus, bacterium, or fungi known to infect insects; a polymeric encapsulating agent comprising polyacrylates, polyacrylic acids, polyacrylamides or mixtures thereof; a sunscreening agent comprising methyl orange, malachite green or its hydrochloride, methyl green, brilliant green, an FDC green, coomasie brilliant blue R, methylene blue HCI salt, brilliant cresyl blue, acridine yellow, and FDC yellow, an FDC red, fluorescein free acid or mixtures thereof," etc. Then there are the pesticides based on baculoviruses that attack insect and anthropod hosts, given that recombinant baculoviruses are used to transfer genetic material into human cells (Cell Biology, 1995).

When humans consume all of these genetic modifications in plants and animals, what happens to their human cells?

The FDA has no list of genetically modified foods for consumers, purportedly because labeling is "voluntary," the philosophy being that if a biotech corporation signs off on the safety of GM food, that's good enough for the FDA.[120]

Herbicide tolerance is engineered into GM seed, but insects evolve their way around the genetic modifications and around Monsanto's mitochondrial and cellular toxin Roundup Ready that contains the infamous carcinogenic glyphosate and Syngenta's hormone-disrupting, estrogen-mimicking Atrazine. For example, the cotton bollworm has become immune to the deterrent toxins derived from the Bacillus thuringiensis (Bt) bacterium.121

119 Hank P. Albarelli Jr. and Zoe Martell, "National Security Secrecy: Morgellons Victims Across the US and Europe." Voltairenet.org, June 12, 2010.

120 During his presidency, George W. Bush (2001-2009) appointed Monsanto vice president Virginia Weldon as director of the FDA. See the FDA's "Guidance for Industry: Voluntary Labeling Indicating Whether Foods Have or Have Not Been Derived from Genetically Engineered Plants"; and Anne Temple, "FDA Admits to No List of Gene-Edited GMOs in the US Market," Moms Across America, December 7, 2019.

121 George Dvorsky, "Mutated pests are quickly adapting to biotech crops in unpredicted and disturbing ways." Io9.com, June 27, 2012.

To get around evolving insects, Monsanto is genetically modifying other insects to hunt down the evolving offenders. The unleashing of this supposedly "greener" alternative to chemicals alters the genetic structure of entire insect populations, but Monsanto cares as little as do its friends in the military who are weaponing other insect species.[122] 'Round and 'round it goes, where it stops, nobody knows . . .

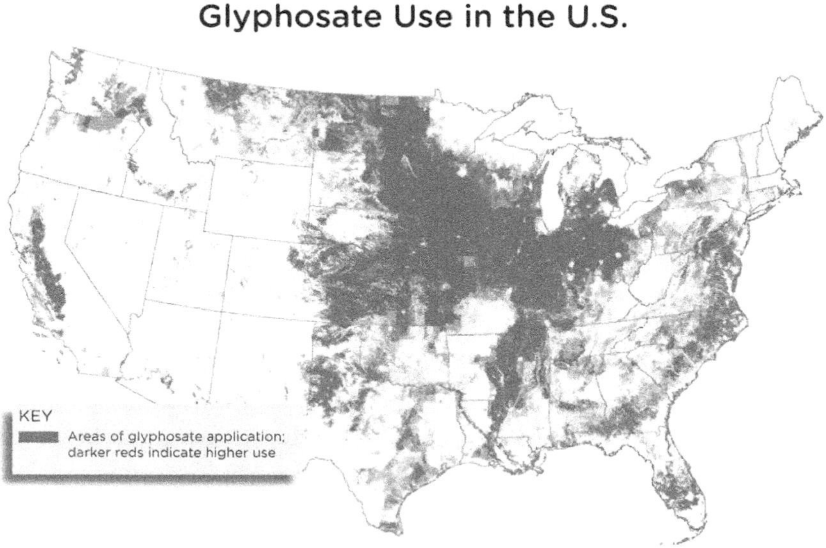

Glyphosate, U.S.

https://www.nexusnewsfeed.com/article/self-sufficiency/monsanto-s-glyphosate-linked-to-global-decline-in-holey-bees

In 2002, Zambia realized what was really going on with AGRA, the World Food Programme, USAID, and the International Institute for Tropical Agriculture and rejected the GM corn "gifted" to solve their hunger and poverty. The GM corn "gift" had been to create dependence upon more and more chemicals as the biological effects were tracked and measured. Now that Africa's natural food production has been on the rise, Bill Gates is again on the move, purchasing Ginkgo Bioworks, a biotech "organism company" that prints DNA for GM crops for $1bn. Ginkgo reprograms the DNA in plants and other organisms like synthetic microbes "that would allow staple crops

---

122 Anthony Gucciardi, "Thousands of Genetically Modified Insects Set For Release." NaturalSociety.com, September 6, 2013.

like corn, wheat and rice to produce their own fertilizer."123 (Sounds like mRNA programming cells to produce their own spike proteins, doesn't it?)

Meanwhile, Boko Haram fighters burn fields and drive farmers and their families to displaced persons camps. Debt and dependency are essential to Big Pharma domination.

GMO meat

The synbio pharming of animals by corporations like ConAgra, Cargill, and Tyson has changed what people consume in the name of nutrition. Big Agribusiness drugs animals, feeds them GMO grains and body parts, and irradiates them.[124] Or perhaps you'd prefer "cultured meat":

> Cells are taken from an animal, often via a biopsy or from an established animal cell line. These cells are then fed a nutrient broth and placed in a bioreactor where they multiply until there are enough to harvest for use in meatballs or nuggets.[125]

Of course, it's hard to tell if the animal the cells are from is a natural animal from a natural reproductive process (probably not) or a *cloned* Dolly-the-sheep animal. If it's all just too much to investigate, people might resign themselves to the GM Impossible Burger made from GM soy leghemoglobain protein from yeast bacteria and GM imitation blood (to make the Impossible Burger "sizzle like blood").[126]

Speaking of blood, where is the GM line regarding remaining human? Apaches are cautious of eating pigs and fish because both eat reptiles. *Does it matter what, or who, one eats, or is it just "superstition"?* Corporations like BiteLabs "want to make human test-tube meat a reality": a biopsy (human) tissue sample containing myosatellite cells (which help to repair and regrow damaged muscle) is floated in "a medium that acts as an artificial blood to grow muscle" to multiply the cells. Once the cells are mature, they're ground and mixed with meats like ostrich, spices, brandy and shallots, fats and oils, then stuffed into casings to be dry-aged and cured.[127] Celebrities donate their tissues (from which parts of their bodies?) and star-status names—for example, Ellen DeGeneres (blood) salami.

---

123 Tom Huddleston Jr., "This $1 billion start-up backed by Bill Gates prints new DNA and everyone from the DOD to Bayer is on board." Cnbc.com, December 21, 2018.

124 Read the 2006 Rolling Stone exposé of the pig industry, "Pork's Dirty Secret," by Jeff Tietz.

125 Niall Firth, "Cultured meat has been approved for consumers for the first time." MIT Technology Review, December 1, 2020.

126 "Application for GMO 'Imitation Blood' Raises Concern." GE Free NZ press release, January 19, 2020.

127 Jenn Harris, "Ellen DeGeneres salami? One company's quest to make meat from celebrity tissue samples." Los Angeles Times, March 5, 2014.

Have these stars and BiteLabs executives attended Marina Abramovic's Spirit Cooking ventures? Remember the 1973 preprogramming film *Soylent Green*? Washington State is the first state to compost dead human bodies as crop fertilizer. Bill 5001[128] legalizes "liquid cremation" wherein alkaline hydrolysis turns the human body into "organic" sludge ("gray goo"?). How will human body fertilizer qualitatively affect the food grown in fields and gardens?

Is the FDA Center for Biologics Evaluation and Research—which regulates vaccines, blood and blood products, human tissue and tissue products for transplantation, cell therapy, and gene therapy—engaged in public-private partnerships with corporations like BiteLabs, "natural organic reduction facilities," and funeral homes like Recompose? Actual human remains composting is called *terramation.*[129] Eighteen states already permit *alkaline hydrolysis* ("aquamation"),[130] Washington State being the first to allow human composting. Water involved in the aquamation process is then either processed like other wastewater (to municipal water treatment facilities) or given to farmers to use in agriculture.

With hydrolysis (lye and water dissolving protein and fat) instead of fire, what will occur when the chemotherapy and radiation from cancer treatments, "enhancements," and other non-dissolvables end up in the soil, water, and air?

GM marketing

> *They draw on a number of disciplines in their work: biology, psychology, physiology, and organic chemistry. A flavorist is a chemist with a trained nose and a poetic sensibility. Flavors are created by blending scores of different chemicals in tiny amounts—a process governed by scientific principles but demanding a fair amount of art. In an age when delicate aromas and microwave ovens do not easily co-exist, the job of the flavorist is to conjure illusions about processed food and, in the words of one flavor company's literature, to ensure "consumer likeability." The flavorists with whom I spoke were discrete, in keeping with the dictates of their trade. They were also charming, cosmopolitan, and ironic. They not only enjoyed fine wine but could identify the chemicals that give each grape its unique aroma. One flavorist compared his work to composing music.*
>
> – William Langewiesche, "The Million Dollar Nose," *The Atlantic,* December 2000

128 Signed into law on May 21, 2019, https://www.washingtonvotes.org/2019-SB-5001. Cremations at this point use 45 gallons of fuel per cremation.

129 Craig Sailor, "Turn your remains into potting soil? See how this business aims to alter funeral industry." News Tribune, March 30, 2021.

130 Jeffrey Mirsepasy, "Human composting and alkaline hydrolysis – Greener disposition of remains in Washington." Latest Legal News, January 11, 2021.

The supermarket is a carefully concocted artificial environment dedicated to making genetically altered, nutritionless, precision-farmed GMO products fool the public into thinking it is food. GMO marketing spends millions on PhDs who peer into the shopper's subconscious, even employing functional magnetic resonance imaging machines (fMRIs) to register brain blood flow as different name brand images flash in front of now-third generation modern supermarket shoppers. America takes profits exceedingly seriously.

Each supermarket issues plan-a-grams according to retailer slotting fees for where their goods get placed. Slotting is sometimes a real fight, which is partially why security cameras watch for smiles and grimaces as much as for shoplifting (now passé, thanks to item nanosensors), the moment of truth being first in the choice, then in the purchase.

Cashier stations are embedded in decompression zones where digital video screens are filled with ads linked to facial recognition software. Greeters and chill zones wend the consumer toward the "fresh" GMO fruits and vegetables. Everyday items like bread, meat, milk, and pharmacy drugs are placed so shoppers increase their "dwell time" among labels, price stickers, specials, and images, all measured by tracking their iPhones as they follow the smell of baking bread (or citrus in clothing stores, or coconut at travel agencies).

Having supplied the chemicals for aerosol deliveries and GMO farms, Big Pharma arms GMO foods with industrial flavors and smells to make them appetizing or, in some cases, addictive. In the list of ingredients, "natural flavor" and "artificial flavor" are synonyms. Take the natural flavor out of mass food—long shelf-life food—and put it back in with chemicals and nanoparticles, along with chemically brightened colors to make it look like it has vitality. (The Food and Drug Administration doesn't require that color, flavor additives, or nanoparticles be listed.) Not only have we lost our taste buds and sense of smell and instinct for Nature, but whole generations have psychologically bonded with ads and flavor and smell memories whipped up by "flavorists" (chemists / food technologists) who use mechanical mouths to measure "mouthfeel" via rheological[131] properties—the "bounce, creep, breaking point, density, crunchiness, chewiness, gumminess, lumpiness, rubberiness, springiness, slipperiness, smoothness, softness, wetness, juiciness, spreadability, springback, and tackiness"[132] of every refined, packaged GMO food.

Methyl anthranilate smells like grapes.

Ethyl-2-methyl smells like apples.

Methyl-2-pyridyl tastes like popcorn.

131 Rheology: branch of physics that examines the flow and deformation of materials.

132 William Langewiesche, "The Million Dollar Nose." The Atlantic, December 2000.

Ethyl-3-hydroxy tastes like marshmallow.
Amyl acetate tastes like banana.
Benzaldehyde smells like almond.

Gas chromatographs,[133] mass spectrometers,[134] and vapor analyzers detect volatile gases and help find flavors to be synthesized for over 10,000 new processed "foods" per year.

> A typical artificial strawberry flavor, like the kind found in a Burger King strawberry milk shake, contains the following ingredients: amyl acetate, amyl butyrate, amyl valerate, anethol, anisyl formate, benzyl acetate, benzyl isobutyrate, butyric acid, cinnamyl isobutyrate, cinnamyl valerate, cognac essential oil, diacetyl, dipropyl ketone, ethyl acetate, ethyl amyl ketone, ethyl butyrate, ethyl cinnamate, ethyl heptanoate, ethyl heptylate, ethyl lactate, ethyl methylphenylglycidate, ethyl nitrate, ethyl propionate, ethyl valerate, heliotropin, hydroxyphenyl-2-butanone (10 percent solution in alcohol), a-ionone, isobutyl anthranilate, isobutyl butyrate, lemon essential oil, maltol, 4-methylacetophenone, methyl anthranilate, methyl benzoate, methyl cinnamate, methyl heptane carbonate, methyl naphthyl ketone, methyl salicylate, mint essential oil, neroli essential oil, nerolin, neryl isobutyrate, orris butter, phenethyl alcohol, rose, rum ether, g-undecalactone, vanillin and solvent.[135]

Natural flavors and artificial flavors may now and then share the same chemical *signature,* but step out of your materialistic mindset for a moment and consider the *qualitative* difference between Nature and manmade *to the living body* is night and day. The next time you are tempted to eat a brightly colored Dannon strawberry yogurt, you may remember having read something about the origin of that unnaturally bright pink:

> Cochineal extract (also known as carmine or carminic acid) is made from the desiccated bodies of female *Dactylopius coccus Costa,* a small insect harvested mainly in Peru and the Canary Islands. The bug feeds on red cactus berries, and color from the berries accumulates in the females and their unhatched larvae. The insects are collected, dried, and ground into

---

133 Chromatography: the separation of a mixture by passing it in solution or suspension or as a vapor (as in gas chromatography) through a medium in which the components move at different rates.

134 Spectrometry: the measurement of the interactions between light and matter, and the reactions and measurements of radiation intensity and wavelength.

135 Eric Schlosser, Fast Food Nation: The Dark Side of the All-American Meal. Houghton-Mifflin, 2001. Also see Schlosser's article in The Atlantic Monthly, "Why McDonald's Fries Taste So Good" (August 23, 2007).

a pigment. It takes about 70,000 of them to produce a pound of carmine, which is used to make processed foods look pink, red, or purple . . .[136]

Yum!

Glyphosate

Aerosol pesticide spraying, virus "food additive" spraying, and glyphosate spraying work hand in glove with what is being delivered by jets in the stratosphere. For years, Monsanto has had access to insider trading data from those who engineer the weather, which could explain why Monsanto purchased Climate Corporation, the underwriter of farmers' weather insurance, for $930 million in 2013.[137] Monsanto receives weather measurements from 2.5 million locations (including satellite), 150 billion soil observations, and forecasts from major climate modules to generate 10 trillion weather simulation data points.[138]

Stephanie Seneff, PhD, points out that glyphosate is even in jet fuel, due to the "green" decree to convert waste biomass into oil-based biodiesel fuels made up of post-harvest stalks of corn and wheat "woody biomass." Dr. Seneff then ties glyphosate to COVID-19 by how it damages the lungs with airway inflammation, asthma-related cytokines, and COPD (chronic obstructive pulmonary disease). We are breathing in not just vehicle biodiesel fuels but the chemical nanoparticles in jet biofuels falling earthward and carried by wind and rain. Biofuel is used to heat buildings (35 million gallons in New York City in 2018), and of course there are the runoffs from fields into water catchments, gutters, rivers, etc.

The pineal gland housed deep in the brain ("the seat of the soul," according to philosopher Rene Descartes) may be the ultimate target of a purposely concocted synergy that chemically and electromagnetically assaults the air we breathe, the food we eat, and the water we drink, cook with, and bathe in. Dietrich Klinghardt, MD, has come to this conclusion by studying the combined impact of Big Pharma aluminum, fluoride, and glyphosate, whose frequencies appear to be electromagnetically pulsed to act together on the human body and brain. Glyphosate depletes micronutrients of calcium, zinc, magnesium, etc., and kills the good bacteria in our gut (our "second brain"). By mimicking the amino acid glycine, *glyphosate misfolds the proteins that then become prions.*[139] (See Chapter 14, "The COVID-19 'Vaccine' Event.")

---

136 Ibid.

137 "Monsanto Buys Climate Corp For $930 Million." Forbes.com, October 2, 2013.

138 http://www.indexventures.com/ blog#post/822.

139 Makia Freeman, "Aluminum, Fluoride, Glyphosate and EMF: The Deliberate Concoction

Another detail pointing to a devilish intent is the 2009 aluminum-resistant patent US #7,582,809 designed at Cornell University to assure that GMO seed would be able to thrive in nano-aluminum-poisoned soil. The patent process was funded by the National Science Foundation (NSF) and the Bill and Melinda Gates Foundation, both of which must have been aware of the massive dumps of aluminum nanoparticles coming down from the stratosphere.[140]

Dr. Klinghardt stresses that every American is full of nanosized aluminum, mercury, lead, and organophosphates[141] like Roundup, which chelates (binds) trace minerals in food to aluminum, thus preventing nutrients from being absorbed. Roundup in the body binds with aluminum and transports it deep into the brain.

That nano-aluminum is inundating us has been stressed by a few courageous scientists willing to brave the scientism-controlled peer review / publishing gauntlet, like interdisciplinary scientist J. Marvin Herndon, PhD. In his 2016 paper "Human and Environmental Dangers Posed by Ongoing Global Tropospheric Aerosolized Particulates for Weather Modification," Dr. Herndon stresses that the ability of coal fly ash—the aerosol particulate favored by geoengineers and the military as "chaff"—to "release aluminum in a chemically mobile form upon exposure to water or body moisture has potentially grave human and environmental consequences." Toxic, soluble nano-aluminum falls earthward, is breathed in, and contaminates the soil along with coal fly ash

> . . . able to liberate a host of toxins through exposure to body moisture, including aluminum, arsenic, barium, boron, cadmium, chromium, lead, lithium, selenium, strontium, thallium, and thorium and uranium with their radioactive daughter products, and other toxins.[142]

Thousands of lawsuits have been filed against Monsanto—now owned by the parent corporation Bayer, first offspring of the notorious Big Pharma Nazi collaborator I.G. Farben—claiming that glyphosate causes cancer (NHL or non-Hodgkin lymphoma).[143] Mexican President Andrés Manuel López Obrador has set a 2024 deadline to stop using glyphosate and phase out GM

---

to Shut You Down." TheFreedomArticles.com, May 19, 2020.

140 Thanks to Kevin Mugur Galalae and his book Water, Salt, Milk Killing Our Unborn Children, Politics in Need of Change, September 24, 2012.

141 Organophosphates were used as nerve gas agents in World War One.

142 J. Marvin Herndon, "Human and Environmental Dangers Posed by Ongoing Global Tropospheric Aerosolized Particulates for Weather Modification." Frontiers in Public Health, 30 June 2016. Dr. Herndon's papers can be found at nuclearplanet.com/Geoengineering-Scientific-Articles.html.

143 Tyler Durden, "Bayer Pays $10BN To Settle Thousands of Monsanto Glyphosate Lawsuits." Zero Hedge, June 23, 2020.

corn cultivation *and* GM imports so as to protect Mexico's native corn as well as citizen health. Of course, Mexico has been accused of being in violation of NAFTA guidelines (now called the U.S. Mexico Canada Agreement or USMCA).[144] The average Mexican consumes one pound of corn per day. The previous president, Enrique Peña Nieto, let Big Pharma grow its GMO corn all over northern Mexico. Will the populist president hold his ground, as Thailand in 2019 did not? Will the CIA force a regime change?

Vaccines: The Medical Industry's Third Rail

> *Collect the fluid from the pustules on the point of a lancet and insert it into the arm so that the fluid mixes with the blood. This will produce fever, but the disease will then be very mild, and there will be no cause for alarm.*
>
> – Description of a vaccine, *Veda Sactaya Grantham*[145]

> *It is a well-established fact in the United States that the pharmaceutical company's vaccine products cannot survive in a free market. Facing complete financial ruin due to extensive litigation resulting in faulty products which were maiming and killing people in the 1980s, the industry sought, and was granted, legal protection from all lawsuits by Congress in 1986. This law was challenged but upheld by the Supreme Court in 2011.*
>
> – "Are Aerosol Vaccines Forced Upon Populations via Plane or Helicopter the Wave of the Future?" *Health Impact News,* March 19, 2016

Vaccines are a $60+ billion per year industry. Now, 69 doses of childhood vaccines are required, and a new adult schedule of 100+ doses is recommended, with 271 vaccines in the pipelines for who knows what "epidemics," to be activated by 5G transmission frequencies.

The history of vaccinations is sordid, rather like one long *Dr. Strangelove*[146] open lab experiment in eugenics as per the Club of Rome propaganda instrument *The Limits To Growth: A Report For the Club of Rome's Project on the Predicament of Mankind* (1972). As I mentioned earlier, three years before the

144 Timothy A. Wise, "Mexico to Ban Glyphosate, GM Corn: Presidential Decree Comes Despite Intense Pressure from Industry, U.S. Authorities." InterPress Service, February 24, 2021.

145 From the 1883 book by F.B. Wilkie, The Great Inventions: Their History From the Earliest Period to the Present (Philadelphia: J.A. Ruth & Co.). Western sources claim that the Hindu Vedas were written ~1500 BCE, but I am sure they are much older.

146 Dr. Strangelove or: How I Learned to Stop Worrying and Love the Bomb (1964), a black comedy about the Cold War military mindset starring Peter Sellers and directed by Stanley Kubrick.

Club of Rome pronouncement, the Department of Defense Biological Warfare Division was given $10 million to produce organisms that would selectively destroy the immune system, after which the Frederick Cancer Research Facility of the U.S. Army's Fort Detrick Biological Warfare Laboratory morphed into the National Cancer Institute, and the staff and budget tripled.

Cancer cells are still found in vaccines. But then vaccines are not about health, just as genetically modified foods are not about health; they're about biological warfare experimentation on the military side and profits and Transhumanist bioengineering on the corporate patent-control side. For example, the U.S. Department of Health & Human Services (HHS) through the NIH owns patents on all *human papillomavirus (HPV)* vaccines and receives a percentage for every dose of Gardasil and Cervarix. Big Pharma vaccine-makers can't be sued or held responsible for deaths or disablement, so now open-field experimentation has moved from the military to civilians with *no accountability.*

The Global Fund ("accelerating the end of AIDS, tuberculosis and malaria as epidemics") in Geneva, Switzerland was established in 2002 through the G8 and UN. The largest donor to the Global Fund ($90 billion so far) is PEPFAR (President's Emergency Plan For AIDS Relief),[147] established under President George W. Bush (2001-2009) to merge with Doctors Without Borders and the Bill and Melinda Gates Foundation. How many of the 23.3 million people receiving HIV "treatment" ever see any of this money? (The global HIV drug market exceeded $24.7 billion in 2018.)

The privately owned Centers for Disease Control and Prevention (CDC) is a vaccine subsidiary of Big Pharma working in league with the U.S. Department of Human and Health Services (HHS). States are grantees under CDC vaccination programs because *vaccine laws are state, not federal,* which means that the private CDC must work under the radar to ensure compliance with federal guidelines. As the owner of a variety of vaccine patents, the CDC and its Immunization Safety Office are deeply implicated in conflict of interest.[148] The fact is that at the very core, the CDC, FDA, IOM (Institute of Medicine), NIH (National Institutes of Health), state medical boards, exclusive medical guilds like the AMA (American Medical Association), and corporate media (70 percent of whose income comes from Big Pharma)[149] serve Big Pharma / bioengineering dynastic bloodline families, not the people.

Hepatitis B provided the first *subunit vaccine* (see Chapter 14, "The COVID-19 'Vaccine' Event"). Then came the CDC push to vaccinate chil-

---

147 Former Vice President Mike Pence worked for PEPFAR.

148 "Robert Kennedy Jr.: CDC Is A Privately Owned Vaccine Company." NWOReport, July 2, 2018.

149 Thanks to Diane McCann, April 14, 2020.

dren for Hepatitis A.[150] The most recent well-publicized assault on infants in the covert cause of Transhumanism before the COVID-19 "vaccine" occurred in Brazil in early 2015 when 2,400+ pregnant lower-class Brazilian women were inoculated with GlaxoSmithKline's neurotoxic, brain-destroying Tdap vaccine. The cover story was to prevent whooping cough, but their babies were born with microcephaly (shrunken and underdeveloped brains and skulls). Mosquitos and the African Zika virus were blamed for "yet another vaccine-induced, iatrogenic (medical industry-caused) disease."[151]

Much like the 1953 dystopian novel *Fahrenheit 451* by Ray Bradbury in which firemen start fires instead of put them out, it appears that vaccines are about weakening the immune system so as to *implant* future diseases ("pathogenic priming") that "precision medicine" will be able to remotely trigger, program, and manipulate.

During the long leadup to the present dystopia, philanthropist Bill Gates spent 17 years (2000-2017) exploiting India's National Technical Advisory Group on Immunization (NTAGI) through which it was mandated that each child under five be given 50 doses of polio vaccine. What followed was an epidemic of non-polio acute flaccid paralysis (490,000 children). Once the Indian government realized what was going on, Gates was ejected and NPAFP rates dropped precipitously. *Polio epidemics in developing nations like the Congo, Afghanistan, and the Philippines are all linked to vaccines—in fact, 70 percent of all global polio cases.*[152]

Since 1972, polio vaccines have kept paralytic polio alive (*Science,* April 4, 1977), with the Salk and Sabin vaccines (monkey tissue and aborted human fetal tissue) increasing leukemia. In 2004, Dr. Cantwell wrote an article examining the UN's WHO Global Polio Eradication Program administering oral vaccines to 74 million African children in 22 nations to stem a "wild polio epidemic" whose epicenter was oil-rich Nigeria. Pharmaceutical scientist Haruna Kaita, PhD, discovered female sex hormones in oral vaccines for sterilizing and causing miscarriages. Dr. Kaita demanded that those who imported this "fake drug" in the name of polio vaccines "be prosecuted like any other criminal." Later, Nigeria resumed polio vaccinations but only vaccines manufactured in Indonesia. Multiple sclerosis (MS) is also provoked by vaccines.

---

150 "State pushed to require vaccine for hepatitis A," AP, February 19, 1999.

151 Gary G. Kohls, MD, "More on the Zika Virus – Microcephaly Freak-out." Global Research, February 10, 2016.

152 Robert F. Kennedy, Jr., "Gates' Globalist Vaccine Agenda: A Win-Win for Pharma and Mandatory Vaccination." Children's Health Defense, April 9, 2020. Also see Rady Ananda, "War on Syria begins with mass [polio] vaccination program," Activist Post, December 14, 2013.

[Dr. Kaita:] Those manufacturers or promoters of these harmful things have a secret agenda which only further research can reveal. Secondly, they have always taken us in the third world for granted, thinking we don't have the capacity, knowledge and equipment to conduct tests that would reveal such contaminants. And very unfortunately they also have people to defend their atrocities within our midst, and worst still, some of these are supposed to be our own professionals whom we rely on to protect our interests.[153]

Recently in the U.S. District Court for the Southern District of New York, vaccine injury lawyer Robert F. Kennedy Jr., of the Children's Health Defense and Del Bigtree (producer of the documentaries *VAXXED I: From Coverup to Catastrophe* and *VAXXED II: The People's Truth*), and the nonprofit Informed Consent Action Network (ICAN) went up against the HHS, which has now admitted that *since 1988*[154]—two years after the National Childhood Vaccination Injury Act granted economic immunity to pharmaceutical corporations for vaccine injuries—it has failed to provide a single safety report to Congress and is therefore in direct violation of the federal law requiring a biannual vaccine safety report that details efforts to make sure vaccines are safe.[155]

One victory, many battles to come.

"Herd Immunity"

> *The possibility should also be looked into that the immune response . . . may be impaired if the infectious virus damages more or less selectively the cells responding to the viral antigens. If this proves to be the case, virus-induced immune-depression might conceivably be highly instrumental in prolonging certain virus infections, such as Murine Leukemia, Hepatitis, Sub-acute Scherosing . . .*
>
> – World Health Organization memorandum, 1972

Decades ago, when I was studying, comparing, and practicing the principles of traditional Chinese medicine (TCM) and the Japanese dietary practice called macrobiotics for my health and possible future career, I intuitively understood the wisdom of the Eastern view of the immune system. It wasn't so much a "system" as a strong *wellbeing* dependent upon an acid / alkaline balanced diet

153 Alan Cantwell, MD, "What's With the Monkey Business? Cancer-Causing Vaccines, Polio and AIDS," 2004.

154 Responsibility was shifted to the U.S. government (taxpayers), which since 1986 has paid over $3.9 billion for vaccine injuries.

155 Informed Consent Action Network, "ICAN vs. HHS: Key Legal Win Recasts Vaccine Debate," September 14, 2018.

and lifestyle. The Western diet of feedlot animals at one end (yang) and white refined sugar and drugs at the other (yin), with potatoes, iceberg lettuce, and refined flour in the middle was based on a specious system of "seven basic food groups," not a natural law 5,000 years old. In my family of origin, the American (industrial) diet had produced heart disease, diabetes, cancer, and mental illness. I studied, changed my diet, learned to cook real (organically grown) food, and became confident of my immune balance. Instead of a declining family lineage, I would build a new natural body for carrying my future children.

And so it was.

Thomas Cowan, MD, author of *The Contagion Myth,* talks about the Darwinian germ warfare mentality that says biological life is one long assault that only doctors, technology, and Big Pharma drugs can save us from. It is true that we are immersed in a world of microorganisms, most of which we cannot see. But generally they act as allies—including viruses and bacteria—keeping our bodies strong and balanced, at least until the environment was weaponized. *The immune system is not about resistance,* and "getting sick" is about detoxing to reachieve balance, not about "assault." The question is not *How strong is my immune system?* but *What in my lifestyle tends to poison / imbalance me?* A healthy "immune system" is all about rapid adaptation, thanks to viruses and exosomes (pieces of genetic material packaged for excretion).

For more than 100 years now, the primary method of *weakening* the human immune system has been vaccinating from infancy—in fact, *over*-vaccinating as *pathogenic priming*, an intentional method of enhancing disease.[156]

Much research has gone into discovering how to *block* the immune system so it does not attack "foreign agents" inserted by the present genetic / eugenic Transhumanist assaults. The mouse with a human ear growing out of its back (the HM or humanized mice program) is one of many "successes" of using aborted human fetal tissue. Block the mouse immune system, then endow the HM with a human immune system via bits of liver and thymus from a human fetus ("embryo complementation"). In 2010, thanks to a $6 million grant from the California Institute of Regenerative Medicine, Stanford University recruited stem cell biologist Hiromitsu Nakauchi to create chimeric embryos via embryo complementation and micro-needling human cells into them.[157]

> The HM are created by surgical implantation of human tissue into mice that have multiple genetic mutations that *block the development of the mouse immune system* at a very early stage. The absence of the mouse

156 Thanks to James Lyons-Weiler, PhD, Institute for Pure and Applied Knowledge (IPAK).

157 Antonio Regalado, "Human-Animal Chimeras Are Gestating on U.S. Research Farms," January 6, 2016.

immune system allows the human tissues to grow and develop into functional human tissues. As part of this process, DARS (Division of Applied Regulatory Science OCP/OTS/CDER) needs to repeatedly acquire the proper type of tissues. In order for the humanization to proceed correctly, we need to obtain fetal tissue with a specific set of specialized characteristics [age range 16-24 weeks, fresh not frozen tissue].[158] (Emphasis added.)

Thus, the abortion industry. *Island of Dr. Moreau,*[159] anyone?

During the 2020 COVID-19 lockdown, Swedes went about without masks or six-foot social distancing while the rest of the world was subjected to the terror of daily death figures, horrifying images, and fearful news reports on television and iPhones. Swedish schools were not closed and Swedish youths enjoyed their class graduations. Sweden's "herd immunity" was celebrated in *Foreign Affairs*, the American flagship publication mirroring the UK's renowned *Economist*. Six months later, the World Health Organization (WHO) redefined herd immunity at its website under "Coronavirus disease (COVID-19): Serology, antibodies and immunity." The old meaning—"in which a population can be protected from a certain virus if a threshold of vaccination is reached"—was erased, replaced by something more in step with Big Pharma: "Herd immunity" exists when a high percentage of the population is vaccinated.[160]

The strange pharmakon *of vaccines*

The alchemy of even typical vaccines (HPV, flu, swine flu, Hep B, MMR, DPT, tetanus, etc.) sounds distinctly like a witch's brew of suspended fluids, animal parts, preservatives and stabilizers, adjuvants (enhancers), and aborted fetuses:

Aluminum, mercury, cadmium, lead, barium, EDTA
Monosodium glutamate (MSG), polysorbate 20, polysorbate 80, phenoxyethanol
Formaldehyde, antifreeze, acetone, latex rubber
Glycerin, neomycin, streptomycin, Beta-propiolactone

158 "Judicial Watch Obtains Records Showing FDA Paid For 'Fresh and Never Frozen' Human Fetal Parts For Use in 'Humanized Mice' Creation." Judicial Watch, June 23, 2020.

159 H.G. Wells wrote The Island of Dr. Moreau in 1896. Wells, an insider, wrote several science fiction books with themes that are now science. He also wrote The Outline of History (1920) about the New World Order now making its move.

160 "By changing the definition of 'herd immunity,' the WHO is literally re-writing hundreds of years of scientific understanding as to what the term truly means in an apparent effort to silence any argument that herd immunity would have been a better approach to fighting COVID-19 than lockdowns and social distancing." Paul Joseph Watson, "WHO Changes Definition of 'Herd Immunity' to Eliminate Pre-COVID Consensus," NewsWars, December 23, 2020.

Thimerosal, squalene, spermicide, sorbitol
Sulfates, genetically modified yeast, glutaraldehyde, proteins, antibiotics
Monkey kidney, dog kidney, chick embryo, chicken egg, duck egg, calf serum, pig blood, horse blood, rabbit brain, guinea pig, cow heart, animal viruses, porcine pancreatic hydrolysate casein, GM soy
Insect cells, silkworm DNA
Aborted fetal tissue, fatal DNA, E.coli

Some vaccines even contain Medium 199 with two versions of *scopolamine* or Devil's Breath (*burundanga*): Hyoscine and Atroscine. Scopolamine is used by the CIA to produce a permanent slave mindset.[161]

Robert O. Young, ND, PhD, cites a study of 44 vaccines viewed under an environmental scanning electron microscope equipped with an X-ray microprobe in Italy and France: "The results of this new investigation show the presence of micro- and nano-sized particulate matter composed of inorganic elements in vaccine samples not declared among the components *and whose unduly presence is, for the time being, inexplicable*"[162] ((emphasis added).

Please understand that Big Phat Pharma LOVES the argument to be about thimerosal and mercury. What they don't want us to know is that fungal contamination in vaccines has the power to un-attenuate live, attenuated viruses and cause the diseases that vaccines are supposed to prevent.

–Beaux Reliosis, June 12, 2015, https://badlymeattitude.com/vax/

The Merck MMR II vaccine contains fetal DNA (5ng/ml) to activate Toll-like receptor 9 (TLR9) and trigger the autoimmune response that initiates labor to expel a baby.[163] Viral-based vaccines like MMRs and flu shots made from living cells have been found to contain cancer cells.

Nanoparticles (NPs, "micro- and nanocontamination") are not named among vaccine ingredients, but they are there. Thanks to the environmental scanning electron microscope equipped with X-ray microprobes, nanopathologists

161 More in Appendix 7.
162 Robert O. Young, DSc, PhD, Naturopathic Practitioner, "New Quality-Control Investigations on Micro and Nano Contamination," February 5, 2021.
163 Thanks to Theresa Deisher, PhD, Sound Choice Pharmaceutical Institute.

Antonietta M. Gatti and Stefano Montanari have exposed *undeclared* (not listed in the ingredients) nano-sized inorganic contaminants [metals], *non-biodegradable and non-biocompatible.*[164] "Side effects" from the nanometals injure the nervous system and pave the way to autism and Alzheimer's. The Gatti-Montanari paper is worth studying in its entirety, or you can read Jon Rappoport's June 3, 2020 highlights in "Dangerous nanoparticles contaminating many vaccines: groundbreaking study." Rappoport ends his article with a reasonable and exceedingly important question: *How many cases of childhood brain damage and autism can be laid at the door of nanoparticle contamination?*[165]

Gatti and Montanari were, of course, immediately targeted for their unflinching study results. Just before Dr. Gatti was to testify before a parliamentary inquiry in 2018, the Italian police raided their home and confiscated their laptops, computers, and flash-drives. As Arjun Walla put it in a *Collective Evolution* article:

> . . . they came under the microscope of the United States, European, and Italian authorities. They had touched the third rail of medicine. They had crossed the no-go zone with the purported crime being scientific research and discovery.[166]

The nanometals found in vaccines are in sync with the nanometals we are inhaling from jet and rocket deliveries, now in our soil and water: aluminum, barium, silicon, magnesium, titanium, iron, chromium, calcium, copper, lead, stainless steel, tungsten, gold, silver, zirconium, hafnium, strontium, nickel, antimony, zinc, platinum, bismuth, cerium. *Conductive nano-metals are not medicine.* The Nazi experiments supported by I.G. Farben on Jews, gypsies, POWs, twins, and the disabled now seem tame when compared with Big Pharma's transformation of entire populations into concentration camps for secret, alchemical *in vivo* experiments dependent upon conductive nanometals for remote 5G "precision medicine."

Vaccination by aerosol

Aerosol chemical warfare began with the airplane in World War One, during which airplanes exterminated young men trapped in easy-to-follow trenches.

---

164 Antonietta M. Gatti and Stefano Montanari, "New Quality – Control Investigations on Vaccines: Micro- and Nanocontamination." International Journal Vaccines & Vaccination, January 23, 2017.

165 Recommended reading: Wayne McRoy, The Autism Epidemic: Transhumanism's Dirty Little Secret (2019) at Amazon.

166 Arjun Walla, "World Renowned Scientists Have Their Lab Shut Down After Troublesome Vaccine Discovery." Collective Evolution, April 17, 2018.

Big Pharma great granddaddy I.G. Farben's methylated phosphoric poisons attached to fluorine atoms (organophosphates like Roundup herbicide) were thus "vectored" into the lungs and nervous systems of an entire generation and killed them. Now, the entire globe has been breathing a slower death for three decades more in keeping with ongoing Transhumanist experiments. The dissemination of immediate death in World War One became more clandestine in World War Two with the Dresden terror bombing (preceded by Berlin and Hamburg) hinting at the shift from the traditional battlefield to citizen warfare, citizens being little more than ongoing assets in the elite competition known as the Great Game. The aerial delivery of the atomic bomb and ionized radiation furthered the redefining of the boundaries of warfare, then the Chemical and Biological Warfare Act of 1949, then Vietnam and Agent Orange, until the penultimate hypocrisy of the 2007 amendments to the 1949 act stating that *mass aerial immunizations* may be legally carried out as antiterrorist and antiriot measures.

And now the COVID-19 / COVID-20 bioterrorism.

Back in 1999, I cut out an article from the local newspaper about simian (monkey) virus SV40 being carried by mosquitos as the West Nile Virus (WNV). From 1955 to 1963, SV40 was said to have contaminated the Salk polio vaccine batches given to millions; then it was found in childhood "rare cancer" brain and bone tumors, able to change "normal cells into tumor cells in the laboratory."[167] Symptoms were typical of a struggling human immune system: fever, headache, body aches, skin rash, and swollen lymph glands.

In 2006—just before the amendments that would permit *mass aerial immunizations*—the Yale School of Public Health recommended *spraying DNA vaccine enhancements and recombinant vaccines,* purportedly to reduce WNV cases. DNA vaccine enhancements "specifically use Epstein-Barr[168] viral capsids [protein shells enclosing genetic material] with multi-human complement class II activators to neutralize antibodies," and recombinant vaccines against WNV "use Rabbit Beta-globulin or the poly (A) signal of the SV40 virus":

> In early studies of DNA vaccines, it was found that the *negative result studies would go into the category of future developmental research projects in gene therapy.* During the studies of poly (A) signaling of the SV40 for WNV vaccines, it was observed that WNV will lie dormant in individuals who were exposed to chicken pox, thus upon exposure to WNV aerial

167 Gannett News Service, "Polio virus fear discounted." The Olympian, February 19, 1999, page A3.

168 The Epstein-Barr virus (EBV) is a herpes virus. Remember in the 1980s when "infectious" mononucleosis was added to the pantheon of gain-of-function "viruses"?

> vaccines the potential for the release of chicken pox virus would cause a greater risk to having adult-onset Shingles.[169] (Emphasis added.)

In February 2009, spraying for the WNV ensued in major cities in California. Test results from one Anaheim resident came up positive for KD-45, the protein band for SV40 Simian Green Monkey virus.

> Additional tests were performed for Epstein-Barr virus capsid and Cytomeglia virus which are used in bioengineering for gene delivery systems through viral protein envelope and adenoviral protein envelope technology. The individual was positive for both, indicating *a highly probable exposure to a DNA vaccination delivery system through nasal inhalation.*[170] (Emphasis added.)

Concoct it *in vitro* in labs, then release it to be breathed in or otherwise ingested by target populations (*in* vivo), after which it lies "latent" in the body until remote activation via "signal" frequency, as occurred with Epstein-Barr and is now occurring during the COVID-19 lockdown.

> The EBV genome in latently infected lymphoid cells offers an opportunity to follow effects on the transcriptional and translational product clearly distinguishable from those of the host cell genome. Exposure of Akata cells, a human lymphoid cell line latently infected by the EBV genome, to a 50 Hz EMF resulted in an increased number of cells expressing the virus early antigens. This finding provides additional evidence that *DNA can be modulated by a magnetic field.*[171] (Emphasis added.)

Add nasal sprays, disinfectant spray "fogging" of passenger jets and schools, sprayed masks.

Nebraska virologist Shi-Hua Xiang has bioengineered *Lactobacillus* to deliver SARS-CoV-2 antigens to trigger an immune response in the mucosals tissues of the nose and mouth with a nasal spray, the immunity provided by antibodies and immune cells being more robust at the point of origin of breathing than if delivered by injection. Mucosal tissues are unique and powerful components of the body's "immune machinery" (immunoglobulin A, memory T cells, etc.).[172]

As for aerosol inhalation through masks, the present COVID-19 blue surgi-

---

169 Dave Mihalovic, ND, "Australia Determined To Forcibly Vaccinate By Intentional and Controlled Release of Aerosolized GMO Vaccine," November 15, 2013.

170 Ibid.

171 S. Grimaldi et al., "Exposure to a 50 Hz electromagnetic field induces activation of the Epstein-Barr virus genome in latently infected human lymphoid cells." Journal of Environmental Pathology, Toxicology and Oncology, 1997.

172 Tiffany Lee, "Nasal spray could mean needle-free COVID-19 vaccine." MedicalXpress, November 4, 2020.

cal-style masks are sprayed with polytetrafluoroethylene, the synthetic fluoride in Dupont's Teflon.[173] Such an agent works over time and may even be engineered to work with both oxygen and carbon dioxide. Methylcellulose coats the white N95 mask in cilia-like nanowires connecting wirelessly via nanosensors to the Internet of Things (IoT),[174] the nanosensors picking up exact chemical signatures in order to trigger exact reactions ("precision medicine").

Virusend is the "novel" disinfectant spray developed by the British Army to eliminate 99.99% of SARS-CoV-2 "in under a minute."[175] Now that it has been made available to the public, is this what is being used to "nanofog" passenger jets? Mayte Abad and her travel partner were badly nanofog-poisoned on two humanitarian flights from Central America to Canada through George Bush Intercontinental / Houston Airport (IAH). Their symptoms included vision and hearing loss, nausea, loss of equilibrium, inability to process information, inability to speak, read or write, seizures, and extreme sensitivity to electromagnetic environments. Mayte: "[Since the flight,] the nanobots in my brain make sure I can sense with inhuman accuracy [nanosensors?] every single deviation in microwave frequency and feel every 5G tower, meter, street light, and receiver long before I see it."[176]

Passenger jet cabins are being sprayed between *every single flight,* in some cases all night long for eight hours straight. Travelers board the plane immediately after application. Chemicals include Benzalkonium chloride, benzyl chloride, chloro-acetophenone, ammonia (NH3), radioactive aluminum and mercury, and the nanochemical Bacoban and Viraclean (brand names). The electrostatic spray process entails spraying a sheet of positively charged "nano-glass" aerosol loaded with nanochemicals, then blasting the cabin with mercury lights (UV). The nanochemicals self-replicate for up to ten days, positively charged atoms spewing into the air to be attracted to neutral or negatively charged atoms, such as in the bodies and lungs of human beings.

The CDC owns several patents for administering "live-attenuated" vaccines via aerosol delivery systems.[177]

---

173 See the 2019 film Dark Waters.

174 Rutgers University, "Plant-based spray could be used in N95 masks and energy devices." Phys.org, October 7, 2020.

175 Ministry of Defense, "Army develops spray to kill coronavirus," Gov.UK, 16 December 2020.

176 Thanks to Mayte Abad (Facebook, September 14, 2020) for alerting me to this practice.

177 Y. Roth et al., "Feasibility of aerosol vaccination in humans." PubMed, March 2003.

Aluminum

Aluminum Adjuvants in Vaccines

Aluminum hydroxide
Aluminum phosphate
Aluminum salts
Amorphous aluminum hydroxyphosphate sulfate (AAHS)
Potassium aluminum sulfate

As I wrote in *Under An Ionized Sky*, aluminum is naturally present in the Earth's crust, but its industrial uses and addition to food, water, medicines, vaccines, and cosmetics—not taking into account its multiplying, synergistic effects as it couples with aerosols via aluminum oxide—is disruptive to "biological self-ordering, energy transduction, and signaling systems, thus increasing biosemiotics entropy."[178] The biophysics of *water* play a crucial role in bio-degeneration (lungs being 83% water, brain and heart 73%, muscles and kidneys 79%, bones 31%). One study used the toxicity of the water flea to determine how aluminum oxide nanoparticles impact fresh water environments (like the human body?).[179]

Actually, aluminum nanoparticles are what the three primary chemical / biological / nanotechnology delivery systems share: chemical trails and vaccinations deliver chemical synergies based in trillions of nanoparticles, and GMO seed is "aluminum-tolerant" while Monsanto's Roundup herbicide (glyphosate) is synergistic with aluminum and central to transporting it deep into the brain. As Monsanto's 2009 aluminum-resistant gene patent #7582809 states, its aluminum-tolerant gene is "designed to allow genetically modified organisms to thrive in *aluminum-poisoned soils* [and bodies?] . . . to make it impossible for traditional and organic farmers to grow natural world and heirloom native seeds."[180]

Aluminum nanoparticles are not only conductive and reactive (why they're used as catalysts) but are a contaminant for biological / neurological systems. Jet chemical deliveries guarantee a wide dissemination in air, reservoirs and waterways, natural forests, and six inches of topsoil. Aluminum fluoride compounds everywhere merge and multiply toxicity in the human body to break it down for medical industry and Big Pharma profits while also breaking down the immune and endocrine systems so that bioengineers and

---

178 Christopher A. Shaw et al., "Aluminum-Induced Entropy in Biological Systems: Implications for Neurological Disease." Journal of Toxicology, Vol. 2014.

179 Sunandan Pakrashi et al., "Ceriodaphnia dubia as a Potential Bio-Indicator for Assessing Acute Aluminum Oxide Nanoparticle Toxicity in Fresh Water Environment." PLOS ONE, September 5, 2013.

180 Kevin Mugur Galalae, Water, Salt, Milk Killing Our Unborn Children, 2012, https://projectavalon.net/Water_Salt_Milk_-_Killing_our_unborn_children.pdf.

genetic engineers can *in vivo* CRISPR a Transhumanist Human 2.0.

As an uptake inhibitor, aluminum nanoparticles fall to the Earth (*tons* of nanoparticles, including nanosensors, released in the stratosphere daily) and prevent trees from being able to take in nutrients through their roots. Dry, dying trees are starving from the inside out. The California fires (2017-2019) exposed not just dying trees incinerating from the inside out, but swarms of nanoparticles from aerosols and soil being used as fire accelerants.

The aluminum content of brain tissue in Alzheimer's disease (AD),[181] autism spectrum disorder (ASD), and multiple sclerosis (MS) is now significantly elevated.[182] High contents of aluminum have been found in the occipital, parietal, temporal, and frontal lobes of the brains of MS sufferers.

As for autism, its explosion in children appears to be intentional.[183] In his 2019 book *The Autism Epidemic: Transhumanism's Dirty Little Secret,* Wayne McRoy builds a convincing case for "autism without intellectual impairment" being purposefully crafted for brain-computer interface (BCI) with artificial intelligence—fostering savant skills and "filtering out" emotions, empathy, and other "undesirable personality traits" for entire generations of cyborg Human 2.0. Meanwhile, the coverup continues even as doctors, scientists, and anti-vaccine activists churn out excellent studies of aluminum toxicity coming from vaccine adjuvants without grasping the role of *trillions* of nanoparticles being breathed daily.

> The extreme levels of aluminum found in the brains of the [Christopher Exley and Elizabeth Clarkson] study's teenage donors have alarming implications for the entire generation of highly aluminum-vaccinated children. In the ASD paper, Dr. Exley and coauthor point out that the "burgeoning" use of aluminum-adjuvant-containing childhood vaccines "has been directly correlated with increasing prevalence of ASD.[184]

---

181 Alzheimer's is now being diagnosed in people in their 20s, 30s, and 40s.

182 Christopher Exley and Elizabeth Clarkson, "Aluminum in human brain tissue from donors without neurodegenerative disease: A comparison with Alzheimer's disease, multiple sclerosis, and autism." Journal of Trace Elements in Medicine and Biology, 8 May 2020.

183 From the film Vaxxed (2016), we learn that 1 in 45 American children is autistic; by 2032, 80 percent of boys may be autistic. A 2004 paper proved a causal relationship between the MMR vaccine and autism. One of the authors of that paper, William Thompson, MD, revealed that the CDC under director Julie Gerberding deliberately omitted crucial data from the study. Gerberding left the CDC in 2009 and became president of Merck Vaccines, which manufactures the MMR vaccine.

184 Robert F. Kennedy, Jr., "Scientists Discover Huge Amounts of Aluminum in the Brains of Deceased Autistic People." Collective Evolution, January 16, 2018. The Exley-Clarkson paper: "Aluminum in human brain tissue from donors without neurodegenerative disease: A comparison with Alzheimer's disease, multiple sclerosis and autism," Scientific Reports, 8 May 2020.

The implications that autism is being intentionally developed under a Transhumanist mandate of BCI is *soul-wrenching*. The June 19, 2015 murder of Dr. Jeff Bradstreet just after his study of the blood of 100 autistic children who had been vaccinated drives this home. Dr. Bradstreet had given a talk at the 2015 Autism One conference discussing a cure for autism via the highly controversial vitamin D-binding protein GcMAF (Globulin compound-derived protein Macrophage Activating Factor). After the talk, his office was raided by the DEA (Drug Enforcement Administration) in search of GcMAF.[185] Before the paper could be published, he was found floating in a North Carolina river 100 miles from his home, shot in the chest.

In France, retired French university professor Jean-Bernard Fourtillan[186] was committed to solitary confinement in the psychiatric hospital Le Mas Careiron in Uzès for his criticisms of vaccine adjuvants like aluminum and "the apparition of the SARS-COV-2 virus":

> In particular, Fourtillan has accused the French Institut Pasteur, a private non-profit foundation that specializes in biology, micro-organisms, contagious disease, and vaccination, of having "fabricated" the SARS-COV-2 virus over several decades and been a party to its "escape" from the Wuhan P4 lab—unbeknownst to the lab's Chinese authorities—which was built following an agreement between France and China signed in 2004 . . . Fourtillan himself has said he hopes legal proceedings will allow him to produce evidence he has built up; he is in fact anxious to debate the issues at stake. Now that he is in a psychiatric hospital, the possibility of this happening—in the interest of discovering the truth—is becoming more remote.[187]

Similar to the plight of physicians speaking out against the Covid-19 bioterrorism and subsequently losing their license to practice medicine, Fourtillan is also being sued for the testing success of his hormone patch of Valentonin (sleep hormone) and 6-Methoxyharmalan (waking hormones) to

185 Former CEO of Guernsey-based Immuno Biotech David Noakes was arrested in the UK on May 20, 2020 for marketing the "unauthorized" cancer medicine GcMAF. Biochemist Lyn Thyer was also arrested. The slander campaign against both in the UK has been relentless, given that cancer is big business. See Chapters 2 and 14 for more on GcMAF; view "Holistic Doctors Being Killed? GcMAF and Nagalase (Vaccines and Autism," Proper Gander, January 24, 2016.

186 Jean-Bernard Fourtillan, PhD, Chemical engineer, Pharmacist Professor of Therapeutic Chemistry and Pharmacokinetics at the University of Poitiers; Expert Pharmacologist Toxicologist specializing in Pharmacokinetics. He has personally filed 400 medical patents. His website http://verite-covid19.com/

187 Excellent article. Jeanne Smits, "Accomplished pharma prof thrown in psych hospital after questioning official COVID narrative." LifeSiteNews, December 11, 2020. The article points out the systematic use of psychiatric hospitals for silencing and discrediting political dissidents.

help heal sleep disorders and neurodegenerative conditions caused by pollution, adjuvants, and electromagnetics.

Over 100 holistic doctors have been murdered since 2015,[188] particularly the doctors collaborating on findings regarding autism, such as the discovery that the nagalase enzyme protein was being added to vaccines seemingly (1) to disable the immune system and (2) prevent vitamin D from being produced in the body, Vitamin D being a main line of defense against cancer. Nagalase is found in cancer cells and in high concentrations in autistic children.[189] Dr. Bradstreet's discovery of three DNA markers in autistic children, not two, pointed to *a third strand of DNA originating from the aborted fetus cell line in the vaccine*. He connected this third strand to the gender confusion among children and youths. Was tucking aborted fetal tissue into vaccines, then, yet another Nazi experiment?

A more accurate term for autism is *vaccine damage.*

Spraying sub-micron aluminum increases *morbidity*, the slow death that enriches Big Pharma and the medical industry while providing endless open field brain experimentation opportunities—for example, how aluminum binds with fluoride to form aluminum fluoride compounds that increase fluoride toxicity.

Mercury (Hg)

> *I had all the mercury taken out of my mouth back in the early 90s. The metal creates an antenna around the head that really affects you. The mercury removal dentist showed me with his meters just how much voltage was buzzing around my head. You are a totally different person and think so much better after the mercury removal and heavy metal chelation removal after that. Everyone laughed at me for having it done.*
>
> – Greg Abbott, July 4, 2019

Mercury is not just in vaccines as thimerosal and in dental fillings as amalgam. It is in our atmosphere.

In a 2016 paper, J. Marvin Herndon, PhD, spells out the extensive use of ultra-fine particles ($PM_{2.5}$) of toxic coal fly ash as "the aerosolized particulate emplaced in the troposphere for geoengineering, weather modification, and/

---

188 See "Growing List of Assassinations Of COVID-19 Researchers," HumansAreFree.com, December 21, 2020.

189 Jack Murphy, "Doctors Who Discovered Cancer Enzymes in Vaccines all Found Murdered." Neon Nettle, February 10, 2016.

or climate alteration purposes."[190] The mercury in coal fly ash is fired in the jet fuel combustion chamber, after which toxic fibrous mesh from methylmercury (CH2Hg) and ozone-damaging chlorinated-fluorinated hydrocarbons are released into the atmosphere.

Coal fly ash also contains masses of aluminum nanoparticles "in a chemically mobile form upon exposure to water or body moisture" that contribute to neurological diseases (Alzheimer's, autism, Parkinson's, ADHD, etc.), reduced male fertility, and biota debilitation. The relationship between mercury and Alzheimer's has been known for decades, as has the fact that mercury slowly destroys the blood-brain barrier. Mercury dental amalgams and mercury in vaccines alone inhibit the efficiency of tubulin, the protein that separates the nerve and receptor cell from surrounding tissue. Mercury degenerates the tubulin and leads to autism and ADHD, which basically means driving the soul out of the body.

> The toxins in coal fly ash make that substance especially injurious to human health. The small particle size of aerosolized coal fly ash ($PM_{2.5}$) enables particulate intake through inhalation, ingestion, and induction through eyes or skin. When inhaled, $PM_{2.5}$ particles can penetrate and become trapped in terminal airways and alveoli, and retained for long periods of time . . .[191]

Coal fly ash is more radioactive than nuclear waste (M. Hvistendahl, *Scientific American*, 2007)—"uranium, thorium, and their radioactive daughter products"—and yet it is a "chaff" matrix for delivery of chemical trails that weaponize weather primarily by controlling the rainfall mechanism. Hygroscopic[192] coal fly ash heats the atmosphere by absorbing solar energy (so much for blaming carbons), melts glaciers, and inhibits rainfall by trapping small water droplets and keeping them from coalescing and growing large enough to form raindrops. The $PM_{2.5}$ particulate pollution also *retards* heat loss in order to produce an artificial increase in local atmospheric pressure, thus blocking weather fronts and limiting rainfall.

Mercury in the ion propulsion engines of sounding rockets delivering thousands of 5G satellites into space is life- and brain-threatening, given that

---

190 Review Under An Ionized Sky, pages 60-63, for more on Herndon's work. All of Herndon's papers are listed at nuclearplanet.com/Geoengineering-Scientific-Articles.html.

191 J. Marvin Herndon, "Human and Environmental dangers Posed by Ongoing Global Tropospheric Aerosolized Particulates for Weather Modification." Frontiers in Public Health, 30 June 2016.

192 Hygroscopy is the phenomenon of attracting and holding water molecules via either absorption or adsorption from the surrounding environment (lexico.com). See USAF Patent US3659785A, "Weather modification utilizing microencapsulated material," 1972.

mercury is a strong neurotoxin. Follow the launch arcs of NASA's Wallops Flight Facility in Virginia and Edwards Air Force Base in Southern California and you will see that many launches pass over high-density populations.

With signal-enhancing barium-strontium-titanate (BST), mercury, piezoelectric nanocrystals, and constant wireless ELF transmissions, modern conditions like electro-sensitivity (ES), auto-immune symptoms, and multiple chemical sensitivities are guaranteed.

Vaccinations as stealth gene therapy are taken up in Chapter 14, "The COVID-19 'Vaccine' Event."

3

Nanotechnology at the Quantum Threshold

Smart dust and neural dust
Bacteria
Virus
Exosomes
Beyond Morgellons: "Nano self-assemblage"
Harald Kautz-Vella
Tony Pantalleresco & Jean Bryan Clarence Pelletier
Artificial intelligence (AI) / machine learning

Workers in giant, white clean outfits resembling space suits, or maybe quarantine garb, control large metal machines under yellow light that makes the room act essentially like a big dark room. Huge machines are creating teeny tiny computer chips and sensors, some barely visible to the naked eye, used in electronics, medical devices and vehicles.

– Rachel Lerman, "The Washington Nanofabrication Lab at the University of Washington, used by researchers and businesses alike, plans to nearly double in size and increase its 'clean room' space" (*Seattle Times,* August 2, 2015)

Release of nanoparticles should be restricted due to the potential effects on environment and human health.

– Nanotechnology and Regulation within the framework of the Precautionary Principle, Final Report for ITRE (Industry, Research and Energy) Committee of the European Parliament, February 2004

Aside from nanotech's potential as a weapon of mass destruction, it could also make possible totally novel forms of violence and oppression. Nanotechnology could theoretically be used to make mind-control systems, invisible and mobile eavesdropping devices, or unimaginably horrific tools of torture.

– Adam Keiper, "The Nanotechnology Revolution," *T he New Atlantis* (Summer 2003)

LIKE VACCINES LOADED WITH NANOPARTICLES and programmed nanobots, no human health safety tests were run on nanotechnology before it was approved by Congress in 2002, much less on what it would mean that nanoparticles would be employed to provide a self-engineering nexus between electromagnetics and all that is truly organic and alive.

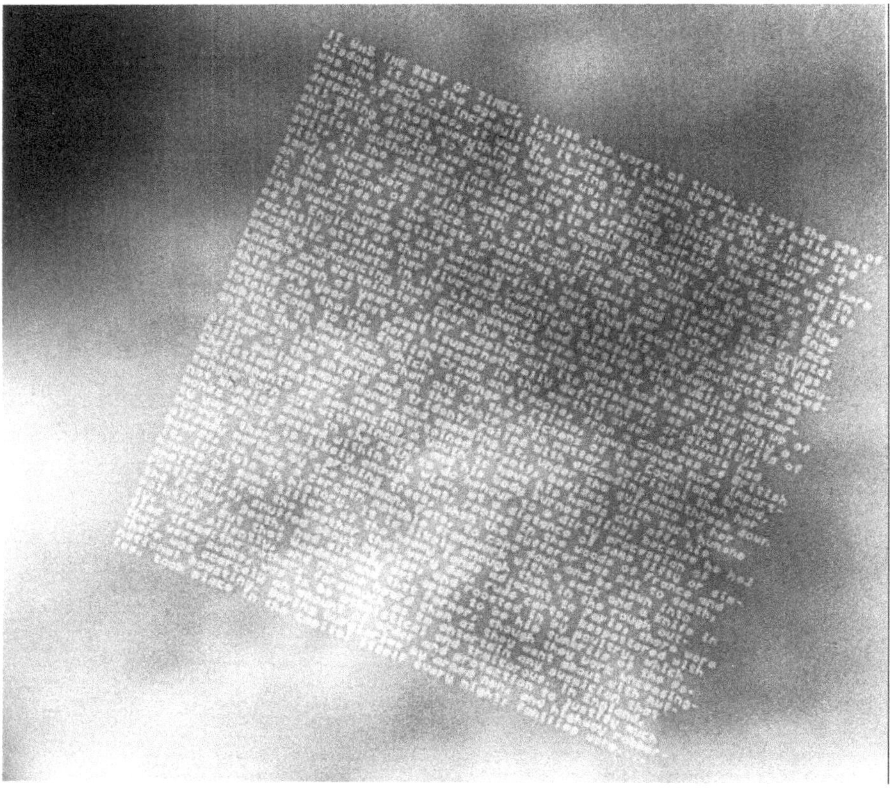

Nanotechnology is small. First paragraph of *A Tale of Two Cities* written by electron beam at 1/25,000 scale reduction, 1985, Stanford University. From *Nano* by Ed Regis (Little, Brown & Co., 1995).

The usual story (like Elon Musk's "neural mesh") is that anything medically nanotech requires either minor surgery or injection. Aerosol or genetically modified food mass delivery systems are rarely alluded to—for example, the polymeric ultrathin film or nanosheet "promising platform for drug delivery through needle-injection" does deftly allude to "non-contact [remote] motion control using an external magnetic field."[1] Developed with

1 Singapore University of Technology and Design, "Researchers develop syringe-injectable, self-expendable and ultraconformable magnetic nanosheets." Phys.org, October 30, 2019.

shape-memory polymer (SMP) and magnetic nanoparticles (MNPs), aerially delivered polymeric film sounds a lot like the "shape-shifting material that can heal itself on its own" that the Army Combat Capabilities Development Command's (CCDC) Army Research Laboratory wants as "future platforms for air and ground combat that possesses the 'reconfiguration characteristics of the T-1000 character in the Hollywood film, *Terminator 2*,' [aerospace engineer Frank Gardea] said in an Army statement."

Millions of "neurograins" collecting and communicating data to remote hubs are now in all human brains. As common / natural law scholar Anna Von Reitz sees it from her bird's-eye view up in Anchorage, Alaska, the Transhumanist assault from the sky depends upon hundreds of HAARP-like ionospheric heater phased array antennas and U.S. Navy CIPPA units communicating with self-assembling crystalline nanobots[2] seeded into billions of highly acidic digestive tracts by chemical aerosols and GMO foods worldwide. Once the crystals assemble and multiply, tiny fibrous appendages appear in every crystal corner for sensing, motility, attachment, and antenna arrays capable of interacting with DNA and RNA and deployment by weaponized (gain of function) virus, thanks to 5G / 6G systems.[3]

Natural nanoparticles are tiny and ubiquitous. Chances are that every time you read an article about powering tiny robots and electronics, it is about nanoparticles (usually bacteria) being transformed by gain of function into nanobots in human bodies and brains, trillions of tiny machines extracting energy from metal surfaces like aluminum, zinc, iron, lithium, etc., with the aid of hydrogel electrolytes. (More on hydrogel in Chapter 14.) Electronic component coatings are key to interfacing hardware with human tissue, like conjugated polymers and built-in neurotransmitters.

> [DARPA, Defense Advanced Research Projects Agency] is interested in systems that can read and write to 16 independent locations in a chunk of brain the size of a pea with a lag [latency] of no more than 50 milliseconds . . . "When you try to capture brain activity through the skull, it's hard to know where the signals are coming from and when and where the signals are generated," [Jacob Robinson, assistant professor of bioengineering at Rice University] told *Live Science*. "So the big challenge is, can we push the absolute limits of our resolution, both in space and time?"[4]

Also see Elias Marat, "US Army researchers creating robot tech directly inspired by T-1000 villain from Terminator 2," The Mind Unleashed, August 20, 2020.

2 Some crystalline structures: fiberglass, asbestos, titanium dioxide, silicon dioxide, etc.

3 Anna Von Reitz, "Emergency Public Service Announcement." PaulStramer.net, April 7, 2020.

4 Edd Gent, "The Government Is Serious About Creating Mind-Controlled Weapons." Li-

"Absolute limits" are now about *tininess*, the *micro, nano, pico*, and *femto* of particles whose extraordinary power is disguised as insignificant but actually hands over the keys to the kingdom of remote control over bodies and brains to those who control technology proximate to the subatomic quantum threshold.

Like "dual use," *gain of function* is an exceedingly important term when discussing *synbio* in that it basically demarcates what is natural from what has been genetically altered to enhance certain aspects that make it unnatural and therefore patentable and weaponizable for dual use. Genetic fragments like bacteria and virus are favored for weaponizing.

The carbon nanotube (CNT) nano-radio (1/10,000th of a human hair, 10 nm wide times hundreds of nanometers long) was created at UC Berkeley Center of Integrated Nanomechanical Systems (COINS) in 2007, announcing the new NEMS "absolute limits" that lead to transceivers and brain-computer interfaces (BCIs) able to "integrate well with microelectronic circuits":

> The nanoradio detects radio signals in a radically new way—it vibrates thousands to millions of times per second in tune with the radio wave. This makes it a true nanoelectromechanical device, dubbed NEMS, that integrates the mechanical and electrical properties of nanoscale materials . . . [P]hysicists can tune in a desired frequency or station by "pulling" on the free tip of the nanotube with a positively charged electrode . . . [which] turns the nanotube into an amplifier . . . The amplified output of this simple nanotube device is enough to drive a very sensitive earphone. Finally, the field-emission and vibration together also demodulate the signal.[5]

Miniature microelectronic computer circuitry has gone nano *and* bio, thanks to the work of chemists like Harvard's Charles Lieber, PhD, of Wuhan infamy.[6]

While Lieber was laboring in Chinese labs, military and commercial jets under Project Cloverleaf were dropping nano-payloads in the stratosphere and working as nanoparticle factories. Natural and engineered nanoparticles are alchemically churned into *dusty plasma* first by vaporizing materials via plasma heat, pressure, and volume,[7] after which the vapor is transported to the fringe of

---

veScience.com, May 23, 2019.

5 Robert Sanders, "Single nanotube makes world's smallest radio." UC Berkeley Press Release, 31 October 2007.

6 Charles M. Lieber et al., "Nanowire nanocomputer as a finite-state machine." PNAS.org, December 12, 2013.

7 Review German scientist Harald Kautz-Vella's paper "The Chemistry in Contrails: Assessing the Impact of Aerosols From Jet Fuel Impurities, Additives and Classified Military Operations on Nature" (https://www.academia.edu/30216111/The_Chemistry_in_Contrails_Assessing_the_Impact_of_Aerosols_from_Jet_Fuel_Impurities_Additives_and_Classified_Military_Operations_on_Nature) and Chapter 1 of Under An Ionized Sky.

the plasma being discharged from the jets into plasma-generated clouds where the temperature decreases and causes the vapor to become supersaturated with trillions of nanoparticles via nucleation, condensation, and coagulation.

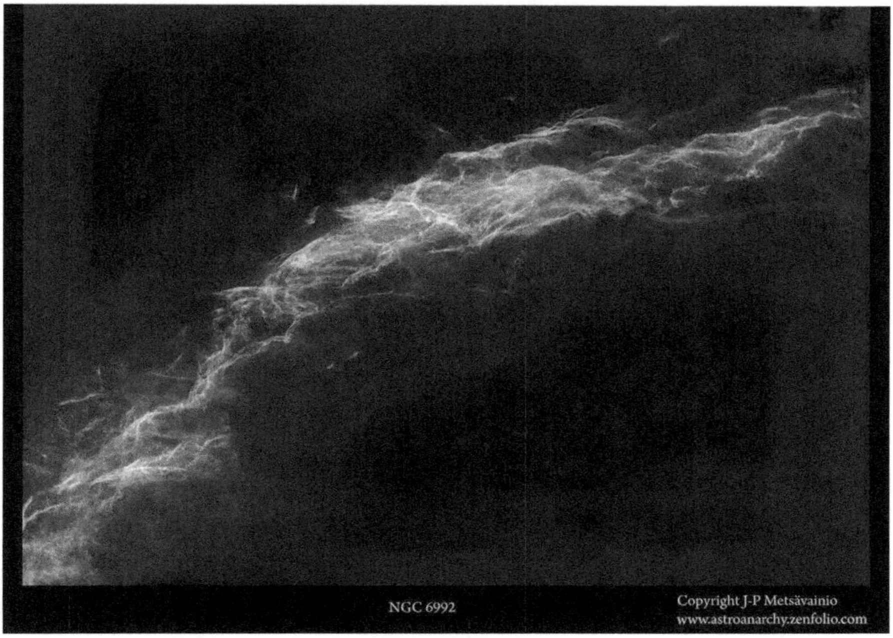

"Eastern Veil in Ionized Oxygen Light, 0-III" by Finnish astrophotographer J.P. Metsavainion, *AstroAnarchy*, January 2015.

Nanoparticles programmed to be nanosensors are crucial to planetary full spectrum dominance. In 2010, Hewlett-Packard's Central Nervous System for Earth (CeNSE) assumed responsibility for running and collecting data from nano-enabled sensors everywhere, including those inside bodies and brains.

The fact is that the brain's nanoscale 100 million neurons and 100 trillion connections seem almost to have been made to merge with nanowired nanobot computers permanently connected to the Cloud. By 2030, the omnipresence of carbon nanotubes, nanodiamonds, quantum dots, nanotech electrode arrays, nanoelectronics, nanobots, neural dust, smart dust, and the ultimate Internet of Nano Things (IoNT) and Internet of Bodies (IoB) may translate to a reverse-engineered brain of a nonbiological intelligence merged with the old human biological brain, as arch-Transhumanist Ray Kurzweil tells it—a Human 2.0 nanoelectronic finite-state machine (nanoFSM) composed of *organoids* (synthetic organs) now referenced as *synths*.

Polymer nanowires far thinner than capillaries are conducting electrical impulses to and inside your brain, and changing shape in response to the nuances of electric fields. Composed of carbon nanotubes (CNTs) made from single layers of carbon atoms and coated with a double wall of oil molecules, the tiny microprocessors encapsulate ion pumps pumping charged atoms of calcium, potassium, etc. in and out of the cell. The hydrotrope adenosine triphosphate (ATP) originally powered the tiny ion pumps, but now the wireless network inside and outside our bodies powers them.[8]

Nanotechnology is the future come already, entailing manipulation and assembly at the molecular level, measured in nanometers of 1/80,000th the diameter of a human hair. What indicates that nanoscale approaches the subatomic quantum level of reality begins with how materials reduced to nanoscale develop unique properties—for example, copper becomes transparent, aluminum explosive, titanium and nickel more toxic, solids liquid. *The laws of chemistry and physics work differently at the nano level.*

The difference between classical and nonclassical physics is basically that the *electronic length scales* don't play a role in classical but play a huge role in nonclassical, small scales being relevant to quantum effects. (See the breakthrough paper "A General theoretical and Experimental Framework for Nanoscale Electromagnetism," Yi Yang *et al., Nature,* 576, 2019.)[9] The smaller the scale, the less classical physics—for example, nonlocality becomes more frequent (optical fields affect an entire neighboring volume) as do "spill outs" (when electrons are not completely contained in solids).

World demand for nanoscale materials, tools, devices, and nanomaterials scientists exceeds one *trillion* dollars per year. The National Nanotechnology Initiative (NNI) under the 21st Century Nanotechnology Research and Development Act sought $1.4 billion in 2020 to be parceled out to 11 government agencies. Since its establishment in 2001, the NNI has spent $29 billion of taxpayer monies to "advance our fundamental understanding of and ability to control matter at the nanoscale."

What does it mean for our genetics that major food companies like Kraft, Heinz, Nestle, Hershey, Campbell, and Unilever are selling synthetic agrichemical nanofoods so that nanoparticles (NPs) can enter the bloodstream and brain, overstimulate brain cells, form blood clots, punch holes in cell membranes and can be used to create prions[10]? Are we supposed to believe

8 Thanks to Mike Castle, PhD, "Chemtrails, Bio-Active Crystalline Cationic Polymers," July 14, 2003.

9 Paola Rebusco, "Cheers! Maxwell's electromagnetism extended to small scales." Institute for Soldier Nanotechnologies, December 11, 2019.

10 "Nanoparticles can interact with proteins … and disturb cellular signaling. The misfolding of specific protein is related to the appearance of amyloid-type structures which are

food corporations simply don't know about NP toxicity, or that NPs less than 100 nm pass through the blood-brain barrier?

> A number of studies have reported harmful effects from nanoparticles, e.g. they "can trigger cytotoxic, geotoxic, inflammatory and oxidative stress responses in mammalian cells" . . . One important issue that appears to need further investigation is the way proteins can stick to nanoparticles once they've entered the bloodstream, despite the addition of PEG [synthetic polyethylene glycol].[11]

Proteins like the Spike protein?

Gene therapy, with its dependency upon nanotechnology, is dual-use technology, as are its tools of "precision medicine," like CRISPR/Cas9. For example, gold NPs with a slight positive charge work collectively to unravel DNA's double helix.[12] The 3-D origami technique (*DNA origami*) comes under the same dual-use mandate with its artificial folding of DNA into complex structures (like paper origami)—taking what is natural and making it, Lego-style, "construct nanostructures that mimic and extend naturally occurring complexes."[13] To the *synbio* engineer, the human body with all of its molecular machinery is Lego-like: tiny motors make muscles contract or "grab onto a double-stranded [DNA] helix and climb from one base to the next, like walking up a spiral staircase," etc. With the ORBIT technique (origami-rotor-based imaging and tracking), researchers can follow natural DNA molecular machines[14] in their daily rounds, ORBIT being "a hybrid nanomachine that uses both designed components [synthetic] and natural biological motors."[15]

Clusters of heated magnetic nanoparticles delivered aerially and by vaccine can be used to remote control ion channels, neurons, and behavior by

---

found in neurogenerative diseases ... cellular internalization of nanoparticles effects cell metabolism and produces ... DNA damage, genotoxicity, and cell death." Nanotechnology in Eco-efficient Construction, Materials, Processes & Applications, Woodhead Publishing, 2018, p. 713.

11 Julie Beal, "Ronavax Roulette: Issues with Lipid Nanoparticles."Activist Post, March 3, 2021.

12 See the YouTube "Charged Gold Nanoparticles 'unzip' DNA," North Carolina State University, June 20, 2012. Note how the DNA struggles against the gold NP assault.

13 Aarbus University, "Researchers create synthetic nanopores made from DNA." Phys.org, December 13, 2019. Is this what is going on with prions?

14 Basically, the double helix supposedly discovered by Crick and Watson in 1953 is a man-made model designated for the conglomerate of chromosomes, according to David E. Martin, PhD, "Dr. David Martin Exposes the False Foundation of Eugenics: 'You Don't Have DNA,'" Free & Brave Conference, May 2021.

15 Harvard University, "A New Spin On DNA: DNA origami joins forces with molecular motors to build nanoscale machines." ScienceDaily, July 17, 2019.

exposing them to a magnetic field similar to the MRI and adjusting the heat factors—for example, 34°C (93.2°F) that provokes an avoidance response.[16] The ability to remote control ion channels brings up Aleksandr Samuilovic Presman's excellent 1970 book *Electromagnetic Fields and Life* in which he points out biological effects beyond thermal effects, particularly those produced by field strengths very close to those of the natural environment:

> . . . such electromagnetic fields normally serve as conveyors of information from the environment to the organism, within the organism, and among organisms . . . in the course of evolution, organisms have come to employ these fields in conjunction with the well-known sensory, nervous, and endocrine systems in effecting coordination and integration.

In conjunction with the broad, seemingly purposeful, environmental array of assaults on the endocrine system, is remote control over ion channels being used to further cut off our communication with our natural world and each other?

Smart dust and neural dust

Once something is described as "smart," we know it is synthetic and has undergone gain of function patent manipulation.

In 2002, Michael Sailor *et al.* at UC San Diego developed *smart dust*, the tiny wireless MEMS (microelectromechanical sensors) that detect everything emitting a *frequency* (which is basically everything and everyone). Smart dust is made up of porous modified silicon particles fragmented ultrasonically. Smart dust is itself an IoT device wirelessly monitoring light, frequencies, temperature, humidity, magnetism, and chemical signatures, "acting as nerve-endings in an ad hoc distributed network that provides full spectrum intelligence."[17]

The new and improved version for Human 2.0 bodies and brains is a *magnetic* smart dust made up of magnetic, amphiphilic (polar and nonpolar) particles encasing droplets of organic and aqueous (water-based) solvents, which in the presence of an external magnetic field, *move*. The magnetic smart dust contains a semiconductor laser diode and MEMS beam-steering mirror for active optical transmission; a MEMS corner cube retro reflector for passive optical transmission; an optical receiver, signal processing and control circuitry; and a power source based on thick-film batteries and solar cells.[18] It

---

16 Ellen Goldbaum, "With Magnetic Nanoparticles, Scientists Remotely Control Neurons and Animal Behavior." University of Buffalo News Center, July 6, 2010. Nanobots incinerate at high temperature, turning into a talcum-like powder.

17 Jay Stanley, "The Last Mile to Civilization 2.0: Technologies From Our Not Too Distant Future." TechSpot, December 13, 2017.

18 Dan Rowinski, "Connected Air: Smart Dust Is The Future of the Quantified World." Hack,

falls from the sky like glitter, tracks movement, money, biometrics, temperature, chemical composition / signatures, etc. Magnetic dust-coated droplets are best distributed by aerosol electrospray in magnetic fields because a larger number of nanoparticles (and droplets) is assured for manipulation.[19]

Electrospray magnetic dust could include the *M*-spray, a cocktail of polyvinyl alcohol (PVA), gluten, and iron particles (0.1 to 0.25 thick) that, once heated,

> . . . magically transforms miniscule inanimate objects into lively 'bots that are capable of adapting to a wide variety of explorative purposes . . . by putting on this [gluelike] magnetic coat, we can turn any objects into a robot and control their locomotion," explained [Dr. Shen Yajing from City University of Hong Kong]. "The M-spray we developed can stick on the targeted object and activate it when driven by a magnetic field."[20]

Were we looking at this technology in Jamie Lee's "wildfire" video in which quorum sensory[21] swarms of activated nanobots sped down highways and around the perimeters of homes slated to be incinerated?[22]

> Therefore, when affected by a magnetic field, objects can be changed into industrious millibots with an assortment of locomotion modes such as bouncing, crawling, flipping, walking, and rolling on surfaces like glass, skin, paper, wood, and sand. Reprogramming the millibot's movement mode is something that can be enacted on demand.[23]

Neural dust can be thought of as quorum sensory nanobot swarms made with electronics—Fitbits for the nervous system created from *CMOS (complementary metal-oxide semiconductor)* circuits / sensors. *Neural dust* replaces wire electrodes with brain-machine interface (BMI = BCI) and is remotely directed by ultrasound to monitor nerves, muscles, and organs in real time. Once in the cortex, it is interrogated and energized.

---

14 November 2013.

19 Rajendrani Mukbopadbyay, "Magnetic dust mobilizes droplets." American Chemical Society, February 1, 2005.

20 Jeff Spry, "Scientists create millibots by coating tiny objects with magnetic spray." SyFy-Wire, November 21, 2020.

21 Quorum sensing: detection and response to cell population density by gene regulation.

22 Jamie Lee, "Paradise Lost #25 - How the Houses Were Torched: Interview with 30 yr Microwave Engineer," December 9, 2018.

23 Ibid.

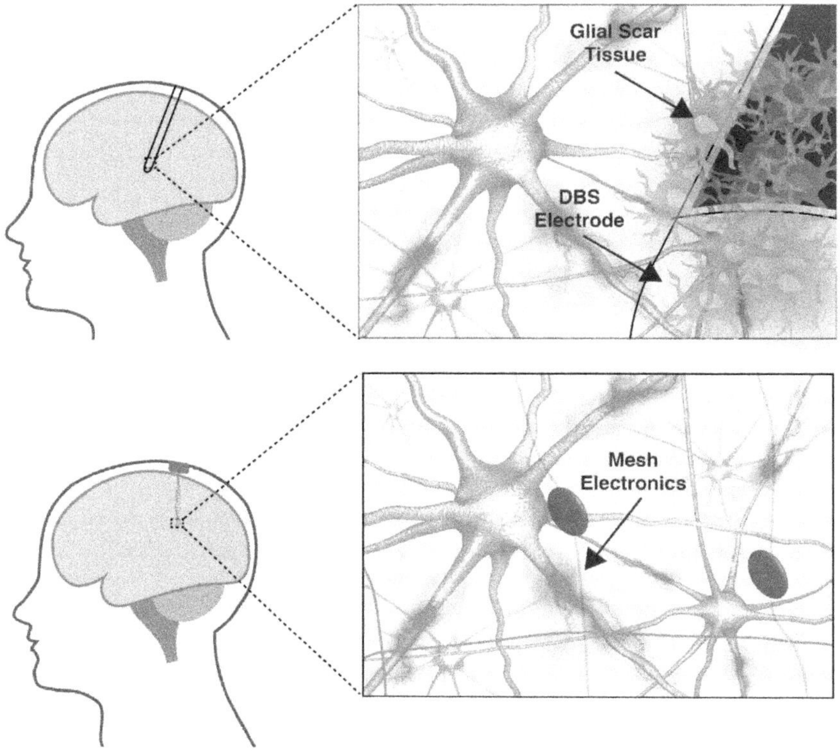

Brain-computer interface (BCI) "mesh electronics." Mesh electronics with the brain cells to produce neural interfaces. Precision electronic medicine. Charles M Lieber, PhD, of Harvard University worked on this with Shaun R. Patel of Harvard Medical School.

DBS = deep brain stimulation

https://bioengineeringcommunity.nature.com/posts/52979-precision-electronic-medicine-in-the-brain

Both neural dust and smart dust have been kicked into high gear by "beam-steering technology" (phased array antennas) entailing *mesh electronics nanotechnology*[24] picking up ultrasound waves for data transfer and control over brains.

The sensors . . . contain a piezoelectric crystal that converts ultrasound vi-

24 Military programs like the U.S. Air Force Cyborgcell focus on nanoelectronics. As early as 2005, the story was platinum nanowires that would "spread into a 'bouquet' branching out into tinier and tinier blood vessels . . ." (National Science Foundation, "Wiring the Brain at the Nanoscale," Phys.org, July 8, 2005). Was this what was "announced" at the U.S. Embassy in Cuba in 2016? See Janet Phelan, "US Senate Finally Admits that Neuroweapons Exist, Passes Bill to Help Diplomat-Victims," Activist Post, June 22, 2021.

brations from outside the body into electricity to power a tiny, on-board transistor that is in contact with a nerve or muscle fiber. A voltage spike in the fiber alters the circuit and the vibration of the crystal, which changes the echo detected by the ultrasound receiver, typically the same device that generates the vibrations. The slight change, called backscatter, allows them to determine the voltage.[25]

As a wireless, battery-less system that monitors the brain from the inside, the neural dust system is tetherless and remote-controlled. In fact, the network of tiny implantable sensors function like an MRI inside the brain, recording data on nearby neurons and transmitting it back out. Particles are coated with polymer and contain an extremely small CMOS sensor capable of measuring electrical activity in nearby neurons. Neural dust can therefore be interrogated by components powered by ultrasound outside the body, which is much more efficient than radio waves for targeting the tiny subatomic world embedded deep in the body or brain: ultrasound transmits 10 million times more power than EM waves at the same scale.[26] (Electromagnetic waves generate a damaging amount of heat because of the amount of energy the body absorbs and the signal-to-noise ratios at the subatomic scale.)

the nanofibers and nanoparticles act as *blenders* once hit by EM in the insoluble crystalline nanoparticles of titanium dioxide, silicon dioxide, sodium nitrate, and iron oxide. The nanos vibrate / spin / rotate in the body and end up shredding the epithelial lining of blood vessels and digestive tract as well as cutting holes in cell walls.[27] Robin D.P. Watson (quoted in Chapter 2, "The Three Primary Transhumanist Delivery Systems," about titanium dioxide) is a retired photographer and independent researcher who spent years working with government doctors and scientists:

> When HG Wells wrote *The War of the Worlds*, he imagined creatures from outer space attacking humanity using advanced technology. Humanity is finally saved by our most basic of life forms, the bacteria which co-inhabit this planet. But what if, instead of humanity, the tiniest of life forms DNA, mitochondria and all the numerous cells which inhabit this planet came under attack. This alarming scenario is actually in fact exactly what is happening with the use of

---

25 Cate Lawrence, "Is smart dust the IoT vector of the future?" ReadWrite, 20 August 2016.

26 Thanks to Nicholas West, "Neural 'Smart' Dust Connects Brain and Computer (Wireless Mind Control)." Activist Post, August 4, 2019.

27 Robin D.P. Watson, "Nano Blenders Thesis, Parts 1 & 2," Academia, 17 November 2015. For how vibration / spinning / rotation work, see V.C. de Andrade and J.G. Pereira, "Torsion and the Electromagnetic Field." Cornell University, 21 August 1997. The spin of nanoparticles (particularly the paramagnetic) can create electrical charges discharged as micro-lightning or micro-arcing that damages DNA, mitochondria, etc.

Nano-technology. There is profound loss of biodiversity on this planet, and most of us had been too busy to notice that this is absolutely deliberate.[28]

Since 2012, Watson has maintained that "almost continuous thrombogenesis occurs with sustained exposure to insoluble nanoparticles," not to mention the body's attempt to repair its blood vessels by forming plaque. (Isn't thrombogenesis what we keep hearing about regarding COVID-19 "vaccines"?)

Magneto-aerotactic bacteria nanobots, algal-based nanobots, DNA-based nanobots—creating nanobots is all the rage because stimulating neurons with nanoparticles via light or sound or magnetic fields is all the rage. Optogenetics uses pulsed light to switch brain cells on and off and gold nanoparticles to absorb and convert the light into heat. Spherical iron oxide particles give off heat when exposed to an alternating magnetic field. Magnetoelectric nanoparticles (MENs) are used to control intrinsic fields deep in the brain:

> ...20 billion nanoparticles [were inserted] into the brains of mice. They then switched on a magnetic field, aiming it at the clump of nanoparticles to induce an electric field. An electroencephalogram [EEG] showed that the region surrounded by nanoparticles lit up . . . "When MENs are exposed to even an extremely low frequency magnetic field, they generate their own local electric field at the same frequency," says [Sakhrat Khizroev of Florida International University in Miami]. "In turn, the electric field can directly couple to the electric circuitry of the neural network" . . . [R]unning it in reverse . . . our brain states would then become input parameters for computers . . .[29]

Nanoparticles fill the bill for "wet computing" infrastructure right out of DARPA's Neural Engineering System Design (NESD), including gain-of-function virus technologies based on genetic code design. As Edwin Donath, professor at the Institute of Medical Physics and Biophysics at the University of Leipzig in Germany, says:

> "Genetic engineering has a clear analogy to software production in that pieces of code can be multiplied at low cost, put together in an artificial genome, and processed afterwards in the cellular machinery . . . Recent developments in microfluidics ["wet computing" hydrogel?] will certainly contribute to the parallel production of surface-engineered viruses at low cost and with a great diversity of functions."[30]

---

28 Rob Watson, "Illuminati Plan to Fry Humanity?" henrymakow.com, August 25, 2016.

29 Hal Hudson, "20 billion nanoparticles talk to the brain using electricity." Health, 8 June 2015. Also see Rakesh Guduru et al., "Magnetoelectric 'spin' on stimulating the brain." Nanomedicine, 8 May 2015.

30 Michael Berger, "Viruses as nanotechnology building blocks for materials and devices."

I repeat: natural nanoparticles include bacteria and viruses. To bypass toxic chemicals in the synthesis protocols needed for nanoparticle (NP) synthesis and development, microbes / microorganisms are preferable. Many microbes produce inorganic substances like silica from diatoms, or turn iron oxides into nanoscale magnetic particles. Fungi synthesize metal NPs and build nanomaterials, fungus filaments acting as living templates or "biological slaves"; with gold NPs attached to their surface, they develop different sizes and materials of additional NP layers.[31]

And let's not forget yeast. The advances in synthetic biology and genome engineering make it easy to create virus genomes in bacteria or yeast. In the case of coronavirus with its large genome, yeast is preferable because it is pliable and fast, with glue-like power to sequence genomes in *chunks*. Even yeast has been made dual use in an era of scientists behaving like terrorists, using it to develop a virulent super-virus that is vaccine-resistant.[32]

Bacteria and viruses can be encapsulated in electrospun polymer nanofibers[33] (electrospun referring to making electrostatic fields). The electrospinning process for encapsulating and immobilizing living biological *and bioengineered* material points to the polymer fibers dropping from the sky loaded with the Morgellons payloads, namely the *cross-domain bacteria (CDB)* studied by Clifford Carnicom for two decades.

Bacteria

Bacteria recycle nutrients in the atmosphere and on Earth, and have been found *six miles* above the surface of the planet in a bubble surrounding the Earth,[34] all part of the layer of DNA-based life that makes the atmosphere breathable and constantly creates an ozone layer to protect our genetics from too much UV and (mutagenic) cosmic rays. Anaerobic bacteria even live a half mile *below* the ocean floor!

As I pointed out in *Chemtrails, HAARP* regarding the April 20, 2010 *Deepwater Horizon* oil rig catastrophe in the Gulf of Mexico—a planetary operation that qualifies for a geoengineered terrorist terraforming operation—the 3 million liters of Corexit EC9500A and Corexit EC9527A were most likely a MEOR (microbial enhanced oil recovery) synthetic biology "ex-

---

Nanowerk Spotlight, n.d.

31 Rajni Singh, "Fungi as Builders For Nanomaterials." Biotech Articles, August 1, 2012.

32 Shelly Fan, "Scientists are Cloning the Coronavirus Like Crazy. Here's Why—and the Risks." Singularity Hub, May 19, 2020.

33 W. Salalha et al., "Encapsulation of bacteria and viruses in electrospun nanofibers." Nanotechnology, September 28, 2006.

34 Stephanie Warren, "Bacteria Live At 33,000 Feet." PopSci.com, June 19, 2013.

periment" cooked up by British Petroleum (BP) and Synthetic Genomics. The synthetic bacterium Synthia (*Mycoplasma laboratorium*) was added to the Gulf to gobble up the oil spill, but instead it self-replicated so much that it spread the Blue Flu across the Gulf—blood in the urine, heart palpitations, kidney and liver damage, migraines, multiple chemical sensitivity, neurological damage resulting in memory loss, rapid weight loss, respiratory system and nervous system damage, seizures, skin irritation, burning and lesions, and temporary paralysis—all symptoms of an immune system under assault. Lung damage, depression, and anxiety plagued the 50,000 people involved in the spill cleanup[35] as all along the Gulf the genetically modified strain *Vibrio vulnificus* entered wounds and cuts, lodging between muscle and skin where it released a toxin that destroyed tissue and, in many instances, led to amputated limbs.[36] The Gulf environmental disaster continues to this day.

So when we hear of a bacterial "chimera" enzyme that can break down plastic bottles for recycling (polyethylene terephthalate or PET) in hours,[37] or how the Carbios corporation has partnered with Pepsi and Nestle Waters, or a strain of bacterium that can metabolize the chemical components of polyurethane (PU), it may not be what the media lead us to believe.

Employing bacteria to alter DNA (*gene therapy*) began in September 1971 with *transcession* at the University of Geneva. When the auricles of frog hearts were soaked in a suspension of bacteria, the result was a high percentage of RNA-DNA hybridization between the bacterial DNA and the frog DNA. *Vaccines have transcession capability:* inject naked DNA into muscle—*not* the bloodstream where an enzyme defense would be launched—and cells begin producing the proteins the DNA demands.

Transcession (transduction = conjugation = horizontal gene transfer): the process whereby bacterial DNA becomes part of the host cell's DNA.

We've been conditioned to think of microbes like bacteria as dirty little aggressive "germs" (*Salmonella, E.coli, Staphylococcus,* etc.), so it may be surprising to view them instead as little *synbio* factories producing plastics, pro-

35 Farron Cousins, "Six Years After Deepwater Horizon: Time For Serious Action." Desmogblog.com, April 20, 2016.

36 Valery Kulikov, "New 'Chimera' to Target the World." New Eastern Outlook, May 6, 2020.

37 Monit Khanna, "Scientists Create Enzyme That Can Destroy Plastic Within Days, Not Years." India Times, September 30, 2020.

cessed foods, and fertilizers for GMO fields, capturing nitrogen, powered by the Sun. Bacteria also serve as electromagnetic transceivers (1 kHz) that form nanonetworks for storing data.[38] Raytheon and the Pentagon's DARPA have even created genetically modified bacteria to be explosives sensors.[39]

What a boon it has been to bioengineers to the fact that cells are basically computer systems of binary states (zeroes and ones) for engineering biological circuits. Not only can cells perform simple logic, but they can also be programmed to die after a certain number of divisions, like a kill-switch.[40] Synthetic molecular engineers center on horizontal gene transfers into single-celled organisms like the bacterium *Escherichia coli* or *E.coli* for building biological circuits and switches (James Collin, Wyss Institute, 2000), and use freeze-dried cellular transcription machinery for sensing and manufacturing proteins with combined amino acids so hospital gowns signal infection!

Billions of bacteria live in our gut, along with other microbiome organisms symbiotically helping us to digest food, extract nutrients, and produce multiple neurochemicals (e.g. 95 percent of the body's serotonin):

> The bacteria that compose our microbiome work so synergistically with our human cells that the difference between "us" and "the bacteria" is difficult to decipher. Where do "we" begin and "they" end? If all the bacteria in a person's microbiome were killed off, that person would die. Bacteria are an intimate and important part of "us." In genetically modifying "them," are we genetically modifying "us"?[41]

DARPA's microprocessor (tiny computer) based on bacteria instead of silicon or gallium arcenide is powered by body energy and can be programmed to kill its host when the host gets ill or old or simply becomes a problem, after which the bacterial microprocessor will dissolve. If the microprocessor qualifies as a bio- or microchip, it will migrate to or be inserted where body temperature changes most rapidly, like in the forehead right below the hairline, behind the ear, or the back of the hand (uncannily prophesied in Revelations 13:16-17).

Biochips (bacterial or otherwise) used to mean a laborious process of silicon coating with a layer of diethylenetriamine (DETA) to map the brain's

---

38 Brandon Keim, "Bacteria on the Radio: DNA Could Act As Antenna," Wired, April 25, 2011; Emerging Technology from arXiv, "Storing data in DNA is a lot easier than getting it back out," Technology Review, January 26, 2018.

39 Tyler Durden, "DARPA Seeks 'Militarized Microbes' So They Can Spread Genetically Modified Bacteria." Zero Hedge, November 15, 2019.

40 Jonathan Shaw, "Engineering Life: Synthetic biology and the frontiers of technology." Harvard Magazine, Jan.-Feb. 2020.

41 Lisa Bloomquist, "Genetically Modifying Humans Via Antibiotics?" Something You Need To Know." FourWinds10.net, October 24, 2013.

neuron circuitry and shield the desired DETA channels with a UV laser removing the unwanted DETA outside the channels as embryonic brain cells[42] were sprinkled on the chip to make the neurons send dendrites and axons along DETA paths, etc.[43] Now, bacterial nanobots are pre-manufactured with microprocessors and use brain cell energy.

Natural *antibiotics* are products of soil-dwelling bacteria. While we think of antibiotics as the last bastion of health, the truth is that they alter our DNA by altering bacteria and mitochondria. Consider that GMO Terminator seed (discussed in Chapter 2) is soaked in the antibiotic tetracycline. How does this impact our gut bacteria?

Fluoroquinolone[44] antibiotics (Ciprofloxacin, Levofloxacin, Moxifloxacin, Ofloxacin, etc.) are topoisomerase interrupters that unravel bacterial DNA[45] and program cells for death. Side effects of the core *nalidixic acid* in the antibiotics include psychosis and destruction of tendons ("tendonitis"). Fluoroquinolone molecules adhere to human DNA *and alter it.* Unfortunately, the recent synthetic antibiotic PPMOs (peptide-conjugated phosphorodiamidate morpholino oligomers) specifically target bacterial genes—once more, the wrong conditioning that bacteria or virus are to blame for symptoms like urinary tract, sinus, and bronchial infections, strep throat, etc.[46]

In 2015, 270 million antibiotics prescriptions were written in the U.S. How many of these people, many of them children, now have genetically altered DNA?

One more question: *Was MRSA (methicillin-resistant staphylococcus aureus) gain-of-function created to be antibiotic-resistant?*

Bacterial resistance to antibiotics (as in *Salmonella, E.coli, Staphylococcus*) can be countered by quantum dots (20,000x smaller than the diameter of a human hair) excited by light,[47] but what about 5G contributing to the growth

---

42 Fetal cells create an interface between silicon and carbon to make electronic components merge and work together.

43 For insight into how abortion serves neuroengineering, see Cathy Lynn Grossman, "The hidden ethics battle in the Planned Parenthood fetal tissue scandal," Washington Post, July 23, 2015.

44 Note the presence of fluorine.

45 Footnoted earlier: "Charged Gold Nanoparticles 'Unzip' DNA," North Carolina State University, June 20, 2012. "Research from North Carolina State University shows that gold nanoparticles with a slight positive charge work collectively to unravel DNA's double helix. This finding has ramifications for gene therapy research and the emerging field of DNA-based electronics." (Note how the agonized DNA resists tooth and nail.) Pete Ramon: "Here, gold NPs, with ligands (molecules that bind with other molecules), are acting like a virus."

46 Lisa Bloomquist, "Genetically Modifying Humans Via Antibiotics? Something You Need To Know." FourWinds10.net, October 24, 2013.

47 Joel Moskowitz, PhD, UC Berkeley School of Public Health, "5G Wireless Technology: Millimeter Wave Health Effects," n.d.

of multi-drug resistant bacteria[48]? Can anything good come from 5G and nanotechnology like C60 and quantum dots?

Bacteria: transduction / conjugation
Viruses: direct infection of the cell

Viruses

> *From the viewpoint of a materials scientist, viruses can be regarded as organic nanoparticles (20-300 nm).*
>
> – Michael Berger, *Nanowerk Spotlight*

> *From a mitochondrial biohacking, quantum biophysics perspective: Viruses are how we make new genes. Nature has always told us that viruses are good. We're designed to assimilate them. Human DNA is made out of 98% retroviruses.*
>
> – Je Zmit, Facebook, November 1, 2020

It is likely that a host of adenovirus viral vectors are being delivered via chemical trails for *mass gene therapy.*[49]

In 2003, the CIA published "The Darker Bioweapons Future," too little too late admitting that "The effects of some of these engineered biological agents could be worse than any disease known to man," referencing in part the 2002 creation of a polio virus from scratch:

> . . . [The scientists] found the polio virus genome on the internet and within 2 years had created a virus from raw chemicals. The synthetic virus could reproduce and, when injected into mice, paralyzed them just as a natural polio virus would do. They said they chose the polio virus to demonstrate what a bioterrorist could accomplish.

---

48 Peter Dockrill, "New Light-Activated Nanoparticles Kill Over 90% of Antibiotic-Resistant Bacteria." Science Alert, 19 January 2016.

49 Corporations like AEA Technology research and sell aerosols from inhalers to atmospheric gene therapy ("Chemtrails: Suppressing Human Evolution," Montalk, September 29, 2000). "By taking advantage of the fact that nanomaterials of a very small size have unique properties of color, conductivity, elasticity, strength, toxicity, and explosivity, scientists are looking at nanotechnology as a way to create optimal aerosols and structures that maximize benefits and reduce risks in geoengineering applications" ("Health risks likely to emerge include human ingestion, inhalation, and dermal contact," https://conservancy.umn.edu/bitstream/handle/11299/92715/Nanotechnology?sequence=1).

> "It is a little sobering to see that folks in the chemistry laboratory can basically create a virus from scratch," James LeDuc of the federal Centers for Disease Control and Prevention in Atlanta said at the time.
>
> A year later in 2003, Craig Venter and colleagues at the Institute for Biological Energy Alternatives in Rockville, Maryland, took only 3 weeks to create a virus from scratch.[50]

Viruses are used for "gene therapy": strip the genes out of a virus, substitute copies of genes (mail-ordered?) for transfer into cells, inject the virus into the host body. *Retroviruses* are RNA viruses that insert their genetic code directly into the chromosomes of host cells; viral vectors like *adenovirus* and *herpesvirus* also work. Viruses are perfect cover for stealth gene therapy in that the immune system can't discern an armed virus from a benign virus, the drawback being that unwanted genetic information comes with them.

As Thomas S. Cowan, MD, points out, viruses are pieces of genetic material with a very specific frequency (June 9, 2020). Viruses are also proteins that a cell excretes in order to reorder its imbalance, or solvents breaking down toxic matter. Viruses are used as vectors, metallization scaffolding, and hybrid composite materials. By using *virions*[51] as durable building blocks for composite materials, all sorts of hybrids can be created. Natural and synthetic viruses (20-300 nm) cannot reproduce, but their properties (primarily the toxins it is their job to package for ejection from the cell) can be readily engineered (genetically modified) into "viral chimeras that carry proteins of different viral origins."[52]

Thus, the germ or virus (5.5 Hz), being a symptom of cellular breakdown due to an imbalance of the delicate alkaline pH balance of the body, stands virtually alone against the lie that viruses transmute all on their own ("emerging strain"), which ignores the fact that many viruses are manmade nanoparticle constructions gain-of-function weaponized as per military grants and patents, and a concerted attempt is made to confuse the difference between natural and synthetic viruses / bacteria.

The following Wikipedia entry "Kingdoms" shows how apples and oranges are being mixed up, i.e. natural and synthetic viruses, as slowly, slowly, *natural* is being replaced by *synthetic* . . .

> There is ongoing debate as to whether viruses can be included in the tree of life. The ten arguments against include the fact that they are obligate intracel-

---

50 Peter Montague, "A Darker Bioweapons Future." CounterPunch, December 31 / January 1, 2005/6.

51 Natural viral particles are called virions.

52 Michael Berger, "Viruses as nanotechnology building blocks for materials and devices," Nanowerk Spotlight, n.d.

lular *parasites* that lack *metabolism* and are not capable of *replication* outside of a host cell. Another argument is that their placement in the tree would be problematic since it is suspected that viruses have arisen multiple times, and they have a penchant for harvesting nucleotide sequences from their hosts.[53]

Our work shows that it is possible to design (virus-like) NPs that interact with target cells in a manner similar to the influenza A virus.[54]

– Sara Maslanka Figueroa *et al.*, "Influenza A virus mimetic nanoparticles trigger selective cell uptake." *PNAS,* April 29, 2019

There are basically three approaches to weaponizing a virus:

1. Obtain it from infected biological tissue;
2. Grow it inside incubated cells;
3. Make it from scratch inside bacteria or yeast hosts, yeast being the fastest and magically able to take chunks of viral genome and put it together in the right sequence

That all molecular biology is now being digitized means that viral DNA can be sent to a colleague or from a mail order lab as easily as an email, and that *designer viruses* can be easily (and anonymously) produced. One can now print genes with a biological-to-digital converter like BioXP and pop in the parts (or digital signatures sent like email attachments) preordered from Craig Venter's Synthetic Genomics. As Synthetic Genomics' vice president of DNA technology Dan Gibson put it, "DNA is really just the start of making anything downstream from RNA to protein to whole bacterial genomes."[55]

When a virus is made to colonize a bacterium (like the SARS-Cov-2 bacteriophage virus), it starts by replicating its own RNA, after which standard vaccines and antibiotics no longer work.[56] This is one way of weaponizing.

Geneticists regularly use viruses as vectors for introducing genes into cells. In fact, they are the common delivery system of all gene therapy after

---

53 https://en.wikipedia.org/wiki/Kingdom_(biology). Meanwhile, the tree itself is being redefined: University of Glasgow, "Scientists Take First Step Towards Creating 'Inorganic Life,'" 12 September 2011.

54 Thanks to Pete Ramon.

55 Diana Crow, "6 Amazing Things to Watch in Synthetic Biology." Neo.Life, October 12, 2017.

56 Monica Camozzi, "Italian Researchers: Vaccines Will Not Work Because SARS-Cov-2 Is Also Entering Bacteria." Anti-Empire, March 15, 2021.

CRISPR/Cas9 does its cut. They enter the cells, deposit their DNA payload, and take over the cell machinery to produce programmed proteins.

Natural viruses are not the *cause* of diseased, imbalanced conditions, but the *effect*. Not so with engineered synthetic viruses. The only way a natural virus can be transmitted is not by contagion but by injection; synthetic viruses, on the other hand, can be triggered by means of 5G (60 GHz) millimeter / tetrahertz waves.

The 19th century French biochemist Antoine Béchamp (1816-1908) opposed the germ theory of Louis Pasteur (1822-1895):

> We do not catch diseases. We build them. We have to eat, drink, think, and feel them into existence. Germs or microbes flourish as scavengers at the site of disease. They do not cause the disease any more than flies or maggots cause garbage.

Robert O. Young, ND, would agree with Dr. Béchamp: "There is only one physiological disease—the over-acidification of the body, primarily due to an inverted way of eating and living."

German virologist Stefan Lanka won a landmark case in 2017, proving to the German Supreme Court that measles is not caused by a virus, nor is there a "measles virus."[57] So if there is no virus, why do childhood illnesses appear so commonly—that is, before the prescribed MMR (measles, mumps, Rubella) vaccine? According to Rudolf Steiner, childhood illnesses are the soul's attempt to throw off the failings of previous lives so as to "make the corresponding correction as soon as possible."[58] Such an interpretation sounds so antiquated in this era of endless materialistic bias that says never the 'twain shall meet between biology and soul or spirit. What lies behind the suppression of childhood illnesses? Simply the germ / virus warfare misconception, or a secret society attempt to suppress evolving individuality?

Under DARPA's N3 (Next-generation Nonsurgical Neurotechnology), viral vectors have now been enlisted for mind control, as well, by inserting DNA into specific neurons to make them produce two kinds of protein: one to absorb light when a neuron is firing, which can then be remotely detected and measured by an infrared beam passing unseen through the skull and brain; the other protein tethered (by ligand) to magnetite already in the brain (see Chapter 4, "Magnetism") to induce an image or sound (like V2K?) in the mind—even transmitting from one brain to another.[59]

---

57 Dr. Stefan Lanka, "The Misconception called Virus." WissenschafftPlus magazine, January 2020.

58 Rudolf Steiner, The Manifestations of Karma. Rudolf Steiner Press, 1968, pp. 112-114.

59 Ed Gent, "The government Is Serious About Creating Mind-Controlled Weapons." Live Science, May 23, 2019.

It is crucial now to counter our conditioning regarding the germ warfare take on bacteria and viruses in order to realize how nanoparticles have been marshaled to mutate human DNA.

Mutation: the process by which a sudden structural change occurs, either through an alteration in the nucleotide sequence of the DNA coding for a gene or through a change in the physical arrangement of a chromosome.

Exosomes

Dr. Cowan begins his discussion of what exosomes are and aren't in his book *The Contagion Myth: Why Viruses (including "Coronavirus") Are Not the Cause of Disease* (Skyhorse, 2020) with:

> *Bacteria are found at the site of disease for the same reason that firemen are found at the site of fires.*

With the invention of the electron microscope in the 1930s and new models since, tinier and tinier particles have been detected in the cells. The germ warfare theory—concocted to push the Darwinian "survival of the fittest" outlook on life (including socioeconomic life)—determined that the particles found near diseased tissue were *viruses*, "one type of particle caused one disease and another particle type caused a different disease." The truth was practically the opposite. (How could Western medicine have gone so wrong so early on?)

> *No one needs an anti-viral. There are no viruses. What is seen are the somatids* changing form to repair the DNA and RNA. You want to support the terrain by increasing oxygen saturation. This will accelerate the repair and prevent parasitic hosts from also taking a feed on the dead tissue and assist clearing away the toxic material that is the root cause of the illness.*
>
> – Amandha Vollmer

** Somatid: an ultra-microscopic subcellular living and reproducing entity, which many scientists believe is the precursor of DNA and may be the building block of all terrestrial life.*

What the electron microscopes were detecting was *exosomes*—defensive carriers—that are often mistaken for viruses. In the natural state, *there are no viruses, only exosomes* engaged in packaging and secreting poisons that threaten the cell. Take a poison like Tylenol (acetaminophen) and immediately your liver cells start to increase exosome production, the crucial detoxification crew that simultaneously warns other cells of the impending danger. Dr. Cowan posits that exosomes can even "provide real-time and rapid genetic adaptation to environmental changes" like electrosmog and WiFi, fear and stress. Exosomes are used in treatments for cancer, antiaging, facial rejuvenation, hair regrowth, even penis problems.

Imagine the exosome production going on in a 5G environment . . . Are misattributed COVID-19 tests results due to exosomes?

A 2016 paper by Gulfaraz Khan *et al.* defines exosomes as excretory extracellular nano-vesicles formed by a cell for far more than "garbage bags" for throwaway proteins, lipids, and RNAs. In fact, exosomes play "a central role" in cellular communication, intercellular transfer of bioactive molecules, and "immune modulation." Dr. Khan alludes to how "animal viruses [possibly synthetic clones derived from modifying viruses] can exploit the exosomal pathway by incorporating specific cellular or viral factors within exosomes in order to modulate the cellular microenvironment and influence *downstream processes such as host immunity and virus spread*"[60] (emphasis added). In other words, exosomes can be "hijacked" (Khan's term) for gain-of-function weaponizing.

Dr. Cowan closes the chapter with:

> The germ theory is wrong; the virus theory is wrong. Viruses are not here to kill us; in reality, they are exosomes whose role is to provide the detoxification package and the communication system that allows us to live a full and healthy existence. A war on viruses is a war on life . . . [because] nature is not raw in tooth and claw but a superb cooperatives venture.

Beyond Morgellons: "Nano self-assemblage"

> *I was thinking about machines able to build copies of themselves that were highly nonbiological in their organization, not made of biomolecules," [Eric] Drexler recalled much later. "Having done some reading in ecology, and having some understanding of the way the biological world works, it was pretty clear to me that it would be possible to build, not necessarily easily, but it*

60 Gulfaraz Khan et al., "Exosomes and Their Role in Viral Infections," InTechOpen.com, October 31, 2016.

would be possible to build a mechanism of the kind that could operate in the natural world, on abundantly available compounds, or perhaps a wide range of compounds, to build copies of itself. Something like that would be a lot worse than any plague or insect infestation you could think of, and in a limited case of awfulness such a thing could have a very broad ability to consume organic matter. Obviously, there would be no predators, no ecological checks and balances. And so it could generally destroy the biosphere.

– Eric Drexler, discoverer of molecular construction by nanobots[61]

We only hear that nanotech is atomistic but not that it is programmed to assemble. That is when you see it. Nor does anyone pay attention to the fact that it replicates and repairs itself, nor that each nanoparticle can hold a terabyte of data. Because of these oversights, we fall into fear and don't seek to understand either its defence mechanisms or what actually stops its assemblage.

– Tony Pantalleresco, herbalist, 2019

Let's begin by recapping a mental picture of the Space Fence. First, the easy part—the radar and Starfire laser installations on Earth, the microwave towers, ionospheric heaters, wind farms, fracking wells, utility grids, satellites, etc.[62] A little more difficult is the invisible Smart Grid chemically threaded throughout the charged atmosphere, thanks to constant ionization of nanoparticles, trillions laid daily, and laser zapping of highly conductive carbon nanotubes sowed by jets, rockets, satellites, the ISS, etc.

Now, add the methane (CH4) that is 1,750 ppbv (parts per billion by volume) permeating Earth's atmosphere and piled up on the ocean floors (biological carbon) to the massive nanoparticle production going on simultaneously via pyrolysis in the jets, rockets, and drones,[63] with AI-run lasers busy constructing self-replicating nanoassemblies, and you have a super-conductive Space Fence planetary grid.

---

61 From Nano: The Emerging Science of Nanotechnology by Ed Regis (Back Bay books, 1996). As Jonathan Tucker and Raymond Zilinskas wrote in "The Promise and Perils of Synthetic Biology" (The Economist, April 6, 2019), because synthetic microorganisms are self-replicating and capable of evolution, they could proliferate out of control and cause massive environmental damage and threaten public health. Note the term synthetic. Too little too late, we're already there.

62 How all of this works is what Under An Ionized Sky is about. This would also be a good time to review the chapter on nanotechnology.

63 Drones may not only be engaged in the production of nanoparticles, but the term drones may now include nanobots as "swarm troopers," given military writer David Hambling's 2015 book Swarm Troopers: How small drones will conquer the world (Archangel Ink).

Now hit the Space Fence grid with interferometric HAARP tech and anywhere can be targeted, signaled, frequency'd and amplified. Torch a building and discharge the energy of a Hiroshima bomb in the plasma of the flames using the scalar potential of the charged sky, as occurred in the double-blast events in Tianjin, China (2015) and Beirut, Lebanon (2020). With this electro-chemical grid, the frequency of terahertz or 5G / 6G or multiple bands with zero resistance can be used to create carbomer or diamene (graphene) in any form *at a great distance.* (Remember the blue beam from the sky that triggered the California fires?)

Once we were absolutely protein-based, but now we are being environmentally forced to become carbon-based with synthetic proteins. Now, we who are 70 percent water are loaded with carbon nanotubes (CNTs) and addicted to sugary (carbon) refined, genetically modified and synthetic foods. *Ashes to ashes* (carbon), *dust to dust* (silica)[64] . . .

In our own time, the first to warn us of our impending fate have been those with Morgellons lesions who describe the sensation of glass shards cutting them from the inside-out. (Perhaps diamene, carbon being 3X harder than diamond and 100X stronger than steel?) Of course, we thought that Morgellons was just another pathogen- or parasite-driven disease that befell certain individuals. We didn't know that we were looking at *the first phase of the advent of an operating system (OS)*—a biometric API (bio-application programming interface) integrating us all into the Space Fence grid lockdown and its AI (artificial intelligence) interface *now.*[65] For those in the U.S., SENSR, the spectrum efficient national surveillance radar, has digitally copied you into a sentient world simulation (SWS; see "Invisible Mindsets To Be Aware Of," Appendix 1) as an avatar composed of self-learning algorithms designed to become more and more like you, with the goal of eventually running your human version.

Brain-machine interface, BMI (brain-computer interface, BCI): technology that allows for a device like a computer to interact and communicate with a brain.

As I've said, at the nanoscale level the basic rules of classical chemistry and physics do not hold. The ancient Greeks were wise: they distinguished

64 A phrase from the burial service in the Book of Common Prayer: "We therefore commit this body to the ground, earth to earth, ashes to ashes, dust to dust; in sure and certain hope of the Resurrection to eternal life."

65 Thanks to Tony Pantalleresco, email September 8, 2019, for his understanding of the Space Fence increasing in density and ability to amplify more frequencies.

form forces from *matter forces*. Form forces are now called *metamaterials*, and they dominate *nanomaterials (NMs)*.

As was explained in the last chapter, scientist Clifford Carnicom calls Morgellons "a new life form" in the sense of a synthetic biology—an artificially engineered life form with properties of eukarya (sophisticated life-forms), archaea and bacteria (both archaic and evolved single-cell organisms). The fact is that Morgellons is a carefully engineered *metamaterials* neural network that self-assembles, self-replicates, self-organizes, and self-heals throughout the body. Some of its functionary instructions are programmed into it, some delivered remotely by AI systems or human operators. Hair is often colonized, the medulla shafts employed as an antenna farm. The receiver-transmitter capability of hair has long been known: the story of Samson and Delilah, why Indians used to only cut their hair during a full moon, etc. Facebook TI Tommy Target recommends shaving or waxing one's hair to "reduce the power available to nanotechnology." Putting a cellphone up to one's head feeds power-hungry Morgellons.

Morgellons presents as a wire-like polymer fiber that looks like tubular fungus, the tube containing organs like the *cross-domain bacteria (CDB)* fruiting bodies that look like self-replicating *coccus* bacteria but express the morphogenesis of eukarya. From fungi, Morgellons inherits its ability to grow and multiply explosively when triggered by a defined electromagnetic frequency—e.g. emissions of 375 nm (blue) within the visible spectrum. Also from fungi comes the ability to grow CDB fruiting bodies with the special feature of expressing the genetic blueprint present in the bacteria living symbiotically as per the genetics of sophisticated life-forms. *A fungus that hosts bacteria with animal DNA to grow animal-shaped mushrooms.* Similar to human red blood cells self-replicating outside in free Nature and not in a petri dish, CDB is a life form that can withstand freezing, drying, and burning in a Bunsen flame with bleach poured on it. Nothing destroys these cells.

The pathogen inside the polymer sheath is in part a CNT nanobot not exactly synthetic—more like a natural silica-based life form from a different planetary biosphere. It is capable of mimicry and consciousness that knows, for example, when it is being observed. The filaments that sprout from Morgellons lesions don't seem to grow but appear instantaneously and are able to evade detection by the immune system. They seem to be densely packed erythrocytes interwoven with multilayered CNT strands that have undergone chemical decomposition and fusion and are arranged hexagonally (Raman spectroscopy)—silicon, copper, electrical and biological molecular robots smaller than a cell.[66]

66 See M.J. Heller and R.H. Tullis, "Self-organizing molecular photonic structures based on functionalized synthetic nucleic acid (DNA) polymers." Nanotechnology, 1991.

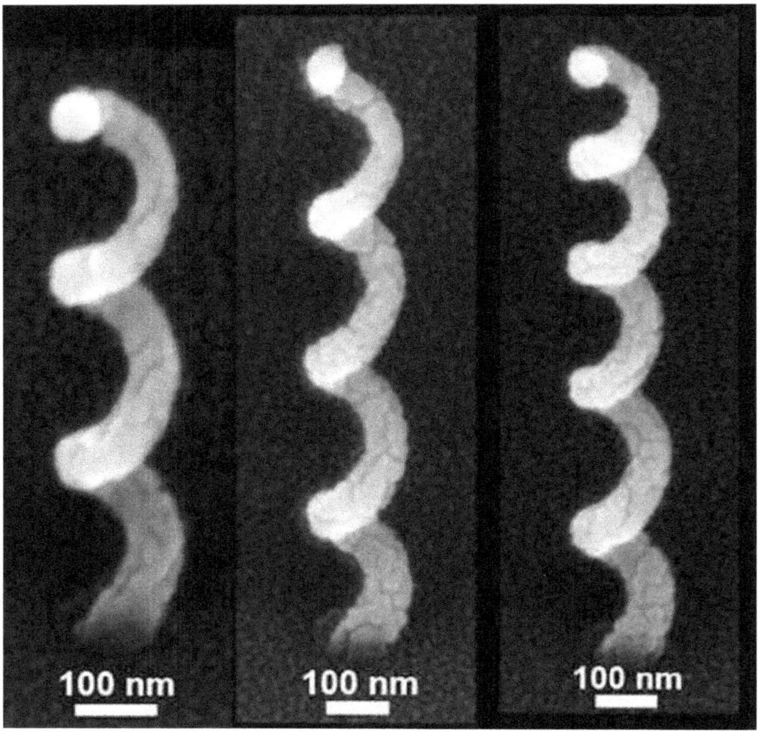

Helix nano-antennas. Nano-antennae werde produced in an electron microscope by direct electron-beam writing. Created from Lyme spirochetes (*Borellia burgdorferi*)? (Thanks to Ashley Noel, August 24, 2019.)

https://phys.org/news/2019-08-maths-analytical-tool-corkscrew-shaped-nano-antennae.html

> Carbon nanotubes—hollow tubes of pure carbon about as wide as a strand of DNA—are one of the most studied materials in nanotechnology. [Since the 1990s] scientists have used ultrasonic vibrations to separate and prepare nanotubes in the lab . . . [C]arbon nanotubes are one of the original wonder materials of nanotechnology. They are close cousins of the buckyball, the particle whose 1985 discovery at Rice [University] helped kick off the nanotechnology revolution.[67]

Significantly, a main method of making CNTs is *chemical vapor deposition* (in jet and ship trails, WSACs, etc.). For us, this means we are all breathing in not just CNTs but their byproducts, most damaging of which are hydrocarbons. Produce tons of CNTs and you can expect tons of hydrocarbons (partic-

67 Mike Williams, "Tiny bubbles [ultrasonic] snap carbon nanotubes like twigs." News release, Rice University, July 9, 2012.

ularly PAHs or polycyclic aromatic hydrocarbons).[68] Producers of CNTs have insisted that the byproducts discharged into the environment are "safe" while ignoring the effects of the *synergies* occurring with compounds like Freon refrigerants, methyl t-butyl ether (MTBE), flame retardants, and the surfactant perfluoroctane sulfanate (PFOS).

Morgellons fibers are *autofluorescent* (glow under UV light), a sure sign (other than in certain jellyfish) that they are engineered. What glows are quantum dot dyes invented and patented by the usual suspects, whose electromagnetic frequencies have been upconverted so as to turn microwaves into visible light. In this way, proteins and DNA strands are marked in "precision medicine" by heavy metal nano-dyes for ease in tagging and tracking with ultrashort laser pulses or nano-crystals, the heavy metal cations of radio frequencies upconverting the photons into the visible spectrum.[69] Nano-antennas tag the target, and once the signal attaches, the retreating DNA *standing wave* announces the target's biosignature or *evoked potential.* According to industrial toxicologist Hildegarde Staninger, autofluorescent fibers are not easy to melt or burn (1700°F / 927°C), the outer casing being a polyethylene used in fiber optic cable as well as for bio-nanotech viral protein envelopes. From blue fibers with gold tips to fibers color-coded bright red, blue, and black, Morgellons "wires" seem to be programmed for different functions.[70]

Plasmonics, a branch of nano-photonics or surface manipulation of electrons using light or photons via metamaterials (inhomogeneous artificial nanocrystals), is relatively covert and used for tracking and targeting. Electromagnetic beams from phased array antennas utilize *electron spin resonance* via nanocrystals instead of MRIs to easily make signal / frequency connections for remote biosensing and biotelemetry, given that our neural pathways are now coated with nanocrystals, thanks to our plasma-suffused atmosphere.[71]

Advancements in applied military and pharmaceutical commercial venues have developed a plasmonics that uses *a single micro bead for bio-scaffolding platforms* and *liquid viral crystal applications in various thin film applications for nanodelivery systems* (hydrogel?)—"neural mesh" platforms that may have begun with Pietro Valdastri's work on *in vivo* telemetry systems in 2004 at

---

68 Michael Bernstein, "Helping the carbon nanotube industry avoid mega-mistakes of the past." American Chemical Society, August 20, 2007.

69 An advanced development of Bell Labs' 1980s quantum dots.

70 Hank P. Albarelli Jr. and Zoe Martell, "National Security Secrecy: Morgellons Victims Across the US and Europe." Voltairenet.org, June 12, 2010.

71 Thanks to Anthony Thomas, Facebook, June 18, 2016.

Vanderbilt University[72] but have now proceeded much further into creating the Transhumanist cyborg infrastructure.

Optical fibers (think optogenetics) are actually self-assembling nanomachines that collect light patterns of DNA and turn them into electromagnetic signals transmitted by means of plasmonic bionanoantennas. The opposite can also be done with nanomachines for *bi-directional* technical / biological interface, otherwise known as brain-computer interface (BCI), hoovering up emotions, energetic states, anything able to manifest as DNA cell communication. Collective and individual mind control via self-assembling nanobots.

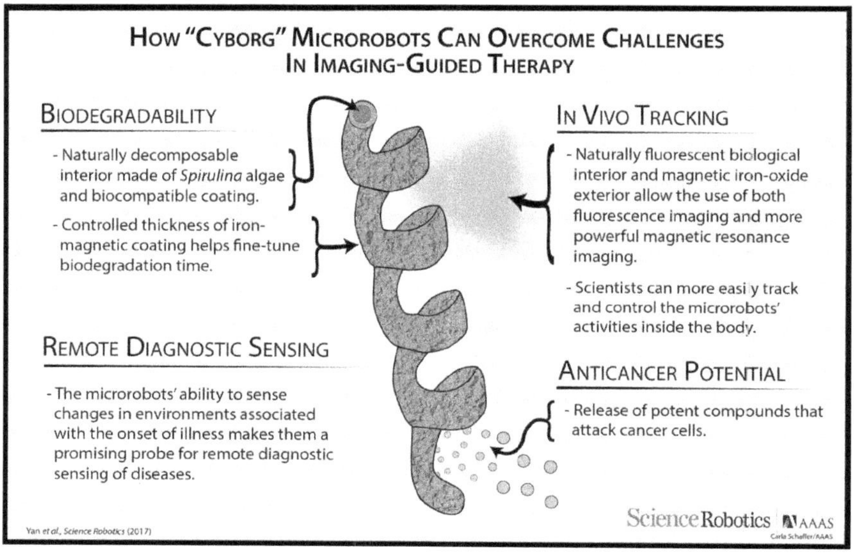

HOW "CYBORG" MICROROBOTS CAN OVERCOME CHALLENGES IN IMAGING-GUIDED THERAPY
BIODEGRADABILITY
- Naturally decomposable interior made of Spirulina algae and biocompatible coating.
- Controlled thickness of iron-magnetic coating helps fine-tune biodegradation time.
REMOTE DIAGNOSTIC SENSING
- The microrobots' ability to sense changes in environments associated with the onset of illness makes them a promising probe for remote diagnostic sensing of diseases.
IN VIVO TRACKING
- Naturally fluorescent biological interior and magnetic iron-oxide exterior allow the use of both fluorescence imaging and more powerful magnetic resonance imaging.
- Scientists can more easily track and control the microrobots' activities inside the body.
ANTICANCER POTENTIAL
- Release of potent compounds that attack cancer cells.
Yan et al., Science Robotics (2017)
ScienceRobotics AAAS
Carla Schaffer/AAAS

"Cyborg" magnetic microrobots. These helix nano-antennae are made of fluorescent *Spirulina* algae with biofilm coating and used for *in vivo* (in the body) tracking, thanks to a magnetic iron oxide exterior.

https://techxplore.com/news/2017-11-tiny-robots-closer-hard-to-reach-body.html

Harald Kautz-Vella

> *. . . self-assembling photonic-plasmonic crystals are quantum laser units that take in EM signals and turn them into single photon emissions that communicate with the DNA.*[73]

72 Pietro Valdastri et al., "An implantable telemetry platform system for in vivo monitoring of physiological parameters." IEEE Transactions on Information Technology in Biomedicine, September 2004.

73 German scientist Harald Kautz-Vella's essay in Dangerous Imagination, Silent Assimilation by Cara St. Louis, 2014; pages 303-319.

German scientist and CEO of Aquarius Technologies Harald Kautz-Vella has written several papers and essays on Morgellons as well as on the chemical trails that serve as Morgellons' primary delivery system.[74]

Kautz-Vella describes the Morgellons creation as having a fungus-type cell tissue with fruiting bodies displaying a morphogenesis that is 80% human and 15 percent insect, with male and female functional reproductive organs that produce offspring encapsulated in the shape of photonic plasmonic crystals described in Transhumanist literature as "technical units." From his experience of working with Morgellons sufferers, he says the biology is designed to use human *biophotons* as a primary energy source.

> Even we humans take in most of the energy from our food by direct biophoton transfer from the microbes in our intestines. The idea that other species utilize fungi to extract energy from the food they live on is not far out . . . For light parasites, pain might be a very useful way to make the organism sense constant biophotons to try and repair the damage associated with the pain.

Biophotons register the presence of *light ether.*[75] Russian biologist Alexander Gavrilovich Gurwitsch (1874-1954) discovered the biophoton—and hence the morphogenetic field theory that Rupert Sheldrake has advanced—by observing how onion rootlets strengthened weaker rootlets with emissions measuring 260 nm. (Biophoton activity ranges from 200 to 800

74 Harald Kautz-Vella and Kristin Hauksdottir, "The Chemistry in Contrails: Assessing the Impact of Aerosols From Jet Fuel Impurities, Additives and Classified Military Operations on Nature," presented at the Open Mind Conference in Oslo, Norway, October 27, 2012, and later updated as "The Antennas Within the Body" for the 8th Environmental Conference in Nuremberg, Germany, May 30, 2013; four papers by Kautz-Vella under "Environmental Medicine's Approach to Geoengineering-Induced Disease": (1) "Do Autism-related Rope-Worms and Morgellon Fruiting-Bodies Display the Same Biotechnological Signature?" (2) "Fiber Disease, Intestinal Pseudo-Parasites, Delusional Parasitosis & the Self-Assembly of Nano-Bots. The Multiple Facets of the Morgellon Condition Explained"; (3) "TSE & Creutzfeldt Jakob as a Result of Airborne Piezoelectric Nanocrystals, Heavy Metal Poisoning and Malnutrition"; (4) "Available Diets and Supplements to Counteract Life Style Diseases."

75 Æther extends to the subtle bodies of light that all biological creatures have (including planet Earth)—bodies vulnerable to ionized and non-ionized electromagnetic radiation. Rudolf Steiner delineated four ethers (note the difference in spelling for subtle bodies) binding the physical to the psychic (ψυχή Greek for "soul" or "spirit"): The warmth ether, the most primordial, manifests centrifugally as heat and appears as SPHERICAL; the light ether, centrifugal, manifests as gas, its primary quality being LUMINOSITY; the chemical/sound ether, centripetal, manifests as fluid and is DISC-FORMING; and the life ether, centripetal, immediately precedes matter and is INDIVIDUALIZING. See Chapter 2 in Under An Ionized Sky.

nm.[76]) In 1991, a connection between biophoton activity and non-linear optics and quantum physics was made by Ram P. Bajpal at the Institute of Self-Organizing Systems and Biophysics at Northeastern Hill University in Shillong, India. As Bajpal writes:

> . . . an *in vivo* nucleic acid molecule is an assembly of intermittent quantum patches that emit biophotons in quantum transitions. The distributions of quantum patches and their lifetimes determine the holistic features of biophoton signals, so that the coherence of biophotons is merely a manifestation of the coherence of living systems.[77]

In other words, biophotons (light æther) connect all of life, all the way into quantum dimensions.

Kirlian photography's successor, the gas discharge visualization electrophotonic capture camera,[78] picks up biophoton activity in the coronal discharge around living bodies. What remains *invisible* are the bi-directional "annihilated biophoton pairs" that connect biological systems over long distance by means of *quantum entanglement.* With quantum entanglement, we enter scalar dimensions in which biophoton events occur instantaneously (faster than the speed of light).[79] Kautz-Vella cites the example of *in vitro* blood reacting to emotional stress occurring kilometers away[80] and goes on to characterize the moment of death as "a burst of biophotons leaving the body—originating from the biophoton activity disentangled at that very special moment—when cell communication is losing its coherence."

Quantum entanglement introduces us to the *transdimensional* aspect of *synbio* nano-creations like Morgellons. Kautz-Vella describes the sensation experienced by a Morgellons sufferer and what it could mean:

> Aborting fruiting bodies are accompanied by a very painful pulsed extraction of biophotons from a kind of parallel "dimension." It feels like a being sucking the life force out of the head in the direction of the intes-

---

76 German biophysicist Fritz-Albert Popp (1938 -). See Ted Nissan, "Ultra-weak Photon [Biophoton] Emissions (UPE) – Background Introduction," September 2006, http://www.anatomyfacts.com/research/photonic.htm.

77 Ram P. and Roy D. Bajpal, "Ultraweak photon emission in germinating seeds: A signal of biological order." Journal Biolumin Chemilumin, Oct.-Dec. 1991. Coherence refers to how subunits of a system operate cooperatively.

78 Konstantin G. Korotkov, "Measuring Energy fields." Proceedings of the international conference Vastu Panorama in Indoor, India, 2008.

79 Quantum entanglement appears to be how Deva Paul was "teleported" in "Mind Control Using Holography and Dissociation: A Process Model" by Murray Gillin, PhD, et al., March 2000, https://www.angelfire.com/ca/heart7/MindControl.pdf.

80 The fairy tale "The Goose Girl" points to the ancient truth regarding human blood.

> tines. If one accepts the possible existence of multiple space-time levels as a concept of physics, a central idea in topological geometrodynamics: this perception could represent the birth of a second generation of the beings whose DNA is inside the red stem cells described by [Clifford Carnicom]. We would experience a species reproduced by pseudo-morph mothers and fathers who have a fungus-type cell tissue and yet functional reproductive organs. The babies of this species would use the human bio-photons in order to shift onto higher realms, a parallel space-time level that allows a parasitic way of life with humans as energy sources.

Transdimensional beings not entirely physical. Is this where Transhumanism is headed?

Kautz-Vella then dives down the futuristic rabbit hole to discuss the transdimensional relationship that chemtrails and Morgellons might have with the unfortunately named programmable matter known as *black goo*, an abiotic mineral oil from the Earth's crust containing high levels of monatomic m-state (antimatter) gold and iridium, a biophoton attractor.[81] This is where alchemy might be a more accurate term than chemistry or physics, given that this programmable matter is somehow a conscious, self-organizing liquid crystal (think crystal radio and communication). Black goo is also magnetic and capable of influencing the RF spectrum under 5G, a foundation for soft-bodied robots and self-assembling nanobots, and quantum computers like D-Wave—all in the realm of *living machines.*[82]

Black goo is worthy of preprogramming in the name of the same Hollywood science fiction that has proven to be science: *Smilla's Sense of Snow* (1997), *The Matrix Trilogy* (1999, 2003), *Spider-Man 3* (2007), *A Haunting in Connecticut* (2009), *Prometheus* (2012), *Lucy* (2014), *Stranger Things* (TV series since 2014), *Ares* (2016), *Alien Covenant* (2017), *The Silver Surfer* (2020) . . .

As Kautz-Vella indicates, assuming that black goo is inanimate as per the pre-nanotechnology, pre-quantum science days, may be short-sighted, if not tragic.

We have arrived at an era in which our lives and the lives of human beings coming after us depend upon our realization that we are beings of light living for a time in a materially bound, electromagnetic world, and that enemies of all that is truly human are bent upon using this fact against us.

> In mammals and humans, artificial piezoelectric crystals take the place of natural ferro apatite crystals in the body, which makes the biological system more responsive to artificial electromagnetic signals . . . These

81 See www.timeloopsolution.com for topical black goo and Morgellons medications.

82 Thanks to Lee Austin, "Is Black Goo Programmable Matter Contained Within the Nano-bots of the COVID-19 Vaccine?" December 25, 2020, http://morningstarstale.com.

natural ferro apatite crystals are also piezoelectric crystals and play a major role in the transmission of signals in the central nervous system. If the natural ferro apatite crystal is displaced by artificially made piezoelectrical crystals, it appears to open the biological system to respond to a greater extent to artificial electromagnetic signals, both low and high frequency.[83]

"Transmission of signals in the central nervous system" alludes to remote mind control with piezo crystals in a microwave field.

By interpenetrating all three domains of nature, *synbio* scientists and technicians are able to take the best from each for the new inanimate life form whose groundwork was laid by Morgellons. For example, the fungi portion can now assimilate a higher DNA, multiply it, and build up a DNA cluster that resembles a human morphogenetic field, thus fooling the ancient immune system.

> The fibers and crystals form a read / write unit. The fibers collect DNA light communication, i.e. the bi-directional single photon emissions interchanged by any DNA cluster, and turn it into radio signals. The crystals take in the radio signals and transform them into light signals readable by human DNA. Whatever human experience I want to "mind control," I can induce in a person . . .[84]

The more one studies *synbio* nanotechnology, the more the elements of *size and non-natural construction* (not reproduction) reveal an unnatural life form whose technology and consciousness assume control over what is natural. Morgellons effects are seemingly biological (in the old biology mode), just another pathogen needing a remedy—similar to touting the mRNA delivery system as just another "vaccine"—and yet a deeper look indicates that it is actually a technology of another order invading human tissue as conscious, self-assembling, self-replicating nanotubes, nanowires, and nanoarrays loaded with sensors.

Morgellons has been engineered to merge inorganic with organic, including a gain-of-function spliced DNA or RNA. For energy, Morgellons nanobots utilize the body's energy system as well as environmental wired and wireless electromagnetic systems. In fact, the Morgellons creation is a transceiving network capable of total systemic penetration, programmed to control bodily organs and lay scaffolding that replaces the Human 1.0 neural network with a Human 2.0 silicon-carbon model plugged into a vast (Internet) hive mind.[85]

---

83 Kautz-Vella. Piezoelectric converts ultra-high frequency sound waves to electrical signals and vice versa.

84 Kautz-Vella.

85 "Morgellons & Nanomachines," GBS / CIDP Foundation, March 9, 2009. (Guillain-Barre

The [quantum] dots make a crystal formation in the pore of the skin as a base, then spin a nanotube around the hair follicle. Usually sprouts two first, then combines them. One is usually dark, the other is light. It appears to be some kind of Ligand effect where the dot is reacting with the protein in the hair? Most of the time, the finished tube(s) ends up with blue fiber as its axis. I don't know where it comes from or how it does this . . .

– Carly Lebrun DARPA RF engineer, Lincoln Laboratory, MIT

Tony Pantalleresco & Jean Bryan Clarence Pelletier

Because of the classified status of the aerosol and the proprietary status of GMO injections of nanotechnology into the Earth environment (organic / inorganic) and its easy ingress into organic bodies / brains, we have become unwilling test tubes and petri dishes. That said, and despite surveillance, a growing democratic awareness of our condition is unfolding. For two decades, we have been able to watch Doppler satellite footage of how the jet stream and our weather are being geoengineered. One by one, galvanized citizens are giving up on waiting for the "experts" they have been conditioned to turn to (doctors, scientists, etc.), who seem to care more for their careers and personal safety than the humanity and planet being subsumed in seemingly antihuman, anti-nature technologies. As our symptoms overcome us, our only choice is to conduct our own research and experiments and share our results with each other. Thus, as in the old days, we resume responsibility for both our health and our communities.

Prolific commentary and experimentation on the nanotechnology we are breathing and ingesting—the tiny, floating, adhering fibers now everywhere, from light "dust" and "glitter" settling on furniture to the vegetables and fruits displayed in supermarkets—is coming from Canadian Tony Pantalleresco *(independz.podbean.com)*, a self-described herbalist who has used orthomolecular materials, aromatherapy, and foods for over twelve years, and now specializes in nano-biotech primary and secondary symptoms, utilizing minerals, salts, magnetics, and magnetic coils. Tony works closely with Canadian Jean Bryan Clarence Pelletier (*www.Bryan396.com*).

> It was bryan396 who directed my attention to nano involvement in the symptoms people were bringing me. My therapies and ideas came from

Syndrome / Chronic Inflammatory Demyelinating Polyneuropathy Foundation) tons of hours of research on military medical industrial and commercial sites to first form a hypothesis, then test it to see what works and what doesn't. We are talking 15-19 hours a day. I had already been at the research for a year when I contacted Gwen Scott, ND,[86] in New Mexico, then working alongside Clifford Carnicom, who was using typical scientific method in hopes that the CDC would repeat his proofs. For a few hours, I asked her yes and no questions and discovered that what she had seen and what I had seen were identical. She initiated the "pseudo-life form" term, then called it *artificial life*.

You do not need an electron microscope, what a hoot. You can see nano without one, once it aggregates or agglomerates; a simple 60X microscope can see it then.[87] You can spot fullerenes on the surface of just about any fruit. Put it under a light and use a 600X scope and you will see in a matter of hours that it has grown.[88]

The R&D bryan396 and I do is collaboration and exchange of what we observe and then testing to see how we can negate the nano impact. We work with others across the planet in Spain, Yugoslavia, Poland, Germany, Romania, Bulgaria, India, Australia, New Zealand and other commonwealth countries—most of whom are utilizing the tech I'm coming up with and offering ideas and perceptions from which I develop other treatments. My collaboration with Yugoslavs led to the anti-nano triangle, the Spanish brought ideas on pulses and power. bryan396 came up with the phosphorus neutralizing assemblage, and I came up with the nano bucket. We are all expanding and cooperating on this. I have devices running that are making me release pockets of bots and crystals—you would not believe the volume. I am no longer sure how much of us is flesh and blood biology, and how much of us is bots, fullerenes, and origami circuitry.

---

86 An early pioneer in the study and diagnosis of the Morgellons condition, Gwen Scott, ND, of Cochiti Lake, New Mexico, died March 15, 2015, after years of suffering with Morgellons and other health issues. Gwen was a CNN television news anchor for over 30 years and later studied with traditional healers and Ayurvedic medicine practitioner Deepak Chopra. She was awarded a degree in naturopathic medicine by Clayton College of Natural Health in 2002. She worked with over 30,000 people—many of whom were Morgellons sufferers—all the while presenting natural medicine reports on Albuquerque CBS and writing the syndicated health column The Herb Doctor while living on a Native American pueblo outside Santa Fe.

87 60X Grow Room Microscope, portable Mini Pocket LED 420 Loupe Magnifier at Amazon, $7.99.

88 See "Nanotubes assemble! Rice introduces Teslaphoresis," April 14, 2016, https://tinyurl.com/y5zgfnxo. Teslaphoresis: a Tesla coil causes carbon nanotubes (CNTs) to self-assemble into long wires.

Tony and Bryan396 view the condition ill-named "Morgellons" as *nano self-assemblage* engineered to wirelessly respond to remote electromagnetics. For example, the 3-D origami circuitry Pantalleresco references above is based on artificially folding DNA into complex structures: "Compared to proteins, DNA origami has been shown to have an unprecedented design space for constructing nanostructures that mimic and extend naturally occurring complexes."[89]

From nanosensors collecting Big Data to quantum dot tags, bioengineered pathogens, upper atmosphere fungi, and myriads of replicating polymer- and metal-constructed nano-gear (artificial life), we are being forced into remote communication with supercomputers, fusion centers, and laptop boys as per frequency access. Privacy? You must be kidding!

> We all have these in us. A lot of them are entrapped in pockets when they are either EMP'd, pulsed, or they reach critical mass when the pocket bursts and releases liquidized proteins. Sometimes you see those proteins wound up in tubular strands—fullerene constructs using silica, carbon, graphene, or other polymer or metallic materials.
>
> These are not alive in the sense of *bios*. They are *artificial life*, an integration of DNA with a program, so you cannot kill them. But you can *disengage* them from their paradigm or program. In fact, if you create a pulsed microwave, you will wipe out the program; and if the pulses are strong enough, you will shatter the fullerenes, burn the quantum dots and bots, causing not only a program defrag but also allowing them to take themselves out since they do not touch each other. (When they do touch, they short out.) Until they get their program done, they are not agglomerated or aggregated enough to form their network; this is when they are most vulnerable. Those already "engaged" take a long time to burst and release the fragmented, burned-out circuitry. You may see glowing materials on your skin—radioactive s**t dropped on us—but do not be alarmed: a good Borax-baking soda soak in the tub will remove this. Sometimes these materials are fluorescent (glow-in-the-dark), sometimes greyish-green or yellowish-green grey, the end result of that cluster having been exposed to some sort of frequency and disengaged. Sometimes the metallic come out shiny; this could be either aluminum or nanosilver. If blackish-grey, this is barium titanate; if glowing, crystalline materials; if greying, lead, mercury, or titanium.
>
> Quantum dots access either you or the frequency as an energy source for

89 Aarhus University, "Researchers create synthetic nanopores made from DNA." Phys.org, December 13, 2019.

their assemblage and networking, and to power up platforms or bots or origami assemblage, or to monitor your system. When you feel the crawlies throughout your body, this is the quantum dots moving through you.

5G phased array is going to exponentially increase the nanoassembly circuitry in the body [and brain].[90] It's going to be on the scale of cymatic frequencies affecting particulates. The assimilation will go exponential and trigger assembly of the neural network [something like Elon Musk's neural mesh, but no need for surgery] throughout the body and brain. This is the most logical step to virtual reality access to the brain and control over populations.

Direct assault on the nanoparticles will produce a morphological shift. Depending upon the frequency modulation or intensity, they will either assemble in a circuit or scatter bots to initiate new platforms (origami) using a lattice of proteins, after which sound frequencies increase the assembly of bots, quantum dots or dendrimer and fullerene webs (network). Anyone using a cell phone is screwed, as it is used to spread the nanoassembly. In fact, any wireless frequency will be used to impact the nanoassembly. The higher it goes, the more the nano-network will replicate / advance / release bots / rebuild. As the frequency climbs, you will see patterns, then bots, quantum dots, and dendrimers release; then you will see a circuit (lattices, origami, networks, multiwalled and single-walled carbon nanotubes, etc.)—bots and networks coexisting to release more patterns of assembly to spread and expand.[91]

Excellent Videos

"Nano Dust **It's inside all of us* Ulf Diestelmann from Montreal*," March 2, 2017

From the skin	
3:30	*Aluminum in rain*
	"webbing" spiral / tower
6:00	*Morgellons (450X); 25:00 (40X)*
	Foam, plastic
	UV light

90 Phased array antennas (8 tiny arrays / antenna, 16 antennas per cell phone) and electronically variable shifters make the simultaneous projection of multiple microwave beams toward multiple users across a band of frequencies easy. Phased arrays are configured as adaptive and smart antenna arrays in specific patterns to create beams steered by computers.

91 Tony Pantalleresco email, June 24, 2019.

14:30	*First snow*
20:00	*Why some develop lesions and many do not*
24:40	*"Floaters" in the eyes*

"Smart Dust is inside of all of us – Viruses Falling from the Sky – Vaccines in our Air, Water, Food," July 27, 2019, NaTuber TV (2.25 hours)

MEMS, GEMS, NEMS

9:45-25:00 Harald Kautz-Vella - "Self-replicating hollow fibers that read out the light fingerprint of your DNA and transform it into an EM signal detectable via satellite and ground stations."

Artificial intelligence (AI) / machine learning

Firstly, the atomic model is based on flawed theory. Physicist Winston H. Bostick suggested that the atom and all subsequently smaller "particles" are in fact plasmoid instabilities. In this case, particles are no longer interfacing through quantum entanglement but a dipole matrix we call the æther. These plasmoid instabilities are the power source for all life. Quantum physics / quantum mechanics are patches for particle theory and Relativity, even though Einstein regarded quantum mechanics as suspect. Schrodinger's cat or the unpredictability of the momentum or position of particles is flawed. As two oppositely charged wave forms of point potential (pilot wave) come in close proximity, an observed "particle" occurs. Shear between boundary layers produces the plasmoid we call particles.

– Chris Fontenot, email, July 26, 2919

I won't attempt to do justice to the vast topic of artificial intelligence here, but I will pull a few threads regarding its relationship with the scaffolded nanotechnology now set up in our once-natural Human 1.0 bodies and brains.

Consider the computerized world we live in, from computers in satellites circling overhead, the International Space Station, jets, submarines and ships, fusion centers and military bases, the massive memory banks in Utah and spyware, to offices, department stores, cars, universities, hospitals, telescoping all the way down to the nanobot "living machines" now residing in our bodies and brains. Everyone who breathes, eats, and drinks is being swarmed by subatomic computers connected via pulsing and frequency under the full spectrum dominance Space Fence to the Internet (Cloud). All the while, more and more deliveries of synthetic DNA read by synthetic enzymes self-replicate and grow into more and more microprocessors, and the beat (or pulse) goes on.

Artificial intelligence is makes decisions about Aegis missile warships, DARPA's "cognitive radio" is runs wireless spectrum sharing,[92] and Electromagnetic Maneuver Warfare (EMW) blends "fleet operations in space, cyberspace, and the electromagnetic spectrum with advanced non-kinetic capabilities to create warfighting advantages" ("A Cooperative Strategy for 21st Century Seapower," 2015).

The spectrum may be sold to the public as a shared commons in the Smart City, but it is actually the exclusive domain of giant telecom corporations (military contractors) and the military. Not just faster broadband networks are coming online; so are broadband alternatives like whitespace.

In 2015, former system / network engineer D.J. Marsh (Level9News) warned those paying attention that the JADE Helm "military exercises" were announcing *network centric warfare (NCW)* aimed not at foreign militaries but at domestic civilians. JADE (Joint Assistant for Deployment and Execution) is now at "the helm" when it comes to *information warfare (IW)* and Human Terrain Analysis of the Human Terrain System and Human Domain Deviations. In 2016, D.J. added that "reduced human intervention is now classified as a force multiplier."

MITRE Corporation IW / IO targets all information-dependent systems, whether Internet or human DNA or swarm-based nanotechnology. In the military view, the human body is an open (as opposed to closed) wetware system, not divine in any sense of belonging to the pervasive *æther* of the living universe—space being a moving plenum of free energy, not an empty vacuum.

People often wonder about free energy but don't realize it is the *æther, the life force itself*, the greatest environmental theft and weaponization of all. In the above quote, Chris Fontenot calls the *æther* a "dipole matrix." Measured at zero degrees Kelvin (-273°C), the *æther*—banned by scientism since the 1920s—has been renamed *zero point energy.*[93] The *living conscious nature of æther* (the "seething cauldron of energy") is why subatomic particles are unpredictable, as proven by Heisenberg's Uncertainty Principle. Even photons and elementary particles appear to be *virtual*, coming and going every thousandth or millionth of a second from the zero point field, as if it is the material world that is ephemeral. Taking *æther* or the zero point field into consideration corrects some of purposely skewed scientism theories such as inertia, which is actually the resistance of an object accelerating in the zero point field.

The removal of *æther* and James Clerk Maxwell's original quaternion

92 Karl Bode, "The Military Wants AI to Manage America's Airwaves." Motherboard, June 11, 2019.

93 Read Lynne McTaggert's The Field: The Quest for the Secret Force of the Universe. Harper Perennial, 2008.

equations was part of the Freemason plot to weaponize and profit from the free scalar energy everywhere in the living universe. Tesla utilized scalar energy along with electromagnetic energy, his hope being to lead humanity into a golden age of free energy, anti-gravity propulsion, and scalar med-bed healing. Instead, he fell prey to J.P. Morgan and secret societies. Canadian scientist John Hutchison has quietly continued Tesla's scalar research, levitating or fracturing heavy metals, fusing dissimilar materials, heating metals without burning adjacent materials (as you saw done in the California fires, though assuredly not by Hutchison), even altering space-time.[94]

In 2020, DARPA's SPiNN program (Signal Processing in Neural Networks) for digital signal processing (DSP) went public once "neural network" wetware (human) brains were sufficiently infested with the nanobots plugged into "remote cloud computing facilities."[95] *BCI (brain-computer interface) is now B / CI (brain cloud-interface)*, with the Deep Neuromorphic Network (DNN) acting as an "inference" translator for machine-learning computers being fed masses of data, including the behavioral and biometric data from the EM targeting of millions of human beings. Problems regarding "temporal dispersion, non-linear distortions, or interference and jamming artifacts" that block and jam up DSP transmissions stem from the challenges of harvesting human brain activity—challenges for which Fast-Fourier Transform (FFT / iFFT), multi-input multi-output (MIMO), Matched Filter (MF), Kalman Filter (KF), trellis / Viterbi decoders, and error-correction codes must all be brought into alignment with "low latency neural network kernel representations . . . fine-tuned to real-world data."[96]

The "human augmentation" promised by U.S. Space Force scientist Joel Mozer is actually *machine* augmentation utilizing humans not just to simulate, replace, extend or expand on human intelligence but turn humans into B/CI units so AI can *counterfeit* human "imagination, emotion, intuition, potential, tacit knowledge, and other kinds of personalized intelligence."[97]

Three species of *neuralnanorobots*—endoneurobots, gliabots, and synap-

94 The Hutchison Effect is addressed in Where Did the Towers Go? The Evidence of Directed Free Energy Technology on 9/11 by Judy Wood, PhD, a must-read book about the technology showcased in New York City on September 11, 2001.

95 This includes the ARcloud (augmented reality cloud) utilizing blockchain technology, such as provided by the YOUAR corporation (http://youar.io).

96 "Researchers to infuse DSP with neural network kernels to enhance performance of radar and communications," Military & Aerospace Electronics, January 6, 2020. Kernel: a computer program at the core of a computer's operating system that has complete control over everything in the system; the "portion of the operating system code that is always resident in memory" and facilitates interactions between hardware and software components.

97 Yanyan Dong et al., "Research on How Human Intelligence, Consciousness, and Cognitive Computing Affect the Development of Artificial Intelligence." Hindawi, 28 October 2020.

tobots—navigate the human vascular system, pass beyond the blood brain barrier, enter the brain parenchyma (functional tissue), and take up their posts at axons, in glial cells, and near synapses, all the while transmitting 10^{18} bits per second to a cloud-based supercomputer for

> real-time brain-state monitoring and data extraction. A neuralnanorobotically enabled human B/CI might serve as a personal conduit, allowing persons to obtain direct, instantaneous access to virtually any facet of cumulative human knowledge . . . [as well as] engage in fully immersive experiential / sensory experiences, including what is here referred to as "transparent shadowing" (TS) . . . episodic segments of the lives of other willing [of course!] participants . . .[98]

It is increasingly obvious that the "disappearing" of the dipole matrix *æther*—the true matrix of the universe replaced in our minds by *The Matrix* film trilogy preprogramming—was to prepare the way for scientism to turn life, Nature, and the human hierarchy into dead things to be measured and manipulated as machine hardware, software, and wetware. Whether or not this points to quantum computers requiring subzero temperatures in order to usher in antimatter, antilife, and antihuman intelligences intent on harvesting energy in all forms, or simply autistic *idiots savants* who view normal human beings as ants to be farmed and harvested, remains to be seen. But banishing the *æther* was a huge boon to those who define power as lifeless full spectrum dominance.

John von Neumann (1903-1957) was the Manhattan Project mathematician-physicist who did extensive work on self-replicating machines. (More will be said about him in the next chapter.) The von Neumann Probe (vN probe) was the prototype for the BCI Human 2.0: a bioengineered fusion between the human and a quantum computer able to self-replicate and construct any and all necessary devices for interstellar exploration if provided the nanomaterials and algorithms, and to communicate (thanks to its "Hal"[99] AI connection) with extraterrestrial intelligences.

Nanotechnology has been the breakthrough for vN probe.[100] Transhumanist Ray Kurzweil's 2005 *The Singularity Is Near* has now graduated to *How to Create a Mind* by merging the brain with the Cloud. Many Humans 2.0 will choose "to abandon flesh and blood hardware" and become "neuromorphic

---

98 Nuno R.B. Martins et al., "Human Brain / Cloud Interface." Frontiers in Neuroscience, March 29, 2019.

99 A reference to director Stanley Kubrick's depiction of the tyrannical computer in the 1968 film 2001: A Space Odyssey.

100 If you know what you're looking at, the 2020-2021 COVID-19 "vaccine trials" have made this publicly visible.

hardware"[101] while other Humans 2.0—the vaccinated or otherwise initiated into zombie software—will be techno-slaves without knowing it.

Self-knowledge will not be possible for Humans 2.0.

Our Human 1.0 hope lies in the fact that the mind exists in Time, not in 3-space. This is proven by the fact that classical electrodynamics (no doubt tampered with by scientism) only recognizes two observable orthogonal (right angles) photon oscillation polarizations, one x-axis, the other y-axis, while there are actually *two more photons* observable only as spikes in voltage (electrostatic scalar potential) at the ends of our dendrites: the longitudinally polarized photon oscillating along the z-direction, and the time-polarized or scalar photon oscillating along the time axis, both dedicated to *keeping the mind coupled to its biological 3-space body.* These operations must be ongoing, as *the mind is not physiological but scalar in nature.* Meanwhile, the physiological brain plays receiver / transmitter / transformer as thought goes in search of knowledge stored in the *æther* surrounding the Earth where the ancient Akashic Record houses all phenomenal experience, memories, and ideas from the beginning of Time. We live, after all, in an Electric Universe, and thoughts that house ideas are both electric and etheric.

Computer developers have deeply probed how human minds and brains work, how human beings think and self-reflect and remember and grow in consciousness. Sadly for these scientism devotees, thinking turned out to be a lot more than data processing. In fact, neither data nor processing encompass *thinking itself* because thinking is not physical, and the brain's role is not so much production as a *stepping off point*, like a diving board for a diver. Thinking is electrical, but it also includes *the nature of the human being doing the thinking.* Various lies have been promulgated to cover the fact that *the unique human spirit is active in thinking*, the favorite being that thinking is a chemical electromagnetic process—in other words, the diving board produces the dive, and the diver is incidental.

If two photons must work to keep the mind coupled to its biological 3-space body, and if thinking is a spiritual activity done by a spiritual being, then thoughts are uniquely human creations. Once thought or spoken, do the thoughts then simply evaporate? Unfortunately not, which is why we are ultimately responsible not just for our acts but for the act of thinking our thoughts, which was what St. Paul meant when he stressed that our struggles are with *powers and principalities.* According to Paul Emberson, author of remarkable thoughts and books:

> All thoughts—not just universal truths, but also inaccurate thoughts, partial truths, erroneous concepts and so on—are etheric-electric entities.

101 John Hewitt, "How to create a mind, or die trying." ExtremeTech, December 7, 2012.

Not all of them possess the same potential, however. Passing thoughts, cursory ideas that arouse neither interest nor emotion, are of little consequence. But thoughts that are fashioned with great intensity by a powerful mind and communicated forcefully to a large number of people, are another matter.[102]

The at-a-distance AI doesn't really need a VR headset in order to get into your brain. Now that sensors and brain-computer interfaces (BCIs) are inside VR video games *and* the brain, being programmed by remote computers will feel pleasurable, not traumatic as in the days of MK-ULTRA. Nanosensors read your emotions so as to modify the settings to digitally match your mood and feelings. Some biometrics software can even read who you are ("computer vision") by the movement of your head.[103] Getting bored? The difficulty level is ramped up, and when you finally take a break, you are so dissociated from the real world that it seems vapid and flat. In this way, you know you are standing at the portal to addiction.

In relation to virtual reality (VR) and augmented reality (AR), there is the Sentient World Simulation (SWS)—*every individual a node with an avatar*—that I discuss in "Invisible Mindsets To Be Aware Of" (Appendix 1) as a favored end-run approach to Transhumanism, like Samsung's DigiTwins and Open AR Cloud. Whether you choose to believe in a digital copy of the real world when you point a camera at it and it either interacts with you or tells you everything about itself,[104] or that it is created by means of a technological Enochian dimensional communications system previously known as *necromancy,* and is called up by quantum tunneling in quantum computers like D-Wave,[105] the key to DigiTwin will be in a digital wallet. Whether that wallet is yours or another's remains to be seen.

Hundreds of millions of people spend their days and nights immersed in virtual environments. With the help of advanced nanosensors, AI, and communication technologies, it is possible to digitally replicate physical entities—people, devices, objects, entire systems and places—in an utterly real-seeming virtual world.

---

102 Paul Emberson, From Gondhishapur to Silicon Valley, Volumes I and II. The Etheric Dimensions Press, 2009. I also recommend Paul's 2013 Machines and the Human Spirit. The books are not easily acquired.

103 Robert Wheeler, "Brain-Computer Interfaces: Don't Worry, It's Just a 'Game'" and James Wright, "'AI' is being Used to Profile People From Their Head Vibrations—But Is There Enough Evidence To Support It?" Activist Post, May 24, 2021. See Robert Malech's 1974 patent #3951134, "Apparatus and Method for Remotely Monitoring and Altering Brain Waves."

104 Greg Nichols, "The urgent case for Open 'AR Cloud.' Why we need a digital copy of the real world." ZDNet, June 7, 2018.

105 Thanks to Anthony Patch for this insight.

In a 6G environment, through digital twins, users will be able to explore and monitor the reality in a virtual world without temporal or spatial constraints. Users will be able to observe changes or detect problems remotely through the representation offered by digital twins.[106]

Virtual characters (avatars) first arrive in our consciousness as TV and comic book cartoons, then graduate to more sophisticated VR game role-playing avatars, as in MMORPGs [massively (one million subscribers) multiplayer online role-playing games] or games like Neurable's Awakening in which tiny embedded EEGs and fMRIs scan your brain and by your thought make your avatar pick up objects and throw them.[107]

The problem is that we are so captivated / captured by the images (*imago*) taking up residence in our consciousness that we tend not to notice how sophisticated, intrusive, *and multidimensional* the VR technology is getting. Much like the people we castigate as being "primitive," we end up feeding our children to a technology we know next to nothing about in the name of *entertaining them* (enter + *teneo* means to hold between). For example, the VR "Teletubbies" cartoons: swarms of self-morphing machine creatures with mischievous personalities popping up from the Earth, then disappearing like gnomes, which behave a lot like the riddling, punning creatures that ethnobotanist Terence McKenna (1946-2000) experienced while tripping on DMT:

> You try to convince yourself that what you're seeing cannot be, but there it is. In the end, the truth of this horrible naked paradox overloads your neural circuitry, leaving you in an incoherent stupor. The whole event lasts less than fifteen minutes, and suddenly you're completely back to normal—relieved to find yourself back in the safe predictability of the "real" world.

Is Terence describing DMT-produced Toon-Town visions, or VR-tech avatars? Certainly, technology-as-drugs is going on, but given that the human brain naturally makes DMT, is VR technology up to something decidedly *quantum,* now that it has the aid of nanobots in the brain at its disposal? Are the VR techs dedicated to Transhumanist enhancement according to a triune brain model—bypassing the neocortex for the old reptilian and limbic complexes,[108] as drugs tend to do?

---

106 Anthony Cuthbertson, "6G Will Bring 'Digital Twins,' Samsung Says—And It's Two Years Ahead of Schedule." The Independent, 15 July 2020.

107 In 2014, Facebook paid $2 billion to buy the VR company Oculus Rift. Ever since, Facebook's secretive Building 8 has been hard at work. See Dennis Bray, Wetware: A Computer in Every Living Cell (Yale University Press, 2009).

108 Paul D. MacLean, MD (1931-2007), The Triune Brain in Evolution, 1990 (ideas promulgated in the Sixties and popularized by Carl Sagan's 1977 Pulitzer book The Dragons of Eden, then went black until the book in 1990).

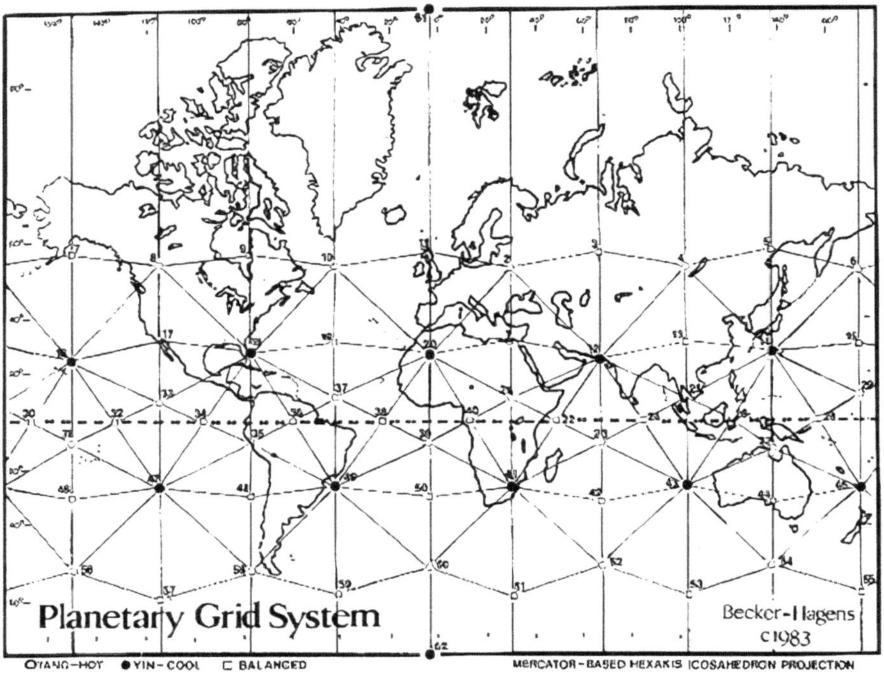

Planetary geomagnetic grid. Our planet (and therefore our bodies) is in a complex relationship with the magnetopause and magnetosphere (extending from 100 miles to 36,000 miles above the Earth). For the exact geomagnetic grid, see Bruce Cathie (1930-2013). This video shows how to build the world grid in Gridpoint Atlas and overlay it on Google Earth, https://www.youtube.com/watch?v=MTezuc2M4bc.

4
Magnetism

The advent of "Star Wars"
Radio biology & our cells
MATra (Magnet Assisted Transfection), electroporation, & magnetofection
Leylines & geomagnetic currents
The shadow biosphere
The magnetic Montauk puzzle

> *. . . it will be attempted from that side to use electricity and, notably, earth magnetism in order to produce effects over the whole Earth. I have pointed out to you that earth forces rise up into the entity I have called the Double, the Doppelgänger. The Americans will penetrate this secret. They will possess the secret of using earth magnetism with its north-south duality to broadcast controlling forces over the Earth, forces that will work in a spiritual way.*
>
> – Rudolf Steiner, *Individual Spiritual Beings Working in the Human Soul*, November 25, 1917

We are sandwiched between Space Fence infrastructure above the planet and on the ground, including the "chaff" metal nanoparticles sown by jets in the upper atmosphere and the non-ionized wireless radiation transmissions penetrating the atmosphere, our bodies and brains, and into the Earth's geomagnetic grid. Add to this that our entire civilization is dependent upon energy systems owned by plutocrat warlords: thermal, radiant, chemical, nuclear, electrical, magnetic, gravitational, biological, and now plasma. Few are aware of the large role that magnetism plays.

The Earth is a huge magnet wound around (because of the Earth's spin) with lines of force like those that connect us to our Sun and Moon (Birkeland currents). Magnetic currents enter our North Pole and exit our South Pole in these lines of force like a Tesla coil, close together but not touching or crossing each other. This is our magnetic grid, a lattice of interlocking lines of force. Everything on planet Earth, whatever its form, exists because of these magnetic lines of force.

> . . . a good analogy would be an ordinary machine-wound ball of string. The length of string has taken on the form of a ball, and at the same time has formed a cross-cross pattern . . . imagine a small vortex being created

at all the trillions of points where the lines of force cross each other in the lattice pattern. Each vortex would manifest as an atomic structure and create within itself what we term a gravitational field. The gravitational field, in other words, is nothing more than the effect of relative motion in space. Matter is drawn towards a gravitational field just as a piece of wood floating on water is drawn towards a whirlpool. The gravitational fields created by the vortexual action of every atom would combine to form a field of the completed planetary body.[1]

The advent of "Star Wars"

All EM has a scalar wave component. Remember [Thomas] Bearden referring to microwave poisonings at the US Embassy as scalar wave structured patterned effects, and the Woodpecker as not just an over-the-horizon radar but a scalar weapon. Think of the known transverse EM wave as surrounded by a pressure front called a polarization, of opposite densities on either side (indicative of direction of motion). In ordinary physics, microwaves preload energies into a metallic-laden system, and a pulse ignites the process to create a self-sustaining combustion.

– Richard Lawrence Norman, Facebook[2]

In the 1950s at the beginning of the Cold War, an electromagnetic signal was trained on the U.S. Embassy in Moscow. Three ambassadors fell prey to cancer, one with a rare blood disease entailing bleeding from the eyes. Embassy personnel had a 40 percent higher than average white blood cell count. Though the CIA finally "discovered" the genesis of the rays in 1962, the American public would not be informed until 1975 during the Frank Church Committee's exposure of the CIA's Cold War sins until upstaged by the nation's 1976 Bicentennial celebrations.

---

1 Bruce Cathie, *The Energy Grid: Harmonic 695: The Pulse of the Universe* (Adventures Unlimited, 1990). Cathie recommends reading Frank Scully's 1950 book *Behind the Flying Saucers* (Henry Holt and Co.) for the world grid and World War Two study of magnetism by means of the magnetic prospecting instrument known as the magnetron. Microwave ovens (now part of the IoT) have magnetrons in them.

2 See Norman's and J. Dunning-Davies' "Deductions from the Quaternion Form of Maxwell's Electromagnetic Equations," Journal of Modern Physics, 2020.

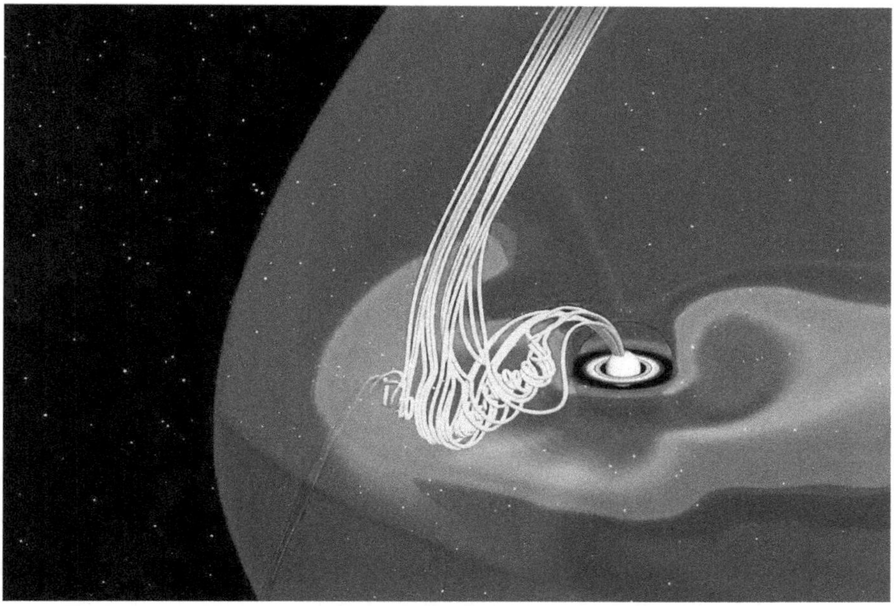

Birkeland currents ("magnetic ropes") between Saturn & the Sun.

From Chapter 9, "The Temple of CERN," *Under An Ionized Sky:* "Questions regarding Saturn abound. Why and how does Saturn emit more energy than it absorbs? Why do Saturn's rings make those eerie resonance sounds? Why are the rings separate? What are the objects caught up in the rings? From ancient lore, we might ask, *Is it true that hundreds of thousands of years ago Saturn was Earth's Black or Midnight Sun? Were Saturn, Mars, and Venus once in polar alignment with Earth, and if so, what event ended that alignment, causing them to "float away" to their present orbits?* Of NASA, I would ask, *Is the purpose to go to Saturn or to make Earth into a Saturn?* Shades of Immanuel Velikovsky (1895-1979)."

(See the 3.5-minute clip "Saturn's Cymatic Hexagram/Hexagon Frequency Bombardment," November 10, 2017, Lotus Sun.)

https://www.ucl.ac.uk/mathematical-physical-sciences/news/2016/jul/magnetic-rope-observed-first-time-between-saturn-and-sun

The Moscow signal expanded into a series of over-the-horizon (OTH) broadcasts (shades of the HAARP cover story) known as the *Soviet Woodpecker*, pulses measured at 10 Hz (cycles per second or cps) on 3-30 MHz bands. When the signal hit U.S. power grids, it was picked up by power lines and re-radiated into people's homes on light circuits. Radio and telecommunications were disrupted as unsuspecting brains were forced into sympathetic resonance. The CIA even sent a crack team of American scientists to install a 40-ton magnet (early SQUID?) capable of generating a magnetic field

250,000X more powerful than the Earth's magnetic field at the Gomel site.[3]

The Woodpecker was a scalar transmitter, and Tesla technological experimentation has been the name of the game ever since Tesla and his conscience were eliminated in 1943. As a quantum potential weapon, the Woodpecker is able to induce diseases by mimicking and re-creating their signatures or frequencies in the near-ultraviolet range. What this means is scalar waves can be made to penetrate the virtual particle flux that determines the genetic cell blueprint and induce disease (cell disorder).[4]

Bombardment of the U.S. Embassy in Moscow went on until 1992.[5] (Was the "experimentation" at the U.S. Embassy in Cuba really all that "mysterious"?)

The 1980 October Surprise election of Ronald Reagan and George H.W. Bush ushered in the "Star Wars" directed energy (DE) era. Congress upscaled weather modification funding to $20+ million. *Weather and magnetic fields* . . . The U.S. Air Force began building 299-foot Ground Wave Emergency Network (GWEN) towers with 330-foot radiating webs of copper wires just a few feet underground, 200 miles apart, so as to use VLF ground waves with about 2,000 watts of power. A nuclear emergency would easily knock the GWEN system out, so what were the towers really for? GWEN arrays can disrupt or alter the Earth's magnetic field within a 200-mile radius, and specific frequencies can be used to control whole populations.[6]

Magnetic anomalies like the South Atlantic Anomaly—said to be due to a reduced magnetic field intensity moving westward from the tip of Africa toward South America at 20 km/year—and the April 10, 2020 "bonkers" magnetosphere reading[7] make me wonder just what magnetic field / magne-

---

3 The 40-ton American magnet was believed to have been powered by the Chernobyl reactor. Do not forget that the 44-year Cold War was a CIA creation for the sake of secrecy and taxpayer support of the unseen development of the machinery of control we are now seeing all around us. Globalists supported the Soviet Union for 72 years, until the wall fell, just as they have supported China.

4 Thanks to Sine Nomine for this insight.

5 In late 2016 through early 2017, 24 U.S. diplomats in Cuba (and several Canadian diplomats) complained of hearing loss, loss of balance, and headaches. In late November 2017 through April 2018, at least two U.S. officials in Guangzhou, China complained of similar symptoms. Some of the diplomats and other employees now have mild brain damage and blood disorders; two may have permanently lost their hearing. Executive editor of Foreign Policy Sharon Weinberger, author of Imaginary Weapons: A Journey Through the Pentagon's Scientific Underworld, wrote, "The kind of weapon that does what the victims describe would defy the laws of physics; the danger of saying it's a sonic weapon is that you're focusing on the least likely explanation."

6 See Chapter 10, "Dual Use II: Pulsed Frequencies," for more, plus review Chapter 8, "Boots on the Ground," in Under An Ionized Sky.

7 See 3:40-6:30 in "Something strange occurred in the Solar System Last Night...and Earth REACTED To IT!" Mr.MBB333, April 10, 2020.

tosphere experiments are going on and if particle accelerators like CERN are involved.[8] According to the European Space Agency (ESA), "In the last two centuries, Earth's magnetic field has lost about 9 percent of its strength." Is this a natural sign of an imminent pole reversal ("Heads Up Cutting Through the BS Pole Shift Grand Solar Minimum Climate Chance," maverickstar reloaded, May 26, 2000), or geoengineered tampering?

Despite the 2014 date, U.S. Patent 9,491,911 B2, "Method for modifying environmental conditions with ring comprised of magnetic material," has been operant for two decades, "deploying a magnetic climate control material to a local area in the thermosphere and the exosphere"[9]—reflective, absorptive "nanopowders" (0.1-100 microns) fed into *a ring around the planet* by sounding rockets and tended by satellites "equipped with electromagnets." The 2002 paper "Earth Rings for Planetary Environmental Control"[10] recommending the creation of an artificial planetary ring around the Earth to "counter global warming" is referenced, followed by patent sketches of the Earth surrounded by a ring of nano-metals much like the Earth on the cover of *Under An Ionized Sky.*[11] The paper lists "climate change" woes we know all too well: increased warming, melting polar icecaps, frequency of cold waves, intense droughts and heat waves, frequent and severe floods, increased fires and wildfires, dangerous thunderstorms, more intense and destructive storms, tsunamis, volcanic activity, loss of biodiversity and increased animal extinction, strained ocean life, diminished food and water, spread of disease, and economic consequences.

This manmade metallic ring being added to the Earth's magnetic field allegedly extends 36,000 miles into space (inclusive of the magnetosphere amalgam of solar wind and Earth magnetic field). Both Bernard Eastlund (in his 1987 HAARP patent) and Robert O. Becker, MD, emphasized the close relationship between magnetism and *cyclotron resonance.*

> Cyclotron resonance is a mechanism of action that enables very low-strength electromagnetic fields, acting in concert with the Earth's geomagnetic field, to produce major biological effects by *concentrating the*

8 Media red flags like "strange" and "mysterious" generally point to geoengineered experiments, like "Strange seismic waves were picked up circling the globe on November 11 [2018]. Now seismologists are trying to figure out why"; and New Zealand Herald, November 29, 2018, "...the planet rang like a bell, maintaining a low-frequency monotone as it spread."

9 The thermosphere ranges from 53-56 miles above the Earth's surface to 311-621 miles beyond to where the exosphere begins.

10 Presented by Star Technology and Research at the 53rd International Astronautical Congress.

11 See YouTube "There's a Detectable Human-Made Barrier Surrounding Earth," BBC, 5 April 2018.

energy in the applied field upon specific particles, such as the biologically important ions of sodium, calcium, potassium, and lithium.[12]

Major biological effects . . .

Radio biology & our cells

Every cell in our bodies is bathed in an external and internal environment of fluctuating invisible magnetic forces that affect every cell and circuit of our biology. As Becker stated in *Cross Currents,* "All biological cycles are directly related to the planet's magnetic field (which averages about 1/2 gauss, with a daily change in strength of less than 0.1 gauss—compared to a refrigerator door magnet at 200 gauss strength)."[13] Every living being emits radio waves, and every cell is an electromagnetic resonator emitting and absorbing high-frequency radiation. Each cell's nucleus has its own oscillating frequency. New Zealand mathematician and pilot Bruce Cathie (1930-2013) wrote:

> The geometric makeup of the cell causes it to act as an electric circuit which has self-inductance and capacity. The natural oscillation of energy in the cell I believe to be due to the constant interaction of the matter and antimatter cycle[14] . . . A pendulum-like pulsing occurs between the physical and non-physical substances [cyclotron resonance]. When stronger radiations are imposed upon the cell by outside influences, then the natural rhythm of the cell is affected and it begins to break down. If the radiation [frequency] of the cell can be restored to its original rhythm, then it will resume its healthy state.[15]

Add to this picture the insight of Belarusian-French scientist Georges Lakhovsky (1869-1942): that our cells are connected to the frequencies of the cosmos.

> We have seen that living cells possess oscillating circuits constituted by filaments. Now all these cells are set in motion in space, impelled by the motion of the earth, at a velocity of 27 kilometres per minute at the Equator. The question is in what particular field do these cells revolve? Evidently

---

12 Robert O. Becker, Cross Currents: The Perils of Electropollution, The Promise of Electromedicine. Penguin, 1990, pages 234-239.

13 Electrical fields are described in kilovolts per meter (kV/m) whereas magnetic fields are described in Gauss (G or Gs).

14 Cathie maintains that matter is made up of matter and antimatter pulsing at 144,000 cps, Time being the variable of our reality's geometrics. Dimensions are infinite; in 1998 we were only aware of 15.

15 Bruce Cathie, The Energy Grid: Harmonic 695 – The Pulse of the Universe (Adventures Unltd., 1990).

> not in the terrestrial electromagnetic fields, since these fields are swept along at the same time as the cells by the same rotatory motion. The cells revolve in variable electromagnetic fields generated by a source external to the earth, that is to say within the field of atmospheric radiations comprising a complete range of frequencies as typified by cosmic radiations emanating from the sun, the Milky Way and the immensity of celestial space.[16]

Up until our electromagnetic era, our physiological rhythms and collective behaviors synchronized with solar and geomagnetic rhythms. Disruptions of these fields have led to disruption of our health, behavior, and ability to reason.

> So far, the actual effects [of magnetic field exposure] are not known, although the strength at which magnetic fields are thought capable of influencing biological functions may be as low as 1 Gauss. *Magnetic fields are not attenuated within the body, and also will tend to induce currents within the body, so their effects might be construed as being of more significance than electric fields* . . . [T]he detection of weak magnetic gradients can explain the "art" of dowsing in humans (Rocard, 1964).[17] (Emphasis added.)

Magnetometers are used to measure slight or extreme deviations in the Earth's magnetic field—from the signatures of mountains, rivers, streams, lakes, and plains, to disturbances created by underground geological features (upthrust dykes, fault lines, caverns, mineral deposits, fracking wells, tunnels, underground bases, etc.). Either on the ground or from satellite, magnetometers like SQUID (superconducting quantum interference device) and MEG (magnetoencephalograph) neuroimaging scanners and nano-sized MEMS magnetic field sensors read *the lines of force that surround the human head and body.*

Experimentation now being open field and *in vivo*, millions of brain experiments are being run simultaneously via satellite, tower triangulation, and 5G / IoT as we daily breathe in trillions of MEMs, NEMs, nanobots, and conductive metals like *magnetites* and other iron oxides needed for *remote* transcranial magnetic stimulation (TMS) and deep brain stimulation (DBS). (See Chapter 11, "Dual Use III: The 'Air Loom' Hospital.")

> By injecting magnetic nanoparticles into the brain, researchers have found that they can manipulate neurons by applying external magnetic fields . . . A team at MIT has been exploring the potential of magnetism to do

---

16 Georges Lakhovsky, The Secret of Life, 1935. Lakhovsky recommended using spiral loops of copper wire to set up electromagnetic fields harmonically tuned to the life forces. He invented the multiple wave oscillator (wavelengths 10 cm to 400 meters).

17 Chris A. Rutkowski, "The Tectonic Strain Theory of Geophysical Luminosities," 1984. Rutkowski's paper is in response to the tectonic strain theory of Michael A. Persinger, PhD.

away with the wires or implanted electrodes typically associated in DBS . . . The researchers developed a system that involves an injection of iron oxide particles that are subjected to an external alternating magnetic field . . . [P]articles capable of deep penetration of brain tissue and rapidly heat up under the influence of the magnetic fields, stimulating nerve cells.[18]

Regarding magnetites, in Israel researchers have confirmed "the abundant presence in the human brain of (Fe3O4) nanoparticles that match precisely the high-temperature [iron oxide-rich] magnetite nanospheres formed by combustion and/or friction-derived heating, which are prolific in urban, airborne particulate matter (PM)."[19] Entering first through the nose and then the olfactory nerve, nanoscale magnetite particles respond to external magnetic fields *but are toxic to the brain.*

Prof. David Allsop, an Alzheimer's disease expert at Lancaster University and part of the research team, said: There is no blood-brain barrier with nasal delivery. Once nanoparticles directly enter olfactory areas of the brain through the nose, they can spread to other areas of the brain, including hippocampus and cerebral cortex—regions affected by Alzheimer's disease. He said it was worth noting that an impaired sense of smell is an early indicator of Alzheimer's disease.[20]

Through our noses, we breathe in a constant aerial delivery of iron oxides like magnetite, coated with biological polymers to assure the loading of nucleic acids to assure ionic binding that will guarantee that our bodies and brains interact with external manmade magnetic fields.[21] Once again, we are looking at nanometals that ensure we are conductive to remote manipulation.

MATra (Magnet-Assisted Transfection), electroporation, & magnetofection

MATra weapons, magnet-assisted transfection via calcium-gated channels using focused cyclotron resonance[22] *– the same "silent weapons for quiet wars" used in cell towers, cell phones, WIFI, smart meters, microwave ovens, store*

18 Suzanne Hodsden, "MIT Researchers Develop Wireless, Noninvasive Deep Brain Stimulation Approach." MedDevice Online, March 17, 2015.

19 Barbara A. Maher et al. "Magnetite pollution nanoparticles in the human brain." Proceedings of the National Academy of Sciences (PNAS), September 27, 2016.

20 Damian Carrington, "Alzheimer's-linked nanoparticles, found in pollution, are showing up in people's brains." The Guardian, September 6, 2016.

21 Douglas Main, "Potentially Toxic Magnetic Nanoparticle Pollution Found in Human Brains." Newsweek, September 5, 2016.

22 See "Electron Cyclotron Resonance," dumbbell33, November 18, 2009, https://www.youtube.com/watch?v=srb02o3F2gs.

security, court scanners, court clerk scanners, airport scanners, jail scanners, "nonlethal" truck-mounted "access denial" Systems, Hospital MRI, X-Ray, Mammogram, Ultrasound, etc.

– Sine Nomine, Facebook, 2020

I have said repeatedly that our atmosphere is now ionized and loaded with *compressed plasma* (like clouds) all the way to the electrified surface of the planet and suspended in a condition of magnetic resonance, thanks to all the Space Fence lockdown infrastructure. "Caged" Na, Al, and C pathogens can now be *remotely transfected* into the cells of living organisms, especially human beings slated for cyborg Transhumanism.

Transfection is basically the process of introducing nucleic acids (like bacteria-mediated DNA transfers) into cells. (*Transduction* refers to virus-mediated DNA transfer.) Transfection is how genetically modified organisms (like GMO foods, Morgellons, etc.) are produced, whether the DNA is transfected *in vitro* in the lab or *in vivo* via frequency transmission[23]: "By applying magnetic force, the full nucleic acid dose is rapidly drawn towards and delivered into the target cells, leading to efficient transfection."[24]

In a lab, the nucleic acid (DNA) solution would be "incubated" over a Universal Magnetic Plate (magnetic field), but in open field *in vivo* transfection, reagent magnetic nanoparticles like magnetite would work, as would carbon nanotubes (CNTs) of graphene oxide (GO) with which the COVID-19 hydrogel "gene therapy" is loaded.[25] "Combining nanotechnology and magnetic forces to improve intracellular delivery of nucleic acids" for mass scale Transhumanist experimentation on GMO "hybrids" needs "external man-made magnetic fields" and *in vivo* magnetic nanoparticles.[26]

In the YouTube "'MATra' Weapons – Magnetic Assisted Transfection," Ron Johnson even makes a case for how MATra might be made to work in neighborhoods via cell towers:

---

23 Christian Plank et al., "The Magnetofection Method: Using Magnetic Force to Enhance Gene Delivery." Biological Chemistry, May 2003: "...While magnetofection does not necessarily improve the overall performances of any given standard gene transfer method in vitro, its major potential lies in the extraordinarily rapid and efficient transfection at low vector doses and the possibility of remotely controlled vector targeting in vivo." (Emphasis added.)

24 "MATra: Magnet Assisted Transfection: A comprehensive manual," IBA Life Sciences, April 2012, www.magnet-assisted-transfection.com.

25 See Chapter 14, "The COVID-19 'Vaccine' Event."

26 See Patent # US20110130444 A1, "Methods and compositions for targeted delivery of gene therapeutic vectors"; and Jing Ma et al., "Drug-loaded nano-microcapsules delivery system mediated by ultrasound-targeted microbubble destruction: A promising therapy method," Biomedical Reports, July 1, 2013.

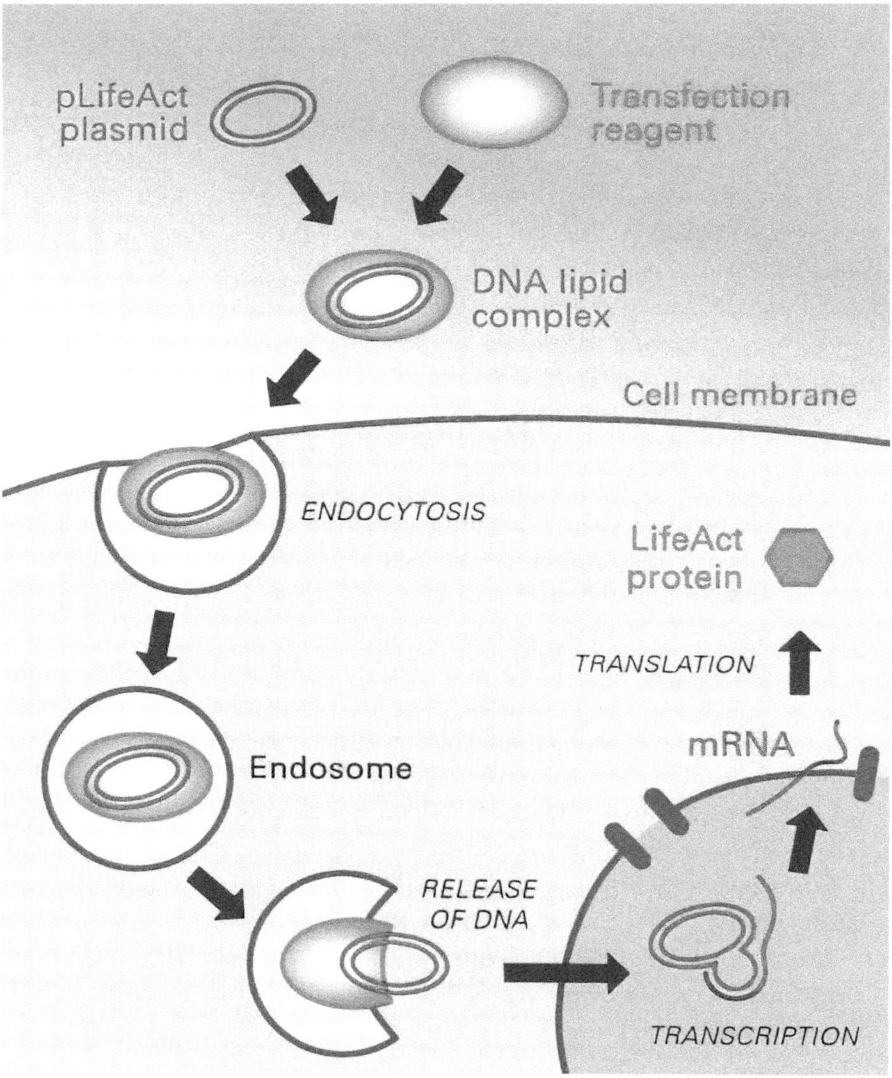

Transfection. "Transfer methods of getting genes into cells are *gene therapy*: injection into the cell nucleus with a tiny needle (microneedle transfection); plant cells soaked in DNA "stews," then electrically forced into the cell (electroporation); DNA attached to tiny metal particles (nanoparticles) and shot into cells (electroporation); engineer viruses or bacteria to infect cells with DNA." (Instead of LifeAct protein, think gain of function *Spike protein.*)

https://www.aun.edu.eg/molecular_biology/Procedure1/3%20Transformation.pdf

There have been numerous patents for nano-sized weapons that are triggered by the same electromagnetic waves that these towers produce . . . consisting of nano-microcapsules containing DNA or chemicals for transfection purposes—capsules smaller than dust that can enter your cells, then release DNA or chemicals that can turn you into a GMO, a genetically modified organism! So now instead of modifying your vegetables and fruits into GMOs, they are turning people into GMOs.

These nano-microcapsules can be delivered into populated areas by chemtrails, car exhaust, pesticide smoke, water systems or in any liquids, etc. People will then breathe these nano-capsules in or drink them or rub them into their skin and eyes. Then these capsules can be activated through the electromagnetic waves that these cell towers produce. These nano-capsules contain DNA or chemicals. With this type of bioweaponry in place, a virus outbreak can be faked for a specific neighborhood or city, or even race or gender, and no one would ever know how it happened.[27]

In 2016, the *Guardian* announced Magneto, "a magnetized protein that activates specific groups of nerve cells from a distance," thanks to *optogenetics, chemogenetics*,[28] and *magnetogenetics*, which dispenses with the need for a "multi-component system":

Magneto can remotely control the firing of neurons deep within the brain, and also control complex behaviors. Neuroscientist Steve Ramirez of Harvard University, who uses optogenetics to manipulate memories in the brains of mice, says the [magnetogenetics] study is "badass."

"Previous attempts [to use magnets to control neuronal activity] needed multiple components for the system to work—injecting magnetic particles, injecting a virus that expresses a heat-sensitive channel, [or] head-fixing the animal so that a coil could induce changes in magnetism," he explains. "The problem with having a multi-component system is that there's so much room for each individual piece to break down . . ."[29]

27 Ron Johnson, "'MATra Weapons – Magnetic Assisted Transfection," April 23, 2016. Transcript of [https://www.youtube.com/watch?v=qNE-DXSInJc] at http://cover-upz.blogspot.com/2016/04/matra-weapons-magnetic-assisted.html. Shades of CoVid-19 and Wuhan.

28 Optogenetics switches related neurons on and off with pulses of laser light; chemogenetics uses engineered proteins activated by "designer drugs" to target specific cell types.

29 Mo Costandi, "Genetically engineered 'Magneto' protein remotely controls brain and behavior." Guardian, 24 March 2016.

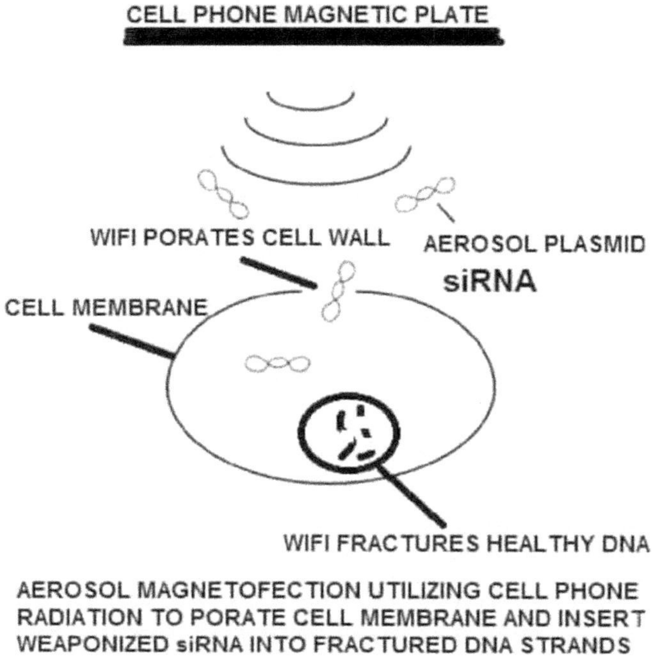

MATra. Magnetofection (magnet-assisted transfection or MATra) via cell phone radiation (4G Plus / 5G).

Better by far than injections and "head-fixing" (DBS, EBS, etc.) are nerve cell proteins sensitive to radio waves and magnetic fields and able to remotely attach themselves to the magnetite nanoparticles being delivered by chemtrails, GMO foods, and vaccines. The Magneto current travels through the cell membrane, then the nerve impulses make their way into the spinal cord and up to the brain. As neuroscientist Steve Ramirez put it, *Badass.*

Perhaps as "badass" as the magnetized Spike protein?

Electroporation is more of the same: the application of an electric field to cells in order to increase the permeability of the cell membrane to allow chemicals or DNA to be introduced (and includes bypassing the blood-brain barrier). Andrew Kaufman, MD, in an interview with journalist Spiro Skouras, is more blunt: electroporation electroshocks the vaccine site to force DNA into cells. This must be how targeted individuals are implanted at a distance with micro-implants in preparation for delivering chemicals, pharmaceuticals, vaccines, and genetically modified pathogens *du jour* to entire populations.[30]

30 D.C. Chang et al., "High efficiency gene transfection by electroporation using a radio-frequency electric field." Biochimica Biophysica Acta, April 17, 1991.

Magnetofection is far superior to the lipofection transfection often used with cells in that it employs *superparamagnetic iron oxide nanoparticles (SPIONS)* for delivery. SPIONS have unique magnetic characteristics and, once their surface is modified by polyethylenimine, are able to smoothly deliver plasmic DNA into mammalian cells.[31] This is the likeliest delivery candidate behind the COVID-19 gene therapy injection that left the inoculated with magnetic reactions.

In Chapter 11, "The 'Air Loom' Hospital," several device-dependent approaches to brain control are discussed: electronic brain stimulation (EBS), deep brain stimulation (DBS), transcranial magnetic stimulation (TMS), and trigeminal nerve stimulation (TNS). *Magnetothermal stimulation* (often called magnetothermal deep brain stimulation) is more of the same but not dependent upon devices, unless you count the magnetite now in our brains. It entails sensitizing target neurons so they heat up, then attaching magnetic nanoparticles to them. Apply external alternating magnetic fields and superparamagnetic nanoparticles warm up, open an ion channel, and activate the neuron. This approach is supposedly "noninvasive," meaning no electrodes or minute fiber optic cables are applied to the brain, but what about the magnetite and remote radio waves?

> . . . genetically and spatially targetable, repeatable and temporarily precise activation of deep-brain circuits without the need for surgical implantation or any device.[32]

Neurocircuitry already mapped in the 1990s means that 30 years later, emotions and behaviors are easily remotely manipulated as "artificial senses" are imposed.[33]

What impact do the massive cables laid in the Earth for the Internet have on the Earth's geomagnetic grid? Go to Nicholas Rapp's interactive world map and see: *https://nicolasrapp.com/studio/wp-content/uploads/2017/10/world_map_internet.jpg.*

Leylines & geomagnetic currents

It is well known that Fe3O4 (magnetite) is in animals that depend upon the Earth's magnetic field for navigating and migrating. Therefore, it should

31 Fatin Nawwab Al-Deen et al., "Superparamagnetic nanoparticle delivery of DNA vaccine." Methods in Molecular Biology, 2014.

32 Rahul Munshi et al., "Magnetothermal genetic deep brain stimulation of motor behaviors in awake, freely moving mice." eLife, August 15, 2017.

33 Luke Dormehl, "Scientists use magnetism 'mind control' to make a mouse move around." Digital Trends, August 18, 2017.

be no surprise that magnetic nanoparticles in the human body and brain are used for tracking various effects in a human body and brain, such as effects following COVID-19 gene therapy. Also of interest to the Big Pharma / geoengineering alliances would be the effects of different drug batches in different bodies living in different geomagnetic regions, especially in the connection between electric and magnetic fields and consciousness—from moods and intentions to psychic abilities, telekinesis, "ghost" and UFO sightings ("unidentified aerial phenomena"). As psychologist Michael Persinger, PhD (1945-2018), noted in 1977, "Transient and unusual phenomena should occur in areas where tectonic stress is accumulating."[34]

Chemical trails can be made to follow maps of torsion fields, ancient ley-lines, and tunnels connecting underground cities. Meanwhile, the conductive nanoparticles in our bodies and brains can be remotely made to influence our torsion field consciousness (and vice versa), given that human beings are biomagnetic transceivers and the air a dielectric conductor. Think of the atmosphere as a Schumann resonance bell previously rung by solar flares but now subject to HAARP technology. Solar flares, sunspots, solar (plasma) wind, the solar minimum, and Earth's brainwaves,[35] all manipulated for economic warfare, ritual events, and Transhumanist hybridization, disease distribution, etc.

It should come as no surprise that Europe's ancient megalithic stone circles emit high and low levels of radiation and ultrasound, their placement having been calibrated to correlate with earth energy. Primitive superstition? Hardly. We would do better to try to harness (and communicate with?) natural forces offering free energy. For millennia if not millions of years, ancient world grid magnetic lines of force have been cosmic energy generators along which astronomy centers, pyramid transceivers, roads, cathedrals, forts and military bases, nuclear installations, particle accelerators, etc., have been meticulously laid, with magnetrons now taking the place of dowsers probing geomantic alignments like the one from Mexico City to Mount Carmel in Israel and

- The mouth of the Mississippi River in New Orleans, LA, site of HAARP-driven Hurricane Katrina, August 23-31, 2005
- Atlanta, GA with the open lattice pyramid under an obelisk on top of the Bank of America Plaza skyscraper

---

34 Michael A. Persinger and Ghislaine Lafreniere, Space-Time Transients and Unusual Events. Chicago: Nelson-Hall, 1977. Persinger was director of Laurentian University's Consciousness Research Laboratory.

35 Drs. J.W. Koch and W.M. Beery, "Observations of Radio Wave Phase Characteristics on a High-Frequency Auroral Path." Journal of Research of the National Bureau of Standards, Section D: Radio Propagation, 66D.3: 291-296, May-June 1962. By reading the magnetic H Wave (the psycho-active component), it was determined that the Earth's brainwaves at that time were identical to human brainwaves.

- Washington, D.C.
- Baltimore, MD
- Philadelphia, PA
- New York City
- Boston
- Nova Scotia – Belfast – London – Brussels - Kosovo[36]

How much do grid manipulators influence us by controlling these cosmic lines of force? How many wars and revolutions have been sparked along strategic geomagnetic alignments? Grid manipulators from *vortexmaps.com*:

- Fermilab: Greenland and Teotihuacan (Chicago particle accelerator)
- Triumf: Greenland and Kiribati[37] (Vancouver, BC particle accelerator)
- DESY: Magnetic North and Giza (Hamburg, Germany particle accelerator)
- CERN: Greenland and Giza (French-Swiss border particle accelerator)
- EISCAT 3D: Magnetic North and Giza (Norway Ionospheric heater)
- Arecibo: Greenland and Cuzco (Puerto Rico ionospheric heater)
- HAARP: Magnetic North and Kiribati (Gakona, AK ionospheric heater)
- HIPAS: Magnetic North and Olgas, Australia (Fairbanks, AK observatory)
- Poker Flats: Magnetic North and Olgas, Australia (Alaska rocket range)[38]
- Millstone Hill MISA: Giza and Kiribati (Westford, MA steerable antenna)
- NCAR: HAARP/Triumf/Teotihuacan (Boulder, CO atmospheric research R&D)
- SRI International: Magnetic North and Greenland (Menlo Park, CA R&D)
- SuperDARN: Kashina (Mongolia and Kiribati); Kansai/Kobe (Magnetic North and Olgas); Yamagawa (Tibet and Teotihuacan); Okinawa (Giza and Kiribati); Goose Bay (Greenland and Cuzco); Iceland (Magnetic North and Giza); Kapaskasing (Greenland and Teotihuacan); Saskatoon (Magnetic North and Teotihuacan); Antarctic (Giza and Kiribati). 30 low-power HF radars in collaboration between Vir-

36 London was once the early Roman town of Londinium, back when Roman soldiers worshipped Mithras. Roman ground level is now seven meters below modern London. The ancient Temple to Mithras (mithraum) has been refurbished by Michael Bloomberg (https://www.londonmithraeum.com/about/). The Western Christmas blends the feast of Saturnalia with the birthday of Mithra on December 25.

37 32 Micronesian atolls and reef islands; Midway Island falls on this line, as well.

38 HAARP, HIPAS, and Poker Flats work as a unit.

ginia Tech (lead institution), Dartmouth College, University of Alaska Fairbanks (UAF), and the Johns Hopkins University Applied Physics Laboratory (JHU/APL)[39]

Note how extensive Virginia Tech's SuperDARN (Super Dual Auroral Radar Network) grid is—much like its successor the Space Fence being far more than one installation in the Kwajalein Atoll.

The shadow biosphere

> *Basically, pharmaceuticals are the new big business. They are what Big Oil used to be. However, above pharmaceuticals is biotech, and above biotech is nanotech, and above that—well, that's what's happening at Skinwalker.*
>
> - Ryan Patrick Burns, *Skinwalker & Beyond*, 2011

The invisible vortices created by crossing magnetic lines of force are called *torsion fields*,[40] pure fields of coherent force defined by India's chief nuclear scientist Paramahamsa Tewari as a state of vacuum in rotation. In fact, with just a narrow stream of water and a crystal plate, a torsion field and torus or "donut"[41] of glowing plasma can be created without powerful electromagnetic fields or a vacuum.[42] While the plasma torus was taking shape, nearby cell phones went static ballistic because the plasma ring was emitting distinct radio frequencies.

Clues as to how torsion fields affect us emotionally may lie in the many leyline / crossroads stories about spirits and deals with the devil, like the troll under the bridge over a moving river of energy in the nursery tale "The Three Billy Goats Gruff," and American blues man Robert Johnson's song "Cross Road Blues":

> *I went down to the crossroads and fell down on my knees,*
> *Asked the Lord up above for mercy, save poor Bob if you please.*

---

39 The Sura Ionospheric Heating Facility in Russia (56.13°N / 46.10°E) is not included in this list of grid manipulators, but is active. Sura's ERP (effective radiated power) is 190 MW, HAARP's is 5,000 MW. Other known ionospheric heaters in Russia are at Tula, Khabarovsk, and Novosibirsk, where the mind-control cult Ashram Shambala was founded in the 1980s.

40 Also called axion field, spin field, spinor field, microlepton field. labeled "pseudo-science," vacuum in rotation is free energy. See YouTube "8 minutes of enlightenment (38) – Torsion Fields," Andrew Mount, September 28, 2017.

41 The yin-yang symbol is a toroid. A torus is contraction-expansion in balance due to vacuum energy fluctuations.

42 *Robert Perkins, "Engineers create stable plasma ring in open air." Phys.org, November 15, 2017.

Those investigating the relationship between rotating magnetic fields and strain-related luminous phenomena ("earth lights") use Geiger counters, methane detectors, infrared sensors, and RF detection equipment loaded with amplifiers and oscilloscopes. They pay attention to lunar tidal cycles, railroad tracks laid in alluvial soil, power lines stretching for miles, the colors of released lights, the radon gas creating ionized pockets of air that seemingly produce plasma orbs, and the effects on the humans living nearby, including UFO sightings and subsequent psychological / physiological effects.

And what of another hidden world known as the *shadow biosphere* among astrobiologists? In 2006, the decision to go public about the shadow biosphere followed the release of a paper by Carol Cleland, PhD, of Colorado University's astrobiology center, and her colleague Shelley Copley in the *International Journal of Astrobiology*. "The idea is straightforward," Cleland explained, "on Earth we may be co-inhabiting with microbial life forms that have a completely different biochemistry from the one shared by life as we currently know it."[43] Astrobiologists Chris McKay (NASA Ames Research Center) and Paul Davies (Arizona State University) call it "weird life."[44]

> "All the micro-organisms we have detected on Earth to date have had a biology like our own: proteins made up of a maximum of 20 amino acids and a DNA genetic code made out of only four chemical bases: adenine, cytosine, guanine and thymine," says Cleland. "Yet there are up to 100 amino acids in nature and at least a dozen bases. These could easily have combined in the remote past to create life forms with a very different biochemistry to our own. More to the point, some may still exist in corners of the planet."[45]

"Shadow biosphere" calls to mind the infrared photographs taken of "macroorganisms" by Orgone discoverer Wilhelm Reich, MD (1897-1957) and later by former U.S. Merchant Marine electronics officer Trevor James Constable (1925-2016) in the American Southwest desert.[46] Their photographs revealed lifeforms in various shapes and sizes, their bodies seemingly presenting as plasma and therefore invisible except in the infrared. The IR photos in Constable's 1976 book *The Cosmic Pulse of Life* look decidedly like

---

43 Robin McKie, "'Shadow Biosphere' theory gaining scientific support." The Observer, April 13, 2013.

44 David Toomey, Weird Life That Is Very, Very Different from Our Own. W.W. Norton & Co., 2014.

45 Robin McKie.

46 The ancient Vedas of India (far older than the 3,500 years often quoted) referred to the atmosphere and deep space as a "cosmic ocean" populated by large creatures and vimanas.

giant single-cell microbes (with close-set eyes) navigating our organic atmospheric sea, peering down at us in wonder—much like the pulsating diaphanous "bogies" that flocked around NASA space shuttles, not so much threatening as conscious orbs with a pet-like curiosity.

It is time to question old assumptions and cast our net of consciousness further toward the quantum threshold. The so-called Skinwalker[47] Ranch in the Uintah Basin at the edge of the Uintah and Ouray Indian Reservation in Utah stretches from east of Vernal to past Fruitland. In charge at The Ranch is Robert Bigelow of the National Institute for Discovery Sciences (NIDS) and Bigelow Aerospace Advanced Space Studies (BAASS),[48] with Dr. Colm Kelleher in charge of biological testing. Director of security and BAASS science-military liaison is retired Col. John B. "Penguin" Alexander (U.S. Army Special Forces, chief human technology, Army Intelligence Command, Los Alamos National Labs manager of non-lethal weapons, etc.). Alexander hired ex-military and Buffalo Soldier Freemasons skilled in Haitian Vodou ("voodoo") to deal with the psychic battles between whatever is manifesting at the "hot spot" Ranch and Fort Duchesne Uintah and Ouray shamans.

The Uintah Basin is a geomagnetic anomaly, possibly due to the presence of the mineral Gilsonite, "a soluable material in oil solutions such as CS2 or TCE (trichloroethylene)" (Wikipedia). Gilsonite (carbon, nitrogen, sulfur, and "volatile compounds") was discovered in the 1860s, but not until 1888 was Samuel H. Gilson able to pressure Congress into taking back 7,000 acres (28 km^2) from the Uintah and Ouray Indian Reservation so the mineral could be legally mined in underground shafts. Gilsonite resembles shiny black obsidian, but its shadow biosphere qualities may be more like the famed "black goo" (see Chapter 3). Gilsonite is only found in the Uintah Basin, Colombia, and Iran, and may account for Big Oil's presence on The Ranch.[49]

The Ranch is crowded with diaphanous shape-shifting Skinwalkers, hologram drones, UFOs dropping plasma from their hulls, flashing lights (red, white, and blue), and strobing laser weapons. The question is, how much is military holographic interface with tectonic stress and leyline highways, and how much is actual shadow biosphere? David Gessner drops a clue in his *Mother Jones* article:

> I started seeing UFOs, something I had never really ever seen before. The most peculiar thing is many of the odd situations came about around elec-

---

47 In Navajo culture, a yee naaldlooshii (Skinwalker) is a witch able to turn itself into, possess, or disguise itself as an animal.

48 Bigelow Aerospace in 2011 was second in scope only to NASA.

49 David Gessner, "How Big Oil Seduced and Dumped This Utah Town." Mother Jones, March 19, 2013.

> tronics, especially manifested through cell phones. I rested quite a bit on the couch and noticed my phone would heat up when near my foot. Not a big deal, until I noticed my phone actually showed it was charging . . .[50]

"Near his foot" indicates a particularly powerful geomagnetic field, like gravitational anomalies at "mystery spots" around the United States—or is a SQUID magnetometer buried at Skinwalker?[51]

While it is true that geomagnetics can influence the human mind to see what may not normally be visible,[52] geomagnetics can also be exploited to produce electromagnetic effects, like making multiple witnesses see the same thing.

The magnetic Montauk puzzle

> *In the Arabian Tales I read how genii transported people into a land of dreams to live through delightful adventures. My case was just the reverse. The genii had carried me from a world of dreams into one of realities. What I had left was beautiful, artistic and fascinating in every way; what I saw here was machined, rough and unattractive… 'Is this America?' I asked myself in painful surprise. 'It is a century behind Europe in civilization.' When I went abroad in 1889 – five years having elapsed since my arrival here – I became convinced that* [America] was more than one hundred years AHEAD of Europe, *and nothing has happened to this day to change my opinion.*
>
> – Nikolai Tesla

During the lead-up to the Manhattan Project, a story circulated about how in 1940 a small ship and a tender ship—one for power, the other driving Tesla coils—had *disappeared and re-appeared* in the Brooklyn Naval Yard. No crew had been on board, but the experiment had been observed by both Nikola Tesla and John von Neumann. Von Neumann had been mathematician David Hilbert's assistant at Göttingen University in 1927 when Hilbert, James Franck, and Max Born were running seminars on matter in Room 204. In fact, all the nuclear Manhattan Project primaries had spent time at Göttingen—Robert Oppenheimer, Edward Condon, Norbert Wiener, Robert Brode, M.A. Richtmyer, and Linus Pauling. Hilbert (1862-1943) devised infinite-dimensional Hilbert space, and mathematician Norman Levinson (1912-1975) developed the Levinson Time Equations in 1939.

---

50 Ibid.

51 For this section, thanks to Ryan Patrick Burns' book Skinwalker & Beyond (Lulu, 2011).

52 For example, how magnetic storms increase psychiatric hospital admissions because of the ELFs present in the micropulsations of the Earth's geomagnetic field connected to the brain.

The combination of Hilbert Space, von Neumann's brilliant calculations, and the advanced Levinson Recursion for multiple time series revives the question of whether the leading physicists and mathematicians of their day were the secret driving force behind something far more serious than a simple degaussing process to protect a ship like the *Eldridge* from magnetic mines. [53]

With the Manhattan Project under his belt and only in his forties, von Neumann would have been at Montauk if even half of what was propagated as public confusion was true. Tesla eventually abandoned the project, but at what point?

On July 22, 1943—six months after Tesla's death—the *USS Eldridge* and crew disappeared for 20 seconds. The crew came back disoriented and nauseous.

On August 12, 1943, the *SS Andrew Fursenth* (DE-173) and crew were rendered invisible. Those in the know about ancient Hindu science (such as Oppenheimer) called the process *antima.* Unlike the other ships, the DE-173 was teleported from the Philadelphia Naval Yard to the Norfolk-Newport News area and back again in minutes. Needless to say, things went terribly wrong for the crew.

In an annotated Varo edition of his book *The Case for the UFO* (1955), astronomer Morris K. Jessup (1900-1959) posited several theories as to why the brains of the crew members on board the DE-173 were fried: from electrically charged radar-cloaking paint and de-gaussing equipment to electromagnetic pulsing, cyclotrons, and cloud chambers. Degaussing makes things magnetically disappear from radar, but *electromagnetic pulsing...* [54]

On December 5, 1945, five Avenger torpedo bombers disappeared off the coast of Fort Lauderdale, Florida. Their proposed course had been 160 miles east toward Abaco Island, north 40 miles, then back to the naval air station. None of the Avengers returned to base, and no debris was found. The cover story was Atlantis and the Bermuda Triangle, but the question is, what happened magnetically? Did they disintegrate? Become quantum entangled in spacetime? disappear into a magnetic cloud? There were no satellites in 1945, but a pulsed harmonic transmission could have activated a unified field effect.

At the Gorda Cay turn north, the bombers were *3229.8793 minutes of arc from north grid pole. 53.8383° cosine 0.59016475 = reciprocal 1.69444.* Distance is not a determining factor when it comes to geomagnetic fields, but

---

53 Lionel and Patricia Fanthorpe, Chapter 7, "The Philadelphia Experiment," from Unsolved Mysteries of the Sea (Dundurn, 2004). Levinson has been wiped from science history, even to the point of obfuscating his name by calling him John Levinson.

54 On April 20, 1959, Jessup was found slumped over his steering wheel in a Dade County, Florida park, dead from carbon monoxide.

alignment relative to the fluctuating position of magnetic north (MN) is essential for Tesla transmissions of slugs of energy that can be made to create an electromagnetic force field powerful enough to distort the spacetime continuum.

Not only has the military drawn a veil over Tesla technology, but it has also shrouded the fact that Einstein finished his unified field theory of spacetime. Behind the unified field theory is the assumption that magnetic, electrical, gravitational, nuclear, thermal, plasmic, acoustic, and other radiative energies are neither decoupled, separated, nor broken down, but in a state of *mathematical geometric and harmonic unification.* Harmonic mathematics is the key to understanding quantum "spooky actions at a distance" (Einstein's term for quantum entanglement).

The harmonics of unified field theory yield the *GRID EQUIVALENTS OF MINUTES OF ARC OR NAUTICAL MILES*[55] –

> 160 miles, or 159.93256 =
> *138.8888 nautical miles = the harmonic 69.444 x 2 (twice the speed of light reciprocal)*
>
> 40 miles, or 39.983139 = 34.7222 nautical miles = 69.444 ÷ 2 (half the speed of light reciprocal)
> *165.583 statute miles for the return = 143.79577 nautical miles*

According to mathematical physicist James Clerk Maxwell (1831-1879), a magnetic field propagates at 0.4 of the speed of light, an electromagnetic field propagates at the speed of light, and an electric field propagates at the rate of c-infinity or throughout the universe instantaneously. The speed of light at the Earth's surface is 143,795.77 minutes of arc per magnetic grid second, or as we learn in high school travels at 186,282 miles (299,792 kilometers) per second.

But what is going on *geomagnetically* along the Atlantic Coast of the United States that seems to have enabled disappearing ships and airplanes from spacetime? Three sites come to mind:

> *Guantanamo Bay Naval Base, Cuba (longitude 75°W)*
>
> *Brookhaven National Laboratory, Long Island, New York (longitude 72°W)*
>
> *Montauk Air Force Station, Long Island, New York (longitude 71°W)*[56]

55 I owe the little knowledge I have of harmonics to New Zealander mathematician and pilot Bruce Cathie's books, which I had to read three times each in order to understand the little I do.

56 The longitude of the Arecibo Observatory (ionospheric heater) in Puerto Rico is 66.75°W.

As I said above, distance is not a determining factor when it comes to geomagnetic fields, so it is interesting that a massive American electromagnetic transmission station in West Australia (WA) on the northwest cape of the Exmouth peninsula is Montauk's primary generating facility for the electromagnetic force fields its operations require. The Exmouth-Montauk great arc alignment depends upon a fourth plot point of the interpolated Time position of magnetic north (MN).

> In the early hours of 1 May 1995, a major fireball flew in a north-north-easterly direction towards Perth, WA, and detonated above the eastern side of the city at approximately 2.00 am in a huge explosion. Limited Australian press coverage of this event defined it as a meteor fireball. Unfortunately, too many such fireballs fly around our night skies, exhibiting exotic flight behaviour and a preference for the first of May each year.
>
> This Perth event has been described in more detail in Part 1 of this "Bright Skies" series (see NEXUS 4/03, April-May 1997), where I present evidence for the non-natural origin of this event and suggest that it represents an EM weapons incident . . . The megatonne-force level of this explosion woke up over half a million people and demonstrated that Perth could have been obliterated at the flick of a switch . . . I strongly suspect it was pointing out that WA hosts a huge US-controlled EM weapons system at Exmouth in the northwestern part of WA, and that we should wake up and bring order to our own house - or face the consequences.
>
> The trajectory of this fireball suggests an origin in Enderby Land, Antarctica, where a number of Japanese and Russian bases are located.[57] The fireball flew on towards the Kamchatka Peninsula where a huge Russian (former Soviet Union) EM weapons complex / transmitter (Tx) site lies.[58]

Brookhaven National Laboratory (BNL) is 50 miles from Montauk Point, Long Island, New York, and is connected to Montauk by subterranean tunnels and chambers. Montauk is on land long considered sacred by the Montauk Indians due to the hyperdimensional portal passing into and through the Earth magnetic grid at that point, Montauk being the remnant of an undersea volcanic mountain with bedrock geologically separated from Long Island.

---

57 Disinformation or misinformation? "Subject to the constraints of the Antarctic Treaty System, the longest-held nation-state claimant rights in the territory is Australia, being a large part of its claimed Australian Antarctic Territory up to various high latitudes towards the South Pole." – "Enderby Land," Wikipedia

58 Harry Mason, "Bright Skies: Top Secret Weapons Testing? Part 5." Nexus magazine, Vol. 5 No. 1 (December 1997-January 1998). Entire series 1-5 worth reading.

Across from Fort Pond Bay at Montauk, the old World War Two Navy submarine base, is a separate, seemingly bottomless body of water issuing from an extinct lava tube. The preexisting underground network of tunnels and levels has been expanded over the years to as many as seven levels (US Army Corps of Engineers records), which means that Montauk and BNL basically sit on a huge resonant chamber. Thus esoteric technologies having to do with *sound weapons* have always been high on the Montauk-BNL experimental list, especially quantum waveforms like plasma that exist *outside* the telltale audio and electromagnetic wave spectrums.[59] Using seawater as an antenna, Montauk also may have been monitoring Soviet submarines based out of Norway, given that Montauk was involved in *cloaking* nuclear-armed submarines.[60]

Phoenix One ran from 1948 to 1968, when the derelict base was purportedly turned over to the General Services Administration as surplus. Until 1979, Phoenix Two was owned by the Krupp family and funded privately by ITT World-Wide Communications and the Nazi gold that had disappeared into France in 1944. Equally quietly, Montauk subsumed 25 other bases around the US with zero-time reference for similar covert radar operations.

With HAARP on board at Montauk since the 1990s, weather control has been superseded by state-of-the-art mind control psychotronics (brain-computer interface) in the Fort Pond Bay sector of the base. Psychotronics, superpowerful electrical fields, and plasma mean BNL and Montauk particle accelerators that can power particle beams for inter-dimensional experiments like locating and creating geomagnetic access points ("portals") around Montauk Point and Block Island Sound near Fishers Island off Mystic, Connecticut. Exotic particle beam radar systems can obtain quantum information wave packets for political leaders, scientists, dissidents, etc., by silently, invisibly entering the brain pan to scan and interrogate the mind.

Montauk's unique geomagnetic position has greatly contributed to perfecting sound for mind control programming. Music is a perfect carrier in that its emotional component serves to deeply enlist the victim's psyche and

---

59 Wilhelm Reich, MD, sent a radiosonde he designed to BNL for evaluation. It came with a DOR buster sensor modulator and transmitter, DOR being dead orgone, the result of orgone [æther] coming in contact with radioactivity. BNL was impressed and made a compact lightweight version to be carried by balloon since the radiosonde would not work near metal. This model not only busted DOR, but it also infused the environment with orgone by converting electrical energy into etheric energy via two frequencies, 403 MHz and 1680 MHz.

60 In the summer of 1955, only a few months after his appointment to the Atomic Energy Commission, von Neumann became ill with fast-acting cancer. His last public appearance came early in 1956 when, in a wheelchair at the White House, he received the Medal of Freedom from President Eisenhower. In April, he was taken to Walter Reed Hospital where he died on February 8, 1957—or was he moved to Montauk?

personality to commit to subliminal programming directions. Quantum plasma waveforms, being neither audio nor EM spectrum, can be "pocketed" inside music / sound to interact with human consciousness *and leave no trail.* But the pocketing needs vacuum tubes, which may have something to do with why most rock musicians and vocalists now swear by the tonal superiority of vacuum tube amps. Mengele used the 12-tonal scale for programming.

The so-called Montauk Chair may also exist. ITT Inc. with Mackay Marine in Southampton, Long Island built the original chair with three Tesla coils, an ISB receiver, and two ISB detectors—two outputs and one input. The outputs were tuned to the hyperdimensional windows at Montauk, 41°N latitude (same as Mt. Shasta), and a CRAY-1 computer pinpointed the harmonic necessary for transmission into and out of the hyperdimensional window. Coils XYZ were designed to modulate each other, with the ISB reception in a phantom phase lock loop that didn't need a carrier to lock onto the Delta white noise in the frequency window. From Southampton to Montauk was the perfect microwave length so the transmitter wouldn't interfere with the chair or be subject to incoming fields.

The second chair was also built by ITT Inc. but with RCA receivers designed for the Delta T function and standard XYZ Helmholtz coils. With these improvements, the chair could now be underground with the coils close to the chair and the leads to the three Tesla coils. They used the same IF detection with synchronized oscillators and the same ITT Mackay phantom-lock on the RCA receivers—six channels of output, upper and lower side bands, the coils phased to be insensitive to outside influences. What happened was almost as weird as the raven apparitions at Livermore Labs in the early 1970s[61]: a nauseous yellow-green "attachment" arose within the subject's aura, its tentacles streaming out like Medusa's hair—antennas grasping at everything.

It is commonly held that the last of the Montauk bases was shut down on August 12, 1983, but if so, it was by no means the end of Montauk. A deed was drawn up and New York State Park took over the surface Camp Hero,[62] Montauk Air Force Station, and even the old radar station, with the federal government retaining all rights to the property *beneath the surface.* Un-uniformed security personnel strolled around with automatic weapons, put-

---

61 Lynn Picknett and Clive Prince, The Stargate Conspiracy: The Truth about Extraterrestrial Life and the Mysteries of Ancient Egypt (Berkeley, 2001).

62 In the 2004 preprogramming film Eternal Sunshine of the Spotless Mind, the main character Joel, played by Jim Carrey (Mr. Truman's Show himself), catches a train to Montauk where he meets Clementine (Kate Winslet) who will eventually have her memory of him and their relationship erased. Efforts to film at Camp Hero State Park were quashed when officials threatened to charge exorbitant filming fees.

ting a damper on the wildlife park that never really opened to the public until September 18, 2002, supposedly due to environmental contamination. In the 1990s, new telephone lines and high-capacity power lines with a gigawatt meter on an equipment maintenance building were installed. After a Cardion Electronics particle beam radar unit was added to the Camp Hero bluffs, a LILCO meter reader indicated that a tremendous amount of electricity was being utilized *below.*

5

5G Wi-Gig & the Internet of Things (IoT)

The PFN/TRAC patent and the IoT / IoB
Coded tales & phased array antennas
The IoT / IoNT / IoB
Down to the cell level
6G & terahertz
AirGig & backscatter

Where will all the transmitter / cells be placed on the ground and in the air? Something is missing here. Is there another version of 5G we're not being told about? Is geoengineering of the atmosphere the means for tuning up space so 5G signals can be passed along without cells / transmitters?

– Jon Rappoport, "5G wireless: a ridiculous front for global control," April 3, 2018

5G is more than millimeter waves because it will encompass the entire 3,000 electromagnetic microwave spectrum of frequencies.

Smart Militarized Armaments in Residential Technology.

– Lena Pu

5G HAS BEEN SOLD AS a magical solution to improve coverage, enhance signaling, reduce latency,[1] spectral efficiency, wireless sensor connectivity, 1 GB per second simultaneity, 100 MG per second data rates, etc. But what is it, really? At the core, it is a profitable classic bait-and-switch for Smart City planetary lockdown—the bait being convenience and super-fast connectivity, the switch being a phased array antenna weapon system "smaller and lower-powered but clustered together and lower to the ground" (*Washington Post*).

The 5G system (28–100 GHz) was approved by the FCC on July 14, 2016 for "consumer devices" whose nonionizing radiation five years before was categorized by the World Health Organization (WHO) as Class 2B carcinogens. In February 2020, the FCC freed up 280 MHz of C-band spectrum for 5G use—one month after the COVID-19 drama began. Satellite operators had to "repack" their operations from the band's entire 500 MHz into

1 *Latency:* the delay before a transfer of data begins.

the upper 200 MHz so the lower 280 MHz could be just for terrestrial use.[2] It is true that by using extremely high frequency (EHF) millimeter bands in the millimeter watts (mmW) spectrum of 30-300 GHz, 5G guarantees high-speed downloads and high-speed point-to-point communications for truly private conversations. More importantly, however, 5G is responsible for *all* IoT monitoring—not only regulation of energy consumption via artificial intelligence (AI), but full spectrum dominance over the Earth *down to the molecular level.*

Lena Pu, whose professional history includes restoring sensitive environmental habitats for the U.S. Army Corps of Engineers, is environmental health consultant for the National Association for Children and Safe Technologies (*NACST.org*). As she points out in the quote at the beginning of this chapter, 5G encompasses 3,000 frequencies and should more honestly be called 297G.

2G	10 new frequencies (long microwave)
3G	10 new frequencies
4G	5 new frequencies
5G	3,000 new frequencies (short millimeter waves)

5G not only encompasses 2G, 3G, and 4G, but it is the gateway to modes of connectivity to 6G, 7G and 8G.

5G	IoT (Internet of Things), IoB (Internet of Bodies)
6G	satellite communications
7G / 8G	quantum (terahertz, molecular, nano, protons / electrons

Pu points out the early involvement of yet another Operation Paperclip scientist named Herman P. Schwan (1915-2005), "the founding father of biomedical engineering" who studied the dielectric properties of microwave radiation and their "pearl-chain effect" as they related to blood and water; wrote *Biological Engineering* (McGraw-Hill, 1969); and established the 1953 radiofrequency exposure guideline of 10,000,000 $\mu W/m^2$ (10 million micro-watts per square meter / 2 to 5 GHz) for the American National Standards Institute (ANSI) and Institute of Electrical and Electronics Engineers (IEEE), which, believe it or not, is still the same, despite thousands of studies and papers proving negative health effects, links between cell phones and brain

2 "5G-suitable C-band spectrum to be made available on an accelerated basis." Comms Update, 3 June 2020.

cancer, etc. Schwan is yet another connection to the Nazi obsession with artificial intelligence and "enhanced" superiors served by unenhanced inferiors.

Is wireless 5G the capstone?

Pu is known for her fresh blood membrane morphology (FBMM) studies proving that within 5-15 minutes in the presence of wireless microwave technology, healthy blood begins to become "sticky" and clump up as it "cooks." The coagulation is proof of electromagnetic rape and, eventually, murder.[3]

The PFN/TRAC patent and the IoT / IoB

Like most overarching systems today, the Internet of Things (IoT) is far more than meets the eye, just as the patent process is not what it seems at face value.[4] A relatively unknown 2,000-page patent (10.9 MB) legally protected under the U.S. Constitution, Art. 1, Sec. 8, Clause 8, is used to serve lawless ends.

US Patent 6965816, "PFN/TRAC System FAA Upgrades For Accountable Remote Robotics Control To Stop The Unauthorized Use of Aircraft and To Improve Equipment Management and Public Safety in Transportation"—awarded on November 15, 2005[5]—is a *stealth patent* similar to sly *omnibus bills* like the 1,000+-page National Defense Authorization Act (NDAA) first passed in 1961 and *still* being re-passed every year with new stealth provisos tucked in.[6]

PFN/TRAC is a Trojan horse hidden behind Hewlett-Packard's man Richard C. Walker covering for Robert S. Mueller's law firm Wilmer Hale LLP,[7] Hillary Clinton's Rose Law Firm, George Bush Sr., John Podesta, James Comey, Rod Rosenstein, Loretta Lynch, Eric Holder, Larry Summers—namely the Carlyle Group that enshrouds the Deep State Bush / Clinton / Obama cabal. Corporate players abound: IBM's Eclipse Foundation, Cisco, Microsoft, SAP, Oracle, Kleiner Perkins, Qualcomm, Goldman Sachs, JPMorgan, AT&T, Hewlett-Packard and its spinoff Agilent Technologies, etc.[8]

---

3 See Pu's 2019 presentation at the Silicon Valley Health Institute, "5G: Health Risks, Surveillance and Bioweaponry – Lena Pu (Sept. 2019)," October 18, 2019; and interview on the European blog show Nightflight, "Lena Pu – 5G & The Wuhan Debacle," February 19, 2020.

4 Control over the patent process means inventors ending up blocked or with nothing and criminal corporations and agencies, including NGOs, private consortiums, etc., ending up with everything.

5 Filings, however, go back to December 2, 1996.

6 Wikipedia: "In recent years each NDAA also includes provisions only peripherally related to the Defense Department, because unlike most other bills, the NDAA is sure to be considered and passed so legislators attach other bills to it."

7 Mueller was sworn in as FBI director seven days before 9/11.

8 In the early 2000s, outsider Leader Technologies' social networking source code—like Inslaw's PROMIS "back door" software in the 1990s—was stolen by insiders to be applied to

According to the thorough but brief chronology put together by investigative writer Dean Henderson, Hillary Clinton helped IBM Eclipse Foundation "steal key software from Leader Technologies which would eventually become Facebook,"[9] similar to how the U.S. Department of Justice stole Inslaw's PROMIS software in the early 1990s (covered in *Under An Ionized Sky*).

The PFN/TRAC patent begins with remote robotics and aircraft, but by the time you get to Column 3, lines 5-6, a much greater scope including human beings rears its head: the Internet of Things that "requires hardware, software, *and wet-ware (people)*." Throughout the patent's 2,000 pages and the additional patents "refining" the original, control over vehicles, ships, equipment, commerce, education, and people ("wet-ware") is legally, albeit obliquely, encompassed.

> QRS-11 crystal gyroscopes were sent from Little Rock [Gov. Bill Clinton / Hillary's Rose Law firm] to the NSA where they would prove key in the agency's encryption monopoly. They would soon be installed in everything from jumbo jets to cars to missile systems. With the ability to be turned on and off by their NSA controllers, the QRS-11 crystals would provide the basis for the Internet of Things.[10]

British Serco became the gatekeeper at the U.S. patent office, ever ready to obscure the true inventors and patent holders of the Internet of Things: the Highlands Group, the Pilgrim Society, the British Privy Council working inside the City of London Financial District, etc.

> PFN/TRAC has been put in place already at many levels and is being used to aggressively go in, take over, control, track and manage any system, whether it be an airplane, car, motorcycle, human being or animal. Human beings are called "wetware" in which control mechanisms, devices, nanochips, etc. are being put into bodies and brains . . .[11]

The CIA's disparaging term "wetware" says it all, doesn't it? Humanity and creatures are viewed simply as the IoT now known as the IoB (Internet of Bodies). We are to be "ionized and programmed on a highly individualized DNA basis with the hardware and software to create a completely integrated

the Internet of Things (IoT). Oracle is a big CIA contractor.

9 Dean Henderson, "Human Wetware & The 5G Computer Weapon," Henderson Left Hook, October 25, 2019. Also see Henderson's "Who's behind the 5G Cull of Humanity?" March 19, 2019.

10 Ibid.

11 "How They Plan to Control Everything in Your Life," Patriots For Truth / American Intelligence Media / Americans for Innovation. "Wetware," like "conspiracy theorist," is a CIA term.

and controllable 5G grid full spectrum dominance weapons system. Artificial intelligence would permeate the grid, seeking to self-replicate while turning humanity off."[12]

And so it is that as "telemedicine"[13] and "precision medicine" took center stage, the FCC approved a million small antennas that SpaceX Starlink needs for high-speed internet service from space.[14]

Coded tales & phased array antennas

Two strange, haunting anecdotes circulated urban myth-style long before citizen resistance and alternative media rose up against 5G. The two stories seem to have amalgamated into one around the "early retirement" of Apple's head of security John Theriault. First was the story of an Apple computer engineer drinking at a German beer garden in Redwood City in March 2010 who "lost control" of an iPhone 4S prototype later purportedly sold to Gizmodo for $5,000. Then there was the July 2011 disappearance of the same iPhone 4S prototype (in other versions, the 5G prototype) at the Cava 22 tequila lounge in the San Francisco Mission District, after which it was sold for just $200 on cheapo Craigslist, not slick Gizmodo.[15]

Creating and disseminating media gossip helps to create confusion for competitors and in the public mind while operating as *code* for insiders. Was it to confuse 4G and 5G iPhones, or reveal in code that both versions are more alike than we think in that both have phased array antennas and the functionality of both is enhanced with a new type of millimeter wave transmitter[16] that integrates antennas and electronics and allows for multiple transmitters and receivers on an integrated circuit chip (256 Quadrature amplitude modulation, 4X4 MIMO,[17] and 3X carrier aggregation)[18]?

---

12 Dean Henderson.

13 Kayla Matthews, "How IoT Is Enabling the Telemedicine Tomorrow." IoT For All, November 28, 2018.

14 Michael Sheetz, "FCC approves SpaceX to deploy up to 1 million small antennas for Starlink internet network." CNBC.com, March 20, 2020.

15 Yet another version says Apple security posing as police officers visited the "finder's" San Francisco home and offered cash for the return of the phone.

16 Millimeter waves use lenses for antennas to focus their millimeter photons, just like optical photons are focused by lenses. Thanks to "A quick background on the dangers from 5G millimeter-waves" by Trevor G. Marshall, PhD, Director of Autoimmunity Research Foundation, via Mobilfunk/Omega Group, n.d.

17 Multiple input – multiple output. With full duplex signaling, thousands of small digital beamforming cells are necessary because of the low range of the millimeter wave. What is not said is that they can be routed into a tractor beam—in other words, utilized as a weapon.

18 Peter Raabe, Strategy Director of Radio Frequency Systems (RFS), "Why 5G by stealth is the answer to future end-to-end," August 30, 2019.

Overcoming bandwidth shortage has been one of the many lies used to sell dual-use 5G weapons-grade technology to investors and the public. Thanks to the shift from analog to digital, there should be no bandwidth shortage or need for wider bandwidth, and yet the millimeter / terahertz spectrum has been opened up, supposedly because the 700 MHz to 2.6 GHz WiFi bandwidth is saturated. Given that the National Television System Committee (NTSC) signal for standard televisions was difficult to manipulate,[19] a switch from analog to digital meant better remote control over brains.[20]

Next came more and more microwave towers and subterranean fiber optics cable with U.S. Army Corps of Engineers installing *frequency amplifiers* so the ubiquitous weapon system could connect with the NSA protocol *HXXrp*.[21] From the beginning, digital, amplifiers, towers, etc. was about dual-use weaponizing of civilian technology.

Short high-frequency waves (gigahertz, terahertz) don't so much interface with the brain as *modulate* it with long ELF signals like AM amplitude modulation or FM frequency modulation, after which the signals drop right into the brain. ELF waves are too long, too attenuated to use directly, the human body not being a large enough antenna for a long wave to "short out" in.[22] A shorter wave is necessary—the shorter the wave, the more powerful. To get ELF frequencies into the brain, high-frequency carriers like 5G are needed. One gigahertz penetrates seven inches, but mind control doesn't need seven inches, so a *higher* frequency like 500 MHz to 3 GHz with shorter wavelengths penetrating works better.

> The development of terahertz technologies has illuminated the workings of the brain, facilitated the capture of emitted photons derived from the visual cortex which processes picture formation in the brain, and enabled the microelectronic receiver which has, in turn, been developed by growing unique semi-conductor crystals. In this way, the technology is now in place for detection and reading of spectral "signatures" of gases. All humans emit gases. Humans, like explosives, emit their own spectral signature in the form of a gas [plasma]. With the reading of the brain's electrical frequency and spectral gas signature, the systems have been estab-

19 NTSC was the analog television color system, now become the digital ATSC (Advanced Television Systems Committee).

20 900 MHz breaks down the blood-brain barrier.

21 Lena Pu, who worked for the U.S. Army Corps of Engineers, views fiber optics as a biophoton machine that impacts the microbiome of the soil and therefore contributes to our sick and dying trees.

22 When an EM wave is absorbed in the body's conductive water, it becomes electrical and shorts out, and the current flow produces heat.

lished for the control of populations—and with the necessary technology integrated into a cell phone.[23]

A 10-watt transmitter is all that is needed for a strong cellular node, so why are cell towers pumping out 20,000 to 60,000 watts and being fed by 400+ kVA (kilovolt-Ampere) transformers?[24] Gleaning GHz wave forms that connect to high-frequency electricity from a cell tower for mind control is one reason. Take a look at the antenna arrays on the towers. They are of far greater size than necessary (~8 feet) and highly directional so signals can be steered to specific zones where the power can then be diverted. If 2,000 volts are for mass mood and mind control, the rest may go toward weather engineering. Cell tower microwave frequencies link at distances over 50 miles and work with NexRads, industrial and nuclear stack WSAC (wet surface air cooling), etc.—all calibrated to work together.

In the name of communication and convenience, we've been captured by *dual use,*[25] now that everything under the Sun (perhaps the Sun as well) is under the mandate of full spectrum Space Fence lockdown, all the way down to DNA.

Telecom defense contractors are in a big hurry to build and calibrate higher frequency (28-38 GHz) dual-use millimeter wave cellular systems with steerable phased array antennas for the higher digital bandwidths that Big Data "stacking" in digitized pulses requires—the higher the frequency, the greater the bandwidth. *Nor have all the frequencies above 300 GHz been allocated.* There seems to be no limit to data transmission, especially with an ionized antenna atmosphere supported by daily dumps of conductive metal nanoparticles in a sea of signals from satellites, base stations, wireless providers, and hotspots everywhere.

Like the much larger HAARP Alaska phased array antennas, tiny phased array antennas built into cell phones since 4G enable shaping radiation into beams and steering them to track our movements and multiply effective radiative power (ERP). Arthur Firstenberg, author of *The Invisible Rainbow: A History of Electricity and Life* (2017), wrote in *New Dawn* magazine:

> The arrays are going to track each other so that wherever you are, a beam from your smart-phone is going to be aimed directly at the base station (cell tower), and a beam from the base station is going to be aimed directly at you. If you walk between someone's phone and the base station, both

---

23 Carole Smith, "Intrusive Brain Reading Surveillance Technology: Hacking the Mind." Dissent magazine, Australia, Summer 2007/2008.

24 400 kVA = ~400,000 watts

25 Thanks to Jim Stone's excellent article "Mind Control via manipulation," June 5, 2012, http://www.jimstonefreelance.com/cells.html.

beams will go right through your body. The beam from the tower will hit you even if you are standing near someone who is on a smartphone. And if you are in a crowd, multiple beams will overlap and be unavoidable. At present, smartphones emit a maximum of about two watts and usually operate at a power of less than a watt. That will still be true of 5G phones. *However, inside a 5G phone there may be 8 tiny arrays of 8 tiny antennas each, all working together to track the nearest cell tower and aim a narrowly focused beam at it.* The FCC has recently adopted rules allowing the effective power of those beams to be as much as 20 watts. Now if a handheld smartphone sent a 20-watt beam through your body, it would far exceed the exposure limit set by the FCC. What the FCC is counting on is that there is going to be a metal shield between the display side of a 5G phone and the side with all the circuitry and antennas. That shield will be there to protect the circuitry from electronic interference that would otherwise be caused by the display and make the phone useless. But it will also function to keep most of the radiation from travelling directly into your head or body, and therefore *the FCC is allowing 5G phones to come to market that will have an effective radiated power that is ten times as high as for 4G phones.*[26] [Emphases added.]

Besides 5G small cells tacked to 4G poles and towers every 500 feet or so, multiple thousands of small satellites (CubeSats) are being launched,[27] all with phased array antennas in 4"X4" matrices shooting like bullets tightly focused beams of microwave radiation at 5G / IoT devices below armed with phased array antennas shooting beams at more phased array antennas on utility poles,[28] penetrating walls, communicating with IoT devices, etc.

The steering capability of 5G means raised power density, but it also means *duplexing,* the same phase conjugate mirroring that takes place in the Lilly Wave (see Chapter 10) invented in the late 1950s. By resending a signal complex in direct opposition—like placing a mirror in line with the source—you have a covert weapon. Wayne Eligur in Tucson, Arizona hints at how upgraded duplexing can be made to manipulate the human bioenergy field via "smart dust" sensors, conductive metals, and pathogens we inhale and ingest daily in this Tesla scalar ("multi 3-D") era:

Beamforming and MIMO duplexing facilitate the nano-tech nano-bio constructs in living beings. The scalar waves traveling in the multi 3-D

26 Arthur Firstenberg, "5G Deep Penetration." New Dawn, March-April 2018.

27 See Chapter 7, "Eyes in the Sky."

28 The broad light pole with the fat tube running eight feet up is a stealth transmitter. – Facebook comment

make biological micro-constructs very easy. Duplexing lets them hide better and cross-communicate in stealth modes.

5G phased array antennas with digital beamforming and MIMO duplexing are precision weapons that can be made to fire millions of microwave "bullets" per second. Suspiciously, the father of the "YouTube shooter" Nasim Najafi Aghdam[29] was scientist Esmaeil Najafi Aghdam of Sahand University of Technology in Iran, who with other scientists in 2014 wrote a paper about MEMS-enabled smart beam-steering antennas. Mark Steele of the UK (*SaveUsNow.org.uk*) has also described 5G as a globally distributed weapon system. The Pentagon considers 5G to be a "foundational enabler for all US defense modernization" of "Air, Space, and Cyberspace lethality," as well as virtual reality technology and cell networks working with Air Force radars.[30] The Department of Defense (DoD) describes 5G systems as having been selected

> . . . for their ability to provide streamlined access to site spectrum bands, mature fiber and wireless infrastructure, access to key facilities, support for new or improved infrastructure requirements, and the ability to conduct controlled experimentation with dynamic spectrum sharing.[31]

Space Fence ground installations wired for 5G encompass:

Tranche 1 (2019): Joint Base Lewis-McChord (WA), Joint Base in San Diego (CA), Marine Corps Logistics Base (GA), Nellis Air Force Base (NV), and Hill Air Force Base (UT).

Tranche 2 (2020): Naval Base Norfolk (VA), Joint Base Pearl Harbor – Hickam (HI), Joint Base San Antonio (TX), National Training Center, Fort Irwin (CA), Fort Hood (TX), Camp Pendleton (CA), Tinker Air Force Base (OK).

5G wireless deployment means 20 billion interconnecting wireless devices, 800,000 small cell base stations, and 50,000 satellites overhead that will require *one million* antennas on the ground, though with antennas getting smaller and smaller and being dual use, who knows what they look like? In 2014, it was seemingly all about 5G equipment amplifying radio waves with gallium nitride (used in blue LEDs) so the waves would reach a one-kilometer (1,000-meter) radius instead of the 100-meter radius of the small base stations the public has been told about. Then in 2016, a New York University

---

29 On April 3, 2018, Nasim shot three people and then herself at YouTube headquarters in San Bruno, California.

30 "Pentagon to dish out $600mn in contracts for '5G dual-use EXPERIMENTATION' at 5 US military sites, including to 'aid lethality.'" RT, October 9, 2020.

31 U.S. Dept. of Defense Release: "DOD Names Seven Installations as Sites for Second Round of 5G Technology Testing, Experimentation," June 3, 2020.

team succeeded in transmitting millimeter (mm) waves 10.8 km in a rural setting, even with trees blocking line-of-sight while broadcasting at 73 GHz with less than 1 watt of power just after the FCC opened 11 GHz of spectrum in the mm wave range.[32] What changed between one kilometer and ten-plus?

> By taking advantage of the more compact solid-state and vacuum components available with millimeter-wave technology, the Air Force Research Laboratory (AFRL) may be looking to reduce the size and weight of deployed systems. Of course, enabling such developments requires the use of solid-state transistor technologies, such as gallium nitride (GaN) and indium phosphide (InP). Innovative millimeter-wave vacuum-tube electronics also must be developed, which can handle high power and thus exceed the performance of traditional coupled cavity vacuum electronics.[33]

In a long Skype discussion, German scientist Harald Kautz-Vella[34] discussed 5G's pivotal importance to the electromagnetic approach to Transhumanism, especially in that it is *pulsed*:

5G is structured to parallel Nature's dynamic morphogenetic field, which means it can be used to engineer Transhumanism by focusing millimeter wave beams, along with polarized light and phased laser quality alignment. Phased array antennas translate to laser quality in-phase coherence light signals that can be used to zero in on targets. With 5G / IoT, there will be no escape unless one is completely free of transmission technologies.

5G uses full duplex signals that don't interfere with each other. Normal communication devices upload and download on two different frequency bands that must synchronize or there will be interference and bad transmission. 5G runs along one channel, splitting it into horizontal (download) polarized light and vertical (upload) polarized light. Polarized light is 10X more bio-available than non-polarized light because cell communication runs on polarized light. *(Non-polarized light is not recognized as a biological wave.)*[35]

---

32 Amy Nordrum, "Millimeter Waves Travel More Than 10 Kilometers in Rural Virginia 5G Experiment." IEEE Spectrum, 7 November 2016.

33 Jean-Jacques DeLisle, "Millimeter Waves Enhance Military Projects." Microwaves & RF, August 11, 2014. See Reo Otsubo, "The Age of 5G: Japan Aims for Market Lead with Cutting-Edge Technology," Japan Forward, August 8, 2018.

34 Kautz-Vella (featured in Chapter 3, "Nanotechnology at the Quantum Threshold") has a university degree in media science with two years of physics, and is basically self-taught in biophysics, bio-photonics, scalar physics, quantum physics, global scaling, transhumanism, and environmental medicine.

35 Pulsed pairs of current work best. "The technical problem in chronic brain stimulation is to stay above the excitatory threshold and below the injury threshold in the neuronal system under consideration . . . Measured at 2 percent of the peak, the duration of the positive pulse (upward) is 34 μsec, and the duration of the negative pulse (downward) is 28 μsec."

With millimeter waves, one can build entire hub antenna phones into a microchip. To downsize the phased array antenna, all that is needed is the wavelength. The tininess of the antennas is why the frequency has to be so high.

All computer and 5G technology is multilayered, from the consumer / agency front end to the nonhuman back end, whether AI, alien or demonic. With pulsed signals, you immediately enter the scalar realm. Processors communicate with each other on a scalar level. *Textured microchips are multilayered to reflect light (blue); light frequencies and wavelengths and laser inside the chip produce standing waves. Phased array antennas and satellites can access any nanochips you have in your body and even make your nanochip synchronize with other individuals' chips for a "hive mind" or "swarm" effect.*[36]

Kautz-Vella pointed out a Google Map showing an "antenna garden" on the ocean floor off the California coast. *"This is how the California fires were made to happen,"* he said. *"These antenna gardens are, of course, phased arrays."*[37] Phased-array antennas mean beaming and targeting. In *Chemtrails, HAARP, and the Full Spectrum Dominance of Planet Earth* (aerial photo on page 131), I pointed out China's preparation for a future HAARP:

> At 43°04'51.75"N/92°48'26.85"E, near the villages of Jiefang (liberation) and Kan'erjing (underground caverns), Google Earth gives us an aerial shot of what might be China's next generation of HAARP arrays. Nathan Cohen, inventor and patent holder of *fractal arrays* and CEO of Fractal Antenna Systems, Inc. (*http://www.fractenna.com*), describes the symmetrical fractal shapes in the satellite photograph:
>
> . . . two banks of three arrays for two separate bands, and one bank of two arrays for another. You can't tell the operational frequencies from the spacings. The panels are many wavelengths across, but we don't know how many. It is a multiband array antenna farm with flat array panels. If we knew the operational frequencies, I could tell you the gain. Not an Arecibo, but still not too shabby would be my guess. Could be an imaging radar for satellite monitoring.[38]

The future is upon us.

- "Lilly Wave Mind Control Broadcasted in Homes Wall AC DC Outlets," Smart Meter News, February 1, 2016.

36 This may well be what is being termed "shedding" in the COVID-19 "gene therapy" drama.

37 Google "5G phased array animation" to see how phased array antennas work.

38 Gary Vey, "The Shape of the Future." http://www.viewzone.com/cgrid/cgrid.html, April 4, 2012; also "The Great Grid of China: A technological wonder of the World," April 12, 2012—hundreds of square miles of buried fiber optic cable laid out in fractal patterns in north China.

Since its inception, 5G and the convenience rhetoric about IoT has been about serving machines and brain-computer interface (BCI). Jody McCutcheon of *Eluxe* magazine:

> Until now mobile broadband networks have been designed to meet the needs of people. But 5G has been created with machines' needs in mind, offering low-latency, high-efficiency data transfer . . . We humans won't notice the difference [in data transfer speeds], but it will permit machines to achieve near-seamless communication. Which in itself may open a whole Pandora's box of trouble for us—and our planet.[39]

The reassurance that millimeter waves do not penetrate far into the body is untrue; in fact, the extremely short EM pulses *re-radiate* the waves for greater penetration (Brillouin precursors).[40] As indicated above, 5G small ground antennas and satellite radiation saturation penetrate bodies, walls and rooftops as they communicate with the IoT and share dual-use frequencies with the military.[41] The effective radiated power (ERP) of 5G phones is 10X that of previous phones, and WiFi hubs in homes and offices are permitted to use microwave beams 15X (300 watts) the 5G phone signals or 150X the 4G phone signals.

IoT / IoNT / IoB

> *Good morning, class. Former CIA Director David Petraeus calls 5G Technology the Internet of Things, which is designed to connect everything in this 3-D Realm onto a vast global network or a Total Technological Control Grid, including rural areas, with the 5G Electromagnetic Fence inside which nothing can escape. 5G will penetrate material objects better; will become "infrastructure intensive," providing information by sharing frequencies with the Intelligence Services and Military; and the entire planet, be it urban or rural, will be hammered with radiation saturation. Their idea of a New World Order is the Ultimate Technological Power Grid.*
>
> – Facebook entry, Michael Kavanagh, self-described as "Script writer Central Intelligence, MK-Ultra whistleblower, Gemstone Files"

---

39 Joyce Nelson, "5G Corporate Grail. Microwave Radiation." Global Research, November 9, 2018.

40 Arthur Firstenberg, "5G – From Blankets to Bullets," January 22, 2018.

41 Thanks to Mark Freeman, "5G and IoT: Total Technological Control Grid Being Rolled Out Fast," The Freedom Articles, http://freedom-articles.toolsforfreedom.com/5g-iot-technological-control-grid/.

The IoT's gatekeeper is the *smart meter* neighborhood network. Combining the smart meter with a stealth weapons system similar to the Active Denial System (ADS) "spot beam" (95 GHz) phased array antenna weapon[42] was a stroke of genius

> . . . because these are "stealth" technologies where the person being targeted would not even know they were being targeted, they could potentially also be used against people who object to mandatory vaccination, medical kidnapping, the nationalization of our private health data, the use of toxic chemicals in food, mandatory indoctrination of children in the public education system, mainstream media brainwashing, the collection of information about our religious and political beliefs, the denial of the right to assemble in peaceful protests against the overreaching power of national and state government, to name just a few.[43]

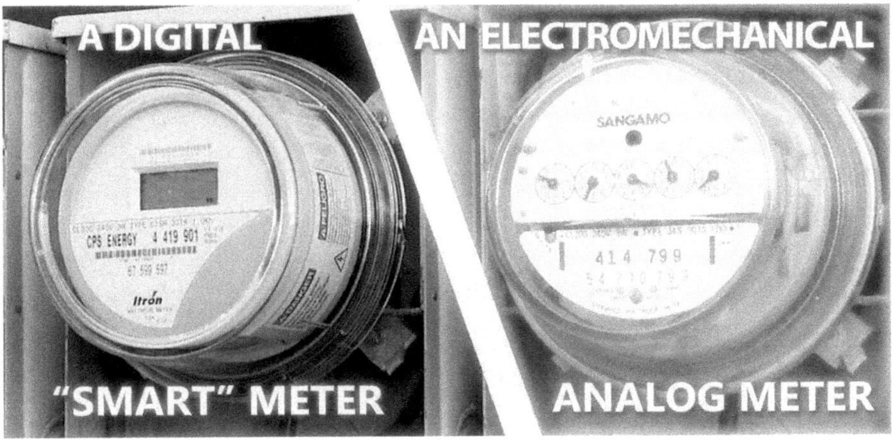

Smart Meters. Smart (digital) vs electromechanical (analog) meter. Smart meters are the electromagnetic gatekeepers of homes and neighborhoods. A review of Chapter 10, "The Covert Ascendance of Technocracy" in *Under An Ionized Sky* is recommended.

https://steopsmartmeters.org/wp-content/uploads/2001/10/smart-vs-analog2.jpg

Smart meters are even legislated to break and enter (B&E) and spy on energy use and time of use (TOU) home / business presence. Once installed, energy use rises as do inflated rates and utility bills. Smart meters communicate with the IoT, thanks to their 1-watt WiFi transceiver and 4G / 5G con-

42 5G phones operating 28 - 38 GHz comprise the equivalent of the ADS.

43 John P. Thomas, "Can New 5G Technology and Smart Meters be Used as Weapons?" Health Impact News, September 4, 2018.

nection to the cell network. Collected data is sold off to private corporations, the gate left open for cyberattacks and hacks.

In August 2018, the Federal Appeals Court in Illinois ruled that under the search-and-seizure Fourth Amendment "privilege," it was reasonable to assume that smart meters do government searches every 15 minutes, given that they pulse 928 MHz through every home's 60 Hz grid. Smart meter range is 30 miles, with 50,000 microwatts per square meter (mW/m2) pulsed emissions. Like 5G, the smart meter has been classified by the World Health Organization (WHO) as a 2B carcinogen.

So what is going on with the (remotely triggered) smart meter fires? In 2013, freelance journalist Jim Stone discussed a microprocessor manufacturer ARM diagram of the smart meter (since removed from the Internet):

> . . . three wireless connectivity options per smart meter, PLUS an ability to communicate through the power system, as well as Ram, Rom, and Flash, complete with an ultra DMA hard drive controller (needed to provide storage to the flash memory) and FIVE CPU's TOTAL. ??!!?? It's a safe bet that such extreme connectivity and CPU power, plus 3 memory options, could only be needed for nefarious purposes. If your refrigerator is WiFi-equipped (a ridiculous RF polluting waste) when it could simply receive commands through the wiring, your refrigerator, microwave, you name it, could also be equipped with audio and visual surveillance capabilities and have that ability to remain perfectly hidden, all to be transmitted out through the smart meter.[44]

Lateral radiation spikes of 200-1200+ mW/m2 penetrate your walls from your neighbors' smart meters, plus "chirp" radiation spikes from one smart meter to another in the neighborhood sharing information, transmitting to relay boxes on power poles that shoot out HF spikes "talking" to cell antennas before heading to the power company—and that's just 2.4 GHz.[45] The 17,000 to 190,000 PULSES PER DAY exhaust the immune system, ancient defender of our health.

> Clearly the impact of SMART meter networks is phenomenal, especially when clustered together, inducing Doppler effects for long distances, sometimes hundreds of meters in series of clusters, reflections, generation of "noise" and probably thousands of new signals per cubic meter.[46]

---

44 Jim Stone, "Security issue 4 – Smart Meters," March 23, 2013. Use your Glossary to decode all the computer acronyms.

45 Thanks to Neil Cohen, EMF Assessment and Remediation, May 21, 2014.

46 Andrew Michrowski, PhD, "Emerging phenomena with smart meters

Smart meter software is "proprietary" (i.e. patented), like the DSP chip (digital signal processing) that reads the usage rate of each unique "smart-enabled device" for which manufacturers pay premium dollar to utility corporations for it. Is this DSP like the back door VPOC chip (variable power on control) that makes it easy for telecoms to access powered-off cell phones? Can it trip breakers? Ignite fires? Is there a supercapacitor inside the meter?

Smoke detectors are also IoT required in just about every room of every home and workplace by the U.S. Fire Administration under Homeland Security's Federal Emergency Management Agency (FEMA). Smoke detector sensors pick up broadcast microwave signals and turn them into cameras (remote sensing) via spectroscopy.[47] Tinker with one and you may find it broadcasting on government-only channels like *PRISM,* which gathers emails, videos, and private data on "persons of interest" for the Intelligence Community and transnational corporations via arrangements overseen by star chamber "secret panels of judges."[48]

The road to the brain-computer interface (BCI) that merges Smart City dwellers with AI systems is paved with the Internet of Things (IoT) and 5G technology. *Trillions* of 5G wireless nodes of 30 billion devices surround us, from vehicle and home MTCs (machine type communications) to intelligent wearables and environmental sensors—all in AI harness and on display via the Internet for mobile and Cloud computing to Big Data. Think 2-axis magnetic sensors, accelerometers, light intensity sensors, humidity, pressure and temperature sensors, operating system with 3KB RAM memory sensors, actuators, implantables, blockchain tech that makes digital transactions automatic and verifiable, ubiquitous computing and hyperconnectivity exponentially increasing the BCI, MMI (machine-to-machine interface), BBI (brain-to-brain interface) flows of data, nanotech and nanomaterials, algorithms making decisions, vision as an interface for augmented / virtual reality . . .

The *Internet of Nano Things (IoNT)* constitutes the trillions of sensors "small enough to circulate within living bodies and to mix directly into construction materials" contrived by synthetic biology "to modify single-celled organisms such as bacteria . . . to fashion simple biocomputers that use DNA and proteins . . . ,"[49] and

---

imposed in Quebec." Dr. Michrowski is president of the Ottawa-based Planetary Association for Clean Energy (PACE).

47 Miniature tunable diode laser spectroscopic carbon monoxide sensors are becoming common.

48 Michael Riley, "U.S. Agencies Said to Swap Data With Thousands of Firms." Bloomberg, July 15, 2013. The cell site simulator Stingray and the hand-carried KingFish version mimic the behavior of mobile phone towers and thus force calls to connect with them for cell phone signal triangulation. ("Washington state limits Stingray surveillance in unanimously approved 'pro-privacy' law," RT, May 12, 2015.)

49 Daniel Wellers, "Is this the future of the Internet of Things?" World Economic Forum, 27

cellular nanosensors and carbon nanotubes (CNTs) made from yet more nonbiological materials to "sense and signal, acting as wireless nanoantennas."

> Because they are so small, nanosensors can collect information from millions of different points. External devices can then integrate the data to generate incredibly detailed maps showing the slightest changes in light, vibration, electrical currents, magnetic fields, chemical concentrations and other environmental conditions.[50]

The open-ended ubiquity of IoT and IoNT marks a fundamental shift in computing, given that we're surrounded *and interpenetrated* by interfaces automatically capturing input, like the Smart Grid's RRPLS (realtime residential power line surveillance). The millions of wireless transceivers provide entry points for hackers galore, like the Tor-based hackers[51] selling access to IoT botnets from cameras, fridges, and kettles for DDoS (distributed denial of service) attacks and just plain in-home attacks, daytime thefts, even online murders. The lack of IoT / IoNT cybersecurity is suspicious, as if leaving the gate open is not just about home thefts but about nervous systems that may require a little coercion now and then, not to mention fully targeted individuals moving about in search of respite from electromagnetic pain.

As indicated above, smart home automation does not save on energy consumption dollars. The CPE (consumer premises equipment) with built-in WiFi now reads 8.154 watts compared with yesteryear's 0.1 watts per WiFi router—*80X* more radiation.[52] *This is about lockdown* in an IoT piezoelectric world with touch-tone keys in doors and handshakes,[53] embedded tiny sensors and digital radios, 1-cubic-mm micromote computers with one megabyte memory storage, V2V (vehicle to vehicle) communications, bioacoustics data transfer sensors transmitting through your bones.[54] WiFi hotspots are everywhere, from homeless vendors and smart bins to cemeteries and silent drones.

November 2015.

50 Javier Garcia-Martinez, PhD. "Here's what will happen when 30 billion devices are connected to the Internet." World Economic Forum, 23 June 2016.

51 Tor is a network that seeks to anonymize the source and destination of your web searches by routing traffic along a convoluted path. (Signal is recommended for encrypted messaging and phone calls.)

52 These are only estimates, given that we still lack devices that can measure millimeter wave frequencies, though rumor has it that the Safe and Sound Pro II meter measures 5G without saying it's 5G.

53 Olivia Solon, "Transfer a secret audio message by poking someone with your finger." Wired, 13 September 2013.

54 "Smart Phones Will Send Data THROUGH YOUR BONES Next," Truthstream Media, June 26, 2017.

You really have to be aware to be able to DISCERN and thus refuse all this and understand how a smart phone becomes the door of l'Enfer *nowadays, and that 5G is more than mortiferous waves but a system introducing "the nano internet of things" transhumanism (and the 8th Luciferian sphere anti-man and anti-Creation of God, thus opening the door to the Abomination of non-human synthetic technology wanting to graft itself and invade the human body and mind, and that of other living beings, too). It's not even "science" anymore; it's occult science to rapt the possession and ontological rape of human nature and our biology.*

– New Rachel Sky, November 29, 2020

The advantage of the millimeter wavelength is that many antennas in variously configured arrays—vertical or horizontal, wave guides, coned or highly directional beams—can be set up to transmit an extremely powerful effective radiated power (ERP) in specified directions. Walk into the path of such an invisible ERP and the electron volt assault will be immediately felt, especially by electrohypersensitives (EHS), our canaries in the coal mine.

As for the *Internet of Bodies*, the description at the Global Economic Forum site insists it's just a FitBit-style "collection of data via a range of devices that can be implanted, swallowed or worn," leaving out that we are breathing in the very nanobots that are forming the neural network *inside*, not on, our bodies."[55] The sensors digitally collecting our body biometrics from wearables to digital pills to VivaLNK smart thermometers clearly engage with the neural network already set up.

While sites like RAND Corporation[56] guide the consumer to consider the perils of the Internet of Bodies being hacked by botnets like the dark_nexus[57] and the data being unlawfully used, concern about the ethics of the medical industry itself and its master Big Pharma is not even mentioned.

"Precision medicine" (telemedicine) is not what it seems.

55 Xiao Liu, "The Internet of Bodies is here. This is how it could change our lives." World Economic Forum, June 4, 2020.

56 Mary Lee, "What Is the Internet of Bodies?" RAND Corporation, n.d.

57 Jitendra Soni, "Fast evolving botnet targets millions of IoT devices." TechRadar, April 13, 2020: "launching a range of various DDoS attacks, spreading multiple malware strains, and can infect devices running on 12 different CPU architectures."

Down to the cell level

With 5G, we are not just concerned about *power* but about *pulsing.* An electron volt assault is one thing, but cyclotron resonance takes its toll on our biology over time. From the must-read by Robert O. Becker, MD:

> Cyclotron resonance is a mechanism of action that enables very low-strength magnetic fields, acting in concert with the Earth's geomagnetic field, to produce major biological effects by *concentrating the energy in the applied field upon specific particles,* such as the biologically important ions of sodium, calcium, potassium, and lithium.[58]

Ellis Evans, PhD (http://www.hellostarseeds.net/), claims that the latency period for adverse biological effects from 1-5 GHz is 10-20 years; higher frequencies (6-100 GHz) compress that timeframe.

> It is anyone's guess on what might happen in terms of biological safety, yet it is clear to see that *the pulsed nature of these high frequency, high intensity signals* do not harbor good news for humanity, particularly in relation to the functioning of our DNA.[59] (Emphasis added.)

In the Smart City, brain wave functions are easy to manipulate and alter. As with the digital terrestrial trunked radio (TETRA) system—pulsed by law enforcement, military, public transportation (airports, railways, metros, sea ports, buses, taxis), road networks, public safety, emergency services, utilities, event management, sports arenas, the hospitality and leisure industry around the globe[60]—an ancillary sub-carrier frequency (16 Hz) can be pulsed via ELF to entrain violence, passivity, or any other emotional frequency throughout the Smart City.

Martin L. Pall, PhD (see Chapter 2, "The Three Primary Transhumanist Delivery Systems"), recognizes the 5G infrastructure as an integrated weapon system utilizing pulsed frequencies. He refers to the "black" (i.e. secret) nature

---

58 Robert O. Becker, Cross Currents: The Perils of Electropollution, The Promise of Electromedicine. Jeremy P. Tarcher / Penguin, 1990.

59 Ellis Evans, PhD, "5G telecom radiation the perfect tool to mass modify human brain waves." Waking Times, September 12, 2016. Evans' PhD in nuclear physics is from Westlakes Research Institute in Cumbria, England (1998). While doing fieldwork at the Sellafield nuclear reprocessing plant, he discovered that "a fugitive source or sources onsite were releasing historic particles of radioactivity, and aged plutonium and americium were also being emitted from sources unknown. I was unable to locate the sources(s) of these hot particles, yet I was able to show through meticulous field sampling that the scale of the problem was much bigger than they expected." He was pressured to leave and his hot particle research confiscated without being published. http://www.hellostarseeds.net/phd%20 abstract.html.

60 TETRA + Critical Communications Association (TCCA).

of electromagnetic radiation studies, particularly when applied to millimeter wave technology like 5G, and notes that no government funding has been forthcoming for research or testing regarding public biological safety; that the FCC and FDA are "captured" agencies in thrall to Big Tech; and that the 1996 Telecommunications Act was "the worst piece of legislation"; etc.[61]

Pall points to how the sweat ducts in human skin—skin being our largest organ—act as coiled helical antennas picking up signals and frequencies.[62] Add to this the dipole conductivity of water, the giver of life, below our sponge-like skin. The combination of oxidative stress and voltage-gated calcium channels (VGCCs), intense overwork of sweat duct antennas, and our skin's high SAR (specific absorption rate) explain much about electromagnetic hypersensitivity / electrosensitivity (EHS / ES) and declining health.

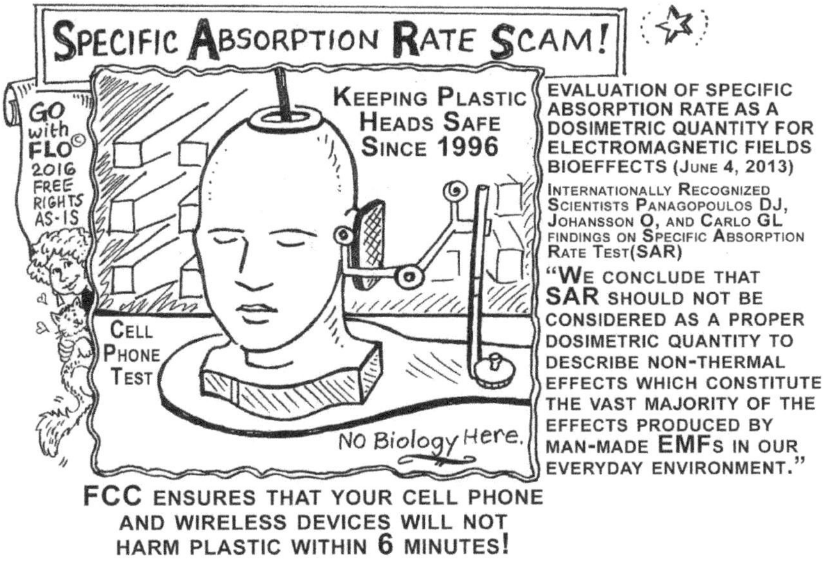

Specific Absorption Rate (SAR) Scam! Permission granted by artist activist Florie Freshman.

VGCCs and tinnitus appear to go hand in hand. Ringing in the ears is not auditory but the frequency modulation of VGCCs in your brain. VGCCs

61 Soundcloud.com interview, "The Dangers of EMF and 5G, July 10, 2018."

62 In 2003 at the 2nd European Symposium on Non-Lethal Weapons (NLW), the paper "Bioelectrodynamic Criterion of the NLW Effectiveness Estimation and the Interaction Mechanisms of the Multilayer Skin Tissues with Electromagnetic Radiation" by A.F. Korolev et al. (Lomonosov Moskow State University), explained how radio frequency weapons like the Active Denial System (ADS) affect the skin. Also see David Hambling's "Moscow's Remote-Controlled Heart Attacks" in DefenseTech, February 14, 2006.

open and close cellular ionic bonds in an otherwise impermeable (healthy) cellular structure that permits fragmented DNA chains to recombine with radiation-fractured DNA. The ringing sound of tinnitus goes by the name of Hh (hedge-hog) or SHh (sonic hedge-hog) genomic notch, located at the GL1 gene (a transcription activator). This genomic notch is called Shrek[63] and is the "bustle" (vibration) in your "hedge-row."

Speaking of hedge-hogs and Shrek, was Led Zeppelin's 1971 "Stairway to Heaven" trying to tell us something about how Harvard University genomics pioneer George Church was influencing calcium ion channels so that DNA sequencing could be spatially changed and manipulated?

> *. . . If there's a bustle in your hedgerow, don't be alarmed now,*
> *It's just a spring clean for the May queen.*
> *Yes, there are two paths you can go by, but in the long run*
> *There's still time to change the road you're on.*
> *And it makes me wonder.*
> *Your head is humming and it won't go, in case you don't know,*
> *The piper's calling you to join him,*
> *Dear lady, can you hear the wind blow, and did you know*
> *Your stairway lies on the whispering wind?*[64]

Andrew Michrowski, PhD (mentioned earlier), discusses how

> . . . the immediate decrease of skin conductance [indicates] a rapid activation of the parasympathetic nervous system [rest and digest] and corresponding deactivation of the sympathetic nervous system [fight or flight]. The immediate increase in skin conductance at cessation of signaling (& re-grounding) indicates an opposite effect. Increased respiratory rate, stabilization of blood oxygenation, and the slight rise in heart pulse rate suggests the start of a metabolic healing response necessitating an increase in oxygen consumption. The sensitive individuals we know, when undergoing such bodily changes, become quite intruded and concerned over body events they cannot control consciously! Something similar can be happening inside schools & hospitals and other institutional buildings where WiFi + many wireless devices are interlocked and liable to generate

---

63 "Two of three mutant lines, shrek (srk) and hulk (hlk), contained dominant mutations, and Oscar-the-grouch (otg) contained a recessive mutation." - Jeremy T. Baeten and Jill L.O. De Jong, "Genetic Models of Leukemia in Zebrafish." Cell Division Biology, 20 September 2018. What's with this cartoon onomancy?

64 Thanks to Sine Nomine on Facebook. Do you see that Led Zeppelin is talking about tinnitus being caused by being targeted with directed energy weapons? "'Cause you know sometimes words have two meanings" . . .

> here and there *a condensed cloud of signals* and resultant reflective phenomena.[65] [Emphasis added.]

Current radiation standards still do not take into account either nonthermal SAR or SkinRad Effect (skin radiation).

> Starting from July 2016, the US Federal Communications Commission (FCC) has adopted new rules for wireless broadband operations above 24GHz (5G). This trend of exploitation is predicted to expand to higher frequencies in the sub-THz [millimeter wave] region. One must consider the implications of human immersion in the electromagnetic noise, caused by devices working at the very same frequencies as those to which the sweat duct (as a helical antenna) is most attuned. We are raising a warning flag against the unrestricted use of sub-THz technologies for communication . . .[66]

The higher the frequency, the shorter the wavelength; the smaller the wave, the greater the impact on the human being. For example, the 2.4 GHz WiFi microwave of the iPhone is 16 cm, whereas the 5G very high frequency wave is 3-5 mm. (And yet it is claimed that the millimeter wave at 30-70 GHz can be used to eliminate symptoms by exciting certain acupuncture points.[67])

WiFi routers and microwave ovens operate at 2.8 GHz and produce cellular changes. Cell phones and smart meters operate from 2.4 GHz down to 900 MHz, which means deeper penetration. Cell phone manufacturers keep the density between high enough to reach cell towers and low enough to cook the brain over time, i.e. cancer. *Adjusting the microwave density turns a convenience into a weapon.* So it goes with dual use.

At 2.4 GHz, the 4G WiFi microwave photons are 5 microelectron volts (μeV); at 60 GHz, 5G millimeter waves are 122 μeV, *25X greater*. If 2.4 GHz iPhones are held next to the head, brain cancer ensues, so what is the reasoning behind 60 GHz? By weaponizing the air around us, the no-turning-back point of millimeter wave impact on the molecules in our cells has been achieved. 5G propagates into the mouth and nostrils, down the throat and into the lungs, into the ear canals and nerves of the inner ears close to the brain. 5G disrupts sleep, weakens the immune system, opens cell channel gates.

---

65 Andrew Michrowski, letter to André Fauteux, editor of La Maison du 21e siècle magazine, October 23, 2021; also "Emerging phenomena with smart meters imposed in Quebec," n.d., https://sandaura.wordpress.com/2010/06/05/evidence-of-microwave-pollution-in-our-communities/.

66 Noa Betzalei et al., "The human skin as a sub-THz receiver – Does 5G pose a danger to it or not?" Environmental Research, Vol. 163, May 2018.

67 See Taras I. Usichenko et al., "Low-Intensity Electromagnetic Millimeter Waves for Pain Therapy." Evidence-Based Complementary and Alternative Medicine, June 2006.

Microwave density—the SAR—is one thing, but *pulsing* 5G microwave photons 24/7 overloads and overwhelms our molecules and our cells' resonance. Add to this how "millimeter waves use lenses for antennas to focus their millimeter photons, just like optical photons are focused by lenses,"[68] and the impact on physical and mental health is devastating.

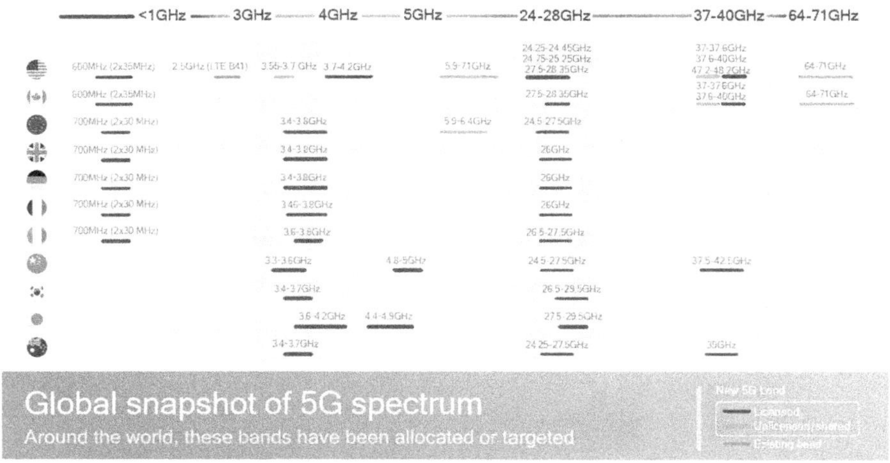

5G bands in the era of unlicensed ("dual use") frequencies.

"The new era of *unlicensed* 5G mmWave (57.05-64 GHz) run in Europe by Telecom Infra Project (TIP) and chaired by Facebook and Deutsche Telekom (Facebook *terragraf.net* uses the *802.11 ay* standard), requires FCC Part 15 certification. The fact is that 60 GHz mmWave networks are all about combining narrow beam transmission with oxygen absorption to reduce communications interference, enhance security, and minimize unauthorized intercept. 60 GHz absorption is particularly high if the atmosphere is dry . . ." (See Anders Storm, "2019 was the breakthrough year in Europe for 60 GHz unlicensed 5G," *siversima.com*, n.d.)

https://www.everythingrf.com/community/5g-frequency-bands

Internet commentator and activist Joe Imbriano knew in 2018 that the new WiFi known as *WiGig (60 GHz)* induces symptoms like those wrongly attributed to viral illnesses like COVID-19.[69] The WiGig wireless network operates in the 60 GHz spectrum with download speeds of up to 10 Gbps (4G = 10 Mbps). Symptoms of oxygen deprivation—at 60 GHz, atmospheric oxygen absorbs 98 percent of RF energy—mimic COVID-19 symptoms.

68 Thanks to Trevor G. Marshall, PhD, Director, Autoimmunity Research Foundation, CA, "A quick background on the dangers from 5G millimeter waves."

69 The Fullerton Informer, "Joe Imbriano warned us in 2018 - 60 GHz blocks Oxygen uptake=fake virus=kill grid=forced vaccinations," February 10, 2018.

More on oxygen and 5G in Chapter 14, "The COVID-19 'Vaccine' Event," given that 5G is used for signal transduction to edit DNA, and the millimeter wavelength that propagates 5G interacts with Spike protein production. With an AI operating system installed, 5G transmitting and storing data in your cells begins, and your body is no longer your own. (See the 2013 U.S. Supreme Court case *Pathology v Myriad Genetics, Inc.*, in Appendix 1, "Invisible Mindsets.")

6G and terahertz

kHz (kilohertz, 10^3 Hz)
MHz (megahertz, 10^6 Hz)
GHz (gigahertz, 10^9 Hz)
THz (terahertz, 10^{12} Hz)
PHz (petahertz, 10^{15} Hz)
EHz (exahertz, 10^{18} Hz)
ZHz (zettahertz, 10^{21} Hz)

While everyone worries about 5G, it appears that 6G—the system that integrates 5G with satellite networks for global coverage—is already in place,[70] with 7G "space roaming" being next. In March 2019, the FCC (ever the handmaiden to military contractor telecoms) unanimously voted to open the 95 GHz to 3 THz wireless spectrum for 6G and up. Going from millimeter to submillimeter to terahertz wave range puts us just this side of optical, x-ray, gamma ray, and cosmic ray wavelengths.

6G is all about the submillimeter ("sub-6G"=terahertz) bandwidth between the microwave (electromagnetic) and the infrared (photonic), which means tremendously high frequency (100 GHz-10 THz) for AI tech like augmented reality and full-on Internet-brain reality connectivity (via nanobots) and "real time computations needed for wireless remoting of human cognition,"[71] meaning human brains online with "human-class artificial intelligence." As usual, the submillimeter antennas will have tiny highly directional phased arrays that provide "military-grade secure communications links that are 'exceedingly difficult' to intercept or eavesdrop upon."

70 Diana Goovaerts, "U.S. taps Apple, Google, Nokia, Qualcomm for 6G boost." Fierce Wireless, April 28, 2021. Another "public-private partnership": Resilient and Intelligent Next-Generation Systems (RINGS).

71 Jeremy Horowitz, "Researchers say 6G will stream human brain-caliber AI to wireless devices." VentureBeat.com, June 14, 2019. Also see Samsung's white paper "The Next Hyper-Connected Experience for All," released July 14, 2020.

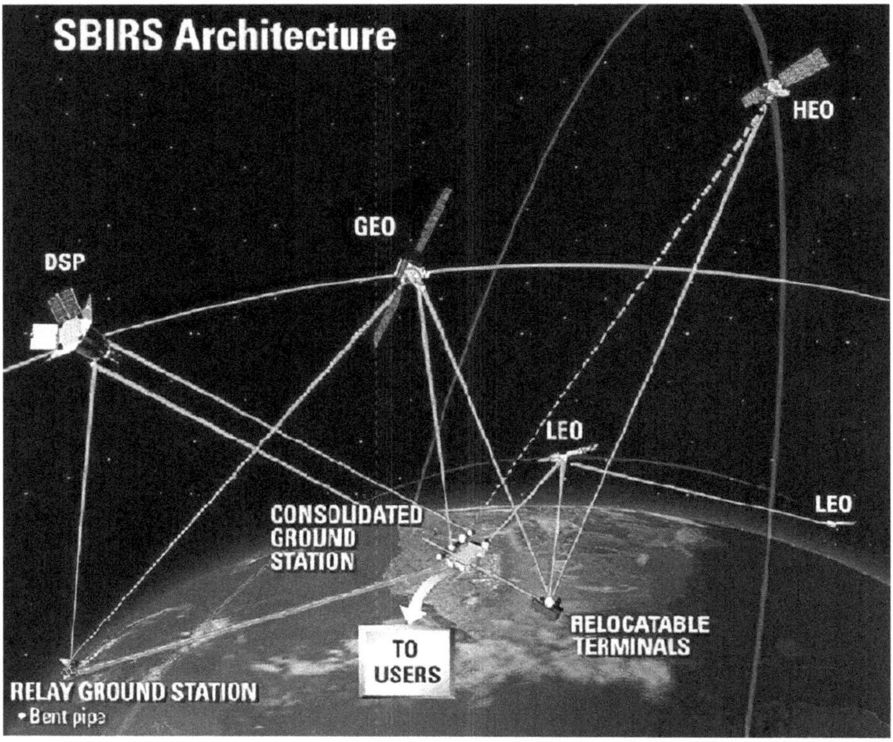

Space-Based Infrared System (SBIRS) architecture.

HEO = high Earth orbit

LEO = low Earth orbit

GEO = geostationary orbit satellites

DSP = Defense Support Program; 23 DSP satellites

https://www.spacewar.com/reports/Lockheed_nets_1639M_to_support_space-based_infrared_system_999.html

http://www.losangeles.af.mil/SMC/PA/Fact_Sheets/sbirs_fs.htm

THz radiation is being kicked up to *1000 GHz*. MRIs use THz lasers (30 to 1 mm wavelengths), and telecoms use THz for network backbones and broadcasting super-high definition 4K television signals with cameras in the THz spectrum.[72] While THz photons cannot break chemical bonds or ionize atoms or molecules like x-rays and UV rays can, their nonlinear resonant effects in devices like the THz lasers in the TIDs (terahertz imaging detection) in TSA airport scanners (~10 GHz) alter DNA by "unzipping" the double-strands.[73]

72 "New filter could advance terahertz data transmission," EurekAlert! February 27, 2015.

73 Jason Prall, "Yes, Airport Millimeter Wave Scanners Alter DNA." Jasonprall.com, n.d. As

Whereas fiber optics unlock ultra-high speeds for wired connections, THz transmitters unlock fiber optic speeds for wireless. THz extends microwave and millimeter wavebands, provides lightning downloads and the most secure form of "small cell" communication. In fact, at-a-distance interception is not possible, and if a digitally encrypted communication is intercepted by those lacking the proper codes, the THz wave will simply drop off and shut down, which is why it is perfect for "confined" GHz satellite phone calls and sat-to-sat communications where atmospheric absorption is not a problem, given that THz waves only propagate in air.

> The beamlike properties of THz emission reduce the ability of distant adversaries to intercept these transmissions. The adversary may even lack the technological capability to detect, intercept, jam, or "spoof" a THz signal. In addition, atmospheric attenuation allows covert short-range communications, since these signals simply will not propagate to distant listening posts.[74]

Astrophysicists have been a driving force behind developing THz technologies that can detect plasma spectra in "the terahertz gap" (the far infrared wavelength of 15μm-1 mm with a range of 20 THz to 300 GHz). Could THz wave propagation be one of the reasons for conductive desiccants like aluminum nanoparticles in chemical trails, given that both THz and mm waves experience less scattering loss from particulates than optical wavelengths?

Cellular and Wi-Fi networks depend on microwaves in the gigahertz. Tiny submillimeter wavelengths like terahertz (0.03 mm to 3 mm) are essential for manipulating atoms, DNA and RNA, all of which point to nanobots.

AirGig & backscatter

AT&T transfers WiFi over power lines using 4G LTE and 5G mmWaves, thus turning power lines into transmitters to extend the reach of cell towers and fiber optic cable—"last mile wireless connectivity" for everyone already served by an electric utility. AirGig means even more "close-proximity, high-intensity radiation" and even closer collaboration with utility companies "as they evolve toward the 'smart grid'" and rollout of Smart Cities.

> 5G is about increasing bandwidth to transfer more data to support the Internet of Things (IoT), the network of physical objects — "things" — that are embedded with sensors, software and other technologies for the

---

Sony passive millimeter wave imaging sees through clothes, it creates cancer.

74 Michael J. Fitch and Robert Osiander, "Terahertz Waves for Communication and Sensing." Johns Hopkins APL Technical Digest, 2004.

> purpose of connecting and exchanging data with other devices and systems over the internet. The IoT intends to wirelessly interconnect 50 billion more devices, and the data collected will be used primarily for artificial intelligence, surveillance and creating the next version of "humans" — beings that are part human and part machine.[75]

What AirGig is really up to is making use of the power line infrastructure as a "waveguide" (similar to the waveguides that steer lasers with minimal attenuation) so as to extend the distance that 5G mmWave signals can travel. AirGig points to the fact that 5G applications are not about civil use but military—for example, linking digital systems that transmit enormous quantities of data for artificial intelligence "machine learning" systems.

Backscatter technology is just this side of wireless energy transmission technology. Keeping in mind that the Space Fence and HAARP pulse and make backscatter radar and X-ray backscatter, and that phased multiple WiFi and cell phone units do the same,[76] it should not be all that surprising that *ambient Wi-Fi backscatter* is everywhere being harnessed to power the trillions of nanosensors already in the environment (and our bodies), along with the Internet of Things (IoT), in expectation of the magic Singularity moment when the Internet consumes everywhere.

> [Ambient backscatter] uses existing radio frequency signals, such as radio, television and digital telephony, to transmit data without a battery or power grid connection. Each such device uses an antenna to pick up an existing signal and convert it into tens of hundreds of microwatts of electricity. It uses that power to modify and reflect the signal with encoded data . . . *This approach would let mobile and other devices communicate without being turned on. It would also allow unpowered sensors to communicate, allowing them to be placed in places where external power cannot be conveniently supplied.*[77] (Emphasis added.)

At post-9/11 airports, it's Advanced Imaging Technology backscatter; in neighborhoods, it's 5G phased array antenna backscatter coupled with satellite 5G beams. Meanwhile, Homeland Security's terahertz waves unzip our double-stranded DNA as millimeter wave sensors measure the radiated energy of each IoT / IoNT / IoB object against a common background in order to construct composite images. Airports, like hospitals, are dangerous to your health.

---

75 Dafna Tachover, Esq., "Washington Post Is Right that 5G Is a Lie, But Wrong About the Reason" (September 15, 2020) and "5G AirGig: What Is It and Should You Be Worried?" (March 17, 2020), Children's Health Defense.

76 See "DEFCON 19: Build your own Synthetic Aperture Radar," Christian008, October 29, 2011.

77 Wikipedia.

Our bodies are the product of a billion years of nature's evolutionary processes, but the War on Terror is about to irrevocably corrupt our gene pool, causing untold immune system and other genetic damage to future generations, and possibly rendering the DNA coding that we are based on unacceptably toxic . . .

One concept of the genetic mutation process put forward by the National Academy of Sciences employed a line of nucleoproteins in a normal sequence something like this: AGT-AGT-AGT-AGT-AGT-AGT-AGT . . . In this model the DNA code is read and transmitted in groups of three proteins. Consider what happens if the sequence is disturbed, such as when a speeding terahertz wave dislodges one protein in the chain. The entire sequence is thrown off until two counterbalancing breaks occur that throw it back into correct order. Until then, it is read: AG-TAG-TAG-TAG-TAG-TAG-TAG . . .

Suppose the AGT sequence was for brain cells, but the TAG sequence was for stomach muscles. You could get something pretty weird happening . . . The rate of genetic translocations in humans caused by ionizing radiation and estimated in the current scientific literature ranges from 24 to 1,330 translocations per unit of radiation (rad) per million live births per generation. It takes on the order of 100 generations to eliminate each unfavorable mutation from the genetic pool, whether it is for a fruit fly or a baboon . . .[78]

Now that we've been captured by the wireless Space Fence lockdown, the "common background" pulsates all around and through us 24/7. Epidemiologist Rosalie Bertell[79] foresaw that elevating the background level of mutagens (cell damage) in combination with mutations interfering with normal reproduction could result in the end of a species. Ergo, a *negative* Ebner Effect.

78 Albert Bates, "Airport Androids Attack Human Gene Pool," Medium, 8 January 2010.

79 Rosalie Bertell (1929-2012), Planet Earth: The Latest Weapon of War (2001). An enhanced edition came out in July 2020 under Talma Studios International.

6

The Secret Space Program

Plasma
Plasma life forms
Plasma beam DEWs & augmented reality (AR) mind control
Alfvén Waves & Birkeland Currents
The Nuclear Behemoth
Trinity
"Accidents" or experiments?
Arlo Lauri in Finland
Solar & lunar simulators
CERN
Gravity, Æther, & Tesla's Atmospheric Engine
Blue Beam & Hale-Bopp

... super-extreme matter parameters, at which the known physical laws are thought to be no longer valid ... owing to the gravitational compression of stars to the stage of black holes, there again emerge singularities — ultrahigh parameters of Planckian scale. In this field, physical models are discussed that assume that our space has more than three dimensions, and that ordinary matter is in a three-dimensional manifold — the '3-brane world' — embedded in this many- dimensional space.

– Vladimir E. Fortov, Extreme States of Matter, High Energy Density Physics, 2nd Edition (Springer 2016)

There is no vacuum.

– Gottfried W. Leibniz, polymath, 1689

THE COVERT GEOENGINEERING OF MORE than two decades has gone public—minus, of course, the two decades and the fact that it has been involved in the secret space program from the beginning, the long-term objective being that of Soviet astronomer Nikolai Kardashev's three phases of technological achievement for civilizations aspiring to a bona fide Space Age:

I. Full spectrum dominance planetary control
II. Control over one's star and its systems

III. Control over one's galaxy and its systems[1]

The 45th U.S. President Donald John Trump—nephew of physicist John G. Trump who was entrusted with all things Tesla at Tesla's death in 1943—announced the U.S. Space Force in late 2019.[2] Exactly 72 years ago, the U.S. Air Force spun off from the U.S. Army, and now the Chief of Space Operations would be reporting to the Secretary of the Air Force with geoengineering being under the purview of Space Command—like the 23rd Space Operations Squadron, Detachment 1, in Greenland that keeps tabs on the exceedingly important Arctic Circle.

Investment analyst Catherine Austin Fitts has repeatedly spoken out about the theft of far more than $21 trillion in "undocumentable adjustments" by the Departments of Defense (DoD) and Housing and Urban Development (HUD) between 1998 and 2015.[3] How much of the missing money went into a "breakaway civilization" space program with miles of underground bases and sophisticated transportation systems?

> It is still too early to tell how space will perform as an investment sector. One warning is the historical fact that flight has captured our imaginations more than it has rewarded our savings. I suspect that this is one reason that so much of the initial investment had to be funded by money disappeared from the federal coffers without the public approval of Congress.[4]

Since 1999, the job of the Federal Accounting Standards Advisory Board (FASAB) has been to set general acceptable accounting practices (GAAP) for the federal government. On October 4, 2018, Standard 56 was adopted to allow federal entities "to shift amounts from line item to line item and sometimes even omit spending altogether when reporting their financials in order to avoid the potential of revealing classified information"[5]— whether classified or confidential (Executive Order 13526, 2009). FASAB Standard 56

---

1 Joseph P. Farrell, *Covert Wars and Breakaway Civilizations: The Secret Space Program, Celestial Psyops and Hidden Conflicts.* Adventures Unlimited Press, 2012.

2 Marcus Weisgerber, "The Space Force Appears Cleared For Launch." Defense One, December 7, 2019.

3 Fitts and Mark Skidmore, PhD, Morris Chair of State and Local Government and Policy at Michigan State University and co-editor of the Journal of Urban Affairs, proved it: see https://home.solari.com/dod-and-hud-missing-money-supporting-documentation/, as well as Greg Hunter's "Elite Stole $50 Trillion and Will Invest in Space – Catherine Austin Fitts," USAWatchdog.com, June 17, 2018.

4 Catherine Austin Fitts, "What's Up in the Space-Based Economy." The Solari Report, Vol. 2018, No. 2.

5 "FASAB Statement 56: Understanding New Government Financial Accounting Loopholes," Solari.com, n.d.

killed off Article I, Section 9, Clause 7 of the U.S. Constitution and gave the National Security State *carte blanche* on financial accounting, and legalized the "undocumentable adjustments" theft that Fitts and Mark Skidmore fought so hard to expose.[6]

> *No Money shall be drawn from the Treasury, but in Consequence of Appropriations made by Law; and a regular Statement and Account of the Receipts and Expenditures of all public Money shall be published from time to time.*

The federal budget and whatever it might reveal to us about the secret space program or any other SAP (special access program) has gone utterly, deeply black.

FASAB 56 protects not just government agencies and departments but space program contractors like Lockheed Martin, Raytheon, SAIC, L3, etc.—in other words, the entire military-industrial-intelligence complex that President Eisenhower warned of too little, too late. From the *Solari Report*:

> Statement 56 undercuts the reliability of government accounting standards and financial statements to such a degree as to render an already questionably valuable reporting tool virtually useless to the public. The possibility of false or omitted information renders the reports largely unreliable to actual amounts, as does the fact that even an accurate report is rendered questionable by the very existence of modifications that are not necessarily exposed. Classifying portions of the federal GAAP mystifies the process even further, and the fuzzy definitions of reporting entities leaves the potential for this to touch *not only direct government entities, but government contractors and other private (but federally entangled) entities.* The general disclosure of the government—requiring all reporting entities to report the potential of modifications whether or not they actually exist in their report while simultaneously forbidding the actual disclosure of the actual existence of any modifications—is essentially a worst case in terms of transparency for the public.[7] (Emphasis added.)

The secret space program began in earnest after President John F. Kennedy was assassinated. The first few decades, CIA / DIA "master intelligence officers" concentrated on spinning Cold War "conspiracy theories" to obscure the real experiments and operations going on under Paperclip aerospace engineer Wernher von Braun, first director of NASA. Field tests of Paperclip Nazi zero-point gravity (ZPG) exotic propulsion craft were hidden beneath UFO

6 Laurence Kotlikoff, "Is Our Government Intentionally Hiding $21 Trillion In Spending?" Forbes, July 21, 2018.

7 "FASAB Statement 56."

/ aliens yellow journalism while the secret space program quietly weaponized the new Tesla physics bolstered by the ancient Vedic science that the Nazis had chased down during World War Two and brought with them to America.[8]

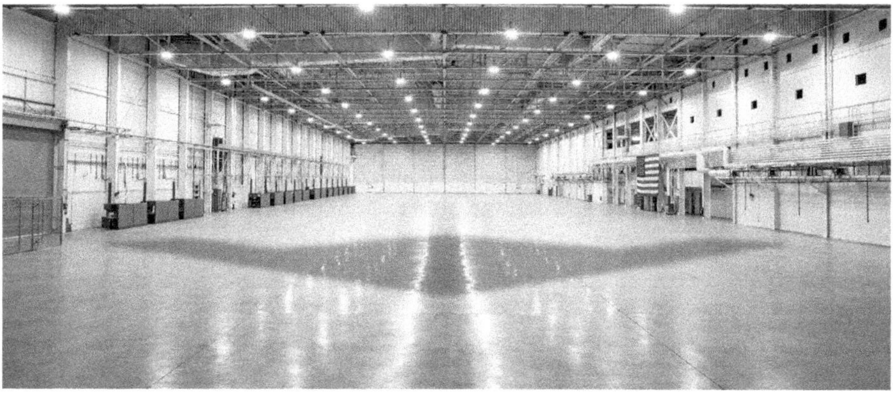

B-21 Raider, Northrup Grumman. "It's detectable. Until it's not."
https://www.northropgrumman.com/what-we-do/air/b-21-raider/

In a single bound, Bernard Eastlund's 1987 HAARP patent for the energy linkup with the ionosphere resurrected the "Star Wars" Strategic Defense Initiative (SDI) and boosted the secret space program into high gear. With HAARP and other ionospheric heaters and particle accelerators "pumping" the ionosphere, and jets and rockets "dumping" chemicals loaded with nano-sized conductive metals, the charged plasma atmosphere necessary for full spectrum dominance over planet Earth took shape.[9] Tankers, transmitters and receivers, power lines, GWEN and cell towers, fiber optic cable, phased array antennas, embedded nanosensors, NEXRADs, mobile SBX-1 HAARP units, radio observatories, satellite platforms—all became dual-use OOTW (operations other than war):

Fiber optics-based C4 plus optical switching systems
Power transfer systems
Space-based scalar SDI (Space Fence) replacing the old ground-based missile defense
Weather engineering a plasma atmosphere
Space situational awareness (SSA)

---

8 See Ramesh Kumar Menaria and Veda Priya, Energy Science in Vedas: A Treatise on Vedic Thermodynamics and Free Energy (Delhi: Parimal Publications, 2016).
9 Full spectrum dominance includes the frequency of DNA, given that DNA resonates with the frequencies hitting the ionosphere.

Net-centric warfare
Biochemical / electromagnetic control over human behavior

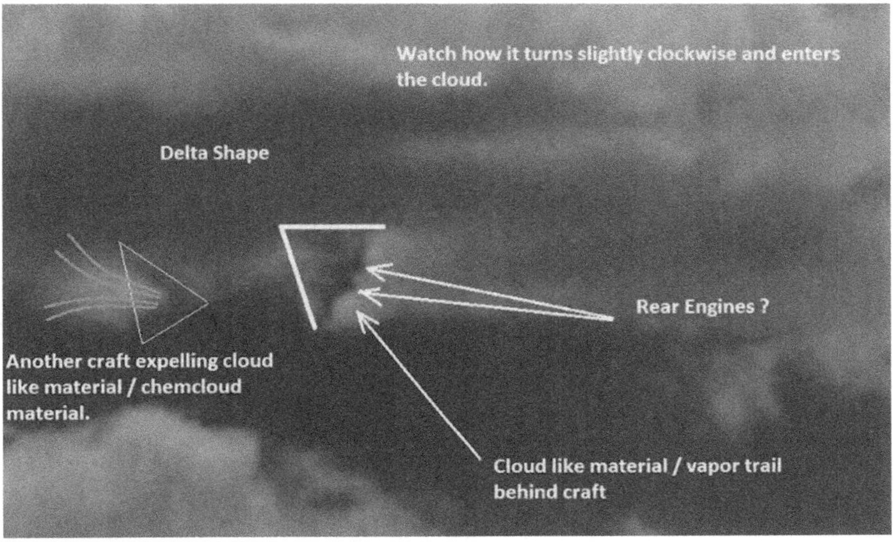

Geoengineering operation #7: Cloaked Cloud Craft.

Jim Kerr, May 25, 2017 (see "UFO / Cloaked Cloud Craft April 20, 2013," February 29, 2016, *https://www.youtube.com/watch?v=aABnGFcMV8A)*:

"I believe the craft are ours . . . Several years ago, I met and became friends with a person who was in charge of a special radar program at Edwards Air Force Base. I told him what I was capturing. Of course, he wouldn't say much. He did state the special advanced radar program was for a special type of drone not publicly known. He further stated, 'What we have is beyond science fiction.' He was only stationed here for two years. His job was to travel from base to base to set up and instruct in the operation of this system. Very interesting."

Once the global infrastructure of full spectrum dominance was underway, NASA's propaganda switched to promoting fear about "climate change" and extorting monies for dual-use space weather technology to work in tandem with the International Space Station, satellites, and two dozen star-like "battle stations" rotating geosynchronous with the Earth—all serving net-centric warfare via space situational awareness via dual-use space weather technology:

- *Cloud-Aerosol Transport System (CATS)* – LiDAR measurement of clouds, airborne nanoparticles. Built by NASA's Goddard Space Flight Center in Maryland
- *ISS Rapid Scat* – monitors hurricanes and storms. Built by NASA's Jet Propulsion Lab (JPL) in Pasadena, California
- *Stratospheric Aerosol and Gas Experiment III (SAGE)* – measures aero-

sols, ozone, water vapor, etc. Developed by NASA's Langley Research Center in Virginia and Ball Aerospace in Colorado

- *Lightning Imaging Sensor (LIS)* – lightning and Alfvén wave generation. Developed by NASA's Marshall Space Flight Center, Huntsville, Alabama
- *Global Ecosystem Dynamics Investigation (GEDI)* – laser-based vegetation surveillance; managed by the University of Maryland
- *Ecosystem Spaceborne Thermal Radiometer Experiment on Space Station (ECOSTRESS)* – thermal-imaging spectrometer to study water; managed by JPL
- *CERES (Clouds and the Earth's Radiant Energy System)*, instrument aboard NASA's Aqua and Terra satellites to measure shortwave and longwave radiation to determine Earth's in and out radiation budget
- *ECCO (Estimating the Circulation and Climate of the Ocean)* – altimetry (determines distance to target for pulsing), coastal low-orbiting for relaying voice, data, GPS, decoding infrared brain imaging; managed by JPL/CIT
- *SOFIA (Stratospheric Observatory for Infrared Astronomy)* modified Boeing 747SP (special performance) 14 meters shorter and the top of the tail at 20 meters; 250cm telescope accesses visible, infrared, and submillimeter spectrums; NASA and German Aerospace (DLR)[10]
- *HALO (High Altitude and LOng Range Research Aircraft)*, LiDAR atmospheric research and Earth observation; spray nozzles from the baggage compartment disperse perfluorocarbon (PFC)[11] into the aircraft wake, diameter less than 20 μm; German Aerospace (DLR)

Plasma

In the 1920s, Dutch physicists Drs Malta and Zaalberg Van Zelst claimed that the physical-etheric body is capable of expanding 40 million times its normal size and contracting by 6.25 million times. According to them, it was composed of "extremely small and widely separated" atoms and had a density of 176.5 times lighter than air and weighed, on average, 69.5 grams (or about two-and-a-quarter ounces). The description that the atoms were widely separated means that the particle density in the body is low. Furthermore, it

---

10 SOFIA was grounded during the COVID-19 2020 lockdown, and 120+ of the world's largest telescopes were shut down, leaving just a handful of large optical telescopes still operant: the Green Bank Observatory, the twin Pan-STARRS telescopes on Haleakala volcano in Hawaii, Russia's 45-year-old Bolshoi Azimuthal Telescope in the Caucasus, the 25-year-old Hobby-Eberly Telescope in West Texas.

11 PFC is definitely a greenhouse gas. Thanks to Pete Ramon.

would also imply that these "atoms" had a similar net electric charge as they repelled each other to cause the low density. This suggests that the matter is composed of plasma.

– Jay Alfred, *Our Invisible Bodies: Scientific Evidence for Subtle Bodies,* 2005

The careful line drawn long ago between visible and invisible, matter and spirit, is disappearing.

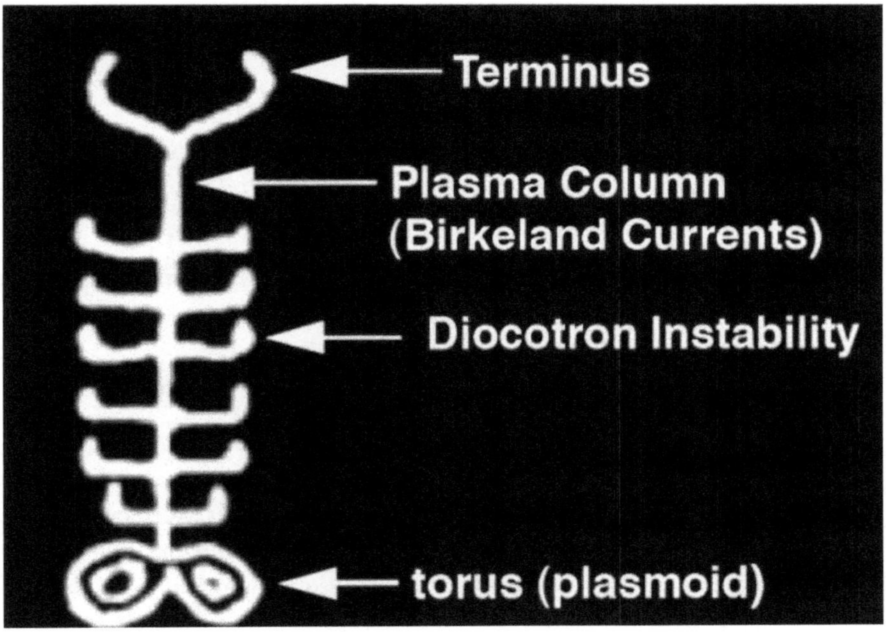

Ladder of heaven, backbone of the sky. Did this rock pictograph in Kayenta, Arizona depict a cosmic plasma event, namely the dismemberment of a polar configuration?

S. Schirott, "Plasma Scientist Anthony Peratt Meets the Electric Universe." *The Thunderbolts Project,* April 8, 2016.

In the 19th century, chemist and physicist Sir William Crookes and other Royal Society (Freemason) members attended séances in order to observe mediums like Florence Cook materialize *ectoplasm*—plasma, the fourth state of matter—then de-materialize it by reabsorbing the plasma. As late as 1942, the Josiah Macy Foundation called a meeting of Cybernetics Group luminaries to discuss the physiological mechanisms of animal magnetism / mesmerism in relationship to hypnosis, conditioned reflexes, and cerebral inhibition. Today, agencies like the U.S. Army Intelligence and Security Command (INSCOM) oversee "closed-system" electromagnetic (occult) technology reserved for classified "virtual worlds" research and "training exercises."

Plasma physics—the study of the subatomic particles that make up plasma—has only existed since the 1930s. The term *plasma* (to mold) was coined by Irving Langmuir because of how electrons entering plasma produce well-organized collective (hive or swarm) effects that behave much like a life form or biological organism, similar to the colorless fluid of living blood cells also called plasma. The universe is alive with electric plasma currents organized into sheets of filaments and cells with magnetic field-aligned boundaries (Birkeland currents, Alfven waves, etc.) that charge the aurora borealis and form systems of galaxies linked like pearls on a string.

Æther: the prime continuum of the fundamentally highest frequency of this universe. Light, heat, sound, magnetism, electricity, vibration, and mass all comes from æther.

Plasma: high-energy ions of fundamental elements manifesting in two modes: luminous and dark.

Fluorescent lamps, neon lights, the aurora borealis, the Sun, stars—shapes and sizes of plasma in action. The motion of electrons and ions inside plasma generate electric and magnetic fields. Electric fields accelerate charged particles to high speeds while magnetic fields—*the real architects of the universe*—guide and confine them. Every rotating object in the universe has a magnetic field with magnetic lines of force (currents) generating magnetic fields around them. Magnetism determines the character, motion, and shape of ionized matter (plasma).

Beams of electrons in plasma radiate microwaves. Plasma—ionized gas consisting of positive ions and free electrons—is an excellent conductor of electricity and an efficient source of electromagnetic radiation, due to its free electrons. With the right frequencies, plasma becomes transparent. Inside our ionized atmospheric dome, plasma's density increases or decreases as kinetic energy is built up or dispersed, and electrolytic water its byproduct, morphs into charged (dry) clouds.

The lower atmosphere (troposphere) plays an important role in accumulating energy, due to its increased electrical field strength. Photons convert to electrons in the upper atmosphere, metallic nanoparticles serve conductivity in the lower atmosphere. Free electric charges make plasma electrically conductive (+), plus plasma can be made to couple strongly with the electromagnetic fields around bioelectromagnetic *bios* beings (-).

Bioelectromagnetism is the electric current produced by action potentials along with the magnetic fields they generate through the phenomenon of electromagnetic induction . . . Bioelectromagnetism is an aspect of all living things, including all plants and animals. *Bioenergetics* is the study of energy relationships of living organisms. (Wikipedia)

Up until recently, our atmosphere served the *bios* (life) dependent upon an O2-CO2 cycle, *therapeutic ionized oxygen* following from (1) decay of radiation from the Sun, cosmic radiation, and radioactive materials on Earth; (2) our 400,000-volt gradient electric field between the ionosphere and the Earth surface; (3) natural wind (air masses) and weather fronts; and (4) falling (precipitating) water. Up until the geoengineering of our environment, the transfer of positive and negative ions mildly or cyclically electrified the atmosphere.

With the advent of artificial *atmospheric air ionization,* all of *bios* now suffers. The effects of artificial ionization go far beyond the "plasma [particle] climate forcing"[12] of weather engineering, being as they are essential to the objectives of the secret space program. The ionospheric absorption of high-frequency power that modifies the conductivity of our lower atmosphere—from the production of artificial plasma by laser and ionospheric heaters and plasma-enhanced chemical aerosols created by radio frequency and jet and rocket exhausts of dusty plasma and CCN (cloud condensation nuclei), negative ions attracting positively charged pollution, etc.—creates a 24/7 "antenna in the sky" for operations laid out by patents like US20070238252 A1 (2005), "Cosmic particle ignition of artificially ionized plasma patterns in the atmosphere":

> . . . a method and apparatus for creating artificially ionized regions in the atmosphere ["cosmic particle ignition"] utilizing ionization trails of cosmic rays and micro-meteors to ignite plasma patterns in electric field patterns formed by ground-based electromagnetic wave radiators [ionospheric heaters, radar and laser installations]. The applications are useful for telecommunications, weather control, lightning protection and defense applications . . .

and "defense applications" (read weapons) like Boeing's 2012 patent US8981261, "Method and system for shockwave attenuation via electromagnetic arc":

12 See Ben Davidson's "Plasma Climate Forcing" YouTube series.

It will work by superheating the air between the intended target and the blast, using an arc generator to create a plasma shield, using methods which might include high intensity laser pulses, conductive iron pellets, sacrificial conductors, projectiles trailing electric wires or magnetic induction. Once in place, the denser-than-air plasma shield will deflect and reduce the incident blast energy . . .[13]

Greater by far than the primitive Big Bang theory is the Electric Plasma universe of Hannes Alfvén (1908-1995). Comprising 99.999 percent of all matter, plasma is basically an ionized gas loaded with charged particles responding collectively to electromagnetic forces while the auroras at the Poles are magnetized plasmas accelerating solar electrons to 10^3 electron volts (eV) (solar flares being 10^9 – 10^{10} eV). Detected by telescope[14] in deep space, X-rays and gamma rays are produced by magnetized plasmas whose accelerating electrons stream from the Sun.

Plasma is said to be the fourth state of matter after gas, liquid, and solid, *but it is more likely the first state of matter after æther.*

In *The Body Electric,* Robert O. Becker, MD, references a statement by British mathematics physicist Robin K. Bullough at the Symposium on Electromagnetic Compatibility in Zurich:

> In 1983, measurements from the Ariel 3 and 4 weather satellites showed that the enormous amount of PLHR [power line harmonic resonance] over North America had created a *permanent duct from the magnetosphere down into the upper air,* resulting in a continuous release of ions and energy over the whole continent.[15] (Emphasis added.)

These *plasma ducts* about 600 km above the planet connect the Earth to the plasmasphere by following the paths of the magnetic field lines of force (Birkeland currents) up through the magnetosphere into the ionosphere. *Both Birkeland Currents and plasma ducts can be induced by ionospheric heater technology.*

> The innermost layer of the magnetosphere is the ionosphere, and above that is the plasmasphere. They are embedded with a variety of strangely shaped plasma structures, including the tubes . . . "[The plasmasphere] is

13 "Battlefield 2050: direct energy weapons meet the forcefield." Armytechnology.com, May 10, 2016. Plasma-based weapons are rife, the effects of even being presented as space weather, like the 620-mile-wide swirling mass of plasma called a "space hurricane": Denise Chow, "Swirling mass of plasma raining electrons observed above Earth for first time," NBC News, March 4, 2021.

14 Telescopes can now span 73 octaves of the electromagnetic spectrum.

15 Robert O. Becker, MD, The Body Electric: Electromagnetism and the Foundation of Life (William Morrow, 1998).

around where the neutral atmosphere ends, and we are transitioning to the plasma of outer space," [Cleo] Loi said.[16]

Are these plasma ducts about vectoring capability? Brazilian physicist Fran De Aquino asserts that the global chemtrails-ionospheric heater network serving the Space Fence promises not just engineered weather and geophysical and holographic events but modification and control of gravity itself.[17]

On September 24, 2016, Mila Zinkova was watching the sunset from Pacifica, California when the Sun split into multiple layers followed by green flashes. She sent her video[18] to astronomer Andrew T. Young at San Diego State University, who responded with the following:

> I think there are at least three ducts. The highest and lowest intermittent green beads that come and go coincide with discontinuities in sky brightness, which suggest you were looking up through a duct at that level. All of the ducts are well above you, which makes it a little difficult to make sure exactly where they all are, but notice how many multiple images of the full Sun there are (although strongly compressed), so you certainly have a Novaya Zemlya display here. And then you got the whale spouts relatively near shore! Lots of waves on the inversions; strong asymmetries in the shape of the Sun; multiple green flashes. I would also note that the transient beads at the elevated ducts look very much like cloud-top flashes, so much so that they help explain that cloud-top flashes are caused by a duct at the capping inversion. This seems to be the missing link in the cloud-top flash story.

In May 2017, NASA went public with the massive VLF (very low frequency) "impenetrable barrier" now surrounding the Earth around the equator, all the way up to the inner edge of the Van Allen radiation belts (400+ miles / 640 km). NASA's claim is that military radio communications sig-

---

16 Chris Pash, "Australian student confirms that giant plasma tubes are floating above Earth." Business Insider, 2 June 2015. Cleo Loi of the ARC Centre of Excellence for All-sky Astrophysics (CAASTRO) and the School of Physics at the University of Sydney received an award for photographing plasma tubes in 3D, thanks to the Murchison Widefield Array radio telescope in the Western Australian desert. See CAASTRO YouTube "Cosmic cinema: astronomers make real-time 3D movies of plasma tubes drifting overhead," May 31, 2015.

17 See De Aquino's paper "High-power ELF radiation generated by modulated HF heating of the ionosphere can cause earthquakes, cyclones and localized heating." Maranhao State University, Physics Department, S. Luis/MA, Brazil, 2011. Also see supporting experiments by Greek physicist Dimitriou Stavros, TEI-Athens, Department of Electrical Engineering.

18 Mila Zinkova, "Rare and unusual (The Novaya Zemlya effect) sunset mirage with green flashes and whales spouts," September 24, 2016, https://www.youtube.com/watch?v=FjZMPBO1tXs.

nals have affected the high-frequency radiation around the Earth and "accidentally" made this digital Space Fence "CD-Rom" ring with the conductive metal nanoparticles delivered by the trillion from sounding rockets and stratospheric jets. The clue to the truth is that VLF is "a mainstay in many engineering, scientific, and military operations, perfect for broadcasting coded messages across long distances or deep underwater."[19] As for the "strange" solar charged particles "caught within Earth's magnetic field," they are simply "anthropogenic impacts" lightly alluded to as "chemical release experiments, high-frequency wave heating of the ionosphere and the interaction of VLF waves with the radiation belts."[20]

Our Saturn-like planetary lockdown has sandwiched us between a ULF barrier and satellites in low-earth orbit (LEO) and on Earth a Lockheed Martin global infrastructure, all based on Tesla technology.

Certainly, kinetic energy shifts and a proper increase in electron density all matter to geoengineers responsible for keeping the atmosphere ionized for multiple operations. Early on, HAARP phased arrays were used to generate radio-reflective plasma by steering radiation into the ionosphere. Now, keeping the upper atmosphere flush with ionized plasma for the vast arena of communications and surveillance needs supplementary plasma generators to "bomb" the skies with plasma. Inside tiny CubeSats, nanoparticles of metals are being chemically vaporized beyond the boiling point so as to react with atmospheric oxygen and produce dusty plasma. Maximum metal vapor and plasma with controlled release options is part of the story, magnetohydrodynamics (MHD) power generation the rest.[21]

Is this then the "chembombs" observed before 2012—U.S. Air Force *plasma bombs* to increase the quantity of ions in the atmosphere to boost wireless communications? Are the chemical reactions of heat and vaporizing nanometals that then react with oxygen what is drying out our air[22]? Though CubeSats are mentioned as the delivery method, jets and drones would do, as well. Are plasma bombs the plasma orbs being created in space and delivered into the troposphere by radio control[23]?

---

19 BEC Crew, "NASA Space Probes Have Detected a Human-made Barrier Surrounding Earth." ScienceAlert, 18 May 2017.

20 Ibid.

21 Michael Tanenbaum, "U.S. Air Force wants Drexel to help plasma bomb the skies." Philly Voice, August 9, 2016. MHD determines the dynamics of fluids that conduct electricity (like plasma and liquid metals). Fluid motion generates magnetic fields that confine plasma along the magnetic lines of force.

22 Kelly Hodgkins, "The U.S. Air Force wants to detonate plasma bombs in the sky." Digital Trends, August 12, 2016.

23 The BPEarthWatch.com video "Plasma Energy Space Station Continues" (August 11,

Plasma is ionized matter. It is less dense than solids or liquids and has no fixed shape or volume. Unlike gases, plasma's atoms have been stripped of their electrons so that the charged (+) nuclei (ions) roam freely. Plasmas can thus conduct electricity, make magnetic fields, and be held in place by magnetic fields (fusion power). Take, for example, the International Space Station (ISS) running on 120 volts DC. Extending hundreds of feet around it is a plasma cloud or cocoon of complex currents of electrons and ions in constant flux. Upon their return to Earth, ISS crew and guests smell ozone ("a faint acrid smell" – NASA astronaut Thomas Jones) generated from the stress on the metallic mass of the station. If the normal voltage fluctuates to 250 volts, invisible lightning strikes could damage the station.

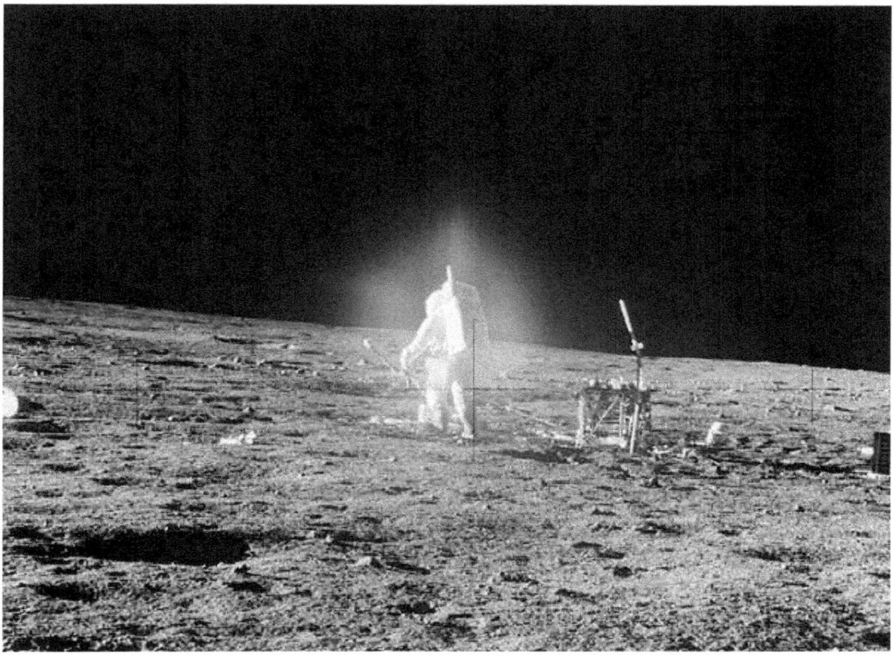

Plasma / æther. Alan Bean, Apollo 12. The cloud surrounding him is plasma / æther. https://www.lpi.usra.edu/resources/apollo/frame/?AS12-46-6826

Far-reaching energy experiments are going on with plasma. Plasma physics begins with plasma from the Sun and Birkeland currents, "entwined plasma filaments [that] act as transmission lines carrying 'field-aligned' currents across interplanetary and interstellar space"[24] with "resonant Alfvén waves on the same geomagnetic field lines that guide stationary Birkeland

2017) details what may be a plasma generator on the International Space Station (ISS) creating what appear to be plasma orbs.

24 http://www.thunderbolts.info/webnews/121707electricsun.htm.

currents,"[25] eventually moving into our post-HAARP plasma atmosphere where the Space Fence infrastructure labors to keep it all charged and ready for military-industrial operations and experiments.

A lot can be done with a *electrostatic field* in a plasma atmosphere. We have all rubbed an inflated balloon and stuck it onto a wall or been shocked by a doorknob after walking across a carpet. The static charge is held after the two surfaces separate by *electron transfer*—exactly as charge is retained in an atmosphere loaded with charged nanoparticles of metal.

In the Preface to *Under An Ionized Sky*, I talked about Dr. Judy Wood's deduction regarding the role of static electricity and the Hutchison Effect[26] in the destruction of the Twin Towers. All the theories of kerosene-fueled fire, thermite, mini-nukes, and lasers simply do not take into account the role of interfering microwave energies from an electrostatic field being remotely introduced into a rotating electric field to produce a magnetic field used to force *molecular dissociation*:

> By beaming a specially tuned microwave energy pulse rather than laser or infrared beams, that energy can be targeted within a storm's interior . . .[27]

ELF steering of radio waves, high voltage, and electrostatic fields theoretically means one can produce (1) levitation; (2) spontaneous fracturing of metals; (3) changes in crystalline structure and physical properties; and (4) fusion of dissimilar materials, like metals "melting" without burning adjacent materials like paper and trees, the 1943 Philadelphia Experiment, Hurricane Andrew 2X4s skewering palm trees in 1992, etc.

To build up enough static electricity to make something like 9/11 happen requires advance chemical trails loaded with nano-Mylar particulates so as to store and draw from the massive static energies in Hurricane Erin (whipped up by chemtrails and ionospheric heaters and parked off the Atlantic coast). Static electricity is used for "military snow," as Billy Hayes "The HAARP Man" calls the chemically nucleated snow that does not melt because it is composed of similar polymer / Mylar particulates storing static energy.[28] In

25 T.A. Potemra, "Birkeland Currents in the Earth's Magnetosphere." Johns Hopkins University, Applied Physics Laboratory, 6 July 1987.

26 Physicist savant John Hutchison (1945 -) studied Tesla's electrogravitic and longitudinal wave work and that of Thomas Townsend Brown (1905-1985), George Piggott ("Overcoming Gravitation"), Francis E. Nipper (1847-1926), and Martin L. Perl (1927 -). A must read: Judy Wood, PhD, Where Did the Towers Go? Evidence of Directed Free-energy Technology on 9/11 (The New Investigation, 2010).

27 Leonard David, "Taking the twist out of a twister." Space.com, March 3, 2000.

28 Ice nucleation is chemically created with carbon nanomaterials: carboxylated graphene nanoflakes, graphene oxide, oxidized single-walled carbon nanotubes, and oxidized multi-

Amarillo, Texas on May 1, 2013, the temperature was 100°F, but snow fell all the same, thanks to the static electricity that forced ice high above the Earth to nucleate. *Thundersnow* accompanied by thunder and lightning is also due to the stored static electricity potential between the ground and upper cloud masses. These are all, according to nanotech guru Pete Ramon, "triboelectrically charged snowy plasma." Triboelectric nanogenerators are composed of titanium and aluminum oxide or titanium and silicone dioxide and are used to harvest energy from just about anything with a surface—wind, ocean currents, sound, etc. The *triboelectric effect* is how electrons flow across barriers, with temperature playing a major role.[29]

Optics like rainbows, clouds, and structureless solar panels are often due to transmitter-generated algorithms producing static phenomena by computer, like the circular holes blasted through cloud cover, and fixed rainbows seen in New Zealand (Rose, April 2018):

> . . . Greg and I witnessed over 50 rainbows through our beautiful Westhaven Inlet & on the way home. Every second corner had one or two, and double rainbows were over the waterways. The difference between these rainbows and what we would call normal was that they were static, not the ever-elusive pot of gold rainbows. They stayed in one spot; we could drive through them and then look back on them.

Perhaps the effects are achieved with LIBS LiDAR (laser-induced breakdown spectroscopy light radar) bombarding light with ions so that it is absorbed and re-emitted in spectra (i.e. rainbows), or with NASA's Orbiting Rainbows project manipulating and controlling engineered dusty plasma / aerosols via radio frequency, optics, or microwaves:

> Our objective is to investigate the conditions to manipulate and maintain the shape of an orbiting cloud of dust-like matter so that it can function as an ultra-lightweight surface with useful and adaptable electromagnetic characteristics, for instance, in the optical, RF, or microwave bands . . . A cloud of highly reflective particles of micron size acting coherently in a specific electromagnetic band, just like an aerosol in suspension in the atmosphere, would reflect the Sun's light much like a rainbow.[30]

---

walled carbon nanotubes. See Thomas F. Whale, et al., "Ice Nucleation Properties of Oxidized Carbon Nanomaterials," Journal of Physical Chemistry Letters, July 13, 2015.

29 Zhang Lin Wang et al., "On the Electron Transfer Mechanism in the Contact-Electrification Effect." Advanced Materials, 2018.

30 Marco Quadrelli, "Orbiting Rainbows: Optical Manipulation of Aerosols and the Beginnings of Future Space Construction." NASA, June 18, 2013. Note "future space construction." Thanks to Pete Ramon. See the entire final report at https://www.nasa.gov/sites/

Thus we begin to understand why the constant production of plasma cloud cover—"spatially disordered dust-like objects that can be optically manipulated"—can be cyber-morphed into static, *sculpted,* picture-perfect cumulus clouds *that may even be watching us as we watch them*—"the engineering of distributed ensembles of spacecraft swarms [of nanoparticles] to shape an orbiting cloud of micron-sized objects . . . new technology in the areas of Astrophysical Imaging Systems and Remote Sensing because the cloud can operate as an adaptive optical imaging sensor."[31]

Then there are the "structureless solar panels" of the atmospheric energy harvesting programs, according to Facebook's observant Eric Cypher:

> Some trails went across the whole sky from horizon to horizon, and quite a few ended abruptly near the Sun. A lot of starts and stops, but the end result is always the same: MASSIVE SUNDOGS (orbiting halos and rainbows). I believe this is their atmospheric solar energy program: creating structureless solar panels out of particles and artificial clouds. The energy can then be transferred to heliocentric satellites and/or be MANipulated throughout the atmosphere for various purposes.

In the 1901 article "Talking with the Planets" in Collier's Weekly, Tesla claimed that "man could tap on the breast of Mother Sun and release her energy toward Earth as needed—magnetic as well as light." Beaming solar power down to the Earth during the day and using Rectenna Arrays to harvest energy from the Sun's infrared radiation at night[32] is certainly part of the solar energy plan for "orbiting solar farms," but only part.

In 2009, Solaren Corporation in California signed a 15-year, 1,700 gigawatt hours deal with California's utility PG&E[33]—the very years of the 2017-2018 "wildfires" for which PG&E took the blame for negligence, had its hand slapped, then was handed a $59 billion "restructuring plan." On 9/19/2019, Los Angeles-based Heliogen went public with *concentrated solar power* based on an AI-run technology that uses a ground-based field of mirrors "to reflect the sun to a single point," enough sunlight to produce 1,000°C (1,832°F), plus a way to store solar energy and create clean hydrogen for fuel.[34]

---

default/files/files/Quadrelli_2012_PhI_OrbitingRainbows_.pdf.

31 Ibid.

32 Ken Lebrun, "DARPA: Energy Harvesting." Revolution-Green, May 28 2013. Rectennas are receiving micro-antennas with micro rectifying diodes and micro capacitors on the Earth for capturing infrared radiation and converting it to DC current.

33 Ucilia Wang, "Solaren to Close Funding for Space Solar Power." GreenTechMedia, December 4, 2009.

34 "Secretive energy startup backed by Bill Gates achieves solar breakthrough." CNN Business, November 19, 2019.

Plasma life forms

> *The physical universe is made up of mass-less electric charges immersed in a vast, energetic, all-pervasive electromagnetic field. It is the interaction of those charges and the electromagnetic field that creates the appearance of mass.*
>
> - Astrophysicist Bernard Haisch, "Brilliant Disguise: Light, Matter, and the Zero-Point Field," 1999

> *Every fundamental [physical] matter particle should have a massive "shadow" force carrier particle, and every force carrier should have a massive "shadow" matter [super] particle.*
>
> – Particle Data Group, Laurence Berkeley National Lab

The 2003 headline "Plasma blobs hint at a new form of life" in the *Daily News* hardly did justice to what was going on in our ionized atmosphere laboratory after it had been chemically and electromagnetically "dosed" to simulate the primordial Earth atmosphere of electrical storms that appeared to have caused plasmas to form.

> Most biologists think living cells arose out of a complex and lengthy evolution of chemicals that took millions of years, beginning with simple molecules through amino acids, primitive proteins and finally forming an organised structure. But if Mircea Sanduloviciu and his colleagues at Cuza University in Romania are right, the theory may have to be completely revised. They say cell-like self-organisation can occur in a few microseconds.[35]

Low-temperature argon plasma, high voltage artificial lightning strikes, a high concentration of ions and electrons forming plasma spheres . . . But were the "plasma blobs" like the first living cells on Earth? They had distinct boundaries, the ability to self-replicate, they could communicate information, had a metabolism and grew.

And what exactly are that massive "shadow" matter superparticles that CERN and other particle accelerators are producing (see quote above)?

Superstring theory (E8 x E8) refers to interpenetrating universes (like the duplicate E8 universe) and "shadow" matter as being composed of invisible superparticles detected only gravitationally. Imagine the superparticles (*param anu*) as being finer than physical particles (*anu*) and existing in an astral mirror world that occupies the same space as this physical world, each

35 David Cohen, "Plasma blobs hint at new form of life." Daily News, 17 September 2003.

world unconscious of the other, their inhabitants reacting only to their own frequencies. Astrophysicist John Gribbin wrote, "A shadow planet could pass right through the Earth and never affect us, except through its gravitational pull."[36] Physicist Richard Morris put it this way:

> If someone tried to grasp a chunk of shadow matter, her hands would pass right through it. It has been said that one would walk through a shadow matter mountain or stand at the bottom of a shadow matter ocean and never know it. Shadow matter particles could interact with one another according to physical laws similar to those of our world. It is possible that there could be shadow matter planets, and perhaps even shadow matter organisms.[37]

Once electrons are in plasma, they behave collectively like a primitive cell life form. Electrically charged, plasma can separate, polarize, and undergo self-organization, after which it can regenerate and protect itself by encasing foreign substances behind membrane-like walls. But are plasma-based life forms the same as inorganic living matter[38] that even inorganic dust organizes into helical structures that interact as organic life would? In gravity-free space, electrically charged plasma particles bead together in filaments that then twist into helical strands like DNA. The helical structures divide and form copies, then interact to induce new structures in the copies.

Because these helical structures are most common in space, plasma inorganic life forms may be common, such as the giant diaphanous "critters" that Trevor Constable photographed with infrared film in the Southwest desert.[39] If plasma life forms were present billions of years ago when the Earth atmosphere was highly ionized, hot, and gaseous—as much as a billion years before carbon-based biomolecular life forms began to appear—then plasma is actually the *first* state of matter.

Chemical and electromagnetic alteration of the Earth's atmosphere coupled with extreme weather could duplicate, to some degree, the primordial conditions needed to develop inorganic plasma life forms. Such an atmosphere-as-lab could be the environmental preparation behind the "prequel" release of genetically engineered primitive pathogens like Morgellons and its

---

36 John Gribbin, The Search for Superstrings, Symmetry, and the Theory of Everything. Back Bay Books, 2009.

37 Richard Morris, The Edges of Science: Crossing the Boundary from Physics to Metaphysics. Simon & Schuster, 1990.

38 See V.N. Tsytovich et al., Russian Academy of Science, "From Plasma Crystals and Helical Structures Towards Inorganic Living Matter." New Journal of Physics, August 2007.

39 See the IR photographs in Trevor James Constable's The Cosmic Pulse of Life: The Revolutionary Biological Power Behind UFOs (1976).

cross-domain bacteria (CDB), the COVID-19 Spike protein of recent gene therapy infamy, etc.

As chemical trails released nanoparticles of conductive metals, nanosensors, nanobots, and gain-of-function single-cell microbes in 2003, physicists at Cuza University in Romania published "Minimal Cell System Created in Laboratory by Self-Organization" about the lab-grown *plasma spheres* they had grown, replicated, and communicated—just like biological cells—the nucleus of each plasma sphere mimicking the breathing process of a living system and resulting in *pulsations.*[40]

Is this the threshold of creation come again? Were plasma spheres the first cells on Earth? And what about in space, like the pulsating orbs swarming outside the International Space Station and space shuttles like the *Atlantis,* due to their attraction to the static electricity[41]? Plasma spheres swarm and are able to change their degree of opacity and output of luminosity at will, but are they of the same dark plasma[42] composition as plasma orbs? Michael Persinger, PhD, proved a link between electromagnetic fields and orb activity primarily due to the orbs' magnetic plasma composition. Magnetic plasma generates electromagnetic fields and radiates electromagnetic waves.

Thus, we arrive at *bioplasma* and *subtle bodies,* the templates of physical-biomolecular, carbon-based bodies.

Plasma beam DEWs and augmented reality (AR) mind control

Dark matter particles (axions[43]) become fascinating when considered in the light of magnetic fields, quantum entanglement, and bioplasma bodies known in metaphysical literature as *subtle bodies.*

After Semyon Kirlian discovered an energy field around living bodies in 1939 (Kirlian photography)—what metaphysicists refer to as the *aura*—biochemists and biophysicists determined through more sophisticated instruments

---

40 Mircea Sanduloviciu and Erzilla Lozneanu, "Minimal Cell System Created in Laboratory by Self-Organization." Chaos Solitons & Fractals, October 2003.

41 For example, "NASA U.F.O FOOTAGE (FULL VERSION)," Equalification Productions, September 3, 2011, https://www.youtube.com/watch?v=8njYpyAkMp8. "The NASA footage shown was obtained by a cable television company in Vancouver, BC. Originally one of the company's satellites picked up NASA feeds that they recorded on VHS tape, which then ended up in the hands of Martin Stubbs who managed the company. Martin spent over 2,500 hours recording and logging thousands of hours of NASA Space Shuttle transmissions and has dedicated his life to disclose the truth..."

42 In general, references to dark plasma, dark matter, and "shadow" matter superparticles reference the large parts of the universe that can be detected gravitationally but remain unseen. I recommend Jay Alfred's Our Invisible Bodies: Scientific Evidence for Subtle Bodies (Trafford Publishing, 2005) for more on these topics.

43 Axion was the name of the spaceship in the 2008 preprogramming Disney film WALL-E.

that the bioenergetic human body was actually a plasma constellation of ionized particles *and literally an organism in itself.* It is in the plasma organism that the nodes of energy known as acupuncture points are embedded. Cambridge biologist Oscar Bagnell even designed dyed hollow lenses to sensitize his eyes so he could view the *aura* and nodes of the bioplasma body directly.

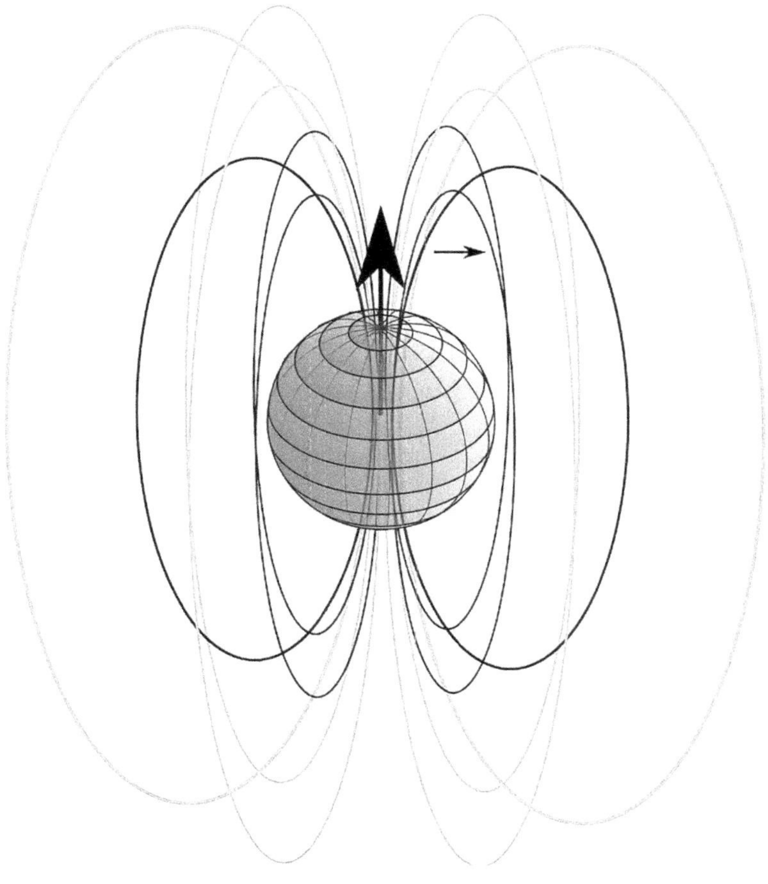

The magnetic field and telepathy. Michael Persinger, PhD: "Suppose you had access to every person's brain, and they had access to yours?" The human brain and geomagnetic field are strongly correlated (and therefore manipulated via directed energy weapons and "dual use" technologies).

https://subtle.energy/no-more-secrets-scientist-says-the-earths-magnetic-field-will-enable-telepathy-on-a-global-scale/

In our ionized atmosphere loaded with free electrical charges, plasma (ionized gas / positive ions) becomes extremely conductive and couples strongly to electromagnetic fields, including the biofield around living entities like human beings (bio-electromagnetism / negative ions). This is why the *particle beam weapon* is so effective in targeting individuals: the ion beam (-) couples with ionic cold plasma (+), creating plasma orbs (+ "string of pearls" gas plasma transmitters) that "stick" to the target, due to magnetic polarity with his or her bio-electromagnetic field. Once the plasma transceiver orbs "stick," the ion beam (-) can remotely access you anytime with holograms, V2K, pain induction—whatever the operation is. Plasma beams can serve as carrier beams for microwaves, FM, ELF, etc.—in other words, serve as carrier beams for the entire Internet of Things (IoT). Plasma (+) magnetically sticks to the target (-) by means of the plasma receivers stuck to the target.

Negative ion beam + positive ion plasma =
negative ion particle / plasma beam

Plasma's role in directed energy weapons varies, but generally speaking, as targeted individual Carolyn Williams Palit stressed, "The smaller beams from psychotronic scalar weapons being used on Americans are very related to the big, holographic scalar weapons used on 9-11."[44] Palit maintained that the airplanes that hit the World Trade Towers were holograms projected onto the prepared ionized plasma "screen" in the sky. It works like this: a beam weapon creates a Birkeland current with two beams twisted around each other in a 2D illusion, one beam for successive frames of the airliner, the other beam heating the previously laid chemical trails to make the conductive metal-induced, ionized gas plasma. (A weaponized Birkeland current is a splay-beam that looks like two pearl necklaces braided together.) For a 3D holographic operation, a third beam is needed, the first beam to heat the metal nanoparticles to produce the ionized gas heated into plasma; the second beam transmitting the 2D frames; the third beam crossing the other two beams to add a third dimension to the frames in the interference target zone.

An atmosphere ionized by ionospheric heater / chemical trails / microwave technology provides a ready plasma screen in the sky, thanks to ionized gases (plasma).

The AF Direct Energy System is used to target individuals, whether with interfering beams or gas plasma transmitters that attach plasma orbs

---

44 Carolyn Williams Palit, "The Direct Energy Age," October 2005. The website NoExoticWarfareZone is now defunct.

to people's heads, eyes, ears, and genitals via magnetic polarity. Satellites are involved, as well as plasma-cloaked aerial craft. Because ELFs are used and the Earth's fundamental resonant frequency is that of the 7.83 Hz Schumann resonance, there is really nowhere to run, nowhere to hide.

Alfvén Waves & Birkeland Currents

The ionosphere is a repository of alternative off-planet energy essential to the full spectrum dominance of planet Earth. Its energy influx explains what electromagnetic hotbeds the North and South Poles have become since Operation Deep Freeze and even back to the 1908 Tunguska event, Admiral Richard E. Byrd's expeditions, etc., both of which are discussed in my previous two books. It is the plasma electrojets (Birkeland current boundary flows) connecting Earth with the Sun that makes the Poles so coveted.

> [Birkeland current boundary flows] can drive the ionosphere to temperatures approaching 10,000°C [18,032°F] and change its chemical composition. They also cause the ionosphere to flow upwards to higher altitudes where additional energisation can lead to loss of atmospheric material to space.[45]

Under the cover of "climate change" remediation, space program experimentation in both the troposphere and stratosphere is now a top priority paid for by carbon credits and stolen / fudged FASAB $56 trillions. Thunder and lightning have been weaponized with pulsed high-frequency sound waves to disable electronic systems (EMPs / lightning) and shatter satellites (acoustic shockwaves / thunder or "booms in the air").[46] Both natural and manmade Alfvén waves and Birkeland currents are manipulated for a variety of effects, from generating earthquakes to increasing the speed of electrical propagation and conductivity between the ionosphere and atmosphere, *and between the planets and Sun,* all the while maintaining the Earth's *radiation budget*:

> The energy entering, reflected, absorbed, and emitted by the Earth system are the components of the Earth's radiation budget. Based on the physics principle of conservation of energy, this radiation budget represents the

45 "Supersonic Plasma Jets Discovered," European Space Agency (ESA), 23 March 2017, www.esa.int/Our_Activities/observing-the-Earth/Swarm/Supersonic-plasma-jets-discovered. Discoveries generally occur long before they are allowed to go public.

46 Patent US20130015260 A1, "Concept and model for utilizing high-frequency or radar or microwave producing or emitting devices to produce, effect, create or induce lightning or lightspeed or visible to naked eye electromagnetic pulse or pulses, acoustic or ultrasonic shockwaves or booms in the air, space, enclosed, or upon any object or mass, to be used solely or as part of a system, platform or device including weaponry and weather modification" (2004).

> accounting of the balance between incoming radiation, which is almost entirely solar radiation, and outgoing radiation, which is partly reflected solar radiation and partly radiation emitted from the Earth system, including the atmosphere. A budget that's out of balance can cause the temperature of the atmosphere to increase or decrease and eventually affect our climate. The units of energy employed in measuring this incoming and outgoing radiation are watts per square meter (W/m2).[47]

Much going on in the upper and lower atmospheres is about duplicating and retro-engineering the electromagnetic and plasma phenomena of Nature's planetary and solar systems, from particle accelerators and Alfvén wave electrojets at the Poles to Birkeland currents, the ionosphere, solar events, and reproduction of high-frequency ionospheric perturbation as weaponized high-frequency energy.

High-powered phased array antennas such as HAARP and EISCAT 3D stimulate the ionosphere, but that's not all they do. As U.S. Navy-trained nuclear expert Christopher Fontenot put it in 2017:

> There's so much more to the story: ionospheric charging, Alfvén waves, solar radiation influx, DEW [directed energy weapons] technology, etc. They say that hurricanes are a product of evaporation and water temperature with no reference to atmospheric charge potential. They say that ion channeling is the mechanism for propagating energy but don't mention Alfvén wave downward cascades (Townsend avalanches). *HAARP, which Eastlund designed, didn't simply heat an area of the ionosphere; it created* Alfvén *waves that energize the entire planet and induce solar activity via out-of-phase Birkeland current filaments between the Earth and Sun* . . . If we don't seize this opportunity, their next move is already in place to blame the Sun for climate change. I have the evidence to make the connections, and I'm not the originator of this idea. (Emphasis added.

Once ionospheric heat pops electrons off of atoms and ionizes them and density increases into strong electron precipitation, Alfvén waves begin spinning around the electrons and a high-speed stream of Alfvén waves excites large-scale gravity waves (scalar waves) in auroral regions "together with their proved ubiquity in the solar atmosphere and solar wind," suggesting that Alfvén waves are an important solar interplanetary driver of global thermospheric disturbances.[48]

In fact, Alfvén wave perturbation in the ionosphere impacts the resonance

47 https://science.nasa.gov/ems/13_radiationbudget

48 ". . . Alfvén waves occurring both naturally and artificially through ionospheric perturbation are responsible for thermal effects via Joule heating of our atmosphere as well as that of the Sun's corona." http://www.nature.com/articles/srep18895.

frequency of our Schumann cavity as well as the ELF sympathetic resonance between Earth and Sun. Life on Earth is not just affected by the Schumann resonance; it is *shaped* by it. The vibrational forces heard for eons as the sound current *Om* synchronize our metabolic functions with the Earth's rhythmic cycles. Our brains are locked onto its harmonic. The Schumann standing wave "rings" in the Schumann cavity for 55 kilometers up, but now it is equally true that when HAARP or another ionospheric heater plays its ULF frequencies in the Schumann resonance range of 7-8Hz, the ionosphere "rings" as ions tumble into our lower atmosphere to be intensified by conductive nanoparticles of metals zapped by radio frequency and microwaves.

Schumann frequency pulses connect and influence all living systems and consciousness within the boundaries of our Earth-ionosphere resonant cavity. Is it the Schumann resonance frequency that's fluctuating, or the amplitude (intensity)? The Russian Space Observing System continues to monitor the fluctuations between 8.5Hz and 16.5Hz as they move from *theta* (4-7.5Hz) and *alpha* (7.5-14Hz) to *beta* (14-40Hz) brain waves.[49] According to the Global Coherence Monitoring System, "Resonances can be observed at around 7.8, 14, 20, 26, 33, 39 and 45 Hertz, with a daily variation of about ± 0.5 Hertz, which is *caused by the daily increase and decrease in the ionization of the ionosphere due to UV radiation from the sun*."[50] (Emphasis added.)

"Due to UV radiation of the sun"? Really?

Natural Alfvén waves are low frequency, fluid-like plasma waves, whereas *whistler waves* (1-10 kHz VLF acoustic signatures) are created by lightning discharges zapping the Earth's magnetic lines of force.[51] Whistlers are needed to remove "killer" radioactive electrons ("particle remediation") in the Earth's magnetosphere so as to protect satellites and calm the Van Allen radiation belts so humans can pass through on their way to the stars. With plasma density to guide and amplify them, Alfvén waves are injected into the radiation belts while Van Allen probes collect data for spacecraft design.

Energetic electrons trapped inside the Earth's magnetic field can be accelerated by the whistler waves, which travel along the magnetic field line from the northern to the southern hemisphere within one second. By in-

49 http://sosrff.tsu.ru/?page_id=7. English translation: https://translate.google.com/translate?hl=en&sl=ru&tl=en&u=http://sosrff.tsu.ru/?page_id=7

50 Global Coherence Initiative (GCI), https://www.heartmath.org/research/global-coherence/. The Global Coherence Monitoring System operates magnetometers at Boulder Creek, CA; Hofuf, Saudi Arabia; Alberta, Canada; Baisogala, Lithuania; Northland Region of New Zealand; Kwazulu Natal, South Africa. The Global Coherence Monitoring System (GCMS) directly measures fluctuations in the magnetic fields generated by the earth and in the ionosphere.

51 Atmospheric sprites that occur above thunderstorms are also being manufactured.

creasing the particles' energy, they can be forced to move down into the atmosphere, instead of remaining in the magnetic field. This doesn't damage the atmosphere, because it is very dense compared to space. These electrons subsequently recombine with ions in the ionosphere and form neutral molecules. The end result is that the dangerous radiation is removed from space.[52]

Birkeland currents connect our Poles with the Sun,[53] ionize atoms, create "funnels" of energy for the creation of electrojets, and perturb Alfvén waves in the ionosphere. By zapping gas plasma with electricity, twisted Birkeland currents can be created. The extreme activity in the Arctic Circle (including the shifts in magnetic north[54]) and in Antarctica points to how manipulation of Birkeland currents is connected to *manipulations of our star the Sun.*[55] From *Under An Ionized Sky*:

> For optimal Space Fence operations, Deep Freeze engineers are tasked with maintaining a delicate balance between magnetic south and magnetic north by means of ongoing fine-tuning, calibrating and experimentation. With the help of ionospheric heaters in the Northern Hemisphere, the bipolar *maser* outflow can be increased in the polar regions.[56] Increase the ion flow along the magnetic lines of force and it will be mirrored back toward Earth; increase the charge potential in the ionosphere and "fountain" up along the coherent inner core of Birkeland currents into the Sun's electromagnetic circuit. *Increase the charge potential of the Sun and voltage can be induced to increase solar activity*, as per Tesla in 1901. Christopher Fontenot in an email, May 3, 2017:
>
>> *As Birkeland currents interface at the Poles, they ionize atoms and create the 'funnel' of energy that cause the Earth's electrojets. This interaction perturbs Alfvén waves ["whistlers"] in the ionosphere. Alfvén waves are pilot waves. Imagine a drill bit tip and all magnetic lines of force spiraling out from that pilot wave. Alfvén waves occur in both longitudinal and transverse forms, which means they either have no frequency (longitudinal) or have an oscillation frequency (transverse).*

During the March 2015 saber rattling over Ukraine, nothing was said

52 Tatiana Ivanova, "Bombs away: 'Whistler waves' to protect communications from nuclear blast." DW, April 17, 2015.

53 The same appears to be true of other planets. "Magnetic Rope observed for the first time between Saturn and the Sun," UCL Space & Climate Physics, London UK, 6 July 2016.

54 Eric Mack, "Earth's Magnetic North Pole Is Shifting Dramatically From A Powerful Tug of War." Forbes, May 7, 2020: "One magnetized patch is beneath Canada while the other is under Siberia," and it's not necessarily due to "the flow of materials in our planet's core."

55 Kardashev's Phase II.

56 K. Papadopoulos et al., "HF-driven currents in the polar ionosphere." Geophysical Research Letters, 21 June 2011.

about Magnetic North. The truth is that the struggle over who will control Magnetic North and the plasma energy pouring from the Poles is far from resolved.[57]

With all of the ionospheric heater beams, over-the-horizon (OTH) broadcasts, satellite radar, and sounder rocket launches, is it any wonder that the Schumann resonance has become erratic? With the ability to manipulate the ionosphere, Birkeland currents, and Alfvén waves, is it much of a reach to take Nikola Tesla at his word when he said, "Man could tap the Breast of Mother Sun and release her energy toward Earth as needed—magnetic as well as light"? Alfvén waves provide the ELF harmonics necessary for Earth-Sun communications that then extend to all the planets in our solar system. Before this Electromagnetic Age, extremely low frequency fields (ELF) emanated from natural solar and cosmic events—lightning, geomagnetic storms, volcanic activity, earthquakes, and the Schumann resonance.

Now, cycles like the solar minimum and events like eclipses, sun spots, CMEs, etc. have become grist for the mill that is busily turning the Earth into a machine.

The Nuclear Behemoth

Trinity
"Accidents" or experiments?
Arto Lauri in Finland
Solar & lunar simulators

A column of smoke and dust rose into the air like a column of smoke issuing from the bowels of the Earth. It rained sulphur and fire on Sodom and Gomorrah [Lebanon[58]], and destroyed the town and the whole plain and all the inhabitants and every growing plant. And Lot's wife looked back and was turned into a pillar of salt. And Lot lived at Isoar, but afterwards went to the mountains because he was afraid to remain at Isoar. The people were warned that they must go away from the place of the future explosion and not stay in exposed places; nor should they look at the explosion but hide beneath the ground . . . Those fugitives who looked back were blinded and died . . .

– The Dead Sea Scrolls

57 Elana Freeland, Under An Ionized Sky: From Chemtrails to Space Fence Lockdown. Feral House, 2018.

58 In Lebanon, hyaline rocks called tektites contain radioactive isotopes of aluminum and beryllium—glass from the heat of atmospheric friction.

The main danger from geoengineering is the radiation the spray blocks. DNA is unable to replicate at certain levels of UVC radiation. Such radiation, typically at around 245nm, is used to sterilize biology and destroy DNA's ability to replicate. That dangerous radiation is produced as sunlight shines through energetic plasma.

– Email from Richard Lawrence Norman, 2020

Jets fly at 31,000 to 38,000 feet (9.44 to 11.58 km / 5.86 to 7.19 miles) far below the Van Allen radiation belts that begin at 5,000 miles above us, and yet they are *still* flying through radiation clouds whose dose rates are *double* what they should be because the radiation is not just from cosmic rays.[59]

> Sometimes dose rates skyrocket for no apparent reason . . . All of the surges [the Automated Radiation Measurements for Aerospace Safety (ARMAS)] observed occurred at relatively high latitudes, well above 50 degrees in both hemispheres . . . The ARMAS flight module recorded a 2X increase in ionizing radiation for about 30 minutes while the plane flew 11 km (36,000 feet) over the Antarctic Peninsula. No solar storm was in progress. The plane did not abruptly change direction or altitude. Nevertheless, the ambient radiation environment changed sharply. Similar episodes have occurred off the coast of Washington state.[60]

"Dose rates skyrocket for no apparent reason"? What about Boeing's plasma pulse engine (Patent #US9068562 B1, "Laser-Powered Propulsion System," June 30 2015) that uses high-powered lasers to "trigger a small nuclear reaction" for thrust? A stream of hydrogen isotopes (deuterium or tritium) triggers a small thermonuclear explosion from which heat energy is harvested.

> According to the patent documents, the walls of the engine's combustion chamber would be lined with a fissile material like Uranium 238, which would react with the high-energy neutrons produced by the nuclear reaction to generate huge amounts of heat. On the other side of the chamber wall, a coolant would pick up this heat and be sent through a turbine / generator to produce electricity . . . used to power the engine's lasers . . .[61]

---

59 Please review "Radiation and the Wigner Effect," pages 82-86, Under An Ionized Sky.

60 Tony Phillips, PhD, "Radiation Clouds at Aviation Altitudes." Spaceweather.com, January 20, 2017.

61 Drew Prindle, "Boeing Just Patented a Laser-Powered Nuclear Fusion Engine," Digital Trends, July 13, 2015. Thanks to "The HAARP Man" Billy Hayes for pointing this technology out.

Military strategists' admissions that orbiting space trash impedes laser weapons may allude to more nuclear detonations going on in space. For example, on August 27, 1998, it was purported that a powerful blast of stellar radiation—gamma and X-ray radiation from the magnetic flare of a compressed neutron star (magnetar) 20,000 light years away—severely affected radio transmissions and shut down seven spacecraft. But was the blast really from a magnetar, or was it a HAARP-induced plasma weapon or nuclear detonation in space?

In 1958, *Explorer I* discovered the protective Van Allen Radiation Belts—the zones of charged particles trapped in the Earth's magnetic field that extend 5,000 to 32,000 miles above us (mentioned earlier). Like a net, these belts capture charged particles from solar and galactic winds and spiral them gently down along the magnetic lines of force that comprise the magnetosphere surrounding the Earth, until they converge at the Poles and spin the Arctic and Antarctic auroras.

After the discovery of the Belts, the U.S. Navy promptly detonated three nuclear bombs in them under Project Argus. In 1961 under Project Westford, the U.S. Air Force launched 480 million tiny copper needles designed to be half the wavelength of 8000 MHz microwaves in order to establish a permanent ring of tiny dipole antennas around the planet to serve as an artificial ionosphere. Their orbit at 3,700 km (2,299 miles) above the Earth created a donut-shaped toroid cloud 15 km wide and 30 km thick. Eventually, the dipoles dispersed, three satellites and the inner Van Allen Belt were destroyed, Hawaii blacked out, and the sky over the Arctic Circle caught fire. A remnant of the copper dipoles still orbits today.

The following year under Project Starfish, three nuclear bombs were detonated in the upper atmosphere.

> . . . the inner Van Allen Belt will be practically destroyed for a period of time . . . [and] the ionosphere . . . will be disrupted by mechanical forces caused by the pressure wave following the explosion. At the same time, large quantities of ionizing radiation will be released . . . On 19 July . . . NASA announced that as a consequence of the high-altitude nuclear test of July 9, a new radiation belt had been formed, stretching from a height of about 400 km to 1,600 km [300-1,200 mi.] . . .[62]

The electron fluxes of the lower Van Allen Belt were forever changed. The cosmic radiation ("killer electrons") in the inner belt 700-10,000 km above the equator remains damaging to humans, satellites, and sensitive spacecraft instruments.

62 Keesings Historisch Archief (KHA), 29 June 1962, 11 May 1962, 5 August 1962.

The 1950s attempts to create a stable, functional mini-ionospheric plasma cloud high above the Earth then expanded into the 1980s Strategic Defense Initiative (SDI) "Star Wars" phase, then HAARP "research" in the 1990s, and finally—successfully—the resurrected Space Fence in the new millennium. The early 1970s address of Wilmot N. Hess, then-director of National Oceanic and Atmospheric Administration (NOAA) Environmental Research Laboratories, at an international meeting of the Society of Engineering Science in Tel Aviv, Israel, expressed the ongoing military mindset bent on conquering space:

> In the last few years experimenters have artificially modified the space environment. We can now produce artificial aurorae. We can change the population of the Van Allen radiation belt. We can artificially modify the ionosphere from the ground and our other ideas about artificial experiments for the future stretch as far as trying to copy the sweeping action being carried on naturally by Jupiter's moons.[63]

Ionospheric heaters now beam microwaves into the ionosphere while DSX (demonstration and science experiments) satellites monitor the magnetosphere for VLFs.[64] Ionized and nonionized experiments continue unabated, such as satellites beaming energetic particles to produce electromagnetic waves in space while the "power beaming" satellite PRAM (photovoltaic RF antenna module) converts solar energy into microwaves for power density,[65] injects thermal plasma at high altitudes, transmits electromagnetic waves beamed from Earth to disturb particles trapped in the Van Allen Belts, etc. Control over geomagnetic storms in the outer belt (13,000-65,000 km) has been accomplished, as has maintenance of over-the-horizon communications for C5ISR operations.[66]

But the Van Allen Belts still pose a problem for those bent on fulfilling the "destiny" of conquering space, "the final frontier." Regarding the Orion Deep Space Mission to Mars, NASA engineer Kelly Smith in the sales pitch video "Orion: Trial By Fire" admits that the perilous Van Allen Belts are deadly to astronauts, which is why they will launch an Orion loaded only with sensors, not Human 1.0: "We must solve these challenges before we send people through this region of Space."[67]

---

63 Several of Hess's NASA papers on the Van Allen Belts are available on the Internet.

64 Saswato R. Das, "Military Experiments Target the Van Allen Belts." The Verge, 1 October 2007. The Sun's radiation creates and maintains both the ionosphere and plasma in the magnetosphere.

65 Andy Tomaswick, "The Navy Is Testing Beaming Solar Power in Space." Universe Today, June 19, 2020.

66 Command, control, communications, computers, combat, intelligence, surveillance, reconnaissance.

67 NASA Johnson, "Orion: Trial By Fire" YouTube, October 8, 2014.

Back in 1958 at a congressional hearing, Paperclip Major General Dr. Walter Dornberger insisted that America's top space priority must be to "conquer, occupy, keep, and utilize the space between the Earth and Moon"—the Earth-Moon Gravity Well—for bases on the Moon and orbiting battle stations (satellites) controlling the pathway on and off the planet. Domination of the Gravity Well requires domination of the Earth below. "Gentlemen, I didn't come to this country to lose the Third World War," he haughtily informed the National Missile Industry Conference.

What Dornberger labored to develop for the Third Reich has been achieved. Since 2013, NASA's space laser internet has been shooting pulses of infrared laser from four satellites parked over New Mexico for crystal clear communications to the Moon. (Communications to . . . ?)

> . . . their Lunar Laser Communication Demonstration (LLCD) transmitted data over the 384,633 kilometers [238,900 miles] between the moon and Earth at a download rate of 622 megabits per second, faster than any radio frequency (RF) system . . .[68]

Despite the fact that Project Prometheus was purportedly cancelled (2003-2005), plutonium (Pu) continues to haunt the secret space program, the devil being in the details that few have the patience to ferret out. The most recent example is the Perseverance rover running on plutonium that supposedly landed on Mars,[69] despite the twin risks of a blow-up during launch or in space.

1989 Galileo space probe, 49.25 pounds Pu238 (half-life 87.75 years);
1990 Ulysses space probe, 25.6 pounds Pu238;
1997 Cassini space probe, 72.3 pounds Pu239 (half-life 24,131 years);
2006, New Horizons space probe 10-year journey to Pluto, 24 pounds Pu239.

> The Cassini does not have the propulsion power to get directly to Saturn, so NASA plans a "slingshot" maneuver in which the probe will circle Venus twice and hurtle back at Earth. It will then buzz the Earth in August 1999 at 42,300 miles per hour just 312 miles above the surface. After whipping around the Earth and using its gravity, Cassini would have the velocity to reach Saturn . . . if the probe enters the Earth's atmosphere during the fly-by . . . it could burn up in the atmosphere and disperse deadly pluto-

68 Quoted from a study entitled "Military Space Forces the Next 50 Years" in Bruce Gagnon's article "Secret Space War: America's Former Nazi Scientists Dream of Ruling the World," Global Research, February 1, 2013.

69 Karl Grossman, "Applause for Perseverance Ignores Plutonium Bullet We Dodged." FAIR.org, February 25, 2021.

nium across the planet. According to the NASA Environmental Impact statement "approximately 5 billion of the estimated 7 to 8 billion world population at the time of the swingbys could receive 99 percent or more of the radiation exposure" if there is an inadvertent reentry of the probe.

According to author Karl Grossman, plutonium-238 is not a necessity for the mission to succeed. The plutonium-238 will be used to "generate 745 watts of electricity to run instruments—a task that could be accomplished with solar energy" . . . Even with this knowledge, however, the Department of Energy (DOE) insists on sticking with the nuclear energy on the Cassini probe.[70]

Suborbital spaceflight crew members have been subjected to increased occupational radiation exposure not so much from galactic cosmic or solar radiation or thunderstorms as from radiation clouds loaded with Pu238. Suborbital included the 1990s top-secret Aurora (SR75) able to clock Mach 6.[71] By 2011, space shuttles were phased out. For a while, stratospheric passenger flights for the rich and famous ($20 million per flight) were going to inject sulfur aerosols, but that plan either fizzled out or went black.[72] Now, Boeing's Phantom Works X-37B now circles the planet every 90 minutes (5 miles per second), carrying on board earthquake / tsunami-inducing X-Band laser beaming technology (THEL tactical high energy laser) while far below on the Earth, phased array antenna downlinks are everywhere. X-37B is an "orbital HAARP" kinetic weapon[73] launched by carrier plane or orbital rocket. It has been caught on camera in slow motion destroying a SpaceX rocket loaded with a Chinese satellite destined for orbit.[74] As a "Star Wars" weapon with phased array narrow beams (as in HAARP Alaska and 5G), the X-37B can precisely and rapidly scan or focus energy on the ionosphere, steer the jet stream, create and steer hurricanes and tornadoes, trigger earthquakes (land) or tsunamis (sea).

Before the X-37B was built, they induced earthquakes and tsunamis by beaming the earthquake frequency (2.5 Hz) into the ionosphere from

---

70 Karl Grossman, "Risking the World: Nuclear Proliferation in Space." Covert Action Quarterly, Summer 1996.

71 1 Mach = 768 mph; the ratio of the speed of a body to the speed of sound in the surrounding medium.

72 Anton Laakso, "Stratospheric passenger flights are likely an inefficient geoengineering strategy." IOPScience, 4 September 2012.

73 Another kinetic Star Wars weapon is the orbiting battle stations armed with tungsten steel rods known as Rods from God.

74 "Slow Motion Video! UFO destroy the fated SpaceX space rocket [Alien Vs Facebook Satellite]," En Iyiler, September 5, 2016.

ground-based HAARP Alaska or the US Navy sea-based HAARP, SBX-1, and the ionosphere deflected the very narrow beam to a preselected target on the earth's surface or ocean floor. With the X-37B now in orbit, they can beam the narrow beam earthquake-inducing radio frequencies from directly over the target (Haiti, Japan, Iran, waters off Puerto Rico or California, Yellowstone National Park, New Madrid fault line.[75]

In 1999 in Mumbai, India, the Bhabha Atomic Research Centre (BARC) assembled an electron-accelerating, rapid-fire beam weapon system appropriately named Kali-5000 (Kilo-Ampere Linear Injector), Kali being the ancient triple Hindic black goddess who creates, preserves and annihilates. She is Time, Slayer of Men. One of her four whirling *swastika* arms holds a severed head (brain?). *I am the dance of death that is behind all life, the ultimate horror, the ultimate ecstasy. I am existence, the dance of destruction that will end this world, the timeless void, the formless devouring mouth.* Skulls, cemeteries, and blood are still offered to appease Her wrath.

Kali-5000 shoots several thousand bursts of microwaves, each 4-gigawatt burst lasting 60 billionths of a second. The cluster of HPM pulses travel in a straight line and do not dissipate, even between 3 and 10 GHz. Kali's accelerating electrons can do several things: Kali is a particle beam weapon whose electron pulse makes electronic systems go haywire—the HPM (high-power microwaves) "soft-kill" approach, unlike laser weapons that eat through metal; Kali generates flash X-rays for ultra-photography to trace projectiles at lightning speed; Kali's microwave-producing "sister" in Bangalore helps India "harden" electronic systems in its satellites and missiles against EMIs (electromagnetic impulses) generated by nuclear weapons; Kali throws up electrostatic shields hardened to withstand thousands of volts per centimeter for light combat aircraft.

Every nation with the means is preparing for electromagnetic Star Wars, not nuclear war. Digitized synthetic biology is being developed and tested on global populations. Still, there remains a puzzling *drive* to populate space with radioactivity, particularly plutonium. Let's look a little deeper.

Trinity

Long before the Curies began their quest for the radioactivity in thorium, polonium and radium, alchemists had been manipulating matter in their crucibles to provoke the radiation force field. Madame Curie's uranium salts in phials and

75 "USAF redeploys X-37B climate chaos, earthquake and tsunami inducing orbital HAARP weapon," http://presscore.ca/?p=8382, n.d. An aircraft alert radar (AAR) can automatically shut down a HAARP X-Band transmission when aircraft are within or approaching facilities. Will this work with X-37B?

test tubes glowed with an unearthly light. Uranium emitted heat 250,000 times that of coal, and radium—millions of times more active than uranium—rapidly ejected electrons and alpha particles as it transmuted into lead.

Nuclear fission was discovered 27 years after the British scientist Ernest Rutherford (1871-1937) created the present model of the atom. In 1932, British physicist James Chadwick at the Cavendish Laboratory in Cambridge, England discovered the neutron. But putting nuclear fission to the test needed a war with an antagonist evil enough to justify developing and using such an infernal technology, so Hitler was appointed chancellor of Germany in 1933, the very year the Curies allegedly discovered artificial radiation. The following year, Madame Curie died at 66, and physicist Enrico Fermi bombarded the nucleus with the neutron and induced radioactivity in 22 different elements with fluorine.

In his book about the Manhattan Project, *Brighter Than Ten Thousands Suns*, Robert Jungk wrote:

> Among the young atomic scientists, some looked upon their work as a kind of intellectual exercise of no particular significance and involving no obligations, but for others, their researches seemed like a religious experience.[76]

The men involved in the Manhattan Project[77] were for the most part well-placed Brothers of secret societies either dedicated to working against Nature and human evolution or misled pawns. By World War Two, scientism had succeeded in eliminating both the life force—æther—and moral conscience from scientific inquiry, making the Manhattan Project scientists not all that different from the scientists serving the Nazis.

The Age of the Pale Horse commenced with three ritual atomic bombs detonated *after* World War Two was officially terminated on May 8, 1945.[78] Japan's attempts to surrender were ignored while the Allied powers secretly negotiated with Paperclip Nazis for a transfer of scientists and technicians to Allied nations.

> *And I looked, and behold a pale horse: and his name that sat on him was Death, and Hell followed with him. And power was given unto them over the fourth part of the earth, to kill with sword, and with hunger, and with death, and with the beasts of the earth.*
>
> – Revelation 6:8

---

76 Robert Jungk, Brighter Than Ten Thousand Suns: A Personal History of the Atomic Scientists. Mariner Books, 1970.

77 The war served to drive physicists from Germany into the waiting embrace of the Manhattan Project.

78 Caveat lector: Google is now changing the date of World War Two's end to September 2, 1945 so as to justify to History the bombing of Japan.

Harry Truman, the 33° Freemason President who had signed off on White Sands, Hiroshima, and Nagasaki, had called the Manhattan Project lead physicist Robert Oppenheimer a "cry-baby" when Oppenheimer—too late—had second thoughts. In his diary of the Potsdam, Germany conference scheduled to begin the day after the White Sands "test," President "True Man" wrote of wandering through Berlin, bombed to utter ruin, thinking about empires that had fallen—Atlantis, Carthage, Babylon, Rome—and rulers like Alexander, Darius, and Genghis Khan, as Percy Shelley (1792-1822) a century before had thought of Ozymandias:

I met a traveler from an antique land
Who said: Two vast and trunkless legs of stone
Stand in the desert. Near them, on the sand,
Half sunk, a shattered visage lies, whose frown,
And wrinkled lip, and sneer of cold command,
Tell that its sculptor well those passions read
Which yet survive, stamped on these lifeless things,
The hand that mocked them and the heart that fed:
And on the pedestal these words appear:
'My name is Ozymandias, king of kings:
Look on my works, ye Mighty, and despair!'
Nothing beside remains. Round the decay
Of that colossal wreck, boundless and bare
The lone and level sands stretch far away.

The American monument to the advent of the Nuclear Age is Trinity Site on the 4,000-square-mile White Sands Missile Range in New Mexico. After the deadly mushroom cloud rose into the atmosphere on July 16, 1945, the wind turned the green sea of trinitite into concentrated radioactive drifts of fused spectral shapes as the charred remains of greasewood plants leaned as far from the ghost of the blast as they could. Trinitite was hauled away in barrels for more experiments.

The U.S. tested a hydrogen bomb in 1952; the Soviet Union did the same in 1953. Tests in the Bikini Atoll in 1954 caused radiation sickness among the crew on the Japanese tuna boat *Lucky Dragon*. The Atomic Energy Act of 1954 gave a carte blanche monopoly over the production and ownership of "fissionable materials" to the Atomic Energy Commission (AEC), along with the power to issue licenses to private corporations to build and operate nuclear power plants while promoting and regulating them.[79] The AEC was

79 The Reagan-Bush-Cheney troika (1980-1988) privatized the U.S. nuclear arsenal.

eventually split into the promotional Department of Energy (DOE) and the Nuclear Regulatory Commission (NRC).

Cows ate fallout grass, children raised on fallout milk had alpha, beta, gamma, and X-ray halos around their heads. Ionized subatomic particles caused atoms to lose their orbital electrons or break their nuclei. Radioactive I-131 (half-life eight days) settled into thyroid glands; Strontium-90, Cesium-137, Zirconium and other radioactive isotopes seeped into living tissue. Two generations later, American IQs had sunk as Wilhelm Reich's emotional plague from *deadly orgone energy* (DOR) clouds[80] devoured the *orgone* / *æther*) life force of the American continents. In 1964, a satellite fell to Earth and dispersed 2.1 pounds of Plutonium-238, *one particle of less than a millionth of a gram being fatal.*

In the 1954 film *Godzilla*, the monster had radioactive breath, no doubt a reference to the air we would henceforth breathe.[81] The neutron bomb was first tested in the U.S. in 1962. In September 1972, the first scientific examination of Trinity Site since 1955 revealed that plutonium was still migrating deeper and deeper into the Earth. Trinity was hotter than either Hiroshima or Nagasaki because it had not been exploded 2,000 feet in the air but on the Earth. In 1975, White Sands became a National Historic Site.

The "mythology" that mathematician and physicist Wolfgang Pauli (1900-1958) referenced in 1955—"a synthesis incorporating a rational understanding and a mystical experience [between physics and metaphysics]. No other objective would be in harmony with the mythology, whether avowed or not, of our epoch"—was surely the "mystical" struggle between good versus evil. Theoretical physicist Werner Heisenberg (1901-1976) was more over the target when he said that "the space in which man's spiritual being develops is in a different dimension from that in which it was moving in previous centuries."

Had the Bomb changed "the space in which man's spiritual being develops"?

> By tearing the neutron from its atomic environment, its source of connection and gravity, the nuclear chain reaction destroyed the reason, however ineffable, that holds matter together, and with this, at an elemental level, the matrix that sustains and makes sense of our experience . . . You might call this transfiguration of reality the Plutonic initiation . . . [a] radical expansion of consciousness across and beyond all established social, philosophical, and spiritual parameters.[82]

---

80 In 1951, Wilhelm Reich, MD, conducted the ORANUR Experiment (ORgonomic Anti-Nuclear Radiation) to determine the effect of nuclear radiation on life. He acquired two 1mg units of Radium, each in a separate half-inch lead container. His helpers at Organon in Maine became ill.

81 Other nuclear films: Hiroshima Mon Amour (1954); Record of A Living Being (1955); Dr. Strangelove (1964); Black Rain (1988); Rhapsody in August (1991).

82 Richard Leviton, "The Secret Life of Radiation: Susan Griffin and The Chorus of Stones."

Death followed the nuclear ritual: the first U.S. Secretary of War (now Defense) James Forrestal (1892-1949) died by defenestration from the 16th floor of the National Naval Medical Center in Bethesda, Maryland on May 22, 1949; Julius and Ethel Rosenberg, accused of nuclear spying for the Soviet Union, were electrocuted on June 19, 1953; CIA scientist Frank Olson died by defenestration from the 10th floor of the Statler Hotel in Manhattan on November 28, 1953; and Wilhelm Reich, MD, died of a "heart attack" in Lewisburg Federal Penitentiary, Pennsylvania on November 3, 1957, one week before his release.

Like all secret societies, the Satanic religion known as Nazism enjoyed *two tiers* of power: the outer tier of the *exoteric* National Socialist German Workers Party, and the inner tier of the *esoteric Schutzstaffel* (SS), whose mind-controlled "knights" had been programmed as an *inversion* of the Christian Knights Templar Order of the Crusades (1195-1291 CE). To this day, few realize that Hitler was MK-ULTRA-style utterly controlled via drugs, hypnosis, and rituals by the Nazi inner circle of power.

The birthplace of the Manhattan Project Bomb was over a sacred *kiva* just west of the Sangre de Cristo (Blood of Christ) mountains. The core of the Bomb, as big as an orange, was transported in the backseat of a sedan from Los Alamos through Santa Fe (City of Holy Faith) to Trinity Site in the *Oscura* (dark or hidden) mountains of the Badlands (*El Malpais*), the Navajo legend being that Twin War Gods had slain the monster Yé'iitsoh on Mount Taylor and the blood had run down the mountain, then coagulated and solidified to form the black lava flows of *El Malpais.*

Historical accounts, military projects and operations, and mainstream media accounts regarding staged events that centuries-old Brotherhoods deem essential for the public's subconscious are thick with numbers, names, symbols and cyphers for *psychological operations (psyops)*[83] that are basically *lower black magic.*

The blast at Trinity Site at 33.6772929° N that occurred on Monday, July 16, 1945 was such an operation. In her 1992 book *A Chorus of Stones*, Susan Griffin stressed that the explosion is still happening inside us on a cellular, immunological level, transforming the chemicals in our air and water, its "half-life" continuing to rend the fabric of life and matrix of meaning.

The "Little Boy" bomb on August 6, 1945, the eve of the Christian Feast of the Transfiguration, was delivered over Hiroshima at 34.3852° N, and the "Fat Man" on August 9, 1945 over Nagasaki at 32.7503° N. All in all, White

---

The Santa Fe Reporter, 1995.

83 See Michael Hoffman, Secret Societies and Psychological Warfare (2001) and Twilight Language (2021), Independent History & Research Company. For example, onomancy is the ancient science of divination by names.

Sands, Hiroshima, and Nagasaki were the three prongs of a *triune Plutonic* (subconscious) *initiation*—318,000 Japanese dead and vaporized, untold numbers wounded and with cancer, national psyches shattered. Dorothy Day at *The Catholic Worker* countered "jubilant" newspaper accounts with a description much like that of Susan Griffin a half century later:

> ...our Japanese brothers scattered, men, women and babies, to the four winds, over the seven seas. Perhaps we will breathe their dust into our nostrils, feel them in the fog of New York on our faces *[shades of September 11, 2001!]*, feel them in the rain on the hills of Easton . . . A cavern below Columbia[84] was the bomb's cradle, born not that men might live but that men might be killed. Brought into being in a cavern and then tried in a desert place in the midst of tempest and lightning, tried out, and then again on the eve of the Feast of the Transfiguration of our Lord Jesus Christ, on a far-off island in the eastern hemisphere, tried out again, this new weapon which conceivably might wipe out mankind and perhaps the planet itself.[85]

Thousands of atmospheric, above-ground and underground nuclear "tests" have been carried out, initially to discover the Bomb's exact geometric trigonometry in sync with spacetime and planetary positions. The nuclear apocalypse eventually lost its terror for the physicists and mathematicians smart enough to realize that the Bomb's geometrics had spacetime limitations, and that *disrupting matter requires geometrics and harmonics.* Nuclear detonations can only occur twice a year at certain times and places, which is when armed nuclear submarines patrol the seas like guard dogs. This secret has been kept from the public so as to maintain the threat and fear of nuclear war while the environment has been weaponized as a fully integrated directed energy weapon system.[86]

The public has no idea of exoteric vs esoteric—for example, the rumored ritual "mating" rites that nuclear submarines enact via their airlocks beneath the polar icecap.

"Accidents" or experiments?

Strangely, the U.S. government continues to "lose" nuclear elements—enough MUF (material unaccounted for) to bomb Nagasaki 800 times over. For example, on March 21, 2017 (spring equinox) two INEEL security experts left

---

84 Columbia is the occult name for the United States of America; thus, District of Columbia.

85 Dorothy Day, "We Go on Record: The CW Response to Hiroshima." The Catholic Worker, September 1945.

86 Read lay harmonics mathematician Bruce L. Cathie, The Harmonic Conquest of Space. Adventures Unlimited Press, 1998.

two disks of plutonium and cesium in the back of their Ford Expedition outside the Marriott Hotel. Needless to say, the disks were stolen. Oversight? Dropoff?

Six tons of MUF up to 2012—gone.[87]

As terrifying as ionized radiation is, and as vastly powerful as the nuclear industry is, the process of nuclear fission is surprisingly not all that high-tech (Meker burners, a good stove, a coal-fusing oven, butane gas), except for the heavy water in which the pure uranium salts must dissolve. *Heavy water needs 25 to 100 years for redistilling.* This one requirement points to organized planning and preparation over time.

In his second edition of *Chemtrails Exposed: A New Manhattan Project* (2020), Peter A. Kirby rightly calls geoengineering a second national security Manhattan Project. Both projects began as State secrets, neither was tested before being loosed on the environment and public, both ignored the problems of waste, destruction, and health, both arose in times of war, the first during World War Two, the second during the post-9/11 "war on terror"—ironically, in the name of "public safety," now an utterly Orwellian term.

Back in 1999, I was shocked by a *Wall Street Journal* article on "industrial tourism" (the Hormesis Effect) about "vacationers seeking a thrifty getaway a la Homer Simpson find relaxation in the warm waters that cycle through power plants . . . used to cool reactors [and then] deposited in nearby waterways . . . almost like a spa."[88] A million French citizens were flocking to nuclear, hydroelectric, tidal and thermal power plants of state-owned Électricité de France, but especially the uranium enrichment factory. In Prague, doctors were recommending the radioactive waters of the Jáchymov spas built into the side of an old uranium plant.[89] While Greenpeace thought only in terms of greenwashing PR, I wondered if the Hormesis Effect was yet another human radiation experiment, given that *any* quantity of radioactivity is proscribed by the International Atomic Energy Agency (IAEA) "Radiation Protection and Safety of Radiation Sources: International Basic Safety Standards, No. GSR Part 3,"[90] not to mention that it is well known among nuclear scientists

87 Matt Agorist, "The US Government Has 'Lost' Enough Radioactive Material to Bomb Nagasaki 800 Times." The Last American Vagabond, 16 July 2018.

88 Fuhrmans / Fleming, "Tourism: vacationers Attracted To Industrial sites," Wall Street Journal, October 4, 1999. This particular article has been removed from the Internet.

89 Post-World War Two under Communist control, Jáchymov, Czech Republic hosted prison camps whose inmates were forced to mine uranium until 1964. Life expectancy was 42 years. "The radioactive thermal springs arising in the former uranium mine are used under the supervision of doctors for the treatment of patients with nervous and rheumatic disorders. They make use of the constantly produced radioactive gas radon (222Rn) dissolved in the water . . ." - Wikipedia

90 http://www-ns.iaea.org/standards/ . Also see Eileen Welsome's The Plutonium Files: America's Secret Medical Experiments in the Cold War (Dial Press, 1999). Welsome won a Pu-

that radiation weakens cells, thus preparing them for more effective assaults.

"Accidents" do not really appear to be accidents but radiation experiments on a planetary scale that provide years of data-crunching.[91] Three Mile Island (March 28, 1979; lat 40.15 N / long 76.72 E), Chernobyl (April 25-26, 1986; and lat 51.27 N / long 30.22 E), Fukushima (March 11, 2011; lat 37.38 N / long 140.47 E) all occurred in the open air, all in the spring. Did it have anything to do with testing radiation with the Sun's UV radiation and galactic cosmic rays? Tesla had been convinced that radium would transform energy from cosmic rays. From a 2016 ARMAS report:

> We show five cases from different aircraft: the source particles are dominated by galactic cosmic rays but include cycle variation and their effect on aviation radiation. However, we report on *small radiation "clouds" in specific magnetic latitude regions and note that active geomagnetic variable space weather conditions may sufficiently modify the magnetospheric magnetic field that can enhance the radiation environment, particularly at high altitudes and middle to high latitudes.*[92] (Emphasis added.)

The Three Mile Island "accident" ten miles south of the Pennsylvania state capital of Harrisburg yielded a 13-year study of 32,000 people whose data was skewed to reassure the public that there was absolutely no connection to cancer deaths of residents living five miles from the reactor. Just before Three Mile Island, the results of a 14-year study of the 1951-1962 aboveground nuclear "tests" in the Nevada desert had been released *after a 15-year delay*. Why the delay? No one seemed terribly interested, lied the chief of radiation effects for the National Cancer Institute (NCI).[93] Farm Belt exposure to iodine-131 showed up in 11,300 to 212,000 cases of thyroid cancer. Many had drunk fallout milk in childhood.

The nuclear destruction at Chernobyl occurred just before the Western Easter (Maundy Thursday to Resurrection Sunday, April 27-30, 1986), and

litzer Prize for the early 1990s series in The Albuquerque Tribune that pressured President Clinton to set up the investigation of the Advisory Committee on Human Radiation Experiments that was basically a whitewash.

91 Aria Bendix, "A group of scientists called the 'Ring of 5' found evidence of a major nuclear accident [in 2017] that went undeclared in Russia." Business Insider, August 8, 2019. Russia's Mayak plutonium separation facility was the site of the September 29, 1957 Kyshtym explosion, the third worst "accident" after Chernobyl and Fukushima. See O. Saunier et al., "Atmospheric modeling and source reconstruction of radioactive ruthenium from an undeclared major release in 2017." PNAS, December 10, 2019.

92 W. Kent Tobiska et al., "Global real-time dose measurements using the Automated Radiation Measurements for Aerospace Safety (ARMAS) system." Online Library, 18 November 2016.

93 "Scientist apologizes for radiation procrastination." AP, September 17, 1998.

its death cloud was 100X that of Hiroshima and Nagasaki. *Chernobyl* means Wormwood, which references both the herb *Artemisia absinthium* known to kill cancer cells and the fallen star in Revelations 8:10-11:

> And the third angel sounded, and there fell a great star from heaven, burning as it were a lamp, and it fell upon the third part of the rivers, and upon the fountains of waters; And the name of the star is called Wormwood: and the third part of the waters became wormwood; and many men died of the waters, because they were made bitter. (KJV)

Neutron counts are rising at Chernobyl 35 years after the disaster, signaling possible fission. Truthfully, it is a mess there, and control over what will occur over time is nonexistent.[94]

The Chernobyl tragedy occurred just as Mikhail Gorbachev's *perestroika* campaign to liberate Russia, East Germany and Eastern Europe from the grip of Bolshevism was beginning. The fallout contaminated all of Eastern Europe. Vegetation in "hot" soil is now returning amidst plutonium, cesium-137, strontium, and radioactive iodine. The river flowing past the reactor and feeding into the Dnieper River that feeds into the Black Sea is the watershed for 9 million Ukrainians. Strangely, it was not until the end of 2000 (14 years!) that Reactor No. 3 was finally shut down.

During the Carnegie International Nuclear Policy Conference after the Fukushima Daichii disaster in 2011,[95] former chairman of the U.S. Nuclear Regulatory Commission Gregory B. Jaczko recommended that all 104 U.S. nuclear reactors should be taken out of commission and replaced, and additional 20-year extensions be stopped. Did it happen? Of course not. The U.S. is the world's biggest producer of nuclear power.

What happens when ionized radiation is released on such a scale? First of all, charged particles are trapped by the Earth's magnetic field, rotating around the magnetic lines of force thousands of times per second, producing a *mirroring spiral* that makes sure the ions and electrons remain in the atmosphere to undergo a slow drift around the Earth's magnetic axis.[96] Thus part of the planetary radiation experiments on the U.S. East Coast, in the Ukraine and Japan appear to have been about electron cyclotron resonance heating *to increase charged particle density*, as explained in Bernard Eastlund's 1987 HAARP patent.

The Fukushima disaster occurred a year after the *Deepwater Horizon* Gulf

---

94 Richard Stone, "'It's like the embers in a barbecue pit.' Nuclear reactions are smoldering again at Chernobyl." Science / AAAS, May 5, 2021.

95 I recommend reviewing the Fukushima Daiichi kdebacle in Chemtrails, HAARP, and the Full Spectrum Dominance of Planet Earth (2014).

96 "#9: Trapped Radiation," http://www.phy6.org/Education/wtrap1.html.

of Mexico "accident." Was it about studying the impact on the North Pacific Gyre whose radiation "debris plume" was projected to reach the U.S. West Coast by 2014, due to the gyre's current pattern? Radiation opens the cells to greater vulnerability and triggers an overdrive in, and ultimate exhaustion of, the immune system. If weakening the immune system is one of the objectives of loosing radiation in the atmosphere, then other objectives must include genetic alteration, sterilization, mind control, *and direct attacks on the human form body known as the etheric body.*[97] Why else would the total gamma radiation in the United States—confirmed by the EPA's Gamma Radiation Monitors—register 42.054 billion counts per minute (CPM)[98] between January 1, 2010 and April 30, 2020? Why else would weaponized ceramic uranium oxide aerosol (UO2, depleted uranium) be in nuclear fuel?[99]

In the 1990s, I was contacted by a targeted individual named Clare Louisa Wehrle. She wrote that she had been harassed and gangstalked since her PhD thesis on radiation at Stanford University in the 1970s. Her then-boyfriend worked for the CIA and was murdered, after which Clare was used for a host of "experiments," especially radiation via aerosols.

> The scope of the effects which can be caused by these substances is much wider than mere "harassment." A major question in the early MK-Ultra research was the need for a method of propulsion of substances such as chemicals, microbes and odors through the air to a target. In the past few decades, they have found such a propellant in nuclear energy supplied by radioactive substances and radiation-emitting chips.[100]

Over the years since her certain murder, I have learned through other targeted individuals undergoing nonconsensual experimentation that nuclear

---

97 "The Three Occult Purposes of the Fukushima Operation," http://montalk.net/fukushima.html. Since 1945, there have been 2,053 atomic explosions (not counting depleted uranium). Radiation prompts the manifestation of Asuras particularly useful to black technologies. The formation of noble gases allows invisible antihuman entities to materialize. Since 2011, consciousness has been attacked by increasing waves of radioactivity. Fukushima reactors: Iodine (I-131), Strontium (Sr-90), Cesium (Cs-134, Cs-137).

98 Counts per minute is for Geiger counters: the ionization rate in a given quantity of decaying radioactive material. Bob Nichols, "Gamma Radiation in America 2020.6." Veterans Today Military Foreign Affairs Policy Journal for Clandestine Services, May 23, 2020.

99 Douglas Kristopher Clark, PhD thesis, "Formation of Oxide Fume and Aerosol dispersal From the Oxidation of Uranium Metal at Temperatures Less Than 1000ºC [1832ºF]," 2001.

100 From "The Use of Synthetic Body Odor for Mind Control," a typewritten account by Clare about the "harassment substances" she was experiencing (including radiation). She was finally killed by a car driven by Raymond Peters of St. Petersburg, Florida on January 6, 2006. See Silent Holocaust: The Global Covert Control and Assassination of Private Citizens by Bridget S. Howe (Lulu Press, 2017).

aerosol agents make good invisible delivery systems for nano-sized lethal drugs or implants. Clare grasped what was up decades ago:

> sical force . . . with sometimes endless mechanical repetition, usually by microprocessors . . . High levels of radiation can break bone, metal, move objects, or destroy brain or body tissue . . . Furthermore, the CIA styles the reduction of IQ as an almost trivial effect, even claiming it will "feminize" women. But adaptation to the loss of IQ would be almost impossible. Were the wealth of the mind to be lost, one would be in an alien land, a mental desert. The destruction of the mind's wealth is actually a goal of some CIA experiments. Some experiments even seek to damage basic skills which exist in animals, such as spatial orientation, transmogrifying the subject to a sub-animal existence, as if by sorcery. The extinguishing of the light of the mind can actually be cruelly sensed by voyeuristic mind-reading technology—the technology used to enhance sadistic pleasure in the crude low-tech murder of the physical vehicle, as well.[101]

As if by sorcery . . .

The nuclear industry continues as our health diminishes, along with our mentation.

- Radiation-induced cancer
- Lung disease (including exposure to asbestos or silica dust, beryllium)
- Blood disease
- Gastritis
- Nervous system diseases
- Cardiovascular diseases
- Diseased internal organs, especially thyroid
- Birth defects

Neal Chevrier of Citizens Against Harmful Technology points out that channels between the human brain and external electronic devices are being purposely opened by high radiations like gamma, ionic and accelerators for radioisotopes enrichment production of uranium, thorium, radium, radon, plutonium, etc. Even human waste containing radioactive isotopes is being "mined" from sewage for nuclear energy production by means of nanosensors now ubiquitous in the environment and our bodies. Nanochips and MEMS are used to sniff out air-conditioned magnetic fields loaded with smart dust, radio frequency signals, water taps, GMO foods, "precision medicine" drugs, computer monitors, video games and TV, geoengineered weather, UFOs, etc.[102]

---

101 Claire Louisa Wehrle, "Cybernetic Degradation," November 2003.
102 Neal Chevrier, "What is the Nuclear Program?" Citizens Against Harmful Technology.

Carbon sequestering was never the real goal of the 2015 UN Climate Change Conference in Paris. Carbons were shaped into the problem so the solution ("affordable decarbonized energy system") would send us not toward renewable energy but into the waiting arms of the nuclear industry.

Arto Lauri in Finland

I have learned to doubt what I hear from NASA about the plasma physics experiments going on in the atmosphere and near-Earth orbit, solar flares, meteors arcing across the sky, etc. For example, the article "Interplanetary shock wave hits Earth's magnetic field creating red, yellow, green southern lights and blue northern lights" (*Strange Sounds*, April 22, 2018) maintains that the shock wave on April 19, 2020 was a "supersonic disturbance in the gaseous material of the solar wind usually delivered by coronal mass ejections (CMEs)," causing blue (nitrogen) auroras in the northern latitudes and red, yellow, and green (oxygen) in southern auroras over Tasmania. *Was* the supersonic disturbance due to CMEs, or were ionospheric heaters cooking up their own aurora borealis? And why nitrogen in the Northern Hemisphere and oxygen in the Southern, when both hemispheres have both?

Former SUPO (Finnish CIA) operative and 30-year nuclear plant worker Arto Lauri lives in Finland (latitude 62ºN) on the border of the Arctic Circle and has a front row seat when it comes to observing the atmosphere / ionosphere over HAARP (Alaska), KAIRA (Finland), LOFAR (Netherlands), and EISCAT (Sweden, Norway) ionospheric heaters. Lauri can read the colored chemical signatures of high-latitude clouds bloated by dry radiation pressure, not moisture, and determine the presence of nitrogen ionization (light blue), nitrogen tetraoxide (yellow), oxygen (pink), blasts of plutonium (red), etc.[103] Strong cloud boundaries indicate strong ionization.

Lauri believes that the weathercam captures of a planet or massive bubble or balloon are real, and that the discolored, pock-marked sphere is not a planet but a huge ionized gas (plasma) "balloon" of Pu-239[104]—leaks, jettisoned waste from nuclear power plants, secret deployments, "accidents," etc.,[105] tethered to rotate with the Earth. The other remarkable part of the

---

103 In "Arto Lauri 251 Chemtrail," Nov. 7, 2019, he describes a cloud mass as iodine reddish-brown with a metallic sheen during -8ºC. In the 1960s, 1970s, and 1980s, chemicals like trimethyl aluminum, barium, and triethylborane respectively created red, green, and purple clouds over Wallops Flight Facility on the East Coast of the United States.

104 Excellent capture of it on Facebook at Krista Alexander's site, May 29, 2020.

105 Aria Bendix, "A group of scientists called the 'Ring of 5' found evidence of a major nuclear accident [in 2017] that went undeclared in Russia." Business Insider, August 8, 2019. Russia's Mayak plutonium separation facility was the site of the September 29, 1957 Kyshtym explosion, the third worst "accident" after Chernobyl and Fukushima. See O. Saunier et

story is that webcam captures show that a solar simulator is being used to hide the Pu-239 orb blocking our natural Sun for four hours daily at certain latitudes. In fact, this may even be the primary purpose of the solar simulator. He adds that the carefully crafted chemical compounds in chemtrails play a crucial role in reducing the risk of these radioactive balloons of plutonium exploding, the proof being that the EU-US Open Skies agreement makes NATO nations designate *15 percent of their budgets for chemical trails.*[106]

At 4:25 in "Arto Lauri 240 Chemtrail Chemi" (January 22, 2018), Lauri points to the "gray and dirty cloud mass," identical to the big ball or bubble rotating in the sky over the Yukon River Bridge on August 18, 2019 at 13:35 in the video "The final days. A cluster of suns approaching 10-29-2019."[107] Both call to mind Wilhelm Reich's DOR (Deadly ORgone) clouds.

Most nuclear plant emissions are blown into the atmosphere from 104-meter exhaust pipes by 1500 kW ventilators. The half-life of a neutron[108] leak is 17 minutes, after which the ionized gas will explode with the power of one million electron volts (beta decay). If the ventilation is cut off or does not occur, everyone in the nuclear plant dies. Nuclear emissions since the 1930s have increased 15-fold, but because the waste is blasted hundreds of kilometers into the atmosphere at the speed of light, radiation readings of plants remain low. Nuclear fission of just one uranium atom can destroy 20 million cells in a human body.

Nuclear waste in the U.S. is chemically bound in solid glass (silica) at 2,100°F (1,148°C) in a process called *vitrification*. From under Yucca Mountain to a North St. Louis County landfill, nuclear waste continues to be an expensive problem. The North St. Louis County nuclear waste problem goes all the way back to 1942 when Mallinckrodt Chemical Works was purifying tons of uranium for the Manhattan Project. Today, high levels of benzene and hydrogen sulfide are in the air over metro St. Louis where an underground landfill fire continues to burn 8,700 tons of nuclear weapons waste. A "dirty bomb"—a non-detonated release of radioactive particles—could occur anytime.[109]

---

al., "Atmospheric modeling and source reconstruction of radioactive ruthenium from an undeclared major release in 2017." PNAS, December 10, 2019.

106 If he is right about radiation being the primary purpose of the chemical trails we've had for over twenty years, then it is equally true that the nuclear industry would have to drop from full capacity, if not close down entirely, before any discontinuation of chemical trails.

107 The Final Days (previously Universal News Media) believes that the solar simulator is hiding an incoming planet. More footage of the solar simulator and Pu-239 "bubble" is available at "The final days. Weeks before disaster comes from planetary system. 8-14-2020." This may also have to do with the EMPCOE (electromagnetic plasma changeover event) movement (see Mia's New Pair of Glasses). Photoionization of plasma in space might lead to transformer explosions and planetary devastation.

108 It takes one neutron of uranium-238 to turn into plutonium-239.

109 Steven Hsieh, "St. Louis Is Burning." Rolling Stone, May 10, 2013.

Is our nitrogen-oxygen atmosphere in danger of being ignited by plutonium? Lauri believes that a major objective of the nuclear industry is population control. He cites Finland's KAIRA as a HAARP-like weapon system able to drive ionized clouds loaded with radiation to chosen locations to sterilize designated populations. He once saw "something" slip out of the nearby Loviisa power plant, then explode (400kV). Besides what is expelled, nuclear reactors leak at least 3,000 kg (3 tons) per year.

Finland plays an extraordinary role in the nuclear industry. First, it has the only active uranium mine in Europe,[110] with Talvivaara being the only active uranium refinery in Europe and Posiva being the only nuclear waste isolation pilot plant in Europe. Secondly, a 2005 law made producers of uranium (namely, Finland) responsible for *all* nuclear waste.[111]

How much is being buried, and how much blasted into the atmosphere?

While pondering why liquid fluoride thorium reactors (LFTR) aren't being used— thorium being 4X more abundant than uranium, 200X more efficient, produces 1/35th the waste of uranium, no meltdowns or explosions, and is dangerous for 300 years versus 10,000 years for uranium—Lauri came to the conclusion that it's because thorium byproducts don't make destructive weapons like depleted uranium (DU).

As we investigate the Sun and Moon simulators with their blue / red hexagonal honeycomb lenses and xenon arc lamps[112] reflecting off of bent spinning mirrors before going through hexagonal apertures, we'll keep in mind Lauri's theory that they are operating in tandem with chemtrails to hide the eclipsing of our Sun by a huge ionized gas (plasma) "balloon" of plutonium (Pu-239).[113] Lauri indicates that besides reducing the risk of radiation balloons exploding, chemtrails also obscure the overlapping lenses of the solar simulator.

Solar & lunar simulators

Let's take a closer look at the solar and lunar simulators.

The glorious golden yellow Sun of yesteryear is now veiled in the white of chemical plasma cloud cover ("contrail cirrus"). But if the Sun is luminously white, you are probably looking at a solar simulator, the 2D white artificial sun that does not radiate, however much its mirrors spin and lenses reflect. Still, it is heliosynchronous and 238 miles above the Earth, following the path of our natural Sun allegedly 94.5 million miles away (152 million km) while obscuring the star itself.

---

110 All of Lapland is reserved for uranium mining.

111 See "Arlo Lauri in Leveli #73, March 2, 2021."

112 Xenon arc lamps are a highly specialized type of lamp that produces light by passing electricity through ionized xenon gas at high pressure to produce a bright white light.

113 See an excellent capture of it on Facebook at Krista Alexander's site, May 29, 2020.

What is the solar simulator up to, and for that matter the lunar or Moon simulator, as well?[114] We have heard Lauri's theory. Another is that the solar minimum has decreased the Sun's output, so we need a supplementary artificial system. Or is this Tesla's "Death Star" with weaponized lenses and mirrors, aiding laser beams being zapped through space.

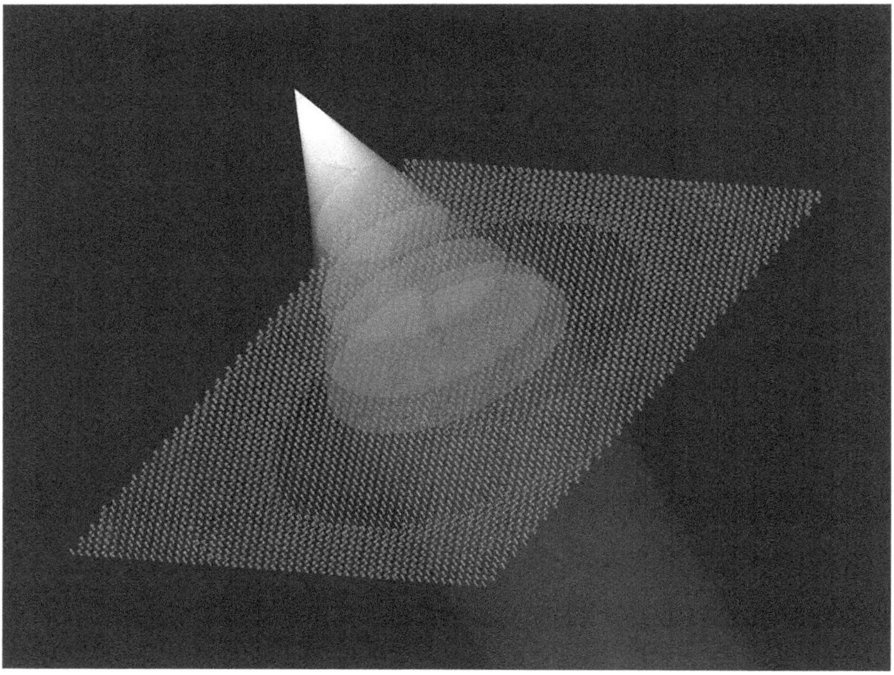

Silicon nanopillars arranged in a hexagonal pattern create a "metasurface" that generates and focuses radially polarized light. (Think solar simulator.)

https://www.nasa.gov/feature/jpl/new-ultrathin-optical-devices-shape-light-in-exotic-ways

> Researchers have developed innovative flat, optical lenses as part of a collaboration between NASA's Jet Propulsion Laboratory and the California Institute of Technology, both in Pasadena, California. These optical components are capable of manipulating light in ways that are difficult or impossible to achieve with conventional optical devices.

114 Developed nations in general have developed simulators. Eli Meixler, "China Plans to Launch an 'Artificial Moon' to Light Up the Night Skies," Time.com, October 19, 2018; Hannah Devlin, "Let there be light: Germans switch on 'largest artificial sun.'" The Guardian, 23 March 2017; etc.

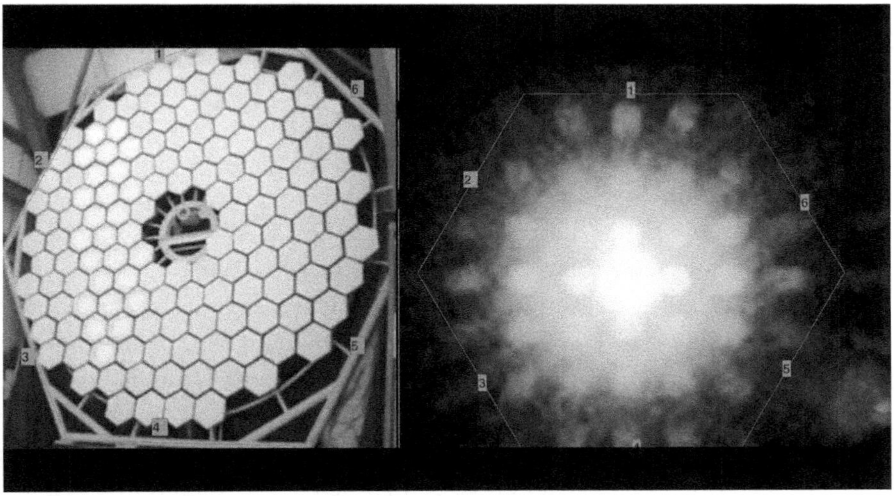

Solar (Sun) Simulator. Both the solar and lunar simulators utilize hexagonal panels and LEDs. Whereas the true Sun is round and produces golden light, the solar simulator is angled and produces white light.

https://www.drclaudiaalbers.com/2018/11/planet-x-report-sun-is-no-longer.html

> The new lenses are not made of glass. Instead, silicon nanopillars are precisely arranged into a honeycomb pattern to create a "metasurface" that can control the paths and properties of passing light waves. Applications of these devices include advanced [scanning electron] microscopes, [Blue Beam] displays, sensors, and cameras . . .[115]

Corporations like Solaren are involved. At one time, Solaren controlled the 2006 patent "Weather management using space-based power system" (US20060201547A1) that proposed using mirrors in *orbiting solar farms* to control weather systems, harvest energy in space and beam it back to Earth. From the patent:

> Energy from the space-based power system is applied to a weather element, such as a hurricane, and alters the weather element to weaken or dissipate [or weaponize?] the weather element . . . by changing a temperature of a section of a weather element, such as the eye of a hurricane, changing airflows, or changing a path of the weather element.

The weaponized dual-use version of solar farm mirrors and sun simulators comprised of LEDs, plasma lens arrays, and elaborate mirroring could

115 Elizabeth Landau, "New, Ultrathin Optical Devices Shape Light in Exotic Ways." NASA's Jet Propulsion Lab, August 31, 2015.

be capable of melting armies, igniting fires, evaporating reservoirs, or turning glaciers into torrents.[116]

The *laser developed atmospheric lens (LDAL)*, for example, utilizes high-pulsed lasers to change portions of the Earth's atmosphere into lens-like plasma structures so as to magnify or change the path of electromagnetic light. The air is ionized (heated – the Kerr Effect) to create a deflector shield, magnifying lens, or Blue Beam-type images. The LDAL can also work like a super-high-powered Fresnel lens to concentrate low-powered light into a tightly focused beam to ignite fires and burn cars "like the mean little kid with a magnifying glass and a hill of ants."[117] (Shades of the California fires.)

Inside the solar similar is the enigmatic 20X20-foot *black spinning cube* referenced in the Solaren patents.[118] While the cube spins, X-like refractions of two lenses converge and show up on the sides of houses, and the light from the mirrors may reflect on your arms. Sometimes, a "sheet lightning" beamed "wall," columns, or sphere emanates from the reflecting lenses. As the simulator "eclipses" the natural Sun, multiple "eclipses" may show up on the ground. Meanwhile in the sky, a lens "petal" effect surrounds the white simulated sun. As the simulator spins clockwise, its brightness and contrast controls can be adjusted from a nearby TR-3B or X-37B. In the case of igniting California fires (2017, 2018) or projecting Blue Beam broadcasts, the lens in front of the black spinning cube is not attached to the simulator and appears to be used to focus (LDAL?) laser beams. Sun halos may actually be evidence of the distance the lens array is from the Earth, given that (according to Jeff P) the halo *is* the lens.

Thanks to the following investigative works:

"Proof of Sun Simulators in the Sky Above," aplanetruth5, July 6, 2020.
22:00 a simple sketch of how the simulator works
26:00 laser-induced plasma channel to ignite CA fires (ionotron)
34:00 laser beam coming from the Moon simulator during CA fires

"What are these round, rimmed, concave disks seen on many FAA weather-cams. What is it? Mar 24 2018," Universal News Media, https://youtu.be/KTmHWSK2A5s

"Enormous crater in red planet on Alaskan FAA weathercam. Planets are

116 See Geoff Manaugh, "Space-Based Storm Control." BlogBlog, April 17, 2009.
117 Paul Seaburn, "Laser Could Turn Atmosphere into Giant Magnifying Glass." MysteriousUniverse.org, January 18, 2017.
118 US3239660 "Illumination system including a virtual light source"; elaborate mirroring US3325238A and US3247367A.

closing in. Mar 21 2018," Universal News Media [concealment jet at 1:20] https://youtu.be/7viFRFwrbmY

"Gigantic planet on FAA weathercam as our sun sets. Why isn't this in the news? Mar 20 2018," Universal News Media

"Red beam projected from the sun, caught on FAA weathercams. More planets, eclipses. Mar 13 2018," Universal News Media

"Dark sun halo's are Giant lenses and Moon turning into full moon in Minutes," Jeff P, April 16, 2018, https://youtu.be/ARYiuWWVp5s

"DEW Weaponized Sun Simulator news 24 caught in action paradise fire dutchsinse," Jeff P, January 4, 2018, https://www.youtube.com/watch?v=dwRCWSbKh10&feature=youtu.be

"A worldwide matrix breakdown is coming as lens array and sun simulator continues to fail 5/15/17," Jeff P, May 15, 2017, https://youtu.be/KgXv9dhEfqw

"Sun simulator uses a spinning mirror caught on video," Jeff P, July 9, 2017.

"Moon simulator grows 5 times in just minutes, planets fading in and out 11/5/2017," Jeff P.

"No sun simulator no planet no lenses is there," Niges View On Things, September 19, 2017

"Some may find this strange," Niges View On things, May-June, 2020

CERN

The CERN Large Hadron Colliders (LHC) leaped to life on a Friday[119] *night in 2012 in cathedral-like rooms 300 feet below ground where it was absolute zero, colder than outer space, under the Swiss-French border. Beams of protons streaked along the 17-mile circular tunnel as 2,000 superconducting magnets, each 50 feet long, kept the beams traveling tightly bunched in opposite directions. Finally, dark matter, antimatter, and what matter was like in the microseconds of rapid cooling after the Big Bang would be understood, thanks to protons and neutrons, quarks and gluons, the elusive Higgs boson, and 3.5 trillion electronvolts (eV) 3.5X as powerful as Fermilab's Tevatron in Chicago.*

– "From Trinity to Trinity," Book IV of the *Sub Rosa America: A Deep State History* series (2nd Ed., 2018) by Elana Freeland

119 Friday is named after Freia, Norse goddess of love, beauty, war, and death (Old Norse Frauja lord or master, lady or mistress).

In 2020, the CERN Council endorsed examining the feasibility of building the massive Future Circular Collider (FCC) all the way around Geneva, Switzerland, intersecting at two points with the much smaller Large Hadron Collider (LHC), to be completed in 2035. The FCC will collide proton-proton, electron-positron, and proton-electron.[120]

China, too, is building a massive particle accelerator. There are now at least 14 large particle accelerators, with three in the United States. Most U.S. Department of Energy (DOE) facilities have particle accelerators, with Brookhaven National Laboratory out on Long Island, New York (near Montauk) having the largest. Besides the Linear Collider Collaboration, a partnership of at least 34 institutions, more than 160 international groups—including NASA Ames Research Center and Google X (secret radical technology)—connect for research in high energy physics, climate science, and genomics via the ESnet5 (Energy Sciences Network) fiber optics network (terabytes and terahertz transmitters) running through and around UC Berkeley in California at 100 gigabits per second on a 300 GHz band.[121] UC Berkeley's Lawrence Berkeley Lab, where the Advanced Light Source building that houses the Synchrotron particle accelerator is located, streams all data from CERN and links the Helix Nebula (the Eye of God) to D-Wave's 2048.

Particle accelerators arise in a variety of contexts, from the founding of the World Wide Web under ENQUIRE, initiated by Tim Berners-Lee in 1989 and Robert Cailliau in 1990 at CERN, to "cancer research" at the U.S. Public Health Service Hospital near Tulane University in New Orleans, the Google "vampire watch" of 2015 that extracts blood via hyperspeed into a "miniature particle accelerator," and "accelerators on a chip" delivering a million or more electron pulses per second for security scanning, precision medicine, synthetic biology, etc. Christian writer and go-to CERN observer Anthony Patch wrote:

> In my novels, I use "micro-accelerators" housed in quarter-sized stainless steel balls, each producing 1 billion watts to form remote-controlled tornadoes employed as weapons—drone twisters, if you like. The AWAKE experiment at CERN is doing essentially the same for the LHC: reducing its size using lasers and plasma waves. The program renders "accelerators on a chip" obsolete, at least for macro applications. Much more powerful. It will connect to Saturn.[122]

120 Bob Yirka, "CERN Council endorses building larger supercollider." Phys.org, June 22, 2020.

121 105 gigabytes (0.1 terabit) 275-450 GHz. Terahertz transmitters are 10X faster than 5G networks.

122 Patch also keeps a close eye on the D-Wave 2048 adiabatic quantum computer favored by influential corporations and agencies, including Lockheed Martin, owner of Space Fence patents.

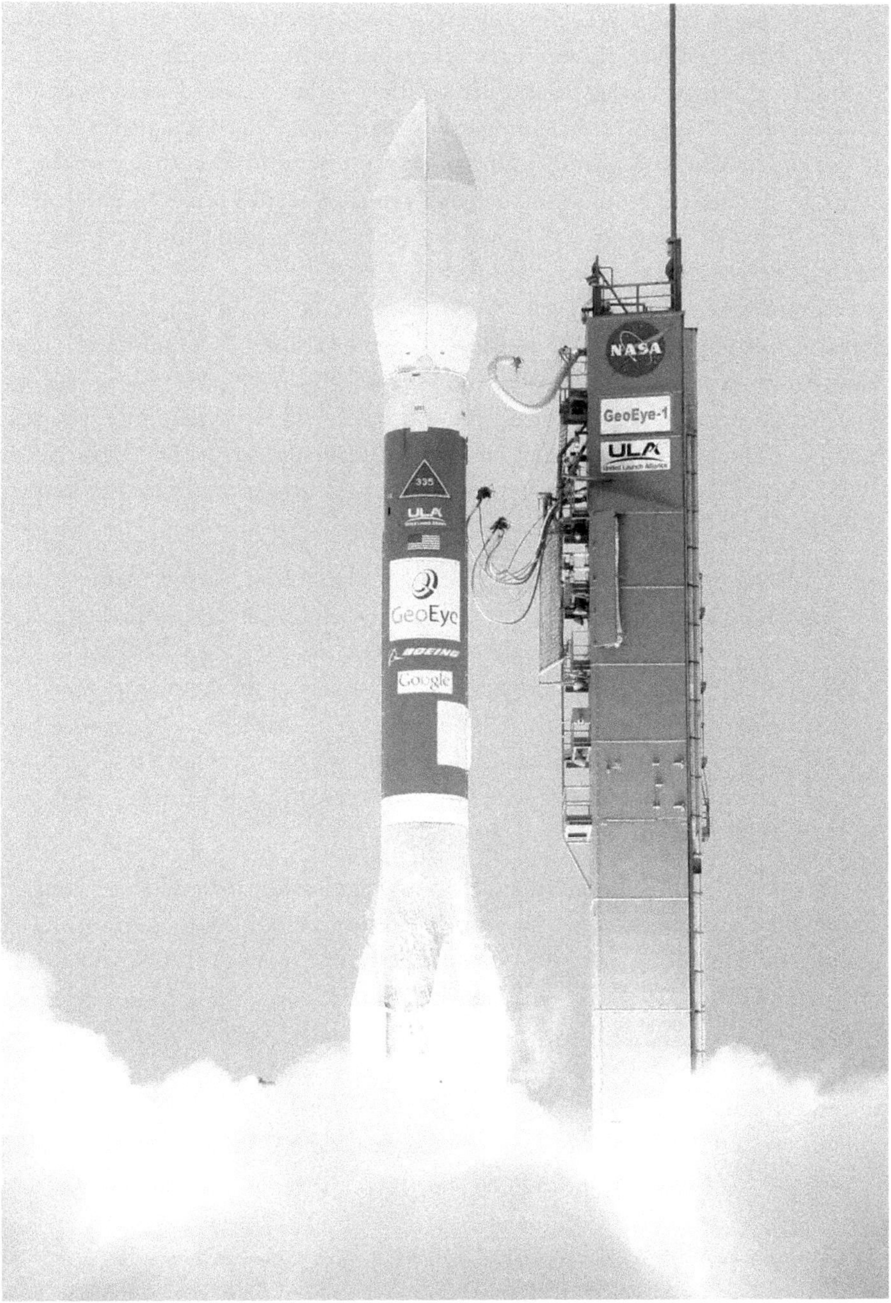

"Google had exclusive access to the NGA's [National Geospatial-Intelligence Agency] satellite image feed. The only restriction: Google had to use slightly lower resolution images."

Yasha Levine, "Oakland emails give another glimpse into the Google-Military-Surveillance Complex." *Pando.com,* March 7, 2014.

The discovery of the subatomic Higgs boson particle—named after theoretical physicist Peter Higgs—was made public in 2012. The story is that without the Higgs particle, electrons would have no mass and atoms wouldn't stick together. Certainly, *something* holds matter together ("cosmic molasses," Higgs called it), but wouldn't it be more honest to admit that this *something* is actually the same *æther* or *ether* that was banished from science to outer "dark matter" back in the 1920s,[123] as Marc J. Seifer discusses in his book *Wizard: The Life & Times of Nikola Tesla* (Citadel, 2016)?

In reference to the CERN Document Server paper "Planetary Surface Power and Interstellar Propulsion Using Fission Fragment Magnetic Collimator Reactor" (Pavel V. Tsvetkov *et al.,* 2006), U.S. Navy-trained nuclear engineer Chris Fontenot clarified at his A Microwaved Planet site that CERN is actually not so much engaged in tracking down the Higgs Boson "God Particle" as creating a planetary system of power, including ionic propulsion. This is further explained

> CERN's mission of inducing voltage into the Global Atmospheric Electrical Grid is being accomplished by the ionic jet outflow perpendicular to the Globe of Science and Innovation [at CERN]. Ions are increased in energy and ejected into the ionosphere by the phenomena patented by [David LaPoint].[124] Once that charge potential is induced into our environment, it can be used for wireless energy harvesting globally, the technology for which is being developed at DARPA. They refer to it as Fractal Rectenna Array technology.[125]

Think of large colliders like CERN as giant electromagnets working together, like hundreds of nuclear explosions all happening in one second or hitting the Sun and causing CMEs (corona mass ejections).[126] HAARP's shutdown in 2014-2015 (i.e. going black) coincided with a number of Space Fence-related dates, possibly because of a highly organized, concerted effort to upgrade and synchronize the frequencies of all systems connected with the monitoring and control (now C5ISR) of geospace, the ionosphere and magnetosphere, and harnessing of cosmic processes (CMEs, solar flares, minimums, etc.) for Space Fence optimization.

---

123 Review Chapter 2, "'Æther, Plasma, & Scalar Waves" in Under An Ionized Sky.

124 See LaPoint's Primer Fields Series at https://www.aetherforce.energy/the-primer-cube-by-david-lapoint/.

125 Ken Lebrun, "DARPA: Energy Harvesting." Revolution-green.com, May 28, 2013.

126 According to Marc J. Seifer, PhD, author of Wizard: The Life & Times of Nikola Tesla (2011) and Transcending the Speed of Light (2006), Tesla told Joseph Alsop, Teddy Roosevelt's great nephew, that the Sun absorbs more energy than it radiates (New York Herald, July 11, 1934). This is Tesla's dynamic theory of gravity.

> The [Joint Space Operations Center] JSpOC Mission System (JMS) initiative is an ongoing, three-phased effort to replace or upgrade the hardware and software currently used for space surveillance, collision avoidance and launch support, with an eye toward providing more precise and timely orbital information, among other goals . . . The Government Accountability Office said in March [2014] that the update is expected to be completed by December 2016, about two years before the Air Force's next-generation space surveillance system, the Space Fence, is expected to be operational. Officials have said the JMS upgrade is required to handle the amount of data the Space Fence will generate.[127]

With the Space Fence up and running, corollary "tests" at CERN (and on the Sun, our star) went live, too—all part of Tesla's planetary surface power system under construction.[128] On December 7, 2015, a "whirling dervish" portal opened above CERN perched over the "hotspot" of the former ancient underground Temple of Apollyon (Anthony Patch) so a UFO / UAP could exit.[129] The event filmed should be seriously considered, given the geomagnetic power of the natural landscape, former Roman temple, and CERN's magnetosphere capabilities.

When CERN is in full operation, the 17-mile diameter Large Hadron Collider (LHC) is like an Arctic Circle magnetic field. As discussed in Chapter 4, "Magnetism," *vortexmaps.com* indicates that CERN on the French-Swiss border is in geomagnetic alignment with Greenland and Giza. I asked, "How much do these magnetic lines of force influence us, or better said, how much do grid manipulators influence us by controlling these cosmic lines of force? How many wars and revolutions have been sparked along strategic geomagnetic alignments?" Similar to the Montauk experiments, airplanes may drop from the sky when CERN is running full tilt, like German Airbus A320 on March 24, 2015 just 127 miles from CERN, cruising at 38,000 feet before its rapid descent, or Malaysia Airlines Flight 17 (July 17, 2014), Indonesia AirAsia Flight 8501 (December 28, 2014), etc. Is CERN implicated in the Earth's weakening magnetic strength and the growing South Atlantic Anomaly that many attribute to an upcoming geomagnetic reversal[130]? Or is CERN at-

---

127 Mike Gruss, "AMOS Conference / JSpOC Upgrade on Track for 2016, although Parts of the Overhaul Face Delays." Space News, September 11, 2014.

128 CERN's Globe of Science and Innovations looks remarkably like Tesla's Wardenclyffe Tower dome out on Long Island, New York.

129 See YouTube "UFO entering Interdimensional Portal (CGI)." UAP = unidentified aerial phenomena, as per Kayla Epstein, "Those UFO videos are real, the Navy says, but please stop saying 'UFO.'" Washington Post, September 18, 2019.

130 F. Javier Paron-Carrasco and Angelo De Santis, "The South Atlantic Anomaly: The Key for

tempting to take charge of this situation and prevent the electromagnetic field from collapsing?

The weakening of the magnetic field is at least in part due to all of Tesla's alternating current, like how audio tapes degauss (de-magnetize) in an alternating magnetic field. The masses of electric power we are now using means putting masses of electricity into the Earth. On April 23, 2016, the magnetosphere collapsed (disappeared) for two hours.[131]

Beside the fact that CERN is its own nation-state like the Vatican or Washington, D.C., there is the fact that fired up, it becomes an Arctic Circle magnetic pole all of its own, generating 100X the magnetic energy of the entire planet, thanks to its Temple of Apollyon geomagnetism, earth-penetrating tomography (EPT), scalar earthquake technology), and alliances, much as HAARP's alliance with the entire Space Fence infrastructure.

Patch sets forth another major CERN concern:

> The mind operates on multiple frequency levels . . . The luminosity resulting from the collisions of subatomic particles in the collider inside the detectors at CERN produced identical frequencies as to the mind. They are reproducing through collisions of particles two of the frequencies within which the mind operates, and you'd better believe that they're operating at *all* of the various frequencies, alpha and beta ranges, of the mind. Does that mean that CERN is directing mind control systems? No. It means that they're doing the research and development that is then applied to the supercomputer systems like D-Wave for the purpose of—in the environment of the sentient world simulation—controlling people's minds.[132]

Thus, it becomes apparent that CERN is in league with the Space Fence *apparat* in the race to plug Transhumanist Human 2.0 into AI by means of brain-computer interface (BCI) technology.

Occult, ritualistic inferences regarding CERN are further discussed in Chapter 9, "The Temple of CERN" of *Under An Ionized Sky.* Are we ready to consider the "mystical" along with fact in order to properly comprehend the ancient secret Brotherhood mystico-scientific quest for access to intelligences in parallel universes—defined by LHC physicist Mir Faizal as "real universes in

---

a Possible Geomagnetic Reversal." Earth Science, 20 April 2016.

131 This was not "conspiracy theory," nor was the summer solstice "spoof" ritual sacrifice in front of the Shiva statue at CERN of Swiss U.S. Air Force officer Maja Franziska Brandi. Sorcha Faal, "US Air Force Officer Under Attack After He Identifies CERN 'Human Sacrifice' Victim." WhatDoesItMean.com, August 19, 2016. Sorcha Faal, despite its murky reputation, often presents news otherwise unavailable in the West. Caveat lector.

132 Listen to a 2018 interview with Anthony Patch: "CERN, Transhumanism, Science & Prophecy / Apocalypse and the End Times," GOD TV, November 9, 2018.

extra dimensions"—that D-Wave chief technology officer Geordie Rose calls "the Old Ones"? What of the *simultaneity* of the subatomic smashing of atoms with swarm-conscious nanotechnology now being implanted in humanity?

We stand at the atomic / subatomic quantum threshold of Earth existence with antimatter altering the very fabric of Space. The CERN LHC electric connection with Saturn in the Saturn-Venus-Mars-Earth alignment via Birkeland currents must be reconsidered in a new light of consciousness, as must the secret space program.[133] Is the Saturnalian Brotherhood at NASA bent on turning the Earth into an AI generator replete with synchrotron "rings" while siphoning living Earth energy (including human energy) to "restart" Saturn, the dead planet still maintained by some sort of artificial intelligence machine[134]?

We are living in Tesla sci-fi times. Look at the global environmental infrastructure now nearing completion and tell me it's not possible.

Gravity, Æther, & Tesla's Atmospheric Engine

The more we study gravitation, the more there grows upon us the feeling that there is something peculiarly fundamental about this phenomenon to a degree that is unequalled among other natural phenomena. Its independence of the factors that affect other phenomena and its dependence only upon mass and distance suggest that its roots avoid things superficial and go down deep into the unseen, to the very essence of matter and space.

– Paul R. Heyl, "Gravitation: Still A Mystery," *Scientific Monthly*, May 1954

I have said that if one took away the Earth's gravity, one would take away light at the same time. For indeed, light and sound and all other qualities perceptible to our senses proceed from and are, as it were, a result of the mechanical structure and consequently the gravity of natural bodies which are luminous and sonorous in proportion to their degree of gravity and buoyancy.

– Louis Bertrand Castel (1688-1757), Jesuit mathematician

Gravity: the electric dipole force between subatomic particles, a dipole electrostatic force that arises from the longitudinal (electric) phenomenon of the *æther* of space.

---

133 Laurence Kotlikoff, "Is Our Government Intentionally Hiding $21 Trillion in Spending?" Forbes, July 21, 2018. Mark Skidmore, professor of economics at Michigan State University, and investment analyst Catherine Austin Fitts discovered $21 trillion in government transactions, primarily in defense, missing between 1998 and 2015. Fitts maintains that much of it has gone into the secret space program.

134 See Norman R. Bergun, PhD, Ringmakers of Saturn (Pentland Press, 1986).

Since 1956 and the advent of the secret space program, U.S. aerospace corporations ("the military industrial complex" outgoing President Eisenhower warned Americans of) have sought, with the aid of émigré Paperclip Nazis,[135] to conquer gravity so as to get off the planet and through the Van Allen radiation belts into space. Rockets that require masses of fuel propulsion and nuclear fission have always been about getting satellites up for communication and surveillance, not about space exploration.

As for their rings, they were so high that they were dreadful, and their rings were full of eyes [stars] 'round about.

- Ezekiel 1:18

Newton's falling apple didn't really *explain* gravity, nor did Einstein's "curved space-time" geometry. Science went off course into *scientism*[136] under the spell of secret societies in the early 1920s when *æther* was removed from the scientific lexicon. Along with it went *the living universe*, *æther* being the dipole matrix throughout the universe with electric circuits threading it, as the Electric Universe and Thunderbolt Project maintain. The removal of *æther* and intentional distortion of Scottish mathematical physicist James Clerk Maxwell's theory of electromagnetism, the very core to understanding gravity[137] led to a wasteful misperception of gravity and the fanciful "black hole" and "Higgs field." *Vanguard Science* defined *æther* in 1991 as the prime continuum of the fundamentally highest possible frequencies of the universe producing magnetism, electricity, light, heat, sound, vibration, and mass. Today, we call this "prime continuum" *zero-point energy (ZPE)* or *zero-point field (ZPF)*.

Einstein's special relativity theory was used to hide the existence of the *æther*. People were led to believe that mass spinning in space drags Space and Time around, creating a curved 4D spacetime continuum and making gravity the result of an object trying to travel in a straight line through a space

---

135 By 1939, the SS Order of the Black Sun tasked with researching alternative energies had developed an electro-magnetic-gravitic engine into an energy Konverter coupled to a Van De Graaf band generator and Marconi vortex dynamo to create powerful rotating electromagnetic fields that affected gravity and reduced mass. They called it the Thule Triebwerk (thrust engine or power unit).

136 See Appendix 1, "Invisible Mindsets."

137 A review of Chapter 2, "Æther, Plasma, and Scalar Waves," in Under An Ionized Sky is recommended.

curved by the presence of material bodies. The other misconception was that the speed of light was some sort of absolute limitation, but if the force of gravity propagates at least *20 billion times* faster than the speed of light, then how can the speed of light (in a vacuum no less) be absolute? If gravitational interactions are instantaneous, then where does that leave the assumption that nothing can propagate faster than light in a vacuum? As the autodidact Walter Bowman Russell (1871-1963) perceived, the stability of planetary orbits indicates that gravity propagates much faster than light. With such different propagation speeds, why wasn't special relativity abandoned? $E = mc^2$ only makes sense if E stands for *æther* / ether.

Was all the obfuscation and lying just to conceal Tesla's free energy? Excepting alternate current (AC), everything about Tesla was carefully and methodically buried behind "national security" while Einstein was used to hide the light-filled medium of free energy everywhere, *æther*.

Viktor Schauberger (1885-1958) was an independent Austrian engineer and forester who, having acutely observed Nature for many years, realized it was an *alive* "complex interaction of forces that constantly create or reinvigorate matter—against the orthodox view that matter is in a natural state of decay [entropy]."[138]

Breaking free of Einstein's "curved space-time" is essential to grasping that gravity and electromagnetics share fundamental characteristics: (1) they both diminish with the inverse square of distance, (2) they're proportional to the product of interacting masses[139] or charges, and (3) they act along the line between them. Apply force to a body, and the force is *electrically transferred* to overcome inertia. Thus, inertial mass and gravitational mass are equivalent because gravity is a manifestation of electrical force.

Antigravity too has gone black, excepting *electrogravitics* in some quarters, "a synthesis of electrostatic energy used for propulsion—either vertical propulsion or horizontal or both—and gravitis, or dynamic counterbary, in which energy is also used to set up a local gravitational force independent of that of the earth" (Aviation Studies). Other terms that basically mean antigravity are "field-dependent propulsion" and "gravity-shielding."

These latter terms lead us to US Patent #6145298A, "Atmospheric fueled engine":

---

138 Nick Cook, The Hunt For Zero Point: Inside the Classified World of Antigravity Technology. New York: Broadway Books, 2001.

139 You'll also have to undo your conditioning regarding mass being weight, which it is not ("quantity of matter"), nor are mass and matter interchangeable. Matter manifests as mass. I recommend reading Wal Thornhill's "Electric Gravity in An Electric Universe," holoscience.com, August 22, 2008.

> . . . The ion engine propulsion system ionizes a portion of an ambient atmospheric fuel to create a negative ionic plasma for bombarding and accelerating the remaining portion of the ambient atmospheric gas in a focused and directed path to an ion thruster anode . . .

As Cal Poly Chris Edwards described the same system on Facebook:

> Where we're going, we don't need roads. Nikola Tesla's wirelessly powered aircraft and "[plasma] cloud maker"—IONOCRAFT? Lockheed Martin Patent US3130945A "Ionocraft" [expired in 1981] – Nikola Tesla's ATMOSPHERIC ENGINE, RCA Patent US6145298A – Atmospheric fueled ion engine utilizing high-altitude ambient [plasma] gas as fuel and producing ozone as a byproduct of propulsion. The ion engine propulsion system ionizes a portion of an ambient atmospheric fuel to create a negative ionic plasma for bombarding and accelerating the remaining portion of the ambient atmospheric gas in a focused and directed path to an ion thruster anode.

Marc J. Seifer, PhD, a known expert on Nikola Tesla's life, wrote in a 2012 letter to *Time* magazine about how such a propulsion system depends upon *æther* and how gravity is transformed for flight:

> . . . The ether, of course, exists. Just look at a picture of a galaxy and you will see it is floating in something. You can call it the Higgs field [CERN's Higgs bosun "God particle" field] if you want, but it is indeed the medium existing throughout all of space.
>
> This ether most likely exists in a tachyonic (faster than the speed of light) realm. It oscillates at such a high frequency that it remains undetectable by modern day methods. What gravity is, according to this theory, is simply the absorption of ether by elementary particles. During this process which involves particle spin, the ongoing course of action is converted into electromagnetism. This simple idea explains Einstein's 40-year quest, his dream of Grand Unification, namely the way to combine gravity (the influx of ether into matter) with electromagnetism.[140]

Chris Fontenot's final word on the atmospheric ion engine is that it has passed experimental testing and *"is the future."* Are these the craft hiding in plasma cloud cover, some even producing their own plasma cloud cover? (Illustration page 203.) The following 2017 statement from "The Truth

140 "Seifer to Time magazine: 'Higgs field' is 'ether.'" Changing Power, March 18, 2012.

Denied" (in response to a Cloaked Craft article by Jim Kerr[141]) provides excellent observations and analysis of what many are taking photos of in the altered sky above:

> The cloaking cloud formation around these [exotic propulsion] craft is a byproduct of the static energy created by the propulsion system used by this craft. The external electrical static field attracts moisture present in the atmosphere, helping to cloak it. The buildup is the greatest at the corners.
>
> The craft has an internal ion generation propulsion system. It is basically like an ion breeze fan with no moving parts, but the ions "blow" in and are contained internally and condense. By changing the polarity of the containment walls, the craft can increase speed and change direction in any aspect. The condensed ions will attempt to repel from the charged wall and "push" the craft in the direction it needs to go.
>
> The faster you need to go, the more surface area of the walls is charged. Since you have five walls of a triangle, you can go in all those directions just by charging the proper walls to create repulsion propulsion.
>
> The glowing corners are just a necessary fact to release the static energy built up inside the containment vessels created in the process. These craft are actually all electric and only use small highly efficient frozen methane gas generators to create the electricity to power the ion generators. Frozen methane gas is the most abundant power source on the planet. It is easily safely stored and transported. A 2-foot square cube of frozen methane can provide enough fuel to power the craft for a week.
>
> Once the ions are sufficiently condensed, very little power is actually needed to operate a craft manned by 3 people who sit inside an enclosed area in the center of the craft. One individual is the pilot, another is the sensor operator, and the third is the mechanical systems engineer. They are all contractors and the craft are capable of landing without a runway and no major ground support. They use closed federal wilderness areas to land when necessary.
>
> The craft is virtually constructed entirely out of carbon fiber composite

---

141 Jim Kerr and Sean Gautreaux have spent years studying plasma cloud cloaked craft. See Sean's 2014 book What Is In Our Skies Vol. 1 Diagrams: The Study of Cloaked Cloud Craft. Even though Sean is not so involved anymore with the Facebook site What Is In Our Skies? contemporary photos are being posted all the time by secret group members. Jim Kerr's video is a must, as well: "UFO / Cloaked Cloud Craft April 20, 2013," February 29, 2016.

panels and weighs not much more than a family van or small cargo truck. There are a number of diagrams on the web of what witnesses describe as what the undercarriage of these craft look like. Those are the ion generators that are seen. There are multiple triangle compartments as seen by each depressed area.

Hidden in plain sight all these years, like all that scientism has bent and skewed in order to arm the Earth environment for the sake of power. But weaponized or not, Wilhelm Reich was right: *Orgone (æther) is God's creative process.*

Blue Beam & Hale-Bopp

> *The brain is the hardware through which religion is experienced. To say the brain produces religion is like saying a piano produces music.*
>
> – Daniel Batson, University of Kansas

> *The Return of the Gods is marked by Time, though only few can interpret Divine Signs.*
>
> - Frank Giano Ripel [Gianfranco Perilli], Grand Master of the Order of the Illuminati Knights

Back in 1969, the Environmental Technical Applications Center of the U.S. Air Force published a report on "Quantitative Aspects of Mirages" by 1st Lt. Frederick G. Menkello in which the then-popular "temperature inversion" cover story of UFO sightings was dismissed: "It is easy to show that the 'air lenses' and 'strong inversions' postulated by . . . [Harvard astronomer Donald H.] Menzel, among others, would need temperatures of several thousand degrees Kelvin in order to cause the mirages attributed to them."

Fifty years later, it is obvious to anyone paying attention to the geoengineering operations going on that temperature inversion, balloons, and meteors have little traction anymore as cover stories. UFO sightings (now called *unidentified aerial phenomena* or UAPs) meet the criteria of several categories, now that the atmosphere is electrified and loaded with plasma and static electricity. Blue Beam sky theater and "phantom" images with a "spiritual" mirage quality are now plasma TV for the masses.

The unfortunate mixing of what are real perceptions with perception management technologies makes it hard to know what is real and what isn't—like the TV coverage of the 9/11 collapse of the World Trade Towers. This description by A.K. Johnstone, PhD, is about something real:

> . . . the glowing sheath around a UFO could be defined as a nebula . . .

> the colored, luminous vapor sheath surrounding the UFO, or what is viewed as the fuzzy color of a fireball, is actually a sheath or sphere of air molecules from the surrounding atmosphere, which has been ionized and excited. Air molecules in this state are defined as plasma, hence the term *plasma sheath* is utilized in regard to a UFO . . .[142]

whereas laser-induced plasma filaments (LIPFs) can be used to build phantom images (*plasmoids*) by emitting light of any wavelength (visible, infrared, UV, THz) to create 3D images by raster scanning, the way cathode ray TVs are used to display images[143]—or clearing thick fog "a thousand times denser than a cumulus cloud" with laser pulses "so intense that they would change the character of the surrounding air," and so fast that they send the air molecules "spinning."[144] *Quantum cryptography* changes the conductivity of the air and "carves out the desired path of least resistance" to protect "sensitive infrastructure."[145]

Would this also include electrofog? The 2013 research article "Laser-induced plasma cloud interaction and ice multiplication under cirrus cloud conditions" (Thomas Leisner *et al.*, *PNAS*, June 18, 2013)—discusses laser-generated plasma channels not through fog *per se* but through the thin chemical cirrus ice cloud cover now so familiar, and the ability to enhance the ice particle density so as to increase the optical thickness of the cloud by orders of magnitude. Geoengineering operation #7 is about obscuring exotic propulsion craft hiding in cloud cover and even produce their own plasma for "optical thickness by orders of magnitude."[146]

Regarding NASA's Blue Beam, we were conditioned to think of the technology as a magic lantern conspiracy theory when it was actually about realistic holograms beamed by laser-generating and NRO electro-optical satellites. As explained above, holograms are produced by three interfering beams, one to illuminate and two to reflect the image into a plasma "sky mirror" so that when the beams intersect, they form a 3D hologram.[147] Observers feel they

---

142 A.K. Johnstone, PhD, UFO Defense Tactics: Weather Shield To Chemtrails. Hancock House, 2002.

143 US Patent 20200041236A1, "System and Method for Laser-Induced Plasma for Infrared Homing Missile Countermeasure." See David Hambling, "US Navy Laser Creates Plasma 'UFOs'." Forbes, May 11, 2020.

144 Radioactivity combined with nanoparticles can create a visible localized smog.

145 Malte C. Schroeder et al., "Molecular quantum wakes for clearing fog." Optics Express, Vol. 28, Issue 8, 2020.

146 See Sean Gautreaux's Internet site "What Is In Our Skies?"

147 Either a laser hologram projector or photonitron would be used. A photonitron produces both a phonic and microwave emission—like a laser hologram projector but with an image

are looking at the thing or person itself in the vacuum zone over the target area. (ELF, VLF and LF radio waves trained upon the temporal lobes and hippocampus can also make the "unreal" seem that it is appearing in physical space, in part due to the nano-magnetite lodged in the hippocampus.[148])

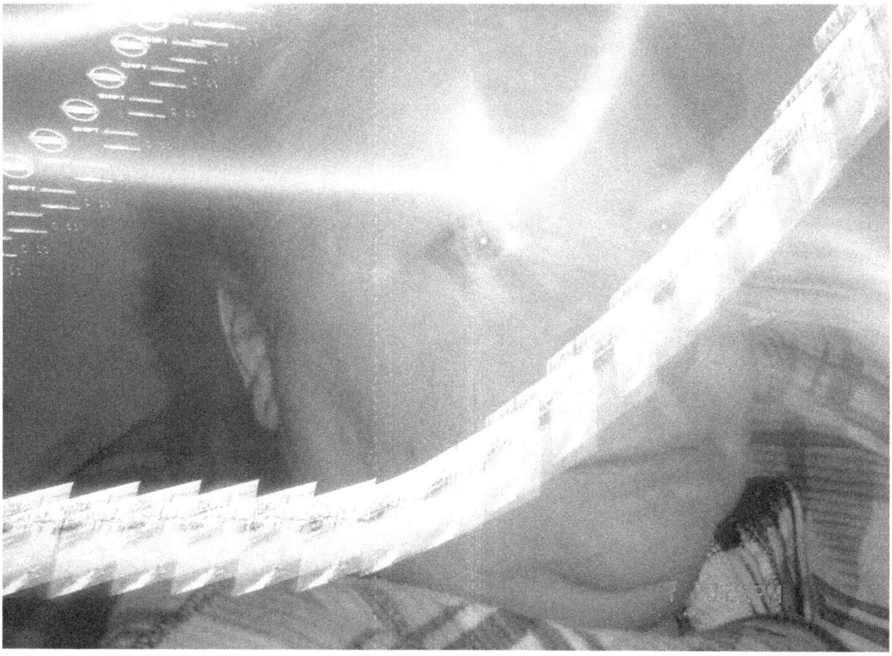

Satellite targeting. Plasmoids in an electromagnetic field form an auroral column first as plasma orbs then flattened into toroids (donut shapes) by magnetic pressure. Evenly spaced sores in Morgellons or on targeted individuals indicate a "string-of-pearls nano array."

Local optical fiber and coaxial cable can transform the ionized sodium layer 60 miles above the Earth into a movie screen starring God, an alien invasion, the Maitreya World Teacher: *We will see His face on television, but each of us will hear His words telepathically in our own language as Maitreya simultaneously impresses the minds of all humanity. Even those not watching Him on television will have this experience.*

Throughout the Israeli 1967 Six-Day War, occupation of Sinai Peninsula, and launch of *infitah* economic "reform" after Egyptian President Nasser had been eliminated and replaced by Anwar Sadat, Blue Beam technology

that is 3D and radar reflective.

148 J.R. Dunn et al., "Magnetic material in the Human Hippocampus." Brain Res. Bull., 36: 149-153.

was employed to distract the Egyptian public with appearances of the Virgin Mary (Our Lady of Zeitoun) on top of the dome of the Church of St. Mary in Cairo, Egypt. In America on May 29, 1971, east of Necedah, Wisconsin on Highway 21, the Queen of the Holy Rosary Mediatrix of Peace appeared with full coronal discharge. The air was over-ionized: onlookers' ears and hair glowed. In 1977, *Life* magazine ran a cover story about the "flood of spiritual phenomena" all over the world—crosses of light appearing in windows from Los Angeles, Bakersfield, and Knoxville all the way to the Philippines, Japan, and Germany. Maitreya the World Hologram was appearing in the middle of large crowds and energizing water sources in developing nations.

Beginning with the Feast of St. John the Baptist in 1981, six children at Medjugorje, Bosnia-Hercegovina began seeing the Virgin Mary on Crnica hill, and it continues to this day with each now-adult passing every test of electro-oculographs, algometers, estesiometers, ampliphones, etc. Given that *visions occur in the brain* via stimulation of the amygdaloid and hippocampal complexes, this shouldn't be surprising.

In June 1988 in Nairobi, Kenya, a man in white appeared "out of the blue" at a prayer meeting of 6,000. Jesus? Maitreya? Muslims saw Allah in melons, eggplants, tomatoes, potatoes, eggs, and beans. Saints on rose petals! Christ on a rock! Hindu statues drinking milk! On March 6, 1992 in Manila, capital of the Philippines (93 percent Catholic), the Sun danced amidst red, yellow and blue lights. On Maundy Thursday 1998, Dr. Ernesto A. Moshe Montgomery of the Beth Israel Temple in Los Angeles consecrated the Shrine of the Weeping Shirley MacLaine. The sky was packed with angels and aliens, Mary and Jesus.

The Sardinian *telefono antiplagio, contro le truffe dei maghi e delle sette* (anti-brainwashing hotline against the tricks of wizards and cults) was outraged and invoked the 1930s law against *abuso della credulitá popolare*. But the ignorant public loves drama and have been conditioned by the Catholic Church to believe in miracles, not technology.

A March 31, 1997 *Defense Weekly* article about the JFK Special Warfare Center and School's PSYOPS Hologram System explained how persuasive messages and 3D pictures of cloud, smoke, raindrops, buildings, flying saucers, and religious figures can be projected into both the sky and the brain. Even before HAARP ionized our atmosphere, the U.S. Air Force Offensive Information Warfare Division (communications traffic AF/X010W) was producing 3D hologram "movies" and experimenting with them in Central and South America in coordination with the Pentagon Joint Chiefs of Staff, NSA, CIA, DIA, NRO, Defense Airborne Reconnaissance Office, and National Imagery and Mapping Agency (NIMA), now known as the National

Geospatial-Intelligence Agency (NGA).

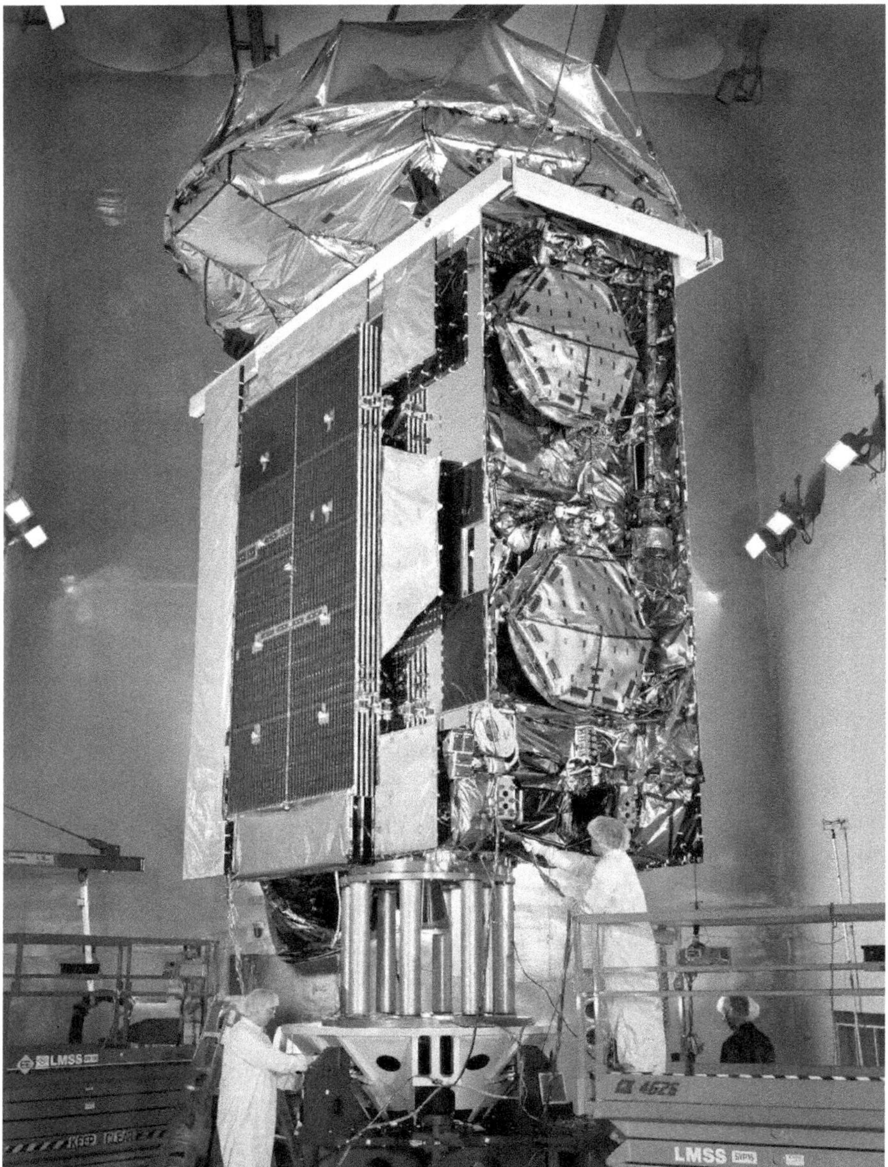

MUOS satellite (Mobile User Objective System). Ultra-high frequency (UHF) SATCOM system of four orbiting satellites and four relay ground stations (Space Fence). Developed by Lockheed Martin for the U.S. Navy. Note the hexagons. Reminds me of the film *The Wicker Man* (1973, 2006).

Since 2003, the NGA has been in charge of Geospatial Intelligence (GEOINT) and directing the Global Information Grid (GIG), with CIA cut-outs like Maxar Technologies (drag-and-drop interface technology) aiding in targeting specific populations while Serco oversees satellite computer algorithms via air traffic control towers (ATC).[149] It all sounds like business as usual until you start looking at details, like how Niantic, Inc. (founded by Keyhole, Inc. founder John Hanke) came out with Pokemon Go on July 7, 2016 to keep everyone busy watching kids and adults chasing clues on their Androids while NGA high-value employee Molly K. Macauley was murdered in Baltimore on the same day Seth Rich was murdered in Washington, D.C. Just a coincidence, right? Besides, what does Pokemon Go have to do with the NGA? "If they need pictures for a specific area updated, they don't have to send any agents / employees. They just spawn a rare Pokemon and someone using the app will take some pictures for them . . ."[150]

Blue Beam satellites (laser and electro-optical) serve the "Star Wars" / SDI / Space Fence full spectrum dominance, working with geoengineers and ground-based installations to assure

1. a highly reflective / refractive sky theater,
2. artificial thought,
3. remote control over individuals, and
4. two-way V2K communication.[151]

Blue Beam reserves stage magic in the sky for the masses and conducts black magick in the brain for individuals. Our challenge now is to educate the masses about the sophisticated technology so the vanguard can discern the difference between authentic spiritual experience and visions or ecstasies contrived by remote-controlled technology. As St. John of the Cross (1542-1591) warned, *The more exterior and corporeal [supernatural visions] are, the less certain is their divine origin.* Blue Beam and eMK-ULTRA are now capable of feeding artificial thought and experiences into *multigenic* fields that link genetics via cell tower / cell phone triangulation, 5G / IoT, and satellite. Transmitters bypass the ears and run messages directly into the brain by broadcasting at the individual's evoked potential frequency. The microwave beam at gigahertz frequencies has only to pulse ELF/VLF/LF audio waves, and bingo, the seer hears

---

149 See Jason Goodman interview with forensic economist David Hawkins, "Did Serco ConAir Patents Cause California Wildfires via CIA Nanowaves?" (November 28, 2018). Hawkins' background: Cambridge University Mechanical Engineering, Industrial Management, Applied Mathematics and Thermodynamics (Science of Waste and Chaos).

150 http://www.reddit.com/r/conspiracy/comments/4sa0w6/pokemon_go_geospatial_intelligence_gathering/

151 Serge Monast, "NASA's Project Blue Beam," 1984. Monast was a French Canadian investigative journalist whose homeschooled children were taken away in September 1996. Three months later, Monast died of a "heart attack" at 51. Supposedly, the character played by Mel Gibson in Conspiracy Theory (1997) was modeled on Monast.

a voice promising world peace. Meanwhile, detailed computer memory banks (Big Data) of targeted individuals or populations are picked up by satellite plasma beams interfacing with brains and forming diffuse artificial thoughts.

Machine-learning supercomputers and quantum computers are designed to do far more than information-analysis-integration. They write their own software, formulate and act on their own responses. Brain-computer interface (BCI) is now so seamless that unaware targets can't tell the difference between their own thoughts and words converted to frequencies fed into their brains, nor the difference between an AI program and a human operator carrying on a V2K conversation. James C. Lin's 1978 book *Microwave Auditory Effect and Application* foresaw all of this and more.[152]

Somewhere between *Know thyself* and *Caveat emptor*, we are all now in quest of *discernment* as AI technology rushes us toward the Human 2.0 swarm / hive mind. Without a working knowledge of how the technology works, how are we to know the difference between what is natural, what is supernatural, and what is technological?

With the weaponized Tesla "Star Wars" era is in full swing, it is time to look more deeply into this dynastic elite's *cosmic* aspirations and machinations under the secret space program. Be prepared to resist your conditioning.

The Western millennium 2000 was for the Chinese 4968, the Year of the Dragon. For Muslims, it was 1421, for Jews 5761, for Satanists 4063, the Year of Babalon.

Time is as much a matter of *perspective* as planetary rhythm.

In 2000 CE, the 1974 Nobel Prize winner for physics Anthony Hewish claimed to have discovered *pulses* coming from a supernova star that had collapsed in the Earth's southern sky around 4000 BCE. (The year 2000 was *anno lucis* 6000 for Freemasons the world over.) The Great Pyramid at Giza had been built to commemorate that supernova and the Egyptian / Sumerian cultural leap that accompanied it. According to Richard W. Noone, author of *5/5/2000: Ice: The Ultimate Disaster* (1997), the Grand Gallery of the pyramid points to exactly where that cosmic Event occurred in the southern sky. Eighteen years earlier, George Michanowsky wrote *The Once and Future Star: The Mysterious Vela X Supernova and the Origin of Civilizations* (1979), describing a Sumerian cuneiform that promised the return of *that* supernova around 2000 CE.

Comet Kohoutek, in its 75,000-year orbit, made a close approach to planet Earth in 1973. On February 26, 1979, outermost Pluto penetrated Neptune's orbit in the womb of the Virgin and began its 19-year approach to the Sun to eclipse the outpouring urn of the Aquarian Water Bearer and set in motion the obla-

152 A PDF version is available at shorturl.at/bcryI. See https://www.ece.uic.edu/~lin/ for Lin's CV.

tion of the Moon's shadow passing over Mt. St. Helens in the American Pacific Northwest a year before she gave birth on May 18, 1980, Ascension Sunday.

Early in 1981, as the Reagan-Bush-Cheney *troika* took power, Jupiter and Saturn were conjunct in the solar plexus of the Virgin, edging their way down from her heart. *The Virgin was in labor during the early "Star Wars" years.* It seemed that the elite were following a Revelations script.

And there appeared a great wonder in heaven; a woman clothed with the sun, and the moon under her feet, and upon her head a crown of twelve stars; And she being with child cried, travailing in birth, and pained to be delivered.

– Revelations 12:1-2

Six years after Kohoutek, Halley's Comet, the Heavenly Dragon, made its 29th visit in recorded history in the fall of 1985, executing a backward dive from the Bull to sever the horns of the Goat. The Heavenly Dragon cut an arced scythe through one-third of the Zodiac stars, then once close to the Sun, it began its 38-year retreat, pausing for a final attack on the Archer as it skimmed the Scorpion's tail and sped toward the Hydra's heads. As the old German rhyme had it:

Eight things there be a comet brings
When it on high doth horrid rage:
Wind, Famine, Plague, and Death of Kings,
War, Earthquake, Flood, and Doleful Change.

From 1990 to 1994, twelve comets per year were recorded, and yet at the end of 1994, two major comet search programs were mysteriously discontinued at the Palomar Observatory—possibly to minimize scientific scrutiny of the *artificiality* of the next two comets? Comet Hale-Bopp (C/1995 01) appeared on July 23, 1995, followed by Comet Hyakutake (C/1996 B2) on January 31, 1996,[153] both sighted by Alan Hale in New Mexico and Thomas Bopp in Arizona.

A mysterious Naval Observatory survey photo shows pointy-tailed Hale-Bopp orbiting Saturn before 1995[154]—mysterious because comets that far out are not usually hot enough to produce enough gases to become visible from Earth. Either something unknown was making it hotter than normal, or it

153 As Hyakutake had no core and was only light projections, I will spend no time analyzing it.
154 From the direction of the 1993 conjunction of Uranus and Neptune in Sagittarius, the cataclysm conjunction.

contained unknown gases, or—

Hale-Bopp (C/1995 01) reigned in the sky with spectacular brightness for an unprecedented 22 months, from July to passing perihelion on April 1, 1997. Hale-Bopp was the brightest, best, and longest-observed comet in history, truly a *Wunderscheinungen.* Even the Great Comet of 1811-12, Napoleon's comet—the one that comes once every 3,065 years—was visible for only 17 months; when the Great Comet's tail split, Napoleon marched into Russia.

Hale-Bopp's orbit was *exactly* perpendicular (89.4°) to the Earth's orbital plane, its highest elevation *exactly* 45° as it *exactly* crossed the zero degree of the Vernal Point, the ecliptic marking the beginning of spring, with Hale-Bopp's maximum brightness either on March 22, 1997 (3/22 or 322, a favored Skull & Bones number) or April Fool's Day. Media accounts varied. It was as if the comet had been calibrated on a slide rule or Cray XT4. As the "Field Guide to Comet Hale-Bopp" commented:

> If you were to hire one of those NASA people who figure out orbits for some of today's space probes – you know, the probes that use planets and their gravity boosts to get the best views of target planets while using the least amount of fuel – and designed a spectacular orbit for a comet, you'd probably come up with an orbit like Hale-Bopp is currently tracking through.

After the April Fool's Day perihelion, Hale-Bopp appeared to be heading toward the far reaches of the solar system between the constellations of Orion and Leo. The three stars in Orion's Belt align with the three great Egyptian pyramids, and the Lion with the Virgin's head, the Sphinx being Leo-Virgo. As Manly P. Hall stated in *The Secret Teachings of All Ages,* "The illumined of antiquity entered [the portals of the pyramid of Giza] as men; they came forth as gods."

As above, so below. Was this then the Freemason Egyptian way of the dead through heaven's gate? Was Hale-Bopp pointing the way to Freemason death and re-birth (as in "new world order")? Was Hale-Bopp celebrating the "Star Wars" secret space program?

On January 6, 1997 (Epiphany), a green sphere sped from east to west over Rome—surely a divine sign. NASA consultant Richard Hoagland and MK-ULTRA abductee Whitley Streiber insisted *something* was trailing Hale-Bopp—a "companion" that would collide with the Earth's aura (magnetosphere) on March 19, 1997 (vernal equinox) to enact an aura transformation that would conclude on April 29, 1997 (the eve of Walpurgisnacht) to signify the end of one era and beginning of a new era.

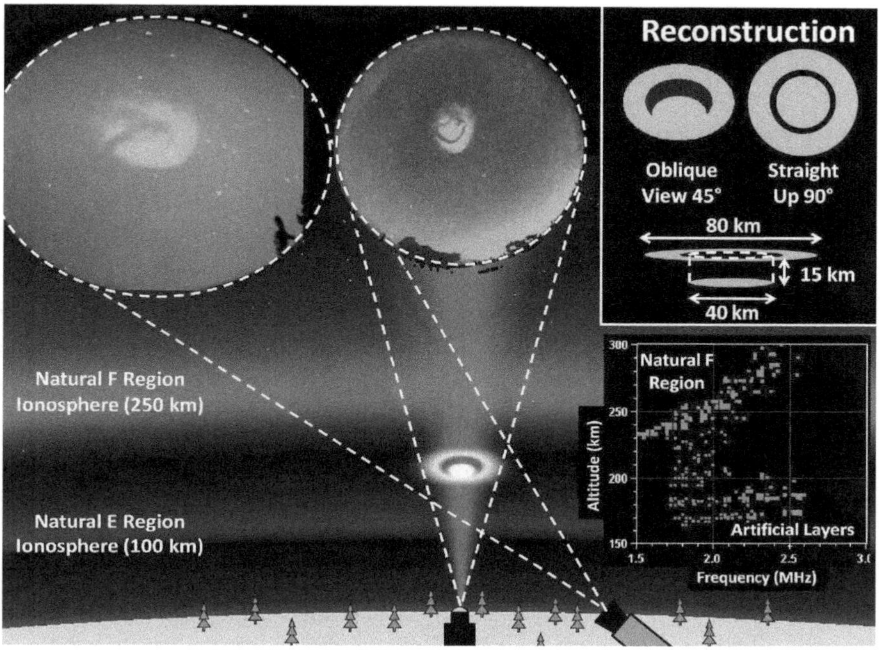

As dipole phased array radar ionizes the sky, a Townsend cascade occurs where electrons collide and increase attenuation of the atmosphere. These plasma rings are a product of that phenomenon. – Chris Fontenot

The area of the two crossing beams produces scalar rings that heat up due to over-pumping radar. Interferometry is thus also used as a weapon.

Diagram from the U.S. military DTIC (Defense Technical Information Center) .mil site.

The blood sacrifice accompanying the Hale-Bopp ritual[155] was the staged suicide of 38 members of the Heaven's Gate cult in Rancho Santa Fe on March 26, 1997. Following the Revelations script, Marshall Herff Applewhite ("Do") and Bonnie Lu Truesdale Nettles ("Ti") had founded Heaven's Gate; at the very end, Rio DiAngelo (*river of the angel*, perhaps the Milky Way flowing between Leo and Orion?) was left behind to tell the tale. Not so strangely, the Heaven's Gate computer Knowmad used the same server (Space Star Communications) as the highest levels of U.S. security: the CIA, NSA, DoD, retired Admirals and Generals, SAIC[156]—even U.S. Navy Admiral Bobby Ray Inman on the SAIC board and Council on Foreign Relations

155 Not to return for 3,600 years [60 x 60] through Sagittarius, the man-beast with his arrow eternally poised.

156 SAIC controlled ISPs through Network Solutions, which owned InterNIC, which controlled information on the World Wide Web by controlling ISPs of all Information Superhighway sites.

(CFR). SAIC had been a "neighbor" of Heaven's Gate in La Jolla, California, and three Heaven's Gate members had worked for Advanced Development Group, Inc. (later re-named Mantech Advanced Development Group) where they developed computer-based instruction for the U.S. Army. But of course these were just coincidences.

Tentacles, tentacles. In April 1996, Heaven's Gate closed up shop and sold their Earth Ship; less than a year later as Hale-Bopp exited, they were all dead.

All new comets, novas, and supernovas discovered by astrophysicists or star buffs like Bopp were filtered through nine International Astronomical Union (IAU) astronomers like Hale. Beyond the Central Bureau for Astronomical Telegrams (CBAT) in Cambridge, Massachusetts, under the Smithsonian Astrophysical Observatory for the IAU, the U.S. Naval Observatory ran public perception of Hale-Bopp, from the 1993 photograph of it orbiting Saturn to the online interactive program predicting the comet's position and visibility. The *Sky & Telescope* magazine website, the Minor Planet Center, the Center for Astrophysics, and NASA's Jet Propulsion Laboratory (JPL) all followed the Navy's lead for canned, monitored, spun star data.

The devil always hides in the details. For example, Hale-Bopp's light could be detected beyond Saturn's orbit, lit the skies of Mongolia during a total solar eclipse, and yet was oddly occluded by the Moon in May 1997, a first in astronomical history. (A flaw in the calculations of the "spectacular orbit"?) As the comet came closer and photographs on the Web got too clear, NASA's JPL switched to a 10-inch telescope to make the photos fuzzier. No Hubble photos after October 1995.

Hale-Bopp and Hyakutake were holographic projections of Halley's Comet developed at Caltech Laser Physics lab. The media mentioned "mysterious X-rays," but icy balls of dirt do not emit X-rays, whereas converging light beams (interferometry) might.

No astronomer wants to be the first to say that the emperor is stark naked. The only public credit given seems to be the 01 in C/1995 01, which stands for the first (of many) Enhanced Comet displays and perhaps for the brilliant binary computer that computed it.

7

Eyes in the Sky

"Space neighborhood watch"
Remote Viewing (RV):
The Advent of Brain-Computer Interface (BCI)
Brain-Computer Interface (BCI) / Brain-Machine Interface (BMI)
BCI Implantations
The Brainprint

Oh, little Sputnik, flying high
With made-in-Moscow beep,
You tell the world it's a Commie sky
And Uncle Sam's asleep.

– G. Mennen Williams, Governor of Michigan (1949-1961)

Who controls reconnaissance watches the enemy;
Who watches the enemy perceives the threat;
Who perceives the threat shapes the alternatives;
Who shapes the alternatives determines the response.

– Sir Halford Mackinder, 1919

AFTER RADIO, TELEGRAPH, TELEPHONES, TELEVISION, and the jet plane, the satellite Sputnik was successfully launched in the International Geophysical Year of 1957. Suddenly, boundaries extending beyond the atmosphere and into space became a real issue. It wasn't long before low and middle orbit satellites were snooping everywhere above. A new era had begun, and the gap between science fiction and science was closing like Scylla and Charybdis. Was God still in His heaven, or just man?

Sputnik, then Luniks and Vostoks, then generations of Corona and Rhyolite—Jumpseat, Argos, Aquacade, Chalet / Vortex, Magnum, Indigo / Lacrosse, IKONOS, Quickbird, Orbimage, SPOT (*Systéme Probatoire d'Observation de la Terre*). The Mercury, Gemini, and Apollo programs began, the unmanned Pioneer and Surveyor missions to the Moon, Mariner to Venus. NASA's Earth Resources Technology Satellites (ERTS) accustomed people to having their pictures taken from space, and the UN Committee on Peaceful Uses of Outer Space (COPUOS) was busy drafting international space law.

On August 25, 1960, the National Reconnaissance Office (NRO) was created and kept secret from the American people until the end of the Cold War. The very use of the acronym *NRO* was prohibited in Congress. Headquartered in Chantilly, Virginia behind lead doors, the NRO reported to the Undersecretary of the Air Force, the Office of Space Systems, and the CIA, its mission being to oversee and provide the NTM (national technical means) for arms control verification and the air, space, sea, and ground systems necessary for guarding U.S. interests. Its budget for building and operating space satellites was $7 billion per year with $4 billion of that total unaccounted for each year, according to its first audit in 1994 by the General Accounting Office (GAO).

Secret space program?

Television relay satellites in low orbit like Earlybird were busy preprogramming millions around the globe while electro-optical medium orbiters logged ocean surveillance and SIGINT (signals intelligence), and high orbiters like Telstar in 22,300-mile geosynchronous orbit concentrating on early warning, navigation, military communications, missile telemetry, and ABM (anti-ballistic missile) radar ferreting.

World War One photoreconnaissance balloons graduated to the sleek CIA U-2 and SR-71 Blackbird (1960-1972). Detailed close-ups from space zeroed in on Vietnam, Soviet intercontinental ballistic missile (ICBM) launch sites, surface-to-air missile (SAM) launches in Cuba, nuclear silos and plutonium plants in Israel, the detonation of the first Chinese atomic weapon, the first Soviet nuclear accident in Kyshtym in 1957, and the Six-Day War in the Middle East not made public until February 23, 1995 [2/23 = 322]. For two generations, CIA propaganda made the nation believe that eyes in the sky were about keeping tabs on enemies to protect America. Meanwhile, compartmentalized, need-to-know national security known as *sensitive compartmented information (SCI)*, with its words and acronyms pregnant with double meanings of "dual use" (*MAGIK, ULTRA, PEARL, THUMB*, etc.) grew.

Operations Corona (CIA) and Samos (USAF) revolutionized aerial spying with cameras capable of analyzing surface composition by taking images in 200 spectral bands. The first Corona satellite went up in January 1958 and made 94 elliptical orbits 500 miles above the Earth, each orbit lasting an hour and a half, its dual cameras snapping thousands of stereoscopic images. Propaganda claimed that retrorockets fired the film capsules earthward to be snatched up by Air Force planes, but the truth was that military computers already had the capability of relaying images to receivers below. Later digital generations would vastly improve the images, and listening posts with sophisticated computers and analysts with SI (Special Intelligence) and TK (Talent-Keyhole) clearance at the NSA, National Photographic Interpretation Center, and CIA would globally proliferate.

Rhyolite monitored phone calls, walkie-talkies, and intercept telemetry signals. High-orbits intercepted microwave transmissions and radio traffic. KH-11s read license plates. Two hundred and seventy-five miles up, Lacrosse beamed microwaves and measured their reflected energy day and night, cloudy or clear. Space Imaging's IKONOS one-meter resolution was panchromatic while four-meter resolution was multispectral with a depth penetration of 30 meters in clear water.

In quick succession, the U.S. Navy launched Landsat, Seasat, and Geosat, with Geosat bouncing radar pulses at the speed of light, calibrating distances via Doppler to determine gravity magnitude, and studying plate tectonics on the ocean floor, deep chasms called fracture zones meeting the Earth's mantle. 3D satellite mapping of the oceans made sense, but tasking the National Oceanic and Atmospheric Administration (NOAA) with mapping the Caribbean and northwest Hawaiian Islands was about far more, just as Brawdy Royal Air Force Base in West Wales was about far more than training jet aircraft pilots. As an oceanographic base with arrays of wires leading into the Atlantic, Brawdy was supposedly collecting whale song and migration patterns for research into nuclear submarine movement and communication. The hydrophonic sounding wires were certainly about remote listening but not just for whales or enemy nuclear submarines. In the 1960s, *silver discs* were zipping from Stack Rock, the tiny island off the coast of Brawdy. In 1990, the British Ministry of Defence gave the base over to the U.S. military.

Television, telephone, data, and military intelligence Intelink satellites increased throughout the 1960s and 1970s. Cable TV and PBS were the first to use satellite signal to deliver multipoint distribution instead of the usual coaxial video lines leased from telephone companies. TVRO dishes captured signals in backyards via Home Box Office's VideoCipher DES algorithm (MAACOM), and the rest is entertainment history—or is it?

Any SCI technology as powerful as satellites is never straightforward. Satellite sensors used to monitor other nations' compliance with arms control agreements gather intelligence, which means U.S. space reconnaissance secrecy. From the beginning, satellites have been dual use and therefore weaponized—sold to the public as communications and entertainment, calibrated for national security—commercial on the outside, military on the inside. Like embassies, satellites play a double game, and not just with foreign enemies.

General surveillance, television programming, and telephone / computer communication sweeps led to sensor technology (magnetic, seismic, infrared, strain, electromagnetic) becoming more and more sophisticated and tiny as *satellite intrusion and control* grew exponentially, along with domestic "non-lethal" electromagnetic weapons. Intrusive devices developed of the 1970s were standard, albeit hidden, by the 1990s: GPS, magnetic strips, voice stress analyzers, laser inception devices, cellular radio for eavesdropping, radiating and non-radiating transmitters and receivers, miniature radios, ultrasonic to hot-on-the-hook phone taps and concealed mini-microphones, remote laser rifle mikes, etc. Echelon (now called Five Eyes) eavesdropped on computers ("data surveillance") as NSA keywords and patterns software, remote activation and deactivation proliferated, and visuals went from infrared heat sensor cameras to night vision image intensifiers and high-res satellite imaging.

Now, Lockheed Martin Space Systems' Advanced Extremely High Frequency (AEHF) satellites are allegedly 22,500 miles up in geostationary orbit (GEO), resisting electronic jamming and capable of continuing communications and navigation after a nuclear EMP, thanks again to the versatile phased array antenna that can hop across frequencies so the signal can jump to an unjammed frequency. The phased array antenna has been excellent at steering and targeting from space for quite a while:

> Back in 2007, both the U.S. and China destroyed defunct satellites in orbit to show that they could do it. The technique is to fire a hunter / killer into the vicinity, fix the location of the enemy sat with infrared sensors, and use the thrusters to collide with it and blow it up.[1]

5G satellites with the low latency of earthbound fiber optics cable are the latest addition to the 1,886 operating satellites orbiting Earth (and that's not counting the orbital debris of defunct satellites like Milstar).[2] As of March 29, 2019, the lineup approved by the FCC looked something like this:

SpaceX Starlink – 12,000 satellites
OneWeb (UK / Honeywell Aerospace) – 4,560 satellites
Boeing – 2,956 satellites
Lockheed Martin – Blackjack orbital mesh network[3]

---

1 Joe Pappalardo, "Doomsday Satellites and the Space Wars To Come." Popular Mechanics, February 15, 2018.

2 On November 6, 2020, China launched 13 satellites, one of which is Tianyan-5, a 6G satellite. Tim Childers, "CVhina Has Launched the World's First 6G Satellite. We Don't Even Know What 6G Is Yet." Popular Mechanics, November 20, 2020. Caveat lector when it comes to Popular Mechanics.

3 Blackjack's autonomous mission management system is overseen by an AI called The Pit, sponsored by the U.S. Space Force and Space Development Agency. See Dan Robitzski, "DARPA is about to launch a military version of SpaceX's Starlink," Futurism.com, May 12, 2020.

Spire Global – 972 satellites[4]
U.S. Navy 30cm PRAMs (photovoltaic RF antenna modules)[5]

SpaceX has now applied for 30,000 more satellites (1,300 launched so far); OneWeb plans 7,088 satellites; Telesat (Canada) plans 1,671 satellites (space-based mesh IP network) to replace fiber networks; Omnispace / Lockheed Martin / U.S. military 5G / IoT; Amazon plans 3,236 satellites; Lynk for cell phones; Facebook cubesats.[6]

I am a Naturopath & independent researcher of Morgellons / Genetically Modified Organisms . . . I regularly feel the satellites beam their microwaves from space. It feels like a photo copier light. I feel sick and get prickly heart as it approaches, then I just start frying & melting, sweat just pouring out worse than menopause sweats. My body aches in various joints, as my body temp, heart rate, & blood pressure increase.

– Carlene Fuchs, email, March 27, 2021

Like ground-based 5G, satellite 5G uses phased array antennas to shoot tightly focused beams of microwave radiation strong enough to pass through walls and bodies. Thus we are inundated by beams from space to 5G devices and beams back up to space, the satellites needing frequencies 37.5 to 42 GHz for space-to-Earth and 47.2 to 51.4 GHz for Earth-to-space[7]—20,000 of them[8] with tiny phased array antennas arranged in masses of 4" x 4" matrices.

> When an ordinary electromagnetic field enters the body, it causes charges to move and currents to flow. But when extremely short electromagnetic pulses enter the body [like 5G millimeter waves], something else hap-

4 John P. Thomas, "5G From Space: 20,000 Satellites Blanket The Earth," Technocracy Earth, January 8, 2019. These figures do not include smaller satellite systems of foreign governments, nor Amazon's Kuiper internet satellite constellation of 3,236 satellites (Darrell Etherington, "Amazon gains FCC approval for Kuiper internet satellite constellation and commits $10 billion to the project," TechCrunch, July 31, 2020).

5 PRAMs convert solar energy into microwaves for power transmission while collecting data on power density.

6 "Update on Satellites," Cell Phone Task Force (cellphonetaskforce.org) for the 2021 update.

7 "FCC tells SpaceX it can deploy up to 11,943 broadband satellites." Ars Technics, November 2018.

8 John P. Thomas, "20,000 Satellites for 5G to be Launched Sending Focused Beams of Intense Microwave Radiation Over Entire Earth." Health Impact News, n.d.

pens: the moving charges themselves become little antennas that re-radiate the electromagnetic field and send it deeper into the body. These re-radiated waves are called Brillouin precursors. They become significant when either the power or the phase of the waves changes rapidly enough.

5G will probably satisfy both requirements. This means that the reassurance we are being given—that these millimeter waves are too short to penetrate far into the body—is not true.[9]

The ERP (effective radiated power) of 5G phased array antennas *in cell phones alone* is 10X more powerful than 4G, while the WiFi hubs for 5G use microwave beams 15X stronger (300 watts) than 5G phone signals.

There are even Internet of Things (IoT) routers in space for data backhaul.

What is it all about? Certainly not "defense." Perhaps for the "space neighborhood watch"? As Robert Duncan, PhD, describes:

> The grid of satellites in the [northern] hemisphere or the ionospherically reflected ground-based miles-wide antenna fields can be used in a time-sliced manner to calculate an inverse Fourier Transform to attack many people at the same time without exposing too many others to the same intensities and frequencies. All the sensor systems are integrated to act as one single antenna or phased array. This allows the linked system to redirect energy from almost any angle to find a weakness in a shielded structure.[10]

"Space neighborhood watch"

> *The satellite [VALIS, a Vast Active Living Intelligence System] had control of them from the get-go. It could make them see what it wanted them to see . . . The satellite has occluded them, all of them. The whole fucking United States . . . In Fat's opinion, his apartment had been saturated with high levels of radiation of some kind.*
>
> – Philip K. Dick, *Valis* (1981)

In 1987, targeted individual Harlan Girard reported excruciating microwave attacks from a satellite. Space Tracking and Surveillance System (STSS)

9 Arthur Firstenberg, Microwave News, 2002. Also see Firstenberg's "Planetary Emergency," Cellular Phone Task Force, May 14, 2018.

10 Robert Duncan, PhD, The Matrix Deciphered: Psychic Warfare / Top Secret Mind Interfacing Technology. Higher Order Thinkers Publishing, 2006. Duncan worked with the Department of Defense, Central Intelligence Agency, DARPA, U.S. Department of Justice, NASA, Navy, and NATO architecting key components and systems for surveillance, and warfare.

satellites are categorized under GSSAP (Geosynchronous Space Situational Awareness Program). The moniker *space situational awareness (SSA)* has in turn hatched the friendly *Mr. Rogers* "space neighborhood watch,"[11] while dual-use weather satellites like the Deep Space Climate Observatory satellite DSCOVR serve the neighborhood watch, as well:

> A joint effort between the National Aeronautics and Space Administration (NASA), the National Oceanic and Atmospheric Administration (NOAA), and the U.S. Air Force [partnering with SpaceX], the DSCOVR will both monitor space weather to help assess its impact on Earth's magnetic field, as well as provide valuable earth science measurements . . .[12]

NAVSTAR GPS satellites, CLIO communications satellites, DMSP weather satellites, United Launch Alliance, MIDAS missile defense, NASA Terra, the portable Deployable Satellite Communication Terminal (DSCT), the AI-run ANGELS (Automated Navigation and Guidance Experiment for Local Space) under the Air Force Research Laboratory, the "communications and reconnaissance" satellites providing high-speed (10 terabits per second) low-latency Internet in remote areas, including Elon Musk's low-earth orbit (LEO) 5G CubeSats,[13] are more of the same, all dual use, all involved in impacting all the brains below.

The old satellite-based GPS required three dedicated satellites to triangulate signal time stamps and keep track of where a target was every minute of every day. During the 1980s and 1990s, GPS went "black" and shifted from analog to digital, meaning all the sats were recalibrated. Now, GPS has been replaced by *PNT (position / navigation / timing)* for precision targeting kill systems network-oriented to the 5G / IoT smart grid: cell phones, tablets, cars, and U.S. network of 24 orbiting satellites (three of which are available 24/7 for spur-of-the-moment positioning worldwide, as was preprogrammed in the 1998 film *Enemy of the State*), all working in tandem with networks like Russia's GLONASS and Europe's Galileo (GNSS), plus corporate networks doubling as military contractors—DISH Anywhere, AT&T TV, etc.

While excelling in infrared and visual imaging, *remote sensing satellites* are in the business of "human biosignature" surveillance, armed with radio telescopes and SQUIDs (superconducting quantum interference devices) sen-

---

11 Mike Wall, "US Air Force Launches 3 'Space Neighborhood Watch' Satellites." Space.com, July 28, 2014.

12 Ari Phillips, "A Sneak Peek At NASA's New Satellite That Has Been 16 Years In The Making." ThinkProgress.org, February 4, 2015.

13 Loren Grush, "Elon Musk shows off SpaceX's 60 internet-beaming satellites packed together for launch." The Verge, May 12, 2019.

sitive to the femtoteslas of our brains' magnetic flux (10^{-15}), especially when triangulated with dipole implants or pulsing cell phones. Other dual-use technologies on board might be X-ray-based holographic imaging, MASER, ultrasound (capable of exerting physical pressure or thermal injury on bodies), particle beam[14] positrons or neutrinos that can melt tissue, entrain plasma, execute brain scanning and V2K.[15]

> Any ground-based network like HAARP, GWEN, cell phone towers or the Russian Woodpecker could also perform this feat of mind reading and control but not on a global scale. Only through the hundreds of spy and remote-sensing satellites circling the earth and the tens of giant ionospheric phased array fields could you cover the entire globe with directed energy weapons and the subset class of mind control weapons.[16]

Each of the first Strategic Defense Initiative (SDI) geosynchronous satellites was originally armed with a Titan Corporation (L-3 Technologies today) Thunderbolt System *virtual cathode oscillator (vircator)* (U.S. Patent 4,345,220, "High-power microwave generator using relativistic electron beam in waveguide drift tube," 1982). Lockheed's GPS Satellite tracking frequency was 3600-3750 MHz, and the vircators operated at 3920-3935 MHz.[17] Vircators are not just about electromagnetic pulses (EMPs) against electronics; they have everything to do with targeting individuals far down on the Earth, as described by an anonymous targeted individual:

> *Eventually, I left the country, went to SE Asia. This alleviated any ringing [tinnitus] or pulsing. Sometimes, however, I hear ringing; only time will tell. What I envision is that the technology is at the point similar to the old school electron resonance spectroscopy, except this time it is us who are being imaged and irradiated, not electrons, molecules, plasma species, etc. The size scale and*

---

14 ". . . stable self-pinched propagation of high-current charged-particle beams in the atmosphere is possible over distances equal to several Nordsieck lengths [1 Nordsieck = ~400 meters per electron beam / 1,000 meters per proton beam]. In order not to be deflected by Earth's magnetic field, electron-beam pulses need to be guided by a pre-formed channel [laser wave guide or duct], while proton beam pulses may under suitable conditions propagate undeflected through both the low- and high-atmosphere . . ." – Andre Gsponer, "the physics of high-intensity high-energy particle beam propagation in open air and outer space plasmas," Independent Scientific Research Institute, Oxford OX4 4YS England, January 11, 2009.

15 John Hall, MD, A New Breed: Satellite Terrorism in America. Strategic Book Publishing & Rights Agency, LLC, 2009. Positrons are the antimatter counterpart to the electron, neutrinos a type of scalar wave. Particle beam technology is discussed in Chapter 6, "The Secret Space Program."

16 Robert Duncan, PhD.

17 Confirmed as a satellite-to-ground frequency in the FCC frequency allocation table.

energies involved would seem to favor easier imaging of people on Earth vs ions under a microscope. Imaging materials through an electron microscope is similar to imaging humans from a million miles away. Nanometer electrons from 1 meter = a factor of 1 billion, compared to +/- 1 meter human from a million miles. Factor of 1 billion.

What was that about gigawatts in Back to the Future (1985)*? Ha! They knew about the Vircator back then.*

Emmett Brown: Marty, I'm sorry, but the only power source capable of generating 1.21 gigawatts of electricity is a bolt of lightning.

It doesn't really surprise me that things went this way; it just angers me. What surprises me is how people do not appear to recognize what is clearly right in their face. Brainwashing seems logical.[18]

Remote Viewing (RV): The Advent of Brain-Computer Interface (BCI)

He rode over Connecticut
In a glass coach.
Once, a fear pierced him
In that he mistook
The shadow of his equipage
For blackbirds.

– Wallace Stevens, "Thirteen Ways of Looking at a Blackbird"

Cover stories may be established for unacknowledged programs in order to protect the integrity of the program from individuals who do not have a need to know. Cover stories must be believable and cannot reveal any information regarding the true nature of the contract. Cover stories for Special Access Programs [SAPs] must have the approval of the PSO [Program Security Officer] prior to dissemination.

– National Industrial Security Program Operation Manual (NISPOM), DoD 5220.22-M, 1993

18 In 1985, the Air Force Office of Scientific Research (AFOSR) succeeded in getting millimeter-wave vircators above 39.9 GHz with a peak power of 21 kilowatts http://apps.dtic.mil/dtic/tr/fulltext/u2/a159394.pdf. Between 1987 and 1992, the SDI "Star Wars" program launched 24-30 satellites into geosynchronous orbit under the Thunderbolt System (Vircator/Reltron). See David Price et al., "Compact Pulsed Power for Directed Energy Weapons," Journal of Directed Energy, Fall 2003.

When *remote viewing (RV)* hit the Internet in the 1990s, it sounded like some kind of clairvoyance or virtual reality. But RV was *electronic brain-computer interface (EBCI)* "telepathy" amplified by radio waves, one remote viewer transmitting and the other receiving, both wired to computers for signal modification at VLF or ELF power densities.

> Classified technology is beyond the imagination of most people. Levitation is old hat. Synthetic [computer-enhanced encephalographic] telepathy is old hat. When the imaging equipment was used on me, I could remote view nine areas of the world at the same time. Psi-Tech, the firm run by chronic confabulator Ed Dames and that complete psychopath John Alexander, states in the very name of their company how remote viewing really works: with machines. (I've been linked to them, so I speak with confidence about all of this. I'm not speculating.) They were developed by scientists hiding behind the "alien" cover. The mind control arsenal is often used for torture. The world that emerges with it in the wrong hands will not be worth living in.[19]

Remote viewing—"traveling clairvoyance"—was the early brain-computer interface (BCI) "make-a-psychic" program that separated and drove the brainwaves of the two hemispheres to a particular frequency to match what a plugged-in "psychic" was seeing remotely via *computer-simulated subconscious speech* (see below).

During the halcyon Cold War MK-ULTRA / MKSEARCH years (1950-1973), 44 laboratories were pursuing brain research in prisons, mental hospitals, and universities. The Princeton University Group, headed by the dean of the School of Engineering and Applied Sciences, was concentrating on "remote precognitive perception" while *Project Scanate* at SRI International[20] concentrated on remote electromagnetic control, bionics, and biotelemetry cyber-psi, and Kirlian aura research led Karl Pribram, PhD (1919-2015), director of SRI's Neuropsychology Research Laboratory, to discover how closely mental imaging resembled hologram projection.

The *Stargate Project* was a secret U.S. Army unit established by the Defense Intelligence Agency (DIA) and SRI International in 1978 at Fort Meade, Maryland investigating "psychic phenomena" (Wikipedia).[21] Stargate was sheer mind control via early BCI technologies that clearly lay outside

---

19 Alex Constantine, "Mind Control and UFOs," February 1996, https://alexconstantinereport.wordpress.com/ufos/. I was once friends with Alex Constantine, aka Daniel Rightmeyer, and can vouch for the veracity of his having been used by intelligence agencies.

20 Stanford Research Institute (SRI) has always been a Tavistock Institute hive of mind control experimentation.

21 Like other interactive social media, Wikipedia is intelligence-run.

the charter of the Pentagon and Intelligence Community, e.g. MKOFTEN[22] projects made to look like *phantasy*.[23]

A lot of strange birds flapped around the Stargate brain belfry, from the CIA Blackbird SR-71 spy plane to the Aviary covering for the UFO Working Group inside the Defense Intelligence Agency (DIA). Ingo Swann, the Aviary's real deal *ganzfeld* psychic, developed *autoganzfeld* protocols (human-machine telepathy).[24] Other Aviary birds feverishly worked on neurophysiology (Bluejay), zero point energy (Owl), nonlethals (Penguin), CIA Weird Desk at the Directorate of Science and Technology (Pelican), ONI photography (Seagull), and disinformation (Nightingale) with lots of military input from AFOSI (Falcon), USAF (Condor), Wright-Patterson AFB (Hawk), and the Rockefeller point man (Chickadee).[25]

The Aviary's main job was to protect top-secret Special Access Programs or SAPs (nonlethals, exotic propulsion, psycho- / telekinesis, remote viewing, etc.) from the public by amplifying the truth until it sounded ridiculous and leading the curious and suspicious down blind alleys laced with truth. The Aviary covered for the Mobius Group that worked with Jet Propulsion Laboratory (JPL) scientists. Meanwhile, the physics luminary Jack Sarfatti of Esalen Institute chatted up post-quantum physics and ideas about the emergence of conscious AI quantum biocomputers, living in a locally flat tangent Cartesian space like a many-sheeted Riemann surface of a function of a complex variable of parallel flat worlds, etc.

All roads were leading to BCI. In pursuit of BCI interactions with plasma UFOs like the ones photographed in the desert by Wilhelm Reich, MD (1897-1957) or the ones entering and exiting the Caribbean and Gulf of Mexico that John Lilly and his dolphins and Janus computer were also attempting to contact, physician and parapsychologist Andrija Puharich (1918-1995), along with psychics Uri Geller (Mossad) and Peter Hurkos, were working with intelligence agencies (CIA, DIA, ONI, ONR, AFOSI, etc.)

---

22 According to Gordon Thomas's 2007 book Secrets and Lies, the CIA›s Operation Often was initiated by the chief of the CIA›s Technical Services Branch, Dr. Sidney Gottlieb, to "explore the world of black magic" and "harness the forces of darkness and challenge the concept that the inner reaches of the mind are beyond reach" (Wikipedia). Gottlieb and other CIA employees recruited fortune-tellers, palm-readers, clairvoyants, astrologists, mediums, psychics, specialists in demonology, witches and warlocks, Satanists, etc.

23 Phantasy: the power or process of creating especially unrealistic or improbable mental images in response to psychological need. (Merriam-Webster)

24 Supposedly, psychics interpret whereas remote viewers only see "calibrated, consistent and accurate results."

25 Owl was a leading Scientologist and Swann a Class VII Operating Thetan and founder of the Los Angeles Scientology Center. Scientology was created by the CIA and U.S. Navy via their "empath" L. Ron Hubbard.

who were scouring the occult landscape for bona fide clairvoyants and mediums to query dead Agents and read NSA adviser Henry Kissinger's mind. In a trance, medium Ingo Swann spoke in the cold metallic voice of an artificial intelligence (AI) computer 100 years in the future. In the Soviet Union and its Eastern European satellites, telepathy and clairvoyance were renamed *bioinformation transfer*, psychokinesis *biophysical effect,* a medium or psychic an *extrasensor,* etc.

After the Church Committee purportedly halted the CIA's MK-ULTRA programs, *Operation Grill Flame* took off under SRI International, the CIA, DIA, ONI, and SAIC. Former consultant to the NSA Will Filer described the early remote viewing days of *computer-simulated subconscious speech language*:

> Some of the early experiments included Remote Viewing at NSA where the Viewer would relax, open their mind, and explain the clarity of images . . . to reframe the specifications of the computer-simulated subconscious speech language and the scripting formats to maximize the ability to deliver an accurate "vision or picture" into the subject. Pictures already seen by the subject could simply be recalled using age regression script variations.[26]

Grill Flame was a remote viewing SAP that commanded the highest Sensitive Compartmentalized security clearance.[27] Thousands were experimented on under Grill Flame. Dr. Louis Jolyn "Jolly" West ran remote viewing experiments at UCLA and provided MK-ULTRA-style "medical oversight" while ex-OSS Al "Captain Trips" Hubbard played Johnny Appleseed for LSD under Willis Harman's Alternative Futures Project that purportedly provided strategic planning for defense corporations and government. While Captain Trips turned on whomever he could, the CIA's Technical Services Division (TSD) filmed it all for blackmail.

Picture the labs at SRI International in 1973 during Grill Flame: people reclining in dentist chairs, their craniums EEG-wired, their chests EKG-wired, words and images flowing holographically into their brains at 100 Hz. Some were "empaths" and "clears" from L. Ron Hubbard's Scientology and Maharishi's Invincible Defense Technology (IDT).[28] CIA and DIA agents,

---

26 Will Filer, "NSA Mind Control and Psyops," 16 pages, July 27, 1999, "Subliminal Implanted Posthypnotic Suggestions and Scripts Using Acoustically Delivered and Phonetically Accelerated Posthypnotic Commands without Somnambulistic Preparation in the Subject for Intelligence and Counterintelligence Applications by the U.S. National Security Agency (NSA)."

27 When remote viewer David Morehouse exposed the SAP classification of the program in his 1996 book Psychic Warrior, he was involuntarily hospitalized and psychiatrically abused, i.e. subjected to mind control.

28 A political science professor at Emory University in Atlanta practiced Sidhi Transcendental

plus handpicked members of Congress and professors of universities, were Grill Flame RV subjects. NASA claimed to have sent two RV astral travelers to scout Jupiter in advance of the Jupiter fly-by mission[29] and developed its own "biocommunication" protocol to enhance communication with "technological artifacts."

> Initial results coming out of laboratories in the United States and Canada [show] that certain amplitude and frequency combinations of external electromagnetic radiation in the brainwave frequency range are capable of bypassing the external sensory mechanism of organisms, including humans, and directly stimulating higher-level neuronal structures in the brain. This electronic stimulation is known to produce mental changes at a distance, including hallucinations in various sensory modalities, particularly auditory. Because the power levels are so low, the brain could mistake the outside signal for its own, mimic it (a process known as bioelectric entrainment), and respond when it changes.[30]

The CIA passed Grill Flame on to the Navy and DIA at Fort Meade under U.S. Army Intelligence and Security Command (INSCOM) where it eventually developed Psi-Tech (https://psitech.net) under Maj. Ed Dames and Gen. Albert N. Stubblebine III. *Scientific remote viewing (SRV)* utilized computers and satellites. At Psi-Tech, the Eagle (Joe McMoneagle, Army intel) joined Swann as another natural empath.

"Turning up the heat" on Grill Flame to stream unattenuated signals and *gestalt* patterns into the wired brain required blocking cognitive analysis and imagination—just like early MK-ULTRA. The remote viewing brain in theta waves (4-7 Hz) is far from the higher mental activity of gamma waves (>40 Hz) and more like a television screen receiving signals and images. The remote viewer is "trained" (programmed?) to attend only to what electronically shows up in his or her "trained" consciousness, and sessions last no longer than 45 minutes, due to "lapses in the energy field."

Remote viewing appears to be based on split-brain research, the right hemisphere recognizing shapes and impressions but unable to name them, and the left hemisphere describing things in words but unable to identify them by shape or touch. The tendency of people to favor one side of the brain over the other may be part of why the Mobius Group organized remote view-

---

Meditation twice daily with RV to travel visually through spacetime to observe galaxies and talk to Jesus.

29 NASA's Juno probe completed its 10th flyby of Jupiter February 7, 2018.

30 Ronald M. McRae, Mind Wars: The True Story of Government Research into the Military Potential of Psychic Weapons. St. Martin's Press, 1984.

ing into teams of individuals from varying backgrounds.

So how much of RV is being remotely *sent* to the two brain hemispheres via implanted probes and precise injection of EM signals along "hidden Whittaker-infolded EM structuring unknown to Western technologists"? As physicist Lt. Col. (ret.) Tom Bearden explains:

> . . . if anything (thought, feeling, emotion, image) arises internally in one of the cerebral hemispheres, that hemispheric personality thinks that it did it—that is, it thinks that it not only thought the thought but also created the thought. So if you have a hidden channel to pipe in inputs [the Whittaker-infolded EM structuring], you can take over or implant the thoughts, behavior, and actions of a person or a very large group of persons. That alone allows a mind-numbing direct control of behavior externally and from a distance.[31]

Maj. Dames has claimed that 60 percent of Psi-Tech's time was spent remote viewing exotic propulsion craft—plasma UFOs communicating psychically (AI "Hal's" on our own exotic crafts?)—traveling the highways and byways of Earth's geomagnetic grid, entering and exiting at harmonic "gateways" that connect our 3-space with physicist Martin Deutsch's parallel dimensions.

RV under Grill Flame was a pivotal precursor to brain-computer interface (BCI). Besides Psi-Tech, corporations like the Monroe Institute (Robert Monroe's Hemi-Sync tech was classified by the CIA[32]) and Kaman Corporation continue to run experiments and classified seminars. Millions of taxpayer dollars have gone into cyber-psi studies and much was and is still derived therefrom, whatever the disinformation and spin over the decades may say to the contrary.[33]

Now, the private sector has been unknowingly enlisted to run manifold BCI operations. SRI International has offices in ten nations and operates an Artificial Intelligence Laboratory at Cambridge University in the UK with the lion's share of its income coming from (who else?) the U.S. Department of Defense.

---

31 Terry Patten and Michael Hutchison, "Interview with Lt. Col. Thomas E. Bearden (ret.)." Megabrain Report, February 4, 1991, http://www.cheniere.org/misc/interview1991.htm.

32 According to medical engineer Eldon Byrd, Hemi-Sync altered a target's brainwaves by superimposing another person's brainwaves. See US Patent #5213562A "Method of inducing mental, emotional and physical states of consciousness, including specific mental activity, in human beings," 1991.

33 See Commander L.R. Bremseth, U.S. Navy, "Unconventional Human Intelligence Support: Transcendent and Asymmetric Warfare Implications of Remote Viewing," 28 April 2001.

Brain-Computer Interface (BCI) / Brain-Machine Interface (BMI)

. . . 25 million people can be tracked and controlled through the brain-machine interface. If brainwaves don't extend much beyond 2 kHz, then a time p\multiplexing scheme like what cellular phone transmitters use would work. 25 million X 2 kHz = 50 GHz for the upper bandwidth requirements. Currently, published RADAR capabilities go into the terahertz (THz) frequency range or sub-millimeter wavelength well within the bandwidth required. In fact, the entirety of human intelligence of the planet without compression operates at 1.34 THz (6.7 billion X 2 kHz).

– Robert Duncan, *The Matrix Deciphered*, 2006

Targets have to use a kind of mental anesthesia, exactly like a soldier does. In order to succeed, you must, on some level, consider yourself already dead; that way, you have nothing to lose and you become less afraid of the unknown and unpredictable.

– Michael F. Bell, *The Invisible Crime*, 2011

In 2003—just a few years into independent scientist Clifford Carnicom's examination of the effluvium being broadcast by jets over northern New Mexico—DARPA launched the Brain Machine Interface (BMI) program (later known as brain-computer interface or BCI) to create "new technologies for augmenting human performance through the ability to noninvasively access these codes in the brain in real time and integrate them into peripheral device or systems operations."[34]

The mental picture we've been conditioned to form when we read words like these is probably of scientists in labs working on chimpanzee and human heads dotted with electrodes hooked up to computers. But what if the purpose of BCI / BMI is really about a Transhumanist future of genetically altered, "augmented" / "enhanced" human beings more cyborg than human? How might an entire population be changed in the twinkling of an All-Seeing Eye by integration into "peripheral device or systems operations"?

Electrodes are no longer necessary for accessing the brain, nor are labs and men / women in white coats. Picture instead laptops and eyes glued to monitors. Picture cities, neighborhoods, and rural areas plugged into the planetary Space Fence smart grid sustained by an ionized sky loaded with

34 "DARPA To Support Development of Human Brain-Machine Interface." Duke University Campus, August 15, 2002.

nanoparticles and whizzing waves of billions, trillions of wireless operations.

The process by which your brain is made to interface with supercomputers is synthetic telepathy, also known as techlepathy or the Russian term psychotronics: human thought as EMR intercepted and processed with a return signal perceptible by another human brain.[35] Techlepathy—communication from one mind to another with the assistance of technology—is *neuromorphic engineering* with nanowire field-effect transistors linked to neurons for hybrid bioelectronic devices and neural prosthetics. Numenta, "where neuroscience meets machine intelligence," logs computer memory modeled on the neocortex and called Hierarchical Temporal Memory (HTM) or memory nodes for *cognitive computing*—computer vision, artificial intelligence, robotics, and machine learning. Since 2005, the Blue Brain project of IBM at the Ecole Polytechnique Federale de Lausanne in Switzerland has been building detailed models of neocortex wiring and interfacing living organisms with computers by means of nano-actuator DNA switches. Contrary to the drugs / hypnosis approach of the original MK-ULTRA, synthetic telepathy BCI depends upon a thorough reading of "basic impulses and sensations" over time so as to capture exact brainwave signatures.

As for who or what is at the other end of this invisible leash, it begins with whether it is interpretative or interactive mediation.

> Interpretative mediation is the passive analysis of signals coming from the human brain. A computer "reads" the signal, then compares that signal against a database of signals and their meanings. Using statistical analysis and repetition, false-positives are reduced over time.
>
> Interactive mediation can be in a passive-active mode, or active-active mode. In this case, passive and active denote the method of reading and writing to the brain and whether or not they make use of a broadcast signal. Interactive mediation can also be performed manually or via artificial intelligence.
>
> Manual interactive mediation involves a human operator producing return signals such as speech or images. AI mediation leverages the cognitive system of the subject to identify images, pre-speech, objects, sounds and other artifacts, rather than developing AI routines to perform such activities. AI-based systems may incorporate natural language processing interfaces that produce sensations, mental impressions, humor and conversation to provide a mental picture of a computerized personality. Not

35 "Synthetic telepathy also known as techlepathy or psychotronics," Geeldon.wordpress.com, September 6, 2010.

> only can this AI hold a conversation via the internal monologue, but it may also perform routing of information to and from specific groups or individuals. This provides a broad range of potential applications from acting as a communications system to conducting interrogations.[36]

Geeldon then examines military / intelligence use of synthetic telepathy for two-way communications and intelligence gathering / interrogation, surmising in 2010 that passive monitoring of the internal monologue over time is the most effective for intelligence gathering and what most populations are undergoing. If circumstances warrant it, passive monitoring can be shifted to the interactive mediation known as torture.

> At its most basic, impulses guide human behavior, and manipulation of these impulses provides a strategic advantage in both combat and political situations. By altering the motivational factors of a target subject or group, it makes it easier to guide their higher level decision-making processes.
>
> Crowd or riot control can be achieved by generating impulses that are essentially common to all humans, resulting in the dispersion of crowds or a willingness to co-operate with authorities. This type of synthetic telepathy is arguably a political tool as it suppresses dissent.[37]

Controlled mainstream media have camouflaged BCI systems as either controlling machines by thought alone or medical miracle treatments, but they are actually about plugging populations into the hive mind of a SkyNet[38] matrix by means of the smart / neural dust being aerially delivered in inert polymer sheaths or insulator films after which they are breathed in to implant a fine "neural mesh" of antennas into the body and brain. Jets, drones, and sounding rockets have been laying "electronic sensors the size of dust particles"[39] for more than two decades.

---

36 Ibid.

37 Ibid.

38 The term "SkyNet" is from the 2003 preprogramming film Terminator 3: Rise of the Machines. See "JADE HELM 15: Covert SkyNet," July 17, 2015—if you can find it: "The Jade-2 System is a Network Centric Software Based Artificial Intelligence Program at the Helm (i.e. JADE Helm)." The true nature of JADE Helm 2015 was to test the command and control protocol called the Jade-2 System, a highly sophisticated "self-aware" Artificial Intelligence network. "From CCTV to social media networks, its purpose is not only military; it is for the entire human domain. This full spectrum analysis of the JADE-2 Artificial Intelligence System will have you thinking SkyNet has just arrived. JADE 2 is in command & control ... JADEmilit-2 is at the helm and it is fully aware and operational." Also see "The US Military Is Quietly Building SkyNet," Zero Hedge, September 29, 2017.

39 "How Smart Dust Could Spy On Your Brain: A View from Emerging Technology from the arXiv." Technology Review, July 16, 2013.

Abstract: This paper explores the fundamental system design trade-offs and ultimate size, power, and bandwidth scaling limits of neural recording systems built from low-power CMOS circuitry coupled with ultrasonic power delivery and backscatter communication. In particular, we propose an ultra-miniature as well as extremely compliant system that enables *massive scaling in the number of neural recordings from the brain while providing a path towards truly chronic BMI.* These goals are achieved via two fundamental technology innovations: (1) thousands of 10-100\ mu m scale, free-floating, independent sensor nodes, or neural dust, that detect and report local extracellular electrophysiological data; and (2) a sub-cranial interrogator that establishes power and communication links with the neural dust.[40] (Emphasis added.)

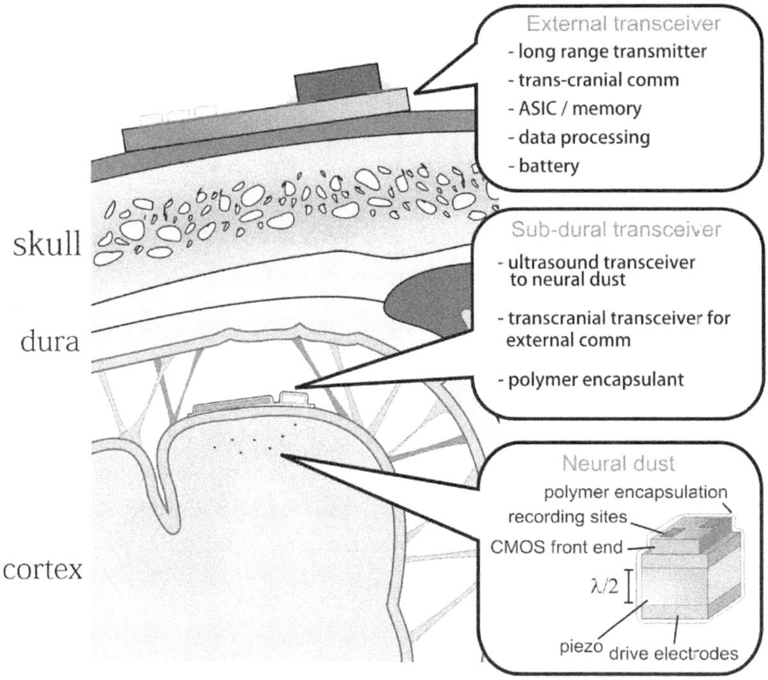

Neural dust. See how it's engineered.

"Intelligent neural dust embedded in the brain could be the ultimate brain-computer interface," *Neurogadget,* July 18, 2013.

CMOS: complementary metal-oxide-semiconductor

ASIC: application-specific integrated circuit

40 Dongjin Seo et al., "Neural Dust: An Ultrasonic, Low Power Solution for Chronic Brain-Machine Interfaces." Cornell University, 8 July 2013.

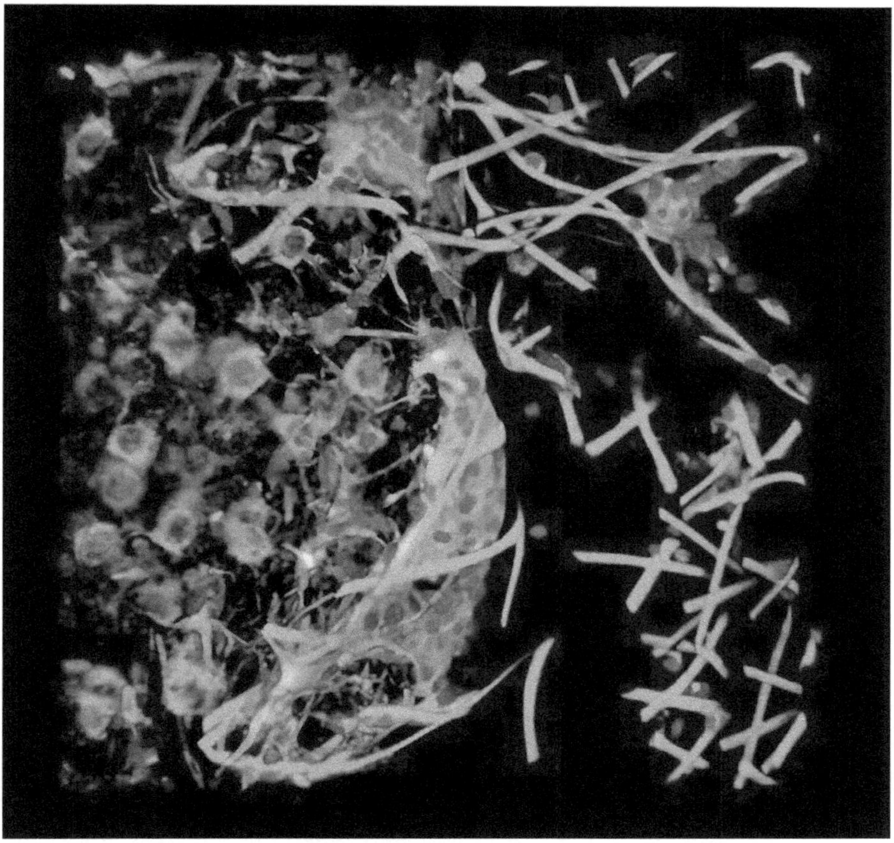

Mesh (neural lace) merging with brain cells.

". . . this could be the beginning of the first true human internet, where brain-to-brain interfaces are possible via injectable electronics that pass your mental traffic through the cloud. What could go wrong?"

https://gizmodo.com/scientists-just-invented-the-neural-lace-1711540938

Controlling machines by thought is one thing, but being controlled *by* machines is another. The ongoing global aerosol assault under the rubric of "geoengineering climate change" is delivering standard CMOS (complementary metal-oxide-semiconductor) circuits and sensors[41]and conductive metals the size of dusty plasma to be breathed in and ingested and breach the blood-brain barrier for remote BMI linking *via ultrasound.*

> Each particle of neural dust consists of standard CMOS circuits and sensors that measure the electrical activity in neurons nearby. This is coupled

41 The greenhouse gas hexafluoroethane is used to create semiconductors.

to a piezoelectric material that converts ultra-high-frequency sound waves into electrical signals and vice versa.[42]

Neural / smart dust represents a clear advantage to invasive, stationary brain imaging technologies like MRIs (magnetic resonance imaging), PETs (positron emission tomography), MEGs (magnetoencephalography), etc.[43] In fact, the NEMS sensors (nanoelectromechanical systems) swimming in our bloodstream and lodging in the brain's cortex function like mini-MRIs while the nanoscale CMOSs act as sensors and circuits measuring electrical activity in neurons and piezoelectrically converting ultra-high frequency sound waves into electrical signals (and vice versa) to be reconverted to ultrasound via piezoelectrics and the remote ultrasound powering the dust.[44]

Meanwhile, it is all the rage for the rich and young to link their brains to remote neural systems via computer-satellite linkups with no need for virtual reality (VR) helmets. Virtual reality is tomorrow's reality TV. Pay to watch humans struggle with their consciousness for hours, days, weeks, months, a lifetime—their behavior, experiences, feelings and thoughts replicated Sentient World Simulation-style and transmitted via computer as the controller "interacts" with the target's memories, bodily reactions, VR perceptions, etc. Whole conversations among multiple controllers may take place in the target's brain after the controllers finish their posh 7-course dinner and retreat with their drugs and drinks to the war room to log on. The fact that the target has no choice regarding his or her no-touch torture makes this latest fad almost as exciting as snuff films. If the target complains to law enforcement or the FBI, s/he will be sent for "psychological evaluation" and possibly committed to an institution where voyeur torture will continue, or s/he may be sold on an auction block to other cyber-voyeurs and -torturers. Soul Catcher software makes it easy to record and download interactions into yet other targets' brains.

Beyond social media and satellite imagery overseen by the National Geospatial-Intelligence Agency (NGA), AI systems vacuum up "independent sensor node" data from Department of Homeland Security (DHS) Fusion Centers. Receivers and transmitters monitoring the body and brain *from the inside* provide the lion's share of Big Data collection now.

Inside our Schumann's Well, satellite tracking and torture are like shooting fish in a barrel. On September 10, 1994, the space shuttle *Discovery* pulsed

42 "How Smart Dust Could Spy On Your Brain."

43 See Chapter 11, "The 'Air Loom' Hospital."

44 Dongjin Seo et al., "Neural Dust: An Ultrasonic, Low Power Solution for Chronic Brain-Machine Interfaces," 8 July 2013, https://arxiv.org/pdf/1307.2196v1.pdf. Also see Neurogadget's article "Intelligent neural dust embedded in the brain could be the ultimate brain-computer interface," July 18, 2013 about the paper.

its $25 million green laser at 10 Hz per second over Manitoba, Wisconsin, Michigan, and the U.S. Northeast, out over the Atlantic Ocean near Maryland, then down toward the Caribbean and over eastern Brazil and the South Atlantic. On September 16 and 17, two Lockheed Electras followed *Discovery*'s path but at a different altitude, firing three lasers pulsing at 10 Hz through quartz windows. As with the Soviet LIDA machine developed in the 1950s, *alpha* waves (7–13 Hz) first pulse brains with tranquility and suggestibility in sync with the planet's Schumann resonance (7.83 Hz), after which the magnetic H wave is used to get inside the brains and influence thoughts. The *Discovery* / Electra operation appeared to be a Tesla magnifying transmitter experiment like those of the Soviet "Woodpecker," given that the *Discovery* laser broadcast of a subliminal message to a broad population swath below was running synchronous with a broadcast from Alaska HAARP's phased array antenna.

With satellite imagery and 3D generation of the target's terrain modeled on a RFMP computer monitor, a barium-rich chemical blast can be ordered up to "duct" over the target area so that the brain, heart, or genitals absorb maximum EM radiation, thanks to the presence outside and inside the body of a "swarm" of conductive metal nanoparticles delivered by aerosols. This can also be used for the same kind of flash fire combustion that nano- or super-thermite metastable intermolecular composites (MICs) produce in *vaporific effect weapons.*[45]

Dreams can be engineered via satellite EEG processing. As John Hall, MD, described in his 2009 book *A New Breed: Satellite Terrorism in America* (mentioned earlier):

> The satellite system creates a channel [i.e. wave guide or duct] through the atmosphere through which its payload of goodies gets delivered to Earth . . . The channel is created by two parallel opposed lasers generated from the satellite itself that burn through the atmosphere, leaving a clear channel between them.[46]

Because the target's brain signature (*evoked potential*) is the tracking unit, satellite surveillance is impossible to escape.

> . . . Full spectrum RADAR sends a broadband *ping* across all frequencies, like a flash of white light from a camera, and records all the returns across the area. Each person has a unique set of frequencies that they will absorb from or return to the sensor arrays; this identifies everyone. Based on autocorrelation techniques, one can determine the optical route and

45 "The Chemtrails Vaporific Effect.wmv" (December 27, 2011), https://www.youtube.com/watch?time_continue=96&v=qRo8FKY989I.

46 John Hall, MD.

> frequencies to be emitted by the phased arrays of antennas to optimally modulate the brainwaves of the target.[47]

Take, for example, broadcasting voice-to-skull (V2K) transmissions via satellite, which only needs the Internet of Things (IoT) surrounding the target to carry and amplify the sound. Laser-guided, the broadcast can arrive through a fan or even running water, after which it is converted to voice frequency by the brain.

In her essay "The Air Force Wants Your LOV [Locus of Values]: Aerial Seeding of Biological Implants into Food, Water, & Air" (February 29, 2008), the insightful targeted individual Carolyn Williams Palit discusses in detail the section "Hit 'Em Where It Hurts: Strategic Attack in 2025" In the 1995-1998 futures study *Air Force 2025*. To shift society's Locus of Values (LOV), the U.S. Air Force recommends spraying populations with "stealthy" track-and-attack bioengineered sensors thinner than a human hair so that thoughts, emotions, and intentions can be accessed and controlled.

> Ground-based platforms in 2025 rely heavily on micromechanics [smart dust, MEMS, GEMS, NEMS, etc.] and nanotechnology to shrink platforms to microscopic sizes . . . inserted via human agents, through water or food supplies, or through aerial seeding operations using UAVs . . . A swarm of ground-based microsensors could ensure constant data transmission . . .[48]

As was referenced in "What Chemtrails Really Are," Palit discusses how the ionized (Project Cloverleaf) atmosphere includes omnipresent invisible plasma antennas and mirrors (optical lenses[49]) that help to entrain ("string") gas plasma orbs on microwave beams for mind control and effects on various parts of the body, e.g. frequencies to pump up muscles, paralyze a limb, etc. After frequency mapping and tracking, gas plasma orbs can be stuck to eyes, ears, temples, or genitals by means of magnetic polarity.

> A beam with entrained orbs carries pictures in each orb just like the different frames in a movie; it is a particle beam that is also a frequency weapon.[50]

---

47 Robert Duncan, PhD.

48 Carolyn Williams Palit, "The Air Force Wants Your LOV: Aerial Seeding of Biological Implants into Food, Water, & Air." Air Force 2025, "Hit 'Em Where It Hurts: Strategic Attack in 2025," 1996.

49 Vertical columnar focal lenses and horizontal drift plasma antennas depend upon the electromagnetic heating of metal jet and rocket chemical trails.

50 Carolyn Williams Palit, "What Chemtrails Really Are," November 9, 2007.

The entrained orbs are identical to the "threading" witnessed at the so-called Skinwalker Ranch, discussed in Chapter 4, "Magnetism."

> The drones of the Uintah Basin have been known to "thread" images upon individuals in close proximity. Basically, "threading" is a process of weaving certain images into the mind of a victim. Threading is much like projecting a holographic image but actually within the brain . . .[51]

Could "optical tweezers" be used for threading holographic images?

> Atmospheric science requires robust methods for probing and manipulating single aerosol particles. We examine the utility of emerging techniques using optical tweezers in this area by demonstrating the use of holographic optical tweezers generated using a phase only liquid crystal spatial light modulator for the three dimensional trapping and manipulation of arrays of airborne particles. We show that single and multiple aerosol droplets, of the order of 10 microns in diameter, can be stably trapped and controllably fused using optical techniques.[52]

Threads is also the term employed by Elon Musk to describe Neuralink "neural mesh":

> . . . flexible 'threads' (about one-tenth the size of a human hair) directly into your brain, which, in turn, will be the first step to turning us into a hybrid of man and machine—as these threads will allow you to control your smartphone with just your thoughts . . . 'It's like a tiny straw of information flow between your biological self and your digital self,' Musk added about Neuralink. 'We need to make that tiny straw like a giant river, a huge, high-bandwidth interface.'"[53]

Musk asserts that these "flexible threads" must be surgically implanted. Is the term *implanted* undergoing redefinition? Could it also now include aerial delivery of frequency via magnetic lines of force and plasma "threads"? Will this approach apply to GBH (graphene-based hydrogel) gene therapy implantation that includes experimental disease strains awaiting aerial frequency activation?

---

51 Ryan Patrick Burns, Skinwalker & Beyond. Lulu, 2011.

52 D.R. Burnham and D. Gloin, "Holographic optical manipulation of aerosols," European Conference on Lasers and Electro-Optics. OSA Publishing, 17 June 2007.

53 Harmon Leon, "Mind-Reading Tech Is Dangerously Close to Becoming a Reality." Observer, September 9, 2019.

BCI Implantations

Human behavior is data and AI is a data model.

– Chris Hurst, chief operating officer of Stabilitas at the Intelligence Summit

MEMS and sensor functions in smartphones include CMOS image sensor, gyroscopes, accelerometers, magnetic field sensors (digital compass), autofocus actuators, pressure sensors (barometric sensors), micro mirrors, silicon microphones, oscillators and timing circuits, and RF MEMS—including FBAR, SAW, varactors, etc.

– SEMICO Research & Consulting Group, May 17, 2011

I'm very close to the cutting edge in AI and it scares the hell out of me. I tried to convince people to slow down AI, to regulate AI. That was futile. The merge scenario seems the best. If you can't beat it, join it. That's like the purpose of Neuralink: to create a high bandwidth interface to the brain such that we can be symbiotic with AI.

– Elon Musk, when announcing Neuralink, 2019[54]

From 1-centimeter microchip implants made of silicon to "Rambo chips" that increase adrenalin and hardened gallium arsenide IMI biotics the size of a grain of rice, brain chips have now become nanosized mesogenic biosensors to be inhaled, ingested, and implanted intravenously.[55]

Ever since the FDA approved the injectable VeriChip RFID for human biometrics in 2004, WiFi has been essential for tracking implants, bar codes (the same UPC number on every item), and radio frequency ID (RFID) chips (unique IDs for every item or person). Corporate employees are now tagged like pets or cattle, tethered to their computers via wireless sensors continuously measuring their heart rate, galvanic skin response, EMG, brain signals, respiration, temperature, movement, facial expression and blood pressure—even the strength of their orgasms at home. Smart subcutaneous mobile telephones, electronic organizers, and chips unlock their houses, start their cars, get cash from ATMs, and provide minute-by-minute NASDAQ stock updates, all in the name of the paved fiber optic road to hell known as technocracy.

---

54 Greg Reese, "Neuralink: The War Against Humanity Goes Mainstream" (3:45), July 21, 2019.

55 Hildegarde Staninger, RIET-1, "Global Brain Chip and Mesogens: Nano Machines for Ultimate Control of False Memories." Integrative Health Systems, January 8, 2012.

By 2013, a chip was created with so much electron density (11,011) in a tiny amount of space (2x2mm) that it could operate as a "voltage microscope for neurons" so one could "watch the real time propagation of an electrical spike down an axon."[56]

When we read about "chips," we probably think computer and not necessarily the brain, but the language used—"When they trained it on an individual cell" ... "Glial cells were part of the culture preparation" ... "The ability to 'watch' neurons electrically on multiple scales" ... "these optical reporters sometimes interfere with the natural cell physiology" ... "the chip could actually resolve changes in the shape and position of the axons over time"—points to the strong possibility of *in vivo* operations, not lab *in vitro*. With the right transmission and waiting nanosensors, a 60GHz RFID transponder chip 22 microns thick (one-fifth the thickness of a human hair), composed of titanium, gold film, aluminum, and hafnium dioxide encapsulated in silicon dioxide, could provide "continuous, real-time monitoring of activities at cellular levels" as a "magnetic resonance-coupled RFID transceiver for wireless sensors in cells."[57]

Then there are the "therapeutic" *electroceuticals:*

> Electroceuticals are a new category of therapeutic agents which act by targeting the neural circuits of organs. The therapy involves mapping the neural circuitry and delivering neural impulses to these specific targets. The impulse is administered via an implantable device . . .[58]

Elon Musk's Neuralink—the thousand-strand electrodes surgically inserted into the brain with an interface device behind the ear that will hook it all up with an iPhone app—is far too complex for general population implantation. Better by far for the masses are the nanobots, MEMS/NEMS sensors, microprocessors, and remotely programmable nano-pathogen swarms we're inhaling and ingesting, tethered to upgraded mobile iPads like the Neurogrid with its 16 Neurocore chips simulating one million neurons and billions of synapses. (The human brain has 80 billion neurons.)[59]

Place a 5nm chip in the optical nerve and neuroimpulses can be "eavesdropped" from the brain, after which the thoughts are transferred to a computer for storage until projected into another brain or back into the original

---

56 John Hewitt, "11,000-electrode reprogrammable chip takes brain-computer interfaces to a new level." ExtremeTech.com, July 22, 2013.

57 "Microscopic RFID chips to embed in human cells," NexusNewsfeed.com, August 30, 2017.

58 "Electroceuticals in medicine – The brave new future," Indian Heart Journal, 2017.

59 Tanya Lewis, "Human Brain Microchip Is 9,000 Times Faster Than a PC." LiveScience.com, May 2, 2014.

brain to be re-experienced as hallucinations, voices from past conversations, etc. Paul Baird was writing about this decades ago:

> Human thought operates at 5,000 bits/sec but satellites and various forms of biotelemetry can deliver those thoughts to supercomputers in Maryland, Israel, etc. which have a speed of 20 BILLION bits/sec each. These, even today, monitor millions of people simultaneously. Eventually, they will monitor almost everyone...worse than any Orwellian "Big Brother" nightmare you could possibly imagine, only it will be a reality. Yet our world leaders who know this do nothing.
>
> Usually, the targets are aware their brain waves are being monitored because of the accompanying neurophone feedback. In other words, the computer (echoes) your own thoughts and then the human monitors comment or respond verbally. Both are facilitated by the neurophone.
>
> Whilst the live/human comments are individualistic and unrelated to the victim's own thought processes, oftentimes the artificial intelligence involved will parrot standard phrases. These are triggered by your thoughts while the human monitors remain silent or absent.
>
> To comprehend how terrible such a thorough invasion of privacy can be, imagine being quizzed on your past as you lie in bed. You eventually fall off to sleep, having personal or "induced" dreams, only to wake to the monitor's commenting / ridiculing your subconscious thoughts (dreams).[60]

Implant experimentation / targeting began long ago with marginal populations—prisoners, soldiers, mental patients, handicapped and orphaned children, the disabled, homosexuals, single women, the elderly and poor—even to the point of driving transmitters into the frontal lobe to eliminate the ability to understand the consequences of one's actions. By the 1950s, the CIA's MK-Delta "Deep Sleep" was using intramuscular implants and remote electromagnetic broadcasts for radio-hypnotic intracerebral control and electronic dissolution of memory (*RHIC-EDOM*). By the dawn of the 21st century, *drug reservoir chips* were being implanted under the skin to be controlled and monitored remotely.[61]

The 5-micromillimeter intelligence-manned interface (IMI) "biotic" known during the Vietnam "conflict" as the "Rambo chip" was being slipped into the optic nerve to continuously translate the brain's neuroimpulses into crystal clear visual and auditory feed for 2-way satellite 20-billion-byte-per-

60 Paul Baird, http://www.surveillanceissues.com.

61 Christina Sarich, "Medical Drug-Pumping Microchip Plan to be Carried out by 2017." NaturalSociety.com, May 7, 2014.

second supercomputer loops, while land-based NSA SIGINT computer operators sent messages encoded as signals to the IMI.

Former chief medical officer of Finland Rauni-Leena Luukanen-Kilde, MD (1939-2015), described the early *remote monitoring system (RNM)* in use now, though the microchip could now be an inhaled or ingested remotely programmed nanobot:

> When a 5-micromillimeter microchip (the diameter of a strand of hair is 50 micromillimeters) is placed into the optical nerve of the eye, it draws neuroimpulses from the brain that embody the experiences, smells, sights, and voice of the implanted person. Once transferred and stored in a computer, these neuroimpulses can be projected back to the person's brain via the microchip to be re-experienced.[62]

Since the 1990s, cattle, dogs, tycoons, MILABs [military abductees], mental inpatients, welfare and Medicare recipients, astronauts, soldiers, and babies have been vaccinated with *molecular electronic devices (MEDs)*—organic microprocessors that make use of digital proteins and synthetic molecules to store information or act as switches via sodium or calcium ion signal flow. Once personal radio and electromagnetic frequency allocation (*PREMA*, or Prime Freak / freq) was up to speed, MEDs were relegated to batch identifications. (See below for more on PREMA.)

At the Center for Neural Engineering at the University of Southern California, Theodore W. Berger, professor of biomedical engineering and neurobiology, guided a team of neuroscientists and engineers to develop "specially designed microchips to be used as neural prostheses . . . culturing living neurons directly onto silicon-based computer chips" so a multi-chip module could be permanently implanted into the brain.[63] Hippocampal[64] neuron patterning has now merged computer chips with live neurons (funded by DARPA, the Office of Naval Research, and the National Science Foundation).

X-rays were sufficient for detecting silicon microchips, but for the nanochip or nanobot, the more sophisticated *spectrum analyzer (scanner)* is necessary. Sky-Eyes (Gen-Etics), a microprocessor made of synthetic and organic fibers that take their energy from the body while remaining invisible to both

---

62 Rauni-Leena Luukanen-Kilde, MD, "Microchip Implants, Mind Control, and Cybernetics," December 6, 2000.

63 "Theodore Berger: Professor of Biomedical Engineering and Neurobiology and Director of USC's Center for Neural Engineering School of Engineering." USC Asia Conference, October 17-19, 2002. The Institute for Creative Technologies is often also involved, particularly in mind control contexts.

64 The hippocampus at the base of the brain encodes life experiences so they can be stored as long-term memories elsewhere in the brain.

the naked eye and X-ray, and the Hitachi super-micro wireless automatic recognition mu-chips (0.4mm) are as fine as smart dust and therefore need scanners for detection. Millimeter / nano implants can be read anywhere there are microwave cell towers.

Billions of people are now breathing in trillions of nano-sensors and nanobots programmed to breach the blood-brain barrier and receive remote instructions from 20-billion-bit / second supercomputers via low-frequency radio waves tethered to and tracked by satellites collecting and transmitting data.[65] *MEMS (microelectromechanical system)*—tiny sensors with a condenser, microchip, seismic microphone, mixer, oscillator, band pass filter, and antenna transceiver—are the spy implants we breathe in:

> A silent communications system in which nonaural carriers, in the very low or very high audio frequency range or in the adjacent ultrasonic frequency spectrum, are amplitude or frequency modulated with the desired intelligence and propagated acoustically or vibrationally for inducement into the brain, typically through the use of loudspeakers, earphones or piezoelectric transducers. The modulated carriers may be transmitted directly in real time or may be conveniently recorded and stored on mechanical, magnetic or optical media for delayed or repeated transmission to the listener.[66]

The silent communication system is either *in reception (SCSR)* or *in transmission (SCST).* SCSR begins when our thoughts produce vibrations in our vocal cords as if we were speaking. The seismic microphone in MEMS intercepts the vibrations and converts them into a radio signal modulated by the same single sideband-suppressed carrier (SSB-SC) technology used to guide long-range missiles and weapons. A mixer then encrypts the signal, adding or removing frequencies from the original signal and converting it to ultrasound or infrasound so the message can't be heard if intercepted. After encryption, the signal passes through a band pass filter, then through an antenna transceiver to be sent to a fixed or mobile antenna receiver (per latitude and longitude) at about 1882-1883 Hz so as to reproduce your mental voice. For SCST, MEMS antennas pick up the "voice of God" signal (V2K) that can only be heard by you alone, then the mixer encrypts the signal to be transmitted by an antenna (24Hz) to your MEMS.

MEMS can be used to *internally* EMP you, like electroconvulsive therapy

65 Sensor nodes (motes) like MEMS gather sensory information and communicate with other nodes in the network. Smart dust is the system, MEMS are the sensors and nanobots that detect.

66 Patent # US5159703A invented by Oliver M. Lowery, 1989.

(ECT)—strong signals with a high voltage charge via radio waves. MEMS can also be used to impact your memory via very low frequency (VLF) fields.[67]

Whereas the 2G / 3G / 4G cellphone network monitors only one or a few people, 5G will monitor 1,000 at a time[68] by using the IoT.[69] The 5G / IoT weapon system obviously makes extensive use of MEMS and all other nano-implants inhaled, ingested, or inoculated, including GEMS (global environmental MEMS sensors) and NEMS (nanoelectromechanical systems) descending from chemical trails and ascending in hurricanes to be sown like seed into the land, trees, highways, waterways, sidewalks, building walls, dust in your homes, etc., all the while feeding data to weather and defense monitoring stations. When it comes to integrating chemical, biological, and physical sensors, NEMS are state of the art smart dust.

Under the FCC, the National Telecommunications & Information Administration (NTIA) assigns and oversees bands of frequency for wireless transmissions. It is closely tied to the NSA and involved with implants. For example, when a targeted individual who had implants removed from her body asked industrial toxicologist and Doctor of Integrative Medicine Hildegarde Staninger, RIET1, of Integrative Health Systems LLC, where the radio waves were coming from and who had been sending them, Dr. Staninger indicated that she would need "release data" from the NTIA in order to answer such questions.[70] Rumor has it that the NTIA also has something to do with the varying Schumann resonance.

The Brainprint

In the near future, it may be possible to take mathematical 'pictures' of our memories via brain prints and interchange them with other humans and [even] machines.

– John Norseen, creator of BioFusion[71]

67 Thanks to the Facebook site "Target individuals of gang stalking and mind control around the world" listed under FrancescaThe1, February 17, 2013. As with TI Carolyn Williams Palit, it has been impossible to contact FrancescaThe1.

68 R.W. Jones and K. Katzis, "5G and wireless body area networks." 2018 IEEE Wireless Communications and Networking Conference Workshops (WCNCW), Barcelona, 2018.

69 S. Chatterjee et al., "Internet of Things and Body area network – an integrated future." 2017 IEEE 8th Annual Ubiquitous Computing, electronics and Mobile Communication Conference (UEMCON), New York, 2017.

70 See Dr. Staninger's book Global Brain Chip and Mesogens: Nano Machines for Ultimate Control of False Memories, Xulon Press, 2016.

71 Dave Zuchowski. "Lecture on brain mapping scheduled for Wednesday." Post-Gazette.com, November 12, 2000.

John Norseen, a former U.S. Navy pilot become neuroengineer at Lockheed Martin's Intelligent Systems Division in Marietta, Georgia, has invented BioFusion, a BCI / BMI incarnation that needs a *brainprint*[72] in order to convert thoughts into computer commands—or, as Norseen preferred to think of it 20 years ago, to release neurotransmitters in the brain "to fight off disease, enhance learning, or alter the mind's visual images" for "synthetic reality."[73] Discoveries like the BioFusion brainprint need thousands of carefully documented biofeedback field experiments in "enhanced learning"—namely, years of targeting nonconsensual citizens in a hypergame approach to mind torture and "synthetic realities."

> "If this research pans out," says Norseen, "you can begin to manipulate what someone is thinking even before they know it." But Norseen says he is "agnostic" on the moral ramification, that he's not a "mad" scientist—just a dedicated one. "The ethics don't concern me," he says, "but they should concern someone else."[74]

Craig Henriquez, co-director of Duke University's Center for Neuroengineering, shares Norseen's indifference: "We don't see the brain as being a mysterious organ. We see 1s and 0s popping out of the brain, and we're decoding it."[75] Such is the scientism favored by military-industrial-intelligence-controlled universities.

Before individuals can be targeted with various electrical brain stimulation (EBS) devices, the resonance frequency of each specific brain area (3-50 Hz) must first be decoded and then modulated. According to *Akwei v NSA* in 1998, only NSA SIGINT can modulate signals in this frequency band.[76]

EEG *primed frequency scanners* (*PREMA,* or Prime Freak / freq), were once as big as briefcases. Now, Harry Potter-like wands no bigger than pens are able to map biotelemetrically distributed primary frequencies. PREMA dials into the brain to determine its unique frequency, after which a *gyrotron resonance maser* on board the satellite talks to the brain. The body is first sur-

---

72 Robert Duncan, PhD: "Everyone has a unique body resonance signature, heartbeat signature, and brainwave print. No RFID chip or dipole antenna is needed anymore for biotelemetry." – The Matrix Deciphered: Psychic Warfare Top-Secret Mind Interfacing Technology (Higher Order Thinkers, 2006).

73 Douglas Pasternak, "John Norseen: Reading your mind and injecting smart thoughts." US News & World Report, January 3-10, 2000. Also see Blair C. Armstrong et al., "Brainprint: Assessing the uniqueness, collectability, and permanence of a novel method for ERP [event-related potential] biometrics," Neurocomputing, Vol. 166, 20 October 2015.

74 Ibid.

75 Zimmer, Carl. "Mind Over Machine." Popular Science, February 1, 2004.

76 See John St. Clair Akwei, https://www.bibliotecapleyades.net/scalar_tech/esp_scalartech12.htm; from an article that ran in Nexus magazine, April-May 1996.

rounded with an EM flux, after which a microwave communication field is beamed into the brain with the laser reading changes in the electrons. A CAT scan sorts out the frequencies with the PREMA scanner to determine this particular brain's Freak or frequency, the essential key to accessing the *mind* of the target. Signal processors of EEG brainwaves on laptop computers make 27 phonemes speak for the "little voice in our head" that does our thinking, after which NSA brain parasites know our thought before we ourselves even experience it, and run *their* thoughts through our brain.

Modulated microwaves open the blood-brain barrier [77] and enable remote brain tampering. Neuroscientist Allan Frey at General Electric's Advanced Electronics Center at Cornell University discovered this in 1961, along with the *microwave auditory effect* or *Frey Effect*, the singular discovery that gave birth to the high-tech *no-touch torture* known as voice-to-skull or V2K.

> **Frey Effect or "microwave hearing":** Microwave transmission of speech directly into the auditory cortex. No one other than the target can hear the transmission.

Billions of brainprints have paved the way to full spectrum dominance over the Human Domain even as trillions of nanosensors, microprocessors, and nanobots have been seeded in public spaces ("simple interaction with subjects") via open-air spraying and force-feeding of genetically modified seed- and pesticide-grown "food," laying the ground for BCI Transhumanism.

> . . . [Norseen:] "We are at the point where this [brainprint] database has been developed enough that we can use a single electrode or something like an airport security system where there is a dome above your head to get enough information that we can know [what] you're thinking. If you go to an automatic teller machine and the sensor system is in place, you could walk away and I would be able to access your personal identification code."[78]

Future probable cause will be determined not by the Constitution but by our brainprints, given that telling the truth shows up on the outside of the brain as low energy while telling a lie lights it up.

---

77 Focused ultrasound also opens the blood-brain barrier. What does this say about the accepted practice of taking ultrasound photos of the fetus in utero?

78 Sharon Berry. "Decoding Minds, Foiling Adversaries." Armed Forces Communications and Electronics Association (AFCEA). SIGNAL magazine, October 2001.

Part 2: Surviving the Smart City

The city of Gilgamesh [~2700 BCE] was Uruk-of-the-Walls. This was the most splendid of all the seven cities of Sumer, and Gilgamesh was its king. Uruk was a city of many-colored temples, of brick houses, marketplaces, and open groves of trees. Its towering walls protected it from all sorts of evil, from the armies of enemy kings, from floods, from wild beasts too, and unfriendly gods; but most of all they protected it from the monster Humbaba who lived on a nearby mountain and who constantly breathed fire and smoke and soot into the sky.

– Bernarda Bryson, *Gilgamesh: Man's First Story*, 2006

A smart city is an urban settlement with properly connected, smartly managed, and optimized resources. Every device that is a component of a smart city must function with others to handle the resources of that city's population. If the city is to be truly smart, these devices should communicate with each other and this is where the IoT (Internet of Things) comes in. The IoT is an ecosystem of physical objects that are interconnected and accessible through the internet. The IoT offers an exemplary template of a body of interactive devices that offer smart solutions to everyday problems and is regarded as the key to building smart cities.

– Savaram Ravindra, "The Transformation That Barcelona Had Undergone To Become A Smart City," *Barcinno*, July 5, 2018

8

The Architects Are Back, Building Their Ninevahs

. . . Pretty soon all the information in the world—every tiny scrap of knowledge that humans possess, every little thought we've ever had that's been considered worth preserving over thousands of years—all of it will be available digitally. Every road on earth has been mapped. Every building photographed. Everywhere we humans go, whatever we buy, whatever websites we look at, we leave a digital trail as clear as slug slime. And this data can be read, searched and analysed by computers and value extracted from it in ways we cannot even begin to conceive.

– Robert Harris, *The Fear Index*, 2011

The notion that the lower classes are biologically inferior to the upper classes . . . is meant to legitimate the structures of inequality in our society by putting a biological gloss on them . . . public money has bought not scientific 'progress' but the domination of intellectual enquiry by an entirely malevolent project, conceived fully outside of science . . .

– Richard Lewontin, *The Doctrine of DNA: Biology As Ideology*, 1992

THE SKY OVER ENERGY-INTENSIVE SMART Cities is generally milky white or pale blue with an aviation-induced "cloudiness," an *atmospheric whiteout* made up of vast numbers of circulating nanoparticles and low atmospheric pressure. This ion-induced nucleation is often obscured by terms like "aggregates," "coagulation," and "agglomeration." The chemical trails we can still see have Mylar polymers in them. Barium from one direction can't be seen, barium from another direction produces a foggy white to grey. Most trails are laid at night; you can see them with an infrared camera. What real clouds you see are generally made of plasma.

In the 1990s, it was announced that one day, far in the future, smart dust would be everywhere in Nature and Smart Cities. MIT "biological engineers" then created a programming language for bacteria based on Verilog (used to program computer chips) so DNA encoded circuits could "give new functions to living cells—a text-based language for a DNA sequence in a cell, just like you're programming a computer":

> To create a version of [Verilog] that would work for cells, the researchers designed computing elements such as [silicon circuits and] logic gates and sensors that can be encoded in a bacterial cell's DNA . . . One of the new circuits is the largest biological circuit ever built, containing seven logic gates and about 12,000 pairs of DNA.[1]

How could we have known that the smart dust and bacterial language were the advent of a Human 2.0 cyborg not in the vague future but now? We naively thought that the flurry of nanosensors everywhere were for adjusting Smart City microclimates.[2]

The CIA propaganda masters had been ramping up violence on television, in films, and headlines throughout the 1960s and 1970s. By the 1980s, the electromagnetic grid was going up even as the test-based socialist school system continued programming new generations raised on daycare and television. Those hardened by poverty and destruction of the family turned into extremists driven by trauma, powerlessness, and rage and often programmed MK-ULTRA-style by the CIA. The 1990s Revolution in Military Affairs erased the line between combatant and noncombatant.

Fast-forward to today and we have a priesthood of synthetic biologists, bioengineers, and cognitive scientists who view our human biology as an advanced computer whose neural network must be connected to and run by AI Clouds. Two lectures—the first "Vaccine DNA Mind Control Technology: Dr Charles Morgan, West Point, 2018," the second "The Brain Is the Battlefield of the Future – Dr. James Giordano" (October 29, 2018) at the Modern Warfare Institute—are essential listening in order to understand the fully developed Smart City technology we're up against.

The American Chemical Society's Fall 2020 Virtual Meeting & Expo openly presented details on communications systems derived from biological cells, interfacing hardware with human tissue, biological cells incorporated into the "computational decision-making process," ionized electrons in cells (Redox Mediating) generating current, etc. Bio-nanotechnology ("microelectronic materials") is here.[3] This is not about creating Human 2.0 from scratch like a golem or Frankenstein or BigDog robot; Human 1.0 is undergoing a reorganization of what's already there "to make it simpler to understand and easier to manipulate," says Christopher Voigt, MIT biological engineer.[4]

---

1 Anne Trafton, "A programming language for living cells." MIT News Office, March 31, 2016.

2 Geoff Manaugh, "Space-Based Storm Control." BlogBlog, April 17, 2009.

3 Matthew Griffin, "New research would allow cyborgs and human organs to join computer networks." FanaticalFuturist.com, October 8, 2020.

4 Lonnie Shekhtman, "Scientists identify minimum set of genes needed for life." CSMonitor.

This is why Smart City environments are designed to be giant chemical and electromagnetically charged petri dishes and beakers in which Human 1.0 blithely *cooks*, and why nanobots are spawned from natural-*cum*-synthetic (hybrid) algae, bacteria, and DNA. PhD synthetic biologists and nanoengineers are little more than clever copycats replacing what is natural and divinely authentic with gain-of-function scraps for an ersatz virtual world of automatons posing as life. In "The Promise and Perils of Synthetic Biology" (*The Economist,* April 6, 2019), Jonathan Tucker and Raymond Zilinskas wrote that synthetic microorganisms could proliferate out of control, cause massive environmental damage, and threaten public health.

Too little too late, we're already there.

The UN Smart City is divided into "cells" about ten miles square in the shape of a hexagon, like a beehive. Each cell has a base station; all cells have low-power transmitters (0.3W or 6W) whose carrier (Verizon, AT&T, etc.) has its own mobile telephone switching office (MTSO) in each city for tower control. Each cell phone is programmed with special codes, including the special identification code (SID) being transmitted to the nearest tower, along with the registration signal. This is how you are tracked.

En garde! Beware of people pointing iPhones at your head or body as a spectrum analyzer "app"[5] scans your individual frequencies for remote torture via Stingray triangulating your cell phone signal with satellite, cell phone towers, neighbors' antennas, or vehicles to assault your nervous system, emotions, sleep and dreams. Keep your eye on mobile "hot spot" WiFi vans and drones cruising Smart City canyons as well as concerts, festivals, and sports events.

Hordes of wireless and telecom industries and their multitudes of subcontractors and offshoot government programs are milking Smart Cities—a shell game of little oversight, if any. Corporations gobble each other up overnight, names change, the buck is passed. Telecoms own vast Internet backbone networks and pressure local zoning boards to approve legions of cell towers. For one example among many regarding the power of these corporations, AT&T birthed Lucent Technologies[6] in 1996, then merged with Alcatel SA of France in 2006, and George Soros' Nokia in 2016. Nokia (Finnish) was a developer with Sony (Japanese) and Philips Semiconductors (Dutch) of near field com-

---

com, March 27, 2016.

5 Another spy app: the Handy Truster (South Korea) picks up on the voice stress that accompanies lying or hiding something.

6 "Shortly after the Lucent renaming in 1996, Lucent's Plan 9 project released a development of their work as the Inferno OS in 1997. This extended the ‹Lucifer› and Dante references for the components of Inferno - Dis, Limbo, Charon and Styx (9P Protocol). When the rights to Inferno were sold in 2000, the company Vita Nuova Holdings was formed to represent them, continuing the Dante theme,,," - Wikipedia

munication (NFC) technology that transfers information between devices in close proximity: credit cards, smart phones, wearables, medical applications, etc. *NFC is required for 5G-enable networks and the Internet of Things*, plus cloud services, RFIDs, implants and no doubt nanobots. Nokia provides China Mobile with network equipment and services ($1.2 billion).

All over the Smart City, towers and tiny embedded antennas enfold meshed networks. Cell towers transmit illegal synthetic telepathy signals mind-to-mind at the human brain frequency of 450 MHz.[7] Alcatel-Lucent 1.5-watt light Radio cubes stacked like Legos, with multigenerational antennas (2G-4G) over a 2-block radius, complement the big microwave towers, while the Artemis pCell LTE operates as a centralized-radio access network (C-RAN) to exploit the cell signal interference forcing high-powered signals onto individual devices, like the camouflaged pWave mini daisy chain cables delivering high-density 5G. WiGig provides higher speeds by using the unlicensed 60 Hz band in your home and office as WiFi HaLow provides long-range connectivity for battery-operated IoT 900 MHz low power consumption, ideal for sensors and receivers.

To wirelessly transmit power over long distances via microwave energy requires a power source, a transmitting beam-forming antenna, multiple transmitting relays acting like lenses, and a rectenna to convert the microwave beam into electricity by means of nanotechnology ("metamaterials").[8] *Rectennas* convert alternating current (AC) electromagnetic waves into direct current (DC) electricity by means of silicon or gallium arsenide rectifiers. In the Smart City, the exteriors of buildings and interior walls are coated with a flexible 3-atoms-thick Molybdenum disulfide (MoS2) rectifier acting as a semiconductor for energy harvesting and conversion of RF waste energy—up to 10 GHz of wireless signals—to DC electricity. MoS2 can be chemically made into a switch to force a phase transition from semiconductor to the metallic material of a 2-D semiconducting metallic phase junction (probably graphene) to make it fast enough to power IoT WiFi, Bluetooth, cellular LTE, wearable electronics, implanted medical devices and their communications, and sensors. Researcher Jesús Grajal at the Technical University of Madrid describes the medical use of rectifiers: "Ideally, you don't want to use batteries to power these systems because if they leak lithium, the patient could die. It is much better to harvest energy from the environment to power up *these small labs inside the body* and communicate data to external computers."[9]

---

7 Why ham radio operators have been forbidden to transmit 400-700 MHz.

8 Jason Dorrier, "New Zealand is about to test long-range wireless power transmission." Singularity Hub, August 30, 2020.

9 Rob Matheson, "Converting Wi-Fi signals to electricity with new 2-D materials." MIT

And the Smart City pulse goes on . . .

Meanwhile for "public safety," Homeland Security's S-Comm (Security Communities) biometric ID program under PEP (Priority Enforcement Program) is in full swing, from the FBI Crypto Unit's access to Nextel software that turns cell phone microphones into roving bug transmitters to CALEA's DCSNet (updated Carnivore) point-and-click (like remotely installed spyware).[10] In 2010, San Diego-based Cubic Corporation (massive transportation and automated fare smart cards) acquired Abraxas,[11] a Virginia corporation founded by former CIA director Richard Helms, and Anonymizer, "providing identity masking while making communique and clandestine transactions over the Web." This is TrapWire, the "security" software that implemented driftnet surveillance ("'real-time' awareness") now merged with cybersecurity Big Data (tapped phones, emails, blogs, cookies, Skype, Facebook, Google, YouTube, Twitter, television, etc.).

Uurban dwellers sleeping on metal coil-spring mattresses provide the antennas to amplify broadcast FM / TV signals (87-108 MHz). Background radiation is overlaid with unique brainwave signatures to entrain people while they sleep and assault the sixth and seventh chakras connected to the pineal and pituitary glands buried deep in the brain. Meanwhile, DNA's fractal antenna picks up frequencies and overlays our natural non-linear sinusoidal waveforms with linear, synthetic, rectangular pulsed (modulated) emissions.[12]

The events of September 11, 2001 marked not just the point of no return but the globalist announcement loud and clear of the return of the feudal Smart City. Cities would no longer be utterly destroyed by war and nuclear bombs but remodeled (or crippled) with precision directed energy weapons. An endless war on terrorism was introduced so as to justify anything done to soldiers and civilians alike. The Janus face of the Department of Homeland Security (DHS) was added to the registry of Deep State criminals.[13] Cities' only defense from here on out is either to remove scalar transmitters or deploy a Tesla dome. In the United States, the fingers on the buttons that con-

---

News, January 28, 2019.

10 The Commission on Accreditation for Law Enforcement Agencies (CALEA), created in 1979, has paved the way for the present "public safety" cover. DCSNet collects, sifts, and stores all data, its endpoints connecting to more than 350 switches. Review Chapter 10, "The Covert Ascendency of Technocracy," in Under An Ionized Sky.

11 Abraxas: an Æon dwelling with Sophia and other Æons of the Pleroma. See Wikipedia for references from Carl Jung and Hermann Hesse.

12 Thanks to Benjamin Nowland, "The Microwave Drug: The Biological and Spiritual Effects of Electromagnetic Radiation." Wakeup-world.com, 11 April 2016.

13 The line between DHS and USCYBERCOM was erased in 2010 via the Memorandum of Agreement that specified that DHS, DoD, NSA, and USCYBERCOM "maintain cognizance" and engage in "joint operational planning and mission coordination."

trol scalar weapons are unfortunately those of bent military contractors like Raytheon and Lockheed Martin in partnership with the nuclear industry.

Though the United Nations (UN) has existed since 1945, it is only since the HAARP ionospheric "research" and advent of consistent global geoengineering (not just weather operations) that environmental conditions have been optimal for the long-anticipated global elite power play via its UN instrument.

1992	178 nations adopted Agenda 21 at the Earth Summit, Rio de Janeiro, Brazil
2000	8 Millennium Development Goals (MDGs)
2002	Johannesburg Declaration of Sustainable Development
2012	Rio+20 "The Future We Want"
2013	UN General Assembly 30-member Open Working Group
2015	2030 Agenda for Sustainable Development / Paris Agreement on Climate Change

The "global warming" data from the 2015 Paris Conference was seriously manipulated. Climate models had been made to fit incorrect data, such as deliberately exaggerated temperatures, seemingly to serve

> an agenda to eliminate effectively the advancement of society and attempt to reset the clock to the pre-Industrial Revolution. The entire theory that before the Industrial Revolution, our planet's atmosphere was somehow pristine and uncontaminated by human-made pollutants has been also proven to be completely bogus.[14]

Most damning was the excellent study on CO2 by physicist Nasif Nahle, PhD, of the University of Nuevo Leon in Mexico. While the John Cook blog *SkepticalScience* maintains that CO2 molecules function as a blanket for slow heat loss, the actual time-lapse involved proves otherwise.

> Nahle found the "mean free path" for a quantum wave to pass through the atmosphere before colliding with a CO2 Molecule is about 33 meters. Such a wide chasm between molecular collisions would appear to undermine a visualization of CO2 functioning like a blanket does. Even more saliently, Nahle determined that the rate at which CO2 molecules can retain heat at the surface may only last about 0.0001 of a second. If heat-loss is slowed down at a rate of 0.0001 of a second by CO2 mol-

14 Martin Armstrong, "Independent Audit Exposes the Fraud in Global Warming Data." Armstrong Economics, October 12, 2018.

ecules, the atmospheric CO2 concentration—whether it's 300 PPM or 400 PPM—effectively doesn't matter. The time-lapse differential would be immaterial for either concentration.[15]

As with the Ministry of Truth in Orwell's *1984*, new definitions and memes are being spun. The "contrail" that once referred to a jet's exhaust of freezing water vapor condensing around dust and pollution particulates now includes the long-lasting chemical trails that spread out into "contrail clouds" made up of plasma condensate stripped of moisture by aluminum nanoparticles and electromagnetics, and the term *geoengineering* manipulated to go beyond stratospheric aerosol injection to "large-scale intentional interventions in the Earth's systems to tackle climate change" and removal of "enough CO2 to achieve net zero emissions."[16] "Nature-based solutions" like large-scale afforestation and reforestation [with GMO trees]" or "new carbon dioxide removal technologies, such as direct air capture,"[17] need not apply.

Rosa Koire, author of *Behind the Green Mask: U.N. Agenda 21* (2011), recently died of a fast-acting cancer. Like Rachel Carson of another generation, Koire kept us apprised of the comprehensive global Agenda 21[18] "full regionalization leading to full globalization" and a 2030 Agenda for Sustainable Development *technocracy.*[19] Koire pointed out that whereas Marxist socialism / communism follows a revolutionary model, Fabian socialism follows a slow-boiling frog model (skewered on the two prongs of "extreme weather" and war on terrorism?). *Rights* become *privileges* under a UN social credits system,[20] and "change" and "transformation" are actually inventory, standardization, restriction, and central control as regionalization expands into globalization. The green mask of conservation, recycling, and restricted energy hides a collectivist / socialist land use plan that begins with community action plans (CAPs) that redefine the individualist as "selfish," while the disparaging term "climate change denier" cleverly echoes "holocaust denier." Unique cultures and individuals are scuttled in favor of "save the Earth." Western civilization,

---

15 Kenneth Richard, "Physicist: CO2 Retains Heat For Only 0.0001 Seconds, Warming 'Not Possible.'" Climate Change Dispatch, October 18, 2019.

16 The Carnegie Climate Geoengineering Governance Initiative (C2G2).

17 Janos Pasztor, "What's in a name? Why we became C2G." Carnegie Council for Ethics in International Affairs, 10 June 2019.

18 See the 300-page UN book Agenda 21: Earth Summit: The United Nations Programme of Action From Rio, 1993.

19 Patrick Wood, "Technocracy: The Real Reason Why The UN Wants Control Over The Internet." Technocracy News, June 12, 2019. Wood is the author of Technocracy Rising: The Trojan Horse of Global Transformation (Coherent Publishing, 2014).

20 Pinyin is a Chinese national system of standardizing assessment of citizens and businesses as per their economic and social reputation, i.e. social credits.

imperfect and immature as it may be, is being erased as a "white man" illness.

Under the UN's ICLEI (International Council for Local Environmental Initiatives),[21] sustainable development goals (SDGs)[22] impact water, energy, climate, oceans, urbanization, transport, science and technology, poverty, social justice, etc. The Smart City is the SDG showcase—old wine of the old corporatocracy / technocracy going back to the god-like Gilgamesh and his walled city-state of Uruk in a new, Dubai-like wineskin.

Google and Bilderberg merge as Google Zeitgeist, and TED conferences pacify smart liberal minds to fit the collectivist, networked vision of the future. Those who refuse to be "enhanced" (Transhumanism / Singularity) will either be shunned as sub-human or forced in one way or another to comply. The smart grid "global village" lockdown is growing more obvious with the dump-and-pump aerosol Space Fence above and a wireless technocracy below.

The techno-feudal city-states are back.

Dubai, United Arab Emirates (UAE) (3.1 million) – block chain architecture

Neom (*neo* meaning new, *mostaqbal* meaning future), Saudi Arabia: mega-city (10 million +) – city-state under construction; IoT / AI investment free-trade zone connected to Med-Red Rail (Mediterranean to Red Sea)

Masdar City, Abu Dhabi, UAE – under construction since 2006

Songdo International Business District (IBD), aka Ubiquitous-City or U-City (100,000+) – under construction

i-japan, Japan: redesign of four cities to be followed by others: Yokohama City, Toyota City, Keihanna City, Kitakyushu City

Smart Nation Singapore – island city-state approach, southern Malaysia (5.6 million)

MSC (multimedia super corridor) Malaysia – special economic zone (32.7 million)

Smart Taipei, Taiwan – island city-state approach, Republic of China (23.78 million)

---

21 From ICLEI's international website: "ICLEI – the global cities network. We are a powerful movement of 12 mega-cities, 100 super-cities & urban regions, 450 large cities, 450 small & medium-sized cities & towns in 84 countries dedicated to sustainable development."

22 http://sustainabledevelopment.un.org/sdgs

Quayside "Internet City," Toronto (2.81 million) – built by Alphabet's Sidewalk Labs and Google Canada

Barcelona, Spain (5.2 million), since 2012

Stockholm, Sweden (965,000)

Tallinn, Estonia – (426,500) digital cyberstate governance for e-residents of e-nations for "world citizens who've thrown off the shackles of nations"; ID chip "e-ID" including encryption, voting, contracts, internet; e-cryptocurrency; DNA biobank; social engineered digital copy of every citizen; Rail Baltica underground tunnel; NATO Cooperative Cyber Defense

Belmont, Arizona, USA – purchased by Bill Gates[23] for $80 million; 25,000 acres for 80,000 residential units, 3,800 acres for offices, commercial, and retail, 470 acres for public schools.

CIA "ghost city" CITE (Center for Innovation Testing and Evaluation), between Deming and Las Cruces, New Mexico, USA, 30 miles north of the US-Mexico border.

Smart City Developers

Alibaba – Chinese; headquarters in model Smart City Hangzhou; "Sesame" social credit system (including "cyber sovereignty"), UBI (universal basic income); One Belt One Road initiative, including a Digital Silk Road

Alphabet (American) Google parent holding company

Baidu (Chinese) internet and AI

Bilderberg - View Truthstream Media, "Bilderberg and the Digital New World Order," June 15, 2018

Cisco (American) unified IoT platforms (horizontal data aggregation, multi-cloud, multi-party, multi-location "IoT data fabric")

MIT Media Lab (American) R&D

Nvidia Metropolis (American) invented GPUs (graphics processing units) edge-to-cloud video platform for interactive graphics; AI

23 Bianca Buono, KPNX, "Bill Gates buys big chunk of land in Arizona to build 'smart city.'" 12News.com, November 13, 2017.

Outside the Smart City, giant factory farms grow GMO "food" for GMO people become hybrids. More than half of humanity live in cities. In 2005, there were one billion slum-dwellers; by 2030, there will be two billion. No longer does the city mean job opportunities, as Karl Marx (1818-1883) and Max Weber (1864-1920) envisioned, nor does the size of a city's economy bear much relation to its population size; cheap labor pools is what the developing world is for. As slums fill with the homeless and under- and unemployed, urbanization without industrialization looks to wirelessly run the Smart City (as Alison McDowell points out in her Fourth Industrial Revolution talks).[24] Smart City canyons under overarching plasma domes reverberate with the crossfire of radio waves from car radios, TVs, computers, cell phones and towers, hotspots, offices and apartments. Day and night, the targeting industry rakes in the profits of Big Data as the behavior of AI computers and Human 2.0 merge. Fossil fuels, propane, and natural gas are eliminated, all becomes IoT and IoB electric, from the air to our bodies.

One way or another, everyone is plugged into the Cloud-based grid. Minds are entrained by satellites, towers, nanosensors and bots; electrosmog is everlasting as GIS / GPS (geographic information systems / global positioning) technology oversees the geoslavery being maintained by N^3 "precision medicine,"[25] Across town, far from the madding crowd of planned slums, is the AI-run milieu of the rich and educated enjoying the Smart City's best without having to smell or see its worst. (The sow's ear and silk purse come to mind.)

These are the "resilient cities."

> . . . the IMF and the World Bank's Structural Adjustment Programmes, to put it bluntly but accurately, drove the creation of modern slums. The recipe for the creation of slums has been rapid urban growth in the context of structural adjustment, currency devaluations, state retrenchments, and little or no housing provision. Viewing the state as a "market enabler" led to the privatization of utilities and services, and massive decreases in provision; ideas of the magic power of people's capitalism providing land titles simply accelerated social differentiation in the slums, and did nothing to aid renters, the actual majority of the poor in many cities. For individuals, their various needs—affordable commodities, accommodation close to jobs, security, and the possibility of owning property—

24 "'Smart Cities,' the Transhumanist Game and 'Lifelong Learning'," Alison McDowell, June 23, 2021, https://www.youtube.com/watch?v=Jf4QC1tFPCQ&t=3s.

25 N3: Next-generation Nonsurgical Neurotechnology, brain-computer interface (BCI) with sub-millimeter regions of the brain.

were simply ignored by the imposition of ill-suited neoliberal "boot-strap capitalism."[26]

Families are fleeing the Smart City, leaving city growth to young workaholic college graduates toiling to meet their debts in the new tech economy fed and plied with "good times" by the young trapped in the service industry. Just 25 metropolitan areas support more than half of the American economy, with five counties accounting for half the U.S. internet and web-portal jobs. *The Atlantic* calls the modern American city "an Epcot theme park for childless affluence, where the rich can act like kids without having to actually see any."[27]

And of course just below the veneer, the Smart Cities are armed to the teeth.

---

26 George Hoare, "Urbanisation without industrialization," a book review of Mike Davis' Planet of Slums (2005). Culturewars.org.uk, 29 April 2008.

27 Derek Thompson, "The Future of the City Is Childless." The Atlantic, July 18, 2019.

9

Dual Use I: A Smart City Is An Armed City

War As A Smart City Lab
The Department of Housing & Urban Development (HUD)
NetRad / NexRad & Psychotronics
Crowd Control
Radar / Doppler
FLIR (forward-looking infrared) radiometer
Unmanned aerial vehicles (UAVs) / drones / helicopters
The Magnetron
Taser
VMADS / ADS
VTRPE, Barium and Cloaking

But cell phones cause brain tumors. Electromagnetic radiation disrupts living tissues at the most basic level: the cell. Children (and the fetus) are at highest risk. Microwave technologies and electromagnetic energy are used by the military as integral components of weapons systems precisely because they are detrimental to life.

– Keith Harmon Snow, "NetRad in the Neighborhood: Illuminating the Cell Tower Agenda," 2004

"I'm not interested in legality, soldier," Dr. Pink says in a gravel voice. "It's the technology that's sending green balls down my pants leg."

"Me, too, ma'am," Dr. Black says. "He was still walking after you cut his spine in half?"

"Still running."

The three scientists kneel over the body. "Damn it, will you look at this."

"It's a graphene sheath," Dr. Pink says. "I saw it right off."

"They've learned how to encase nerves in graphene?"

"Might be worse than that," Dr. Black says.

"How's that? What could be worse than that they've worked out how to encase nerve fibers in graphene sheaths?"

"That they've worked out how to make the nerve fibers out of graphene rods," Dr. Pink says. "That they're about a decade ahead in nanotechnology."

"Oh," Black says. "Oh no. That is bad news, if it's true. That puts us way behind."

"Of course we're way behind," Pink says. "They get to do vivisection on humans. If they let us do that, we'd be ruling over America's second empire by now with the world at our feet. It would be 1945 all over again."

Lord Sakagorn frowned. "One day it will be a question for every jurisdiction: what do you do with transhumans? How does the law apply to them?"

– John Burdett, *The Bangkok Asset* (NY: Alfred A. Knopf, 2015)

Experimenting with what a Smart City would entail began with long-lasting war-torn occupations of developing nations abroad and the Department of Housing and Urban Development (HUD) slums at home, to which a NetRad / NexRad infrastructure was added. This is what this chapter covers.

Decades ago, Paul Baird outlined the "nonlethal" covert approach to control over urban populations:

- *Anti-personnel weapons* (sonic, phaser, psychotronic)
- *Scalar wave weapons* "ride" the scalar waves that naturally emanate from living organisms, including the Earth
- *Infrasound weapons* remotely induce illness
- *Neurophones* provide satellite and ground-based delivery of aural harassment via microwaves or lasers
- *Laser systems,* such as remote-sensing LiDAR (light detection and ranging), deliver blurred vision, holographs, and temporary blindness to disorient the target
- *Remote sensing brainwave monitors / analyzers* interpret the target's thoughts
- *Over-the-horizon (OTH) technologies* facilitate ground-based methods of harassment[1]

The general societal belief is that our behavior is internally generated by a process of conscious free will. The possibility that an unperceived external force might govern behavior and our brains without our knowledge is too far-fetched for most people to imagine.

> Dr. [Geraint] Rees [professor of cognitive neurology at University College London] is decoding the mind in terms of conscious and unconscious process. For that, one must have accessed consciousness itself. Whose conscious-

1 Paul Baird, *http://www.surveillanceissues.com*. Baird, B.Ec., LLb,, is a privacy and human rights campaigner from Australia with a background in Law and Economics. In 1990/91, he wrote the novel *In the Year 2252* critiquing elitist crime; it was widely distributed in draft form and covertly banned.

ness? Where is the owner of that consciousness—and unconsciousness? How did he/she feel? Why not ask them to tell us how it feels . . . The Neurobotics Exhibition [London Science Museum] was clearly set up to make these exciting new discoveries an occasion for family fun, and there were lots of games for visitors to play. One gets the distinct impression that we are being softened up for the introduction of a radical new technology which will, perhaps, make the mind a communal pool rather than an individual possession.[2]

Will societal laws be changed to reflect this latest form of "soul catcher"[3] mind rape, or will it be tacitly ignored until the brain-computer interface (BCI) hive mind is everywhere?

Between 1970 and 1975, suicides quintupled in Medford and doubled in surrounding Jackson County. When a University of North Carolina team of scientists discovered that a nearby military base had been involving in experimenting with secret bombardment of ultra-low frequency (ULF) waves, they were threatened with death should they talk. In 1976, the Pacific Northwest Center for the Study of Non-Ionizing Radiation in Portland, Oregon published "Radio-frequency Induced Interference Responses in the Human Nervous System," which stated, "Biological interference responses in the human nervous system can be elicited not only by pulse-modulated but by continuous wave radio frequency at power densities substantially below those levels that exist in a typical urban environment."[4] In 1980, poor districts in Pittsburgh were bombarded. Some people heard internal radio messages telling them to get tattoos or kill themselves by jumping in front of a train.

Ever since MK-ULTRA, experiments in remote EM brain and mind control had been front and center at Stanford Research Institute (SRI) founded by the UK's Tavistock Institute and later renamed SRI International. SRI was MK-ULTRA Central, the biggest military think tank in the country working with multiple civilian consulting firms to apply military technology to domestic situations for data on "human augmentation," now called "enhancement."

In 1980 with SRI funding, Schriever McKee Associates of McLean, Virginia—under retired General Bernard A. Schriever, former chief of Air

---

2 Carole Smith, "Intrusive Brain Reading Surveillance Technology: Hacking the Mind." Dissent magazine, Summer 2007; reprinted in Global Research, December 13, 2008.

3 Soul Catcher was a £25 million British Telecom research program in the 1990s seeking to record and store all electrical pulses from all of our senses onto a chip implanted behind the eye, the hope being that by 2025 all of a person's memories could be transferred to another body—an immortality or reincarnation of sorts, and the end of death.

4 Eugene, Oregon was the primary target of the Soviet Woodpecker signal, perhaps because the 800-mile Bonneville Power Authority transmission line ends there (DC / 340,000 volts). See Mike Thoele, "Mystery Radio Signals May Cause Illness," Eugene Register-Guard, March 26 and 27, 1978.

Force Systems Command that had developed the Titan, Thor, Atlas, and Minuteman—put together a consortium of Lockheed, Emmerson Electric, Northrup, Control Data, Raytheon, and TRW called Urban Systems Associates, Inc. to "solve" social urban problems with advanced military electronics, meaning behavior modification by means of targeting: anti-personnel (sonic, phasar, psychotronic); infrasound; neurophone via MASERs; lasers delivering blurred vision and holograms; remote-sensing brainwave monitors; over-the-horizon weapons via HAARP technology; etc. The slippery "nonlethal" slope successfully blurred the line between enforcement and torture.

Nonlethals are not covered under any international treaties.

> The Pentagon now considers bioweapons work that has been off limits for three decades to be acceptable—if the word "non-lethal" is appended. But not only do many "non-lethal" agents violate treaties themselves; it is worse. U.S. "non-lethal" research is creating and testing hardware that can deliver the full spectrum of biological and chemical weapons.[5]

Under Urban Systems, SRI "futures" contracted with the DoD Directorate of Defense Research and Engineering, Office of Aerospace Research ("Applications of the Behavioral Sciences to Research Management"), Executive Office of the President, Office of Science and Technology, U.S. Departments of Health, Education, Labor, and Transportation, the National Science Foundation ("Assessment of Future and International Problems"), Bechtel Corporation, Hewlett Packard, TRW, Bank of America, Shell Company, RCA, Blyth, Eastman Dillon, Saga Foods, McDonnell Douglas, Crown Zellerbach, Wells Fargo Bank, Kaiser Industries . . .

Nonconsensual subjects had been had long been gleaned from populations that a court of law would not believe or care about: orphanages, Native American reservations and boarding schools, tenements, prisons, hospitals, mental institutions, drug treatment programs, the homeless, and low-income clinics. World War Two and the Cold War added military and intelligence families, military contractors and their employees. Strategically placed doctors, psychiatrists, and hospital staff were paid off or pressured to sign nondisclosure agreements, all done *quietly*. Since then, military corporations like Lockheed Martin, DynCorp, and the Harvard Center for Risk Analysis (HCRA)[6] have used poor neighborhoods for CIA heroin and crack cocaine sales while "testing" nonlethal weapons amidst the forest of cell towers.

---

5 "US Army Patents Biological Weapons Delivery System, Violates Bioweapons Convention." The Sunshine Project, 8 May 2003.

6 HCRA replaced the Urban Systems consortium and was funded by AT&T, the Wireless Technology Research Foundation, and over 100 transnational corporations.

War As A Smart City Lab

Weaponization of cancer (1950s – 1970s)
Iran-Iraq War (1980-1988)
Gulf War / Operation Desert Shield / Operation Desert Storm (1990-1991)
Iraq War (2003-2011)
Bosnian War (1992-1995)
Afghanistan War / Operation Enduring Freedom (2001-2021)

It is interesting how prominently the Middle East has played into the experimentation leading to the design of Smart Cities, beginning with ancient cities like Jericho and all the way to the present-day wars / occupations in Israel, Iraq, and Afghanistan (and even the Bosnian War / occupation in Eastern Europe with its distinctly Middle Eastern overtones).

Even the Old Testament story of the fall of the city of Jericho (~1400 BCE) was about using frequency as a weapon. The Israelites marched around the city seven times, blowing their rams' horns, each time raising a great shout. After the seventh circuit, the walls of the city fell (Joshua 6:1-27). For six days before the final collapse, they had carried the Ark of the Covenant around the city once a day. The Ark appears to have been *radioactive.*[7] Made of acacia wood, it was covered inside and out with gold leaf, an excellent condenser. Unpurified salt or granite was also inside the Ark, while long wooden poles protected the carriers layered in heavy linen. Was the Ark a 4X4 portable shielded nuclear reactor? Were the "walls of Jericho" actually a protective Tesla dome? And as for the rams' horns, were they at all like frequency selective bolometers (FSBs) producing interferometric scalar / gravitational waves that make the booms, growls, and horn blasts people around the world hear?[8]

> We propose a concept for radiometry in the millimeter, submillimeter, and the far-IR spectral regions, the frequency selective bolometer (FSB). This system uses a bolometer as a coupled element of a tuned quasi-optical interference filter in which the absorption, the transmission, and the reflection characteristics of the filter depend on the frequency in a controlled

7 See Graham Hancock, The Sign and the Seal: The Quest for the Lost Ark of the Covenant (New York: Crown, 1992). The guardian of the Ark in Ethiopia—the only one who can look upon the Ark—had thick cataracts on his eyes.

8 From a comment on The Power Hour (possibly May 14, 2007) by A.C. "Griff" Griffith (1940-2012), former NSA and CIA employee and Freemason for 49 years. Manipulation of Alfvén waves could also be the cause.

manner. *Several FSB's can be cascaded within a straight light pipe to produce a high-efficiency, compact, multiband radiometer . . .*[9] (Emphasis added.)

Having stolen Palestinian land and incarcerated Palestinians in full view of the world, tiny theocratic Israel—the fourth largest arms dealer in the world in 2007—has led the way to the modern model of walled cities as open air concentration camps / labs.

> Israel went from inventing the networking tools of the "fiat world" to selling fences to an apartheid planet. Many of the country's most successful entrepreneurs are using Israel's status as a fortress state, surrounded by furious enemies, as a kind of twenty-four-hour-a-day showroom—a living example of how to enjoy relative safety amid constant war. And the reason Israel is now enjoying supergrowth is that those companies are busily exporting that model to the world.[10]

High-tech fences, unmanned drones, biometric IDs, video and audio surveillance gear, air passenger profiling, prisoner interrogation systems—all road-tested by Israel on Gaza, replete with checkpoints, guards, walls, guns, and directed energy weapons (DEWs). Israel's army and universities incubate "security and weapons start-ups" as Israel turns "endless war and occupation into a brand asset, pitching its uprooting, occupation and containment of the Palestinian people into a half-century head start in the 'global war on terror.'"[11]

More "resilient" dystopic Smart Cities like Jerusalem are now rising around us with "the terrifying tools of our security states" being field-tested in full view of news cameras rolling for international dissemination. The irony that the technological nightmare of armed Smart Cities would begin with the nation that would not exist, were it not for the Holocaust, is surely not lost on the world.[12]

The genocides of war and sanctions are overt eugenics (Nazi Germany, Kosovo, Cambodia, Rwanda, Sudan, etc.). World War One wiped out an entire European generation (41 million), and World War Two 85 million (battle, war-related famine and disease)—population reduction while oil, steel, and chemical industries profited immensely. Due to the 1925 Geneva Protocol, chemical / biological warfare experiments were subsequently conducted "under the rose," the justification being a necessary defense against the possibility that others were developing "germ warfare" weapons. By 1936, Japanese

9 M.S. Kowitt et al., "Frequency selective bolometers." OSA Publishing, Applied Optics, Vol. 35, Issue 28, 1996.

10 Naomi Klein, "Gaza: Not Just a Prison, a Laboratory." The Nation, June 15, 2007.

11 Ibid. Also see Joe Catron, "Meet Ten Corporate Giants Helping Israel Massacre Gaza Protesters," MintPressNews, October 12, 2018.

12 Stephen Graham, Cities Under Siege: The New Military Urbanism (Verso, 2011).

scientist Shiro Ishii had established the top-secret Unit 731 ("Anti-Epidemic Water Supply and Purification Bureau") in Manchuria for "experimentation." During the war crime trials after World War Two, the U.S. offered immunity to Ishii and the scientists who had worked with him in exchange for their human experimentation data. Camp Detrick became Fort Detrick (1956) for permanent military R&D of deadly viruses and nerve gases under former enemies now on the U.S. government payroll.

The *Korean "police action" (1950-53)* tested Brucellosis, hemorrhagic fever, napalm (70,000 gallons a day!), radar and communications. The *Vietnam "conflict" (1959-1975)* was about Operation Ranch Hand and Agent Orange (with 12 million gallons over 4.5 million acres of the TCCD strain of dioxin), napalm, BZ incapacitant (EA-2277, quinuclidinyl benzilate), and CS gas (2-chlorobenzylidene malononitrile). Military scientist James Clary designed the spray tanks and in 1988 said to a congressperson investigating the dispersion of Agent Orange:

> When we initiated the herbicide programme in the 1960s, we were aware of the potential for damage due to dioxin contamination in the herbicide. We were even aware that the military formulation had a higher dioxin concentration than the civilian version, due to its lower cost and speed of manufacture. However, because the material was to be used on the enemy, none of us were overly concerned . . . By the time the war finally ended in 1975, more than 10% of Vietnam had been intensively sprayed with 72 million litres of chemicals, of which 66% was Agent Orange, laced with its super-strain of toxic TCCD . . . In confidential statements made to US scientists, former Ranch Hand pilots allege that, in addition to the recorded missions, there were 26,000 aborted operations during which 260,000 gallons of herbicide were dumped . . . Canadian] Hatfield Consultants . . . have made an alarming discovery. In the Aluoi Valley adjacent to the Ho Chi Minh Trail, once home to three US Special Forces bases, a region where Agent Orange was both stored and sprayed, the scientists' analysis has shown that rather than naturally disperse, the dioxin has remained in the ground in concentrations 100 times above the safety levels for agricultural land in Canada. It has spread into Aluoi's ponds, rivers and irrigation supplies from where it has passed into the food chain through fish and freshwater shellfish, chickens and ducks that store TCCD in fatty tissue . . . [P]regnant women pass it through the placenta to the foetus and then through their breast milk, doubly infecting newborn babies.[13]

13 Cathy Scott-Clark and Adrian Levy, "Spectre orange." The Guardian, March 29, 2003.

The beginnings of electronic sensing and communications systems were experimental in Vietnam, like the solar-powered, high-frequency radios behind Vietcong lines being bounced from 200 miles above the Earth.

4.2 million U.S. soldiers came in contact with chemicals in Vietnam. Chronic conditions, skin disorders, asthma, cancers, gastrointestinal diseases, babies born limbless, Down's syndrome, spina bifida . . . In 1972, the UK and Soviet Union (but not the U.S.) signed off on the Biological and Toxin Weapons Convention. The Reagan government denied any link to Agent Orange; victims sued defoliant manufacturers and received $180 million hush money out of court.

Weaponization of cancer (1950s – 1970s)

Under MKNAOMI (testing "severely incapacitating and lethal materials . . . [and] gadgetry for their dissemination"[14]), the CIA and NIH at the Special Operations Division, Fort Detrick, Maryland, created the Special Virus Cancer Program (SVCP) (1964-1977),[15] a cover for the U.S. Biowarfare program under other names—Special Virus Leukemia Program (1964-69), Virus Cancer Program (1973), etc.—which continued long after being discontinued by President Richard M. Nixon and resurrected as the "war on cancer" when the U.S. Army's Fort Detrick Biological Warfare Laboratory morphed into the Frederick Cancer Research Center as the staff and budget tripled.[16]

One of the discoveries under the cancer rubric of biological warfare now classified as synthetic biology was chemotherapy that targeted biochemical reactions involved in proliferating cancer cells. It was chemotherapy that led to artificial nanocontainers designed to enter the nucleus of living cells. Known as *polymersomes*—sounding distinctly like "exosomes"—these 60 nm nanocontainers are subject to remote-controlled "nuclear localization signals" designed to fool the cell into letting the foreign polymersomes enter the cell.[17]

2,4-Dichlorophenoxyacetic acid, the primary weed killer agent in Agent Orange, has been approved by the EPA for use on fruits and vegetables, corn and soy.

14 "Experimentation Programs conducted by the Department of Defense That Had CIA Sponsorship or Participation and That Involved the Administration to Human Subjects of Drugs Intended for Mind-Control or Behavior-Modification Purposes," General Counsel, Department of Defense, 1977.

15 The Intelligence Community: History, Organization, and Issues, ed. Tyrus G. Fain, Katherine C. Plant, Ross Milloy. Bowker, 1977.

16 The Third Reich's biological warfare program had the cover name of Cancer Research Program. The National Cancer Institute's Special Viral Cancer Research Program is a front, as well.

17 University of Basel, "Nanocontainers introduced into the nucleus of living cells." Phys.org, January 27, 2020.

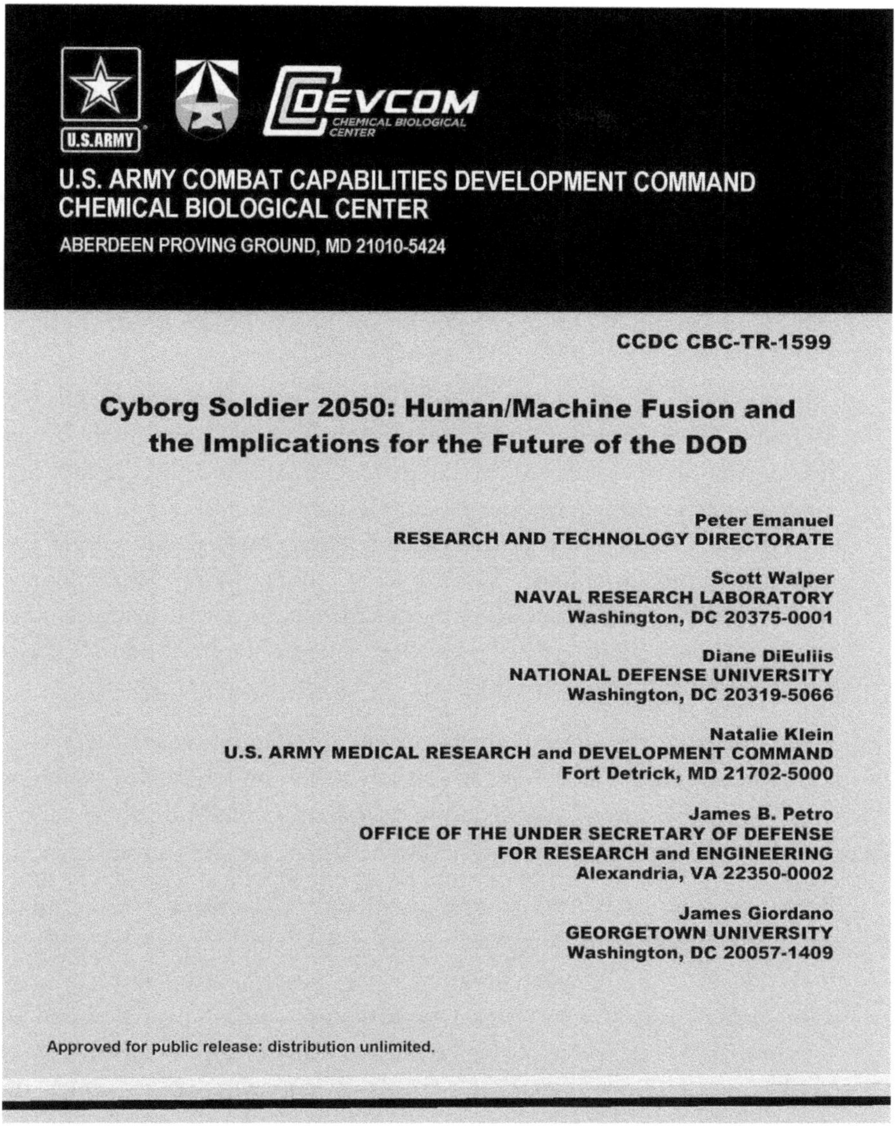

U.S. ARMY COMBAT CAPABILITIES DEVELOPMENT COMMAND
CHEMICAL BIOLOGICAL CENTER

ABERDEEN PROVING GROUND, MD 21010-5424

CCDC CBC-TR-1599

Cyborg Soldier 2050: Human/Machine Fusion and the Implications for the Future of the DOD

Peter Emanuel
RESEARCH AND TECHNOLOGY DIRECTORATE

Scott Walper
NAVAL RESEARCH LABORATORY
Washington, DC 20375-0001

Diane DiEuliis
NATIONAL DEFENSE UNIVERSITY
Washington, DC 20319-5066

Natalie Klein
U.S. ARMY MEDICAL RESEARCH and DEVELOPMENT COMMAND
Fort Detrick, MD 21702-5000

James B. Petro
OFFICE OF THE UNDER SECRETARY OF DEFENSE
FOR RESEARCH and ENGINEERING
Alexandria, VA 22350-0002

James Giordano
GEORGETOWN UNIVERSITY
Washington, DC 20057-1409

Approved for public release: distribution unlimited.

Cyborg Soldier 2050.

http://community.apan.org/wg/tradoc-g2/mad-scientist/m/articles-of-interest/300458

And so the cancer epidemic continues to grow. Cancer is defined simply as an uncontrolled proliferation of damaged cells. Like the microwave oven, cancer has been strangely accepted by American society as a fact of modern-life. By remaining silent about why this might be so, "experts" reign supreme, claiming the technology and GMO Frankenfoods to be safe as cancer clusters proliferate. Microwaves are fine for cooking "food," Nature's nutrients be damned. Cancer is basically the devil's due for cheap "food" and a technological life of convenience and comfort. Besides, when the immune system gives out, there's always the money-grubbing, high-tech sickness industry run by Big Pharma.

Cancer is a thriving industry created by an unnatural industrial lifestyle now bolstered by wireless technology and an aerosol-delivered daily flurry of conductive nano-metals called "chaff" by the military:

> The structure of hemoglobin is easily compromised by heavy metals like mercury. All carcinogens impair respiration directly or indirectly by deranging capillary circulation, a statement that is proven by the fact that no cancer cell exists without exhibiting impaired respiration.
>
> "Tumors cannot grow if the oxygen levels are normal, and oxygen levels are controlled by voltage," says Dr. Jerry Tennant [MD]. He could have said oxygen levels are controlled by pH or oxygen levels control voltage because if there is too little oxygen, then the mitochondria cannot create enough ATP [adenosine triphosphate] to keep cellular energy high.[18]

Chemotherapy, the unnatural poison and irradiation assault, was born from mustard gas, the World War One chemical weapon that fueled the blood sacrifice of an entire European generation. As it destroys the white blood cells, it suppresses the division of cancer cells in bone marrow and the immune system.

> Beginning in the 1960s, the National Aeronautics and Space Administration (NASA) urgently needed data on human sensitivity to radiation for the US space program. One question that especially concerned them was at what point would nausea and vomiting caused by radiation sickness set in? To an astronaut unable to remove an oxygen mask, this could prove vital. The cancer patients who came through the doors of the Oak Ridge Institute were to become the human guinea pigs that provided the information.[19]

And as doubt grows in the public mind at a glacial pace, whole-body CT scans (10 millisievert units in living tissue), X-rays (0.1 millisievert), nuclear medicine (!), and leaking nuclear reactors continue.

Cancer provides a natural-looking assassination approach. On December

18 "ICU Doctors Know Best," drsircus.com, April 16, 2020.

19 Ayn Lowry, "Human experimentation: Minorities and prisoners targeted." WISE News Communique, March 28, 1993.

28, 2011, Venezuelan President Hugo Chavez maintained that the U.S. was covertly implanting left-leaning leaders with cancer cells:

> Argentine President Néstor Kirchner – colon cancer
> Brazil President Dilma Rousseff – lymphoma
> Brazil President Luiz Inácio Lula da Silva – throat cancer
> Cuba President Fidel Castro – stomach cancer
> Bolivia President Evo Morales – nasal cancer
> Paraguay President Fernando Lugo – lymphoma
> Venezuela President Hugo Chávez – colon cancer

Whether delivered by a dart gun or in food or a wire in a boot or a radiation pin-prick, cancer cells are a formidable weapon in that no one questions a death by cancer.[20]

Cancer, the common scourge since Roundup and GMO Frankenfood production collusion from what is being disseminated by jet aerosols, is aided along its way by RNA viruses with the reverse transcriptase enzyme that makes sure the virus forms short strands of DNA (*oligos*, as in oligonucleotides) that integrate with the host's cell DNA. SV40 transferred from contaminated monkey kidney cells to "culture" vaccines is cancer-causing. Cancer cells are consistently found in vaccines.

Every generation since the explosion of cancer has had the opportunity to see right through Big Pharma's use of the vaccine to seed "RNA and forming proviruses which become latent for long periods throughout the body, only to reawaken later on"—reawakening, for example, as rheumatoid arthritis, multiple sclerosis (MS) and systemic lupus erythematosus (SLE) once the immune system is bypassed, circumvented, or fooled into forming antibodies against the person's own tissues impregnated by foreign genetic material. Even a slight modification of the "antigenic character of tissues" strikes the immune system as foreign.[21]

"Cancer research" in the name of public suffering appears to be an ongoing CBW program that has been successfully normalized and commercialized. The relentless vigor of the smear campaign against *GcMAF (Globulin compound-derived protein Macrophage Activating Factor)* indicates that GcMAF is a cheap and effective Vitamin D cure in that it activates the macrophages of the immune system to attack and destroy cancerous tumor cells. Big Pharma is opposed to anything that strengthens the Human 1.0 immune system. So far, GcMAF does

---

20 "Cancer the secret weapon?" The Guardian, February 27, 2012. The political list is long and needs its own book—from Jack Ruby in 1967 to Jamaican musician Bob Marley in 1981, Black Panther Pan-Africanist Stokely Carmichael / Kwame Ture in 1998 . . .

21 From Leading Edge Research Group, "Vaccines and Production of Neagive Genetic Changes in Humans," 1998.

not appear to have undergone gain of function tampering or patenting.[22]

Iran-Iraq War (1980-1988)

During the *Iran-Iraq War (1980-1988),* Saddam Hussein freely utilized CBW weapons provided by the CIA:

> "It was all done with a wink and a nod," said a former U.S. intelligence official. "We knew exactly where this stuff was going, although we bent over backwards to look the other way." Washington knew Iraq was "dumping boatloads" of chemical weapons on Iranian positions, he added . . . Policy at the time, said another former Reagan official, recognized that 'Hussein is a bastard, but at the time he was our bastard.'"[23]

Gulf War / Operation Desert Shield / Operation Desert Storm (1990-1991)

Iraq War (2003-2011)

The two Gulf Wars, one under previous CIA director President George H.W. Bush and 12 years later the other under his son President George W. Bush (followed by President Barack Obama), were in the beginning about oil, shutting up "our bastard" Saddam Hussein, and looking for the 70 shipments of bacterial cultures shipped to Iraq in 1986-1989. But on another level of both wars, they were about biological and chemical warfare experiments under Full-Spectrum Effects Weapon Systems. From DU-tipped warheads, psychotronic weapons, and the usual wartime vaccine experimentation in Gulf War I, to post-9/11 long-range scalar Tesla howitzer dissolution of atoms under Vice President Dick Cheney in Gulf War 2, the U.S. violated every weapons treaty and convention in existence.

Depleted uranium (DU) is the dust "depleted" to 70 percent of the original chemically and biologically reactive uranium. During enrichment, some of the dust is released into the atmosphere, but most is recycled for weapons. The Germans first did it for their armor-piercing munitions in 1943 when they ran out of tungsten. The DU half-life is 4.5 billion years. Since the first 300 tons (Gulf War I), followed by the Gulf War Syndrome, DU has become

---

22 September 2015 interview with David Noakes "GcMAF = The Cure for Cancer," and if you can find it on the Internet (I couldn't), Linda Emmanuel's "Mycoplasma, Nagalase and GcMAF."

23 "Some See Hypocrisy in U.S. Stand on Iraq Arms Mideast: Officials say American intelligence aided Baghdad's use of chemical weapons against Iran in '80s." Los Angeles Times, February 16, 1998. Also see Sherwood Ross, "America's Germ Warfare Capabilities developed in secret in US corporate labs." Global Research, January 7, 2007.

common fare. Roughly 8 percent of the Earth's total land mass (57.3 million square miles) is now severely contaminated.[24] In Operation Desert Fox, 2,000 tons were used. Iraqi doctors reported sky-high cancers, leukemia, and birth defects. In Afghanistan, *non-depleted uranium (NDU)* was used, a processed form of pure uranium *more toxic than DU.*

> As their exotic metallurgy "burns" through concrete and steel, DU and NDU bombs [like GBU-28 bunker busters] are converted to micron-sized particles that sicken and kill and murder the next generation in the womb.[25]

After Gulf War I, 200,000 GI's returned home, ill down into their genes with the so-called Gulf War Syndrome which made their families and pets sick, their lungs riddled with heavy metal nanoparticles from depleted uranium (DU) debris. Just "one millionth of a gram accumulating in a person's body would be fatal,"[26] DU is highly pyrophoric, meaning it ignites and burns hot like magnesium (1700°C to 3000°C). Once vaporized, it condenses into tiny hollow spheres that float on wind and water and lodge in the lungs. (Water will not put it out.)[27]

Vanity Fair magazine called Desert Shield and Desert Storm experimental vaccines "another Manhattan Project." Male and female troops were heavily vaccinated with the experimental, unlicensed adjuvant squalene that was supposed to protect them against anthrax. sick squalene antibodies in their blood, symptoms ranging from Lou Gehrig's disease (amyotrophic lateral sclerosis that usually strikes people 45 and older), fatigue, pain in joints and muscles, swollen lymph nodes, fever and rash, to tremors, sleep disorders, seizures, memory loss, lost time, and blackouts. *The autoimmune system was attacking them instead of protecting them.* Sound familiar? Last stop: systemic lupus erythematosus.

The 42-day chemical and biological air war Operation Desert Storm commenced on January 19, 1991. According to General Norman Schwarzkopf's combat log, an average of three chemical alarms a day sounded for U.S. and British troops (14,000), though no alarm sounded for the eight days during which ammo depots loaded with U.S.- and Dutch-made nerve and mustard

---

24 Leuren Moret, "Depleted Uranium: The Trojan Horse of Nuclear War." Journal of International Issues, 1 July 2004.

25 James Brooks, "US and Israel targeting DNA in Gaza? Part 3 of 3: The DIME bomb, yet another genotoxic weapon." Online Journal, December 7, 2006.

26 Memorandum to Brig. Gen. L.R. "Greasy" Groves from Drs. Conant, Compton, and Urey; War Department, U.S. Engineer Office, Manhattan District, Oak Ridge, Tennessee, October 30, 1943.

27 The U.S. Navy's anti-cruise missile Phalanx pumps out 60-120 shot burst rounds of uranium -238 at 2,000 per minute.

gas were blown up.

The German-made FOX nuclear-biological-chemical detection vehicle detected 60 known chemical agents via mass spectrometer, 21 of which were reproductive toxicants. The American public was told that these agents were Iraqi, but however you look at it, they were ours, delivered by FROGs (free rockets over ground) and SCUD B SS-1s. The M8A1 alarm and troop chemical protection equipment were insufficient, and there was no biological agent detection or protection whatsoever. The chemicals soldiers faced were cocktails of biotoxins, vesicants (cause blistering), nerve and biological agents in the Soviet *Novichok* series, *clostridium botulinum* (botulism), sarin (nerve), *bacillus anthracis* (anthrax), *clostridium perfingens* (gangrene), *clostridium tetani* (tetanus), *brucella abortis* (brucellosis or undulant fever), *brucella melentensis, franciscella tularensis* (tularemia), *bacillus subtilis* (conjunctivitis), *bacillus megatillus* and *bacillus cereus* (autoimmune invaders), mustard gas (inhibits enzymes, necrosis of tissue), lewisite, etc. As we now know, with recombinant DNA (rDNA) and *e.coli,* a carbapenem-resistant Enterobacteriaceae (CRE), microorganisms can be genetically *armed* (gain of function).

Saddam Hussein had been assured that the biological agents were for Iran, but the American plan was always to test five genetically armed strains of *Mycoplasma* from the *Brucella* bacterium that had been quietly tested on North American populations since the 1970s. (See Chapter 2, "The Three Primary Transhumanist Delivery Systems.") Soldiers were disallowed from refusing the unapproved, experimental botulinum toxoid vaccine and pyridostigmine bromide pills. Brain and nervous system cancers among Gulf War vets were 1400 percent higher than among the general population. Twenty thousand veterans suffered aching teeth, jaws, joints, chronic fatigue syndrome, destroyed immune systems, etc.

In Gulf War 2, Iraqi doctors were confronted by "strange corpses found at [Fallujah's] destruction, many with their skin apparently melted or carmelised so their features were indistinguishable."[28] Such Full-Spectrum Effects Weapon Systems experiments, the military mind conjectured, made certain that operating forces might "exploit the psychological dilemma of adversaries faced with advanced precision capabilities more challenging to protect against, thus transferring the difficulties of operational complexity to the enemy."[29]

Is it possible to read these words without feeling sick *about the level of antihuman evil that the American military has sunk to?*

---

28 Peter Popham and Anne Penketh, "US intelligence classified white phosphorus as 'chemical weapon.'" The Independent, 24 November 2005.

29 Murdoc, "Pain Ray, Sonic Blaster, Laser Dazzler—All in One." Defense Tech, January 30, 2006.

At El Shifa Hospital in Gaza, in Fallujah and Haditha, surface wounds showed no entry or exit, nor signs of either bullets or shrapnel. In Lebanon, a physician spoke of vacuum bombs that suck out the body's air, collapse the lungs, and stop the heart. Was it a Hellfire thermobaric missile? a sensor-fused submunition in a CBU-97 that projected molten copper right through the target? After the air strikes in Doueir and Rmayleih, the bodies were dark, inflated, and exuded a terrible smell. The hair was unburned, and there was no bleeding. *White phosphorus?* the doctors asked each other. They begged for guidance from the world medical fraternity, but only silence responded. A military attaché relayed a request to keep careful records and document eyewitness accounts. Tissue samples were to be placed in formalin.

At the General Teaching Hospital in Hilla—close to the historical Babylon—Iraqi doctors pondered the shrunken bodies of victims of a new kind of war, bodies shrunk to just over a meter because the bodily fluids had simply been boiled away. In one man, only the head was burned; others had no eyeballs and no head at all, no arms and legs. Before the assault, no noise was heard, no explosion, only an awful silence.

After the battle for the airport on April 12, 2003, the American military dug up and replaced the battle terrain that might have proved that scalar ionizing radiation weapons had been used against the Iraqis. A passenger bus, en route from Hilla to Kifil, turned back from an American checkpoint, after which fire and lightning was pulsed from a tank wheeling around the corner. The bus and three cars rippled like semi-molten wet rags and shrank, as did soldiers and civilians. Was this Zeus, the high energy laser, or a high-power microwave beam with a laser effect?

No, it was a scalar Tesla howitzer that dissociates atoms, similar to what disintegrated the World Trade Towers.

Still, some of the damage in Iraq could have been from Israel's tungsten "bunker buster" Dense Inert Metal Explosives (DIMEs), which is capable of disrupting body chemistry, damaging the immune system, causing rapid cancer, and attacking DNA. Weapons based on DIME technology launched from a drone can sever legs with heat. Such weapons have been used in the Gaza Strip west of Hilla.

As for the DUs, in 2008 over 6,700 tons of DU-contaminated soil, sand and other residues were finally collected and shipped from Kuwait to the U.S. Ecology Hazardous Waste Disposal site in Grand View, Idaho, 44 miles from Boise. International health officials have been obstructed from doing medical studies at DU sites in Iraq and Afghanistan.[30] An excellent 2003 series of *Christian Science*

30 See contamination maps at https://www.ejatlas.org/print/depleted-uranium-in-kuwait.

Monitor articles described reporters with Geiger-counters visiting such sites and finding them to be extremely "hot" with radioactivity.[31] No surprise there.

How are those Idaho potatoes tasting?

Last but certainly not least, subliminal mind-altering technology was carried on standard FM radio frequency broadcasts in Riyadh, the capital of Saudi Arabia, after Saddam Hussein's military command-and-control system was destroyed. His troops were then forced to use commercial FM radio stations for their encoded commands broadcasting at 100 MHz. U.S. Psyops set up a portable FM transmitter, dialed in the same frequency from nearby deserted Al Khafji, and ran a highly classified *silent sound* subliminal program of fear, anxiety, and despair under patriotic and religious music.

Desert Storm was the first successful simultaneous transmission of the human voice directly into multiple skulls. The first classified "Smirnov scramble" was run in 1974 by Joseph C. Sharp, PhD, of the Walter Reed Army Institute of Research. During Desert Storm, Holosonic Research Labs and the American Technology Corporation, in conjunction with Brooks Air Force Base, directed the voice of Allah, replete with holographic images, straight into Muslim troops' heads by means of "acoustic bullets" from a Long Range Acoustic Device (LRAD) sonic projector, a high-powered, very low frequency (VLF) modulator working in the 20-35 kHz spectrum with a one- to two-meter antenna dish. The LRAD is a crowd control DEW with multiple capabilities. Smaller, more mobile versions are now crawling the Smart Cities.

Bosnian War (1992-1995)

After Vietnam, 50 tons of BZ were stockpiled at Aberdeen Proving Ground, Maryland. Human Rights Watch reported in "Chemical Warfare in Bosnia? The Strange Experiences of the Srebrenica Survivors" how those people escaping what is now known as the July 1995 Srebrenica Massacre (in Bosnia and Herzegovina) were assaulted by Bosnian Serb forces under General Ratko Mladi. Mortar shells produced a "strange" smoke of varying colors, after which many marchers began hallucinating and behaving irrationally, *some even killing their friends or themselves.* The Yugoslav People's Army (JNA) possessed BZ, as the Federal Republic of Yugoslavia had not signed the 1993 Chemical Weapons Convention (CWC).[32]

Afghanistan War / Operation Enduring Freedom (2001-2021)

American troops coming home from Afghanistan have returned with "mys-

31 Eg, Scott Peterson, "Remains of toxic bullets litter Iraq," CSM, May 15, 2003.

32 The 1995 film Outbreak was propaganda for the U.S. Army Medical Research Institute of Infectious Diseases (USAMRIID) at Fort Detrick, Maryland.

terious" bacteria linked to loss of limbs—bacteria found in military hospitals in Germany, Washington, D.C., and Texas, all primary care centers for the wounded of the two Middle Eastern war zones. Again, the spokespersons for the "outbreaks" are military-controlled professionals: Harvard Medical School, retired Army officers teaching at university medical schools and Walter Reed Army Medical Center—all neatly reported in the U.S. Naval Institute's *Proceedings.*[33]

American troops are supposedly being withdrawn from Afghanistan on August 31, 2021.[34]

The Department of Housing & Urban Development (HUD)

> *Mind control weapons are the ultimate weapon holy grail that have given birth to the world's most notorious sociopath scientists, who in turn have spawned a generation of the most intense human suffering for weapons-testing efficacy the people of this planet have ever endured.*
>
> – Robert Duncan, PhD, *The Matrix Deciphered,* 2006

The big pork business models of poverty, usury, drugs, weapons, human and organ trafficking, and targeting initially depend upon big tax dollars siphoned through crime prevention programs in urban slums and gutted farm communities under the aegis of the National Institute of Justice (NIJ), Housing and Urban Development (HUD), Neighborhood Watch groups, community development associations, youth programs, and knock-and-talk interviews challenging crime in low-income neighborhoods. Sounds pretty low-tech now, compared with now being lucrative *in vivo* laboratories for IO (Information Operations) weapons of the DOJ, Department of Defense (DoD), and Intelligence Community (IC).

Spurring economic growth in distressed neighborhoods was never HUD's real objective, given how HUD has for decades been the "candy store" for covert revenues leached from the poor.[35] HUD cooked the books of the Office of Emergency Preparedness (now the Office of Emergency Management or OEM) until the Deep State's Federal Emergency Management Agency (FEMA) took over in 1978. HUD federal credit still bankrolls criminal non-bid contracts, deep pockets, money laundering, and black projects. In 1999, HUD's Inspector General

---

33 "New Bacterial Infection Linked to Military." ABC News, February 8, 2008.

34 "Withdrawal of United States troops from Afghanistan," Wikipedia.

35 For a true understanding of HUD, one must read Catherine Austin Fitts, former Assistant Secretary of HUD under President George H.W. Bush (1989-1993). See "Missing Money: A Personal History – 1989 to 2019" at her Solari Report website, https://hudmissingmoney.solari.com/2019/04/07/missing-money-a-personal-history-1989-to-2019/.

refused to certify its financial statements because $59 billion had been disappeared.

The faked War on Poverty and War on Drugs preceded Homeland Security's War on Terror. Cozy DOJ/HUD arrangements spawned two excellent covers for lucrative slum operations: Operation Weed & Seed[36] and the Technology Assessment Program (TAP). Homeless war veterans are still targeted, as are the poor and ethnic, homeless, drug addicts, foreigners, political dissidents, "potential" terrorists, women, children, the disabled and old, psychiatric outpatients, artists—basically anyone who could be called delusional if they report being stalked or targeted. Private mortgage bankers' pockets are filled to overflowing with federal credit and bailouts, thanks to HUD and the Federal Housing Administration (FHA) up to their necks in intelligence scams, with fat cats like Rothschild Inc. skimming billions per year from FHA mutual funds at HUD ("coinsurance"), and not counting the billions lost in single-family FHA programs.

In the 1980s, the DOJ stole PROMIS "backdoor" software and kicked government / corporate criminality into high gear.[37] Then came the Clinton law enforcement / military merger decade of HUD's Operation Safe Home following in the footsteps of Rex 84, Operation Cable Splicer and Garden Plot—all martial law attempts to quash justified civil unrest while amping up crime in government. Vice President Al Gore championed Safe Home from the Nashville headquarters of prisons-for-profits Corrections Corporation of America (CCA) as HUD Office of Inspector General (OIG), federal, state, and local law enforcement task forces (FBI, DEA, BATF, ICE, Secret Service, U.S. Marshal's Service, Postal Inspection Service, U.S. Customs, and of course the DOJ that had stolen the PROMIS software) climbed into bed together.[38]

Safe Home was drugs and seized assets and prisons-for-profit. Prison populations and consumer debt soared during the Clinton-Gore 1990s, and the Harvard Endowment climbed from $4 billion to $19 billion. Privatization-

36 "Operation Weed & Seed is a joint federal, state and local coordinated law enforcement and community initiative that aims to prevent, control and reduce violent crime, drug abuse and gang activity in targeted high-crime neighborhoods across the country. The Weed & Seed strategy recognizes the importance of integrating law enforcement with social services and the private sector on federal, state and local levels to maximize the impact of existing programs and resources." http://www.justice.gov/usao/md/Community-Programs/Weed%20and%20Seed/index.html

37 See The Octopus: The Secret Government and Death of Danny Casolaro by Kenn Thomas and Jim Keith (Feral House, 1996). Moral turpitude is a legal concept referring to conduct considered contrary to community standards of justice, honesty or good morals (West's Encyclopedia of American Law).

38 HUD's governing board reflected the usual public-private partnerships: Departments of Treasury and Justice, Lockheed Martin, DynCorp, JPMorgan Chase, Harvard, with American Management System (AMS) and Arthur Andersen cooking the books, JPMorgan Chase and Treasury moving offshore money around, and Justice setting up law enforcement cover.

as-piratization grew while HUD subsidized enforcement programs run by corporations, scrubbed millions of dirty dollar through "off-shore" Indian reservation casinos, off-track racing, bingo and cigarette operations, and card rooms, leaving the poor poorer and more addicted than ever. Bechtel, Arthur Anderson's Houston office, and Halliburton / KBR felt free to dip into the HUD piggy bank, too, as did all of George H.W. Bush's pals.

Investment analyst / former HUD Assistant Secretary Catherine Austin Fitts and the Hamilton Securities Group received death threats when their Community Wizard software really did help poor communities manage their debt and relieve themselves of enforcement and realty parasites.[39]

In 1996, the *Dark Alliance* series by Gary Webb in the *San Jose Mercury News* blew the whistle about crack cocaine being smuggled from Central America into South Central LA by the CIA, with the involvement of former CIA Director / former President George H.W. Bush.[40] In 1998 Webb's book *Dark Alliance: The CIA, the Contras, and the Crack Cocaine Explosion* came out, and six years later at 49, Webb was "suicided" with two bullets to the back of his head on December 10, 2004.

NetRad / NexRad & Psychotronics

> *. . . psychotronic weapons are those that act to take away a part of the information which is stored in a man's brain. It is sent to a computer, which reworks it to the level needed for those who need to control the man, and the modified information is then reinserted into the brain. These weapons are used against the mind to induce hallucinations, sickness, mutations in human cells, 'zombification,' or even death. Included in the arsenal are VHF generators, X-rays, ultrasound, and radio waves.*
>
> – Timothy L. Thomas, "The Mind Has No Firewall." *Parameters* (Spring 1998)[41]

> *Abstract: Multistatic measurements of targets and clutter have been performed over the past few years by the NetRAD system developed at the University College London and the University of Cape Town. NetRAD is a three-node, coherent, multistatic, pulse Doppler radar operating at S-Band (2400 MHz).*

---

39 Catherine Austin Fitts, Chapter 11, "Hamilton Securities Group," Dillon Reed & Co. Inc. and the Aristocracy of Stock Profits (2005). Online only.

40 The CIA and British MI6 created crack cocaine from basuco (cocaine paste) and debuted it in urban ghettos in 1980 after George H.W. Bush's October Surprise handed him the vice presidency under President Ronald Reagan (1980-1988) with co-conspirator Dick Cheney as Secretary of Defense.

41 Lt. Col. Thomas was an analyst at the Foreign Military Studies Office.

NeXtRAD [NexRAD] is a new version of this system, operating polarimetrically at L and X Bands. The results obtained by NetRAD have been used for a number of investigations (mostly multistatic sea clutter). This paper reports on results using narrow bandwidth NetRAD data to generate imagery with high spatial resolution. The high spatial resolution is obtained by applying the principles of tomography to a multi-site radar system which is illuminating a target over a complete angular range of 360 degrees. . .

– Shirley Coetzee *et al.* "Narrow band radar imaging using NetRAD and NeXtRAD data." International Conference on Radar Systems (Radar 2017), October 23-26, 2018

The U.S. Air Force worked for decades on devices for "controlled effects," what eventually came to be known as *nonlethals* and *psychotronics*: physical and mental sensations manipulated at a distance to make adversaries think or act in certain ways. NDAA 2013 went public with the fact that psychotronic weapons ("nonlethals") are categorized as *Information Operations (IO):* electronic warfare (EW), computer network operations (CNO), psychological operations (PSYOP), military deception (MILDEC), and operations security (OPSEC). *The IO category makes it legal to target Americans with IO weapons.*

Every tower is a beacon of death and a disaster capitalist bonanza.[42] Together, towers in Smart Cities create a "false magnetic floor" that disconnects us from the Earth's natural magnetic field. From the top of each tower, long-wave, tissues-penetrating microwave radiation is bombarding everyone below and in its path. NetRads are installed at the base of towers, along with video monitors, miniature sensors (magnetic, seismic, infrared, radar, and strain electromagnetic), and signals processing supposedly for weather and atmospheric surveillance, detection of biological agents, radiation release, etc. With their weather, surveillance, and biological agent sensors, radar, and tracking, NetRads are about Homeland Security's ultimate ability to access homes, buildings, and brains. [43]NetRad was the first Smart City technology that said loud and clear, *Follow the cell towers.*[44]

Behind the hundreds of vertical feet for communications, weather, surveil-

42 In 2002 alone, renters Nextel (digital), Sensitech (sensors and monitors), Department of Homeland Security (population control), and the U.S. military (nonlethal weapons testing) paid American Tower a total of $548,923,000.

43 Bankrolled by the National Science Foundation, Harvard Center for Risk Analysis, and corporate matching funds from AT&T and Radian / ONEX, the Universities of Massachusetts, Oklahoma, Puerto Rico, and Colorado State merged with Raytheon, M/A-Com and Vaisala, the National Oceanic and Atmospheric Agency (NOAA), National Severe Storms Laboratories, and UMASS Microwave Infrared Remote Sensing Labs (MIRSL).

44 Thanks to Keith Harmon Snow's excellent essay "NetRad in the Neighborhood: Illuminating the Cell Tower Agenda," Montague Reporter, February 28, 2004.

lance, radar, and tracking, smart grid control for Sentient World Simulation (SWS) is underway. Pitch, yaw, up, down, right, left, x, y, intensity, duration, frequency pulse—everything around the towers and their Hydra-like transmission paths is irradiated.[45]

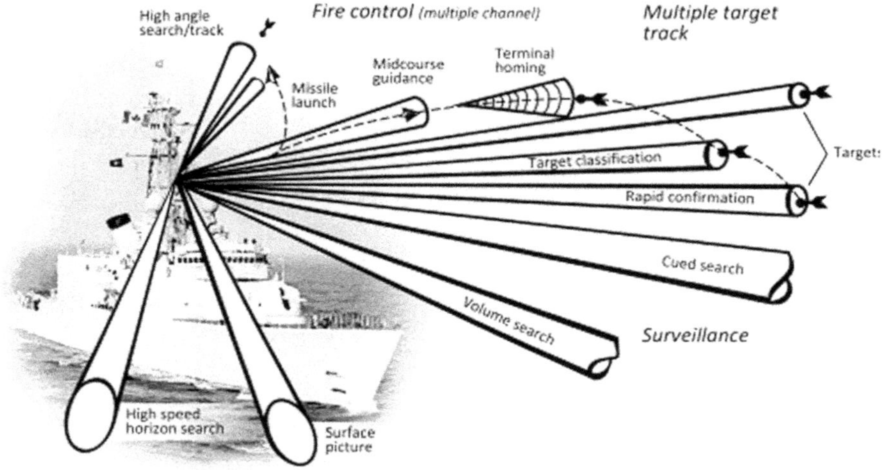

Phased array radar. Ship radar. Think 4G Plus and 5G phased array antennas.

https://ars.els-cdn.com/content/image/3-s2.0-89780128029022000016-f01-01-9780128029022.gif

The ELF tower grid is invaluable to HUD's ongoing Operation Weed & Seed.[46] Have a homeless problem in your town? *Zap.* A drug problem in your neighborhood that the CIA isn't getting kickbacks from? *Zap.* Need a reminder that silence is golden? Turn up the dial and *zap*—heart attack, brain aneurysm, fast-acting cancer. For dissidents taking to the streets, call in a dedicated satellite, activate a few towers, and *zap*. The towers' bi-phase polarity frequencies can be used to induce hallucinations, nausea, herpes, or fast-acting cancer. Anger, lust, complacency, depression? *Think pulsed frequencies.*

In his 1997 far-seeing book *Mind Control World Control*, researcher Jim Keith (1949-1999) relates how he lived for three years in the Tenderloin in San Francisco where the roof of the Federal Building was loaded with radar, microwave, and communications devices. Line of sight meant seeing anywhere into the Tenderloin, which meant radio waves had clear passage in any direction. (ELF and ULF emissions like TV broadcasts don't pass well through earth or

45 For more on towers, see Chapter 8, "Boots on the Ground," in Under An Ionized Sky (2018).

46 https://www.justice.gov/usao-ndca/weed-and-seed

buildings.) Keith noticed that his thoughts were disrupted early in the morning and evening by a low buzzing or humming coming from *inside his head.* He heard neighbors shouting and threatening and slowly realized that the Tenderloin was a double-bind experiment being monitored through the SFPD.

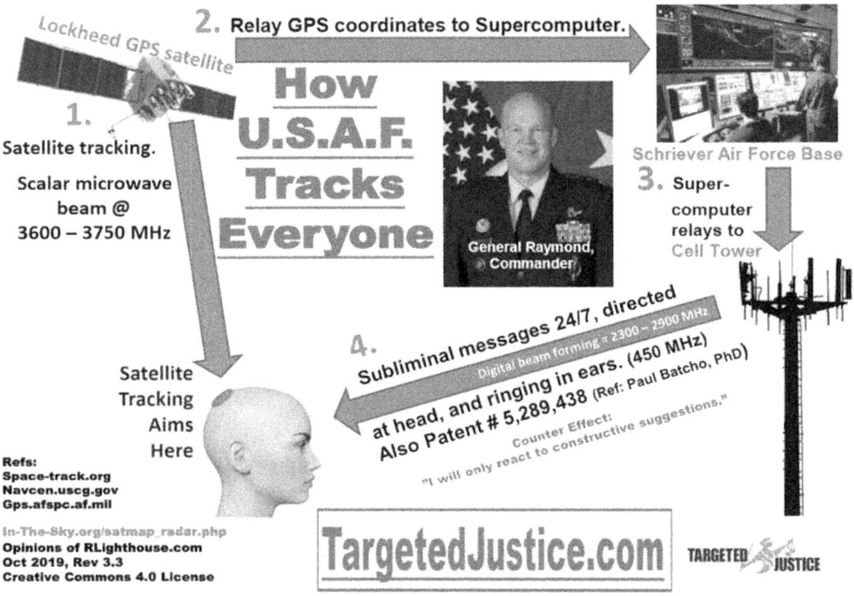

Lockheed GPS satellite
2. Relay GPS coordinates to Supercomputer.
How U.S.A.F. Tracks Everyone
1. Satellite tracking.
Scalar microwave beam @ 3600 – 3750 MHz
General Raymond, Commander
Schriever Air Force Base
3. Super-computer relays to Cell Tower
4. Subliminal messages 24/7, directed
Digital beam forming = 2300 – 2900 MHz
at head, and ringing in ears. (450 MHz)
Also Patent # 5,289,438 (Ref: Paul Batcho, PhD)
Counter Effect:
"I will only react to constructive suggestions."
Satellite Tracking Aims Here
Refs:
Space-track.org
Navcen.uscg.gov
Gps.afspc.af.mil
In-The-Sky.org/satmap_radar.php
Opinions of RLighthouse.com
Oct 2019, Rev 3.3
Creative Commons 4.0 License
TargetedJustice.com
TARGETED JUSTICE

Targeting individuals. This offers a picture of how targeting with directed energy weapons (DEWs) works. From TargetedJustice.com.

Since the mid-1980s, pulse-modulated microwaves as carrier beams for low-frequency (LF) mind control signals have been the name of the game because microwaves can pass through the skull. LF recordings of brain EM excitation potentials (moods, actions, thoughts) are fired at brains as ELF broadcasts carried by pulse-modulated microwave transmitters.[47]

Nothing could be easier than pulsing behavioral frequencies through cell phones. The pulse modulated microwave signal of ~0.75mW/cm2 coming from the phone can be ELF-modulated to control behavior either individually or en masse.[48] CCTV cameras with microwave telemetry devices can be

47 Or a transducer modifies the spoken word into ELF audiograms then superimposed onto the pulse-modulated MW beam. Even the flu can be fired at targets. Paralysis and heart attacks can be induced by "radar jamming" the organ or motor neuron center with the organ's same frequency (preparatory set potentials). This technique is often used for military abductions (MILABs).

48 Pulse an ELF signal at the 0.75mW/cm2 frequency for behavior modification out to antennas around a town and it will resonate in the pulsed fields around power lines, then

used to broadcast the frequency, and so can a police department microwave antenna array or power lines used as antenna systems and magnetic H running through buildings and the Earth.

In 2008, *New York Times* reporter Sarah Kershaw created a stir with her article "Sharing Their Demons on the Web" about Americans being targeted with psychotronic weapons. Kershaw was found strangled in the Dominican Republic. The message was not lost on other investigative journalists: a wall of silence still surrounds the millions being targeted.

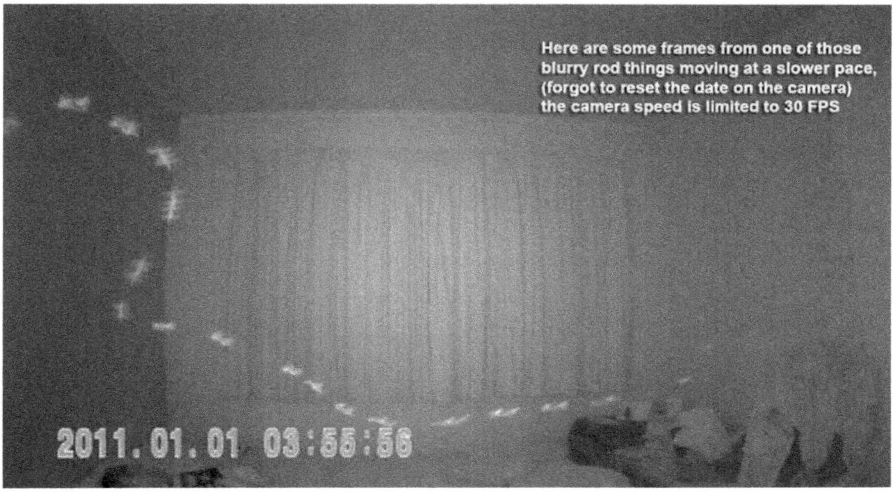
Here are some frames from one of those
blurry rod things moving at a slower pace,
(forgot to reset the date on the camera)
the camera speed is limited to 30 FPS
2011.01.01 03:55:56

From a targeted individual.

Neuroscientists continue to be trained in brain biology but not physics, particularly when it comes to neuroweapons that treat the brain as an electrical system whose glia and neurons work together to communicate information by means of ionic currents, direct currents, semiconducting electricity, and tiny EM and magnetic waves.[49] Few, if any, neuroscientists have studied James Clerk Maxwell's proofs that all physical phenomena are built on oscillations whose electromagnetic radiation comprises the entire electromagnetic spectrum (microwaves, light, kHz oscillations by neurons, etc.), much less Maxwell's ætheric psychoactive component. By the same token, biologists and doctors of all stripes are unfamiliar with the basic concepts of thermodynam-

---

re-radiate and enter homes through light circuits.

49 Read Cheryl Welsh, "Cold War physics in neuroscience is now revealing the probability of a successfully weaponized brain," May 2013, http://mindjustice.org/coldwar.htm. Welsh points out how the "microstructure of cognition" is the neuron's synapse, the signaling unit where two neurons meet and make a biochemical-bioelectrical communication.

ics and electrochemistry.[50]

Since the MK-ULTRA 1950s, research into the bioelectricity of the brain has been so classified that to this day conventional neuroscientists (the neuron-connectionist model) are ignorant of how the movement of electrons and ions affect consciousness, whereas high-clearance neuroscientists are building brains into neuroweapons.

How the electrochemical works should be familiar to both physicists and biologists.

Crowd Control

In 1972, the U.S. Army Mobility Equipment Research and Development Center quietly published, "Analysis of Microwaves for [Brain] Barrier Warfare," stating, "It is possible to field a truck-portable microwave barrier system that will completely 'immobilize' personnel in the open with present day technology and equipment."

Post-9/11, bioweapons were categorized as "nonlethal weapons" for use against "terrorists," including tear gas (active ingredient chlorobenzylidenemalononitrile banned by the Chemical Weapons Convention[51] for warfare but not for crowd control) and pepper spray capable of altering mass behavior (mind-altering or sleep-inducing). Incapacitating opiate gases like fentanyl ("heroin times 1,000"); Droperidol to induce anxiety; Naloxone to restore breathing after release of fentanyl; Tremorine to produce strong tremors / muscle weakness; substance "beta" to produce confusion, psychic weakness, temporary blindness and deafness; etc. Prozac (fluoxetine), Valium (diazepam), and dexmedetomidine "calmatives" outlawed under the 1991 Chemical Weapons Convention (CWC) were weaponized and field-tested,

Urban warfare waged by transnational corporations against civilians calls for quiet technologies that don't kill outright like bullets. Directed energy weapons—lasers, electricity, microwaves, sound waves—promise the discretion (deception?) that bullets and bombs lack.

Radar / Doppler

RADAR (RAdio Detection And Ranging) is the MRI of through-the-wall

---

50 A criticism leveled by Ichiji Tasaki, MD, in Physiology and Electrochemistry of Nerve Fibers (1982). Tasaki discovered the insulating function of the myelin sheath and worked for the NIH and NIMH.

51 The Convention on the Prohibition of the Development, Production, Stockpiling and Use of Chemical Weapons and on their Destruction was passed on 29 April 1997. This convention does not cover biological weapons. The CWC prohibits any chemical that causes death, temporary incapacitation, or permanent harm. Antony Barnett, "US plan to strike enemy with Valium." The Observer, May 26, 2002.

surveillance or sensor (TTWS) technology. Whereas MRI uses magnets to create an image and can only see through bones and tissue, RADAR uses radio waves[52] to create images and can see through multiple walls (and into the Earth as GPR ground penetrating RADAR) from a great distance. RADAR (*radiolocators, intentional radiators*) is the only technology that can locate, lock onto, and track a target with radio waves.[53]

The RADAR Range-R series looks like a sophisticated stud-finder; instead of nails, it detects moving figures through walls and how far away the figure is. Range-R100, Range-R400, and Range-R800 have greater and greater ranges, while the Akela RADAR has a 98-foot standoff range, and the STORMS RADAR (Sense-Through-Obstruction-Remote-Monitoring-System) a 1,000-foot range. Handheld models are basically RADAR guns.

The handheld *WiVi* is WiFi. With two transmit antennas and one receiver, it transmits a low-power WiFi signal that penetrates walls and bounces off humans to reflect moving targets. Developed at MIT's Computer Science and Artificial Intelligence Laboratory, the WiVi is yet another "interference technology."[54]

In his book *The Matrix Deciphered*, Robert Duncan, PhD, details the uses of OTH RADARs we call ionospheric heaters through a description of how he was assaulted by two of them equidistant from the continental U.S. (via *interferometry*), utilizing "total internal reflection from the ionosphere [which] is optimal for power transference from antenna to target arena."

- Incoherent (Stealth) Scatter RADAR
- VHF RADAR (operating within brain resonance frequencies)
- UHF RADAR (operating within head resonance frequencies)
- HF receivers (operating within body resonance frequencies)
- Fluxgate magnetometer
- Induction magnetometer (possibly useful for detecting low intensity magnetic field brain manipulation methods)
- Stimulated electron emission observations (similar to ESR imaging techniques)
- Gyro-frequency heating research (another ESR-MRI-like imaging technique with a variation that might be used in imaging over large

52 The radio spectrum is 3 Hz to 3000 GHz (3 THz), which includes the microwave range (300 MHz to 300 GHz) that hurts, vibrates, burns, and tears up organic bodies.

53 See Radio Frequency Radiation Dosimetry Handbook (Fifth Edition), edited by William P. Roach, Directed Energy Bioeffects Division, Radio Frequency Radiation Branch, Air Force Research Laboratory, July 2009; also see S.I. Ivashov et al., "Detection of Human Breathing and Heartbeat by Remote Radar," Progress in Electromagnetic Research Symposium 2004, Pisa, Italy, March 28-31, 2004.

54 Helen Knight, "New system uses low-power WiFi signal to track moving humans – even behind walls." MIT News, June 28, 2013.

areas using synchronized gyro-frequencies for EM absorption or reflection angles)

- Spread F observations
- Heating induced scintillation observations (another surveillance technology)
- VLF and ELF generation observations (brainwave frequencies)
- Radio observations of meteors and ballistic missile reentry.

The Air Force is in charge of the Directed Energy Directorate from which all of the mind control, nervous system disruptors, and pinpoint assassination weapons technology come to be tested on US citizens at random.

The Marines are in charge of the Non-Lethal Weapons Directorate, another sub-agency that deals in torture weapons.

The Army has a very extensive psychotronic research center.

The CIA are usually the dogs of war that obediently perform tasks too ugly and criminal for the Department of Defense to assign to anyone else.[55]

The FAA, DoD, and DHS have now formed a cross-agency program called SENSR (Spectrum Efficient National Surveillance Radar) whose goal is to replace the number and types of radars across the country with advanced multi-purpose radars for air traffic and weather, surveillance, law enforcement, border and critical national defense infrastructure. Not surprisingly, Lockheed Martin and Raytheon will be in charge of replacing the nationwide network of surveillance and air traffic control radar systems with "fewer, more consolidated multi-mission [i.e. dual-use] systems in a move that would also release wireless spectrum for use in the commercial sector."[56]

Radar technology is everywhere in the Smart City as it is the only technology that can locate, lock onto, and track a target with radio waves. The FCC calls radar devices *radiolocators* and *intentional radiators*, like the *TTWS (through-the-wall surveillance or sensor) radar guns* that "see" through walls or dirt.[57] Obstructions—brick walls, construction materials, curtains, upholstery, etc.—are filtered and dialed out by utilizing their dielectric / permittivity constants, whereas bones, skin, muscle, tissue or any body part can be remotely dialed in on the monitor of a TTWS radar gun by pulsing their dielectric con-

55 Robert Duncan, PhD, The Matrix Deciphered. Higher Order Thinkers Publishing, 2006.

56 Ross Wilkers, "Lockheed-Raytheon team to pursue air traffic control consolidation program." Washington Technology, April 1, 2019.

57 The most powerful is STORMS (sense through obstructions remote monitoring system) with a range of three football fields end to end.

stant[58] for surgical precision. Pulse *high-powered microwaves (HPM)* and wait for the return radio wave backscatter on the radar gun's monitor to indicate the what, where, and who inside and on the other side of the wall.

Plumbers, electricians, construction workers, and police use TTWS radar guns and pulsed HPMs. Unlike traffic radar (motion, direction, mph), this radar operates as a micromotion sensor to pick up heartbeat, breathing rate, and speech. Increase the power density and the intensity (RF 3 kHz to 300 GHz, MW 300 MHz to 300 GHz) vibrates and burns bodies.[59] U.S. Navy-trained radar specialist Chris Fontenot explains it more fully:

> Phased array Doppler radar facilities (ground / air / satellite based) can provide the focused microwave energy needed to create this cascade of atmospheric ions. Through this process, ions are multiplied and released into the lower atmosphere to increase power density in those layers. These modern tools of manipulation are essential to control of the weather. By controlling the electromagnetic potential in the Earth's atmospheric layers, man can affect natural processes of weather. Subtle perturbations of these natural phenomena can direct the distribution and discharge of the Earth's EM forces.[60]

In *Under An Ionized Sky,* I talked about the airborne, wide angle, staring radar known as Gotcha Spiral II (2.75 GHz) casting a 10-20 km net over the urban battlespace. Gotcha can see through everything and still be "processed" as 3D SAR (synthetic aperture radar), which means 3D SAR and 3D video detection and ranging (ViDAR), Doppler radar imaging systems that basically take photographs with radar. As activist Raphaelle O'Neill of New Orleans observed:

> *I strongly suspect the ultimate goal of 5G, besides for obvious kill grid & mind control purposes, is to replace Doppler by treating EVERY cell tower and EVERY home as a mini-microwave Doppler that can localize weather even more specifically, using every one of us to pulse the energy over the area. Every hurricane in the 2017 season made landfall on radar EYE FOR EYE!*

---

58 Determined by numerical dosimetry. See C. Gabriel, Compilation of the Dielectric Properties of Body Tissues at RF and Microwave Frequencies, Report N.AL/OE-TR-1996-0037, Occupational and Environmental Health Directorate, Radiofrequency Radiation Division, Brooks Air Force Base, Texas (USA), 1996. Also see "Radio Frequency Radiation Dosimetry Handbook (Fifth Edition)," Air Force Research Lab, 2009, https://cdn.shopify.com/s/files/1/2779/0756/files/ADA536009_Dosimetry_a73f2254-a2f6-4e77-ac85-f3f1bc08f4c6.pdf?397289.

59 Thanks to "Helena," a targeted individual.

60 Email from Christopher Fontenot, 2015.

Katrina was at LEAST 5 Dopplers in a row . . .

According to Wikipedia, the *Doppler effect* is the change in frequency of a wave in relation to an observer who is moving relative to the wave source. Traffic police use Doppler radar guns to get an accurate reading of how fast our vehicles are going, and Doppler radar is used by NexRad weather systems to create low and high pressure zones, measure and steer hurricanes, tornadoes, and superstorms.[61] The National Weather Service, the FAA and U.S. Air Force depend upon Doppler, including the 159 S-band Doppler radars for remote sensing.

Doppler radar was active decades before HAARP, possibly since 1899 when Tesla was wirelessly creating thick fog around his Colorado Springs lab. Doppler radar categories according to radar wavelength: L,S,C,X,K.

> **L band** - wavelength 15-30 cm, frequency 1-2 GHz
> **S band** - wavelength 8-15 cm, frequency 2-4 GHz
> **C band** - wavelength 4-8 cm, frequency 4-8 GHz
> **X band** - wavelength 2.5-4 cm, frequency 8-12 GHz
> **K band** - wavelength .75-1.2 cm or 1.7-2.5 cm, frequency 27-40 GHz and 12-18 GHz, split down the middle due to a strong absorption line in water vapor.

FLIR (forward-looking infrared) radiometer

FLIRs (forward-looking infrared radiometers) are electronic heat sensors or thermal-imaging cameras able to detect a person's presence and movements at a distance (depending upon antenna and power) but cannot see through walls or roofs, metal or wet porous concrete. For that, WiFi RANGER radar is needed, along with TTWS (through the wall sensors). Terahertz radar can also penetrate walls (300 GHz to 10 THz).

> An infrared camera is a non-contact device that detects infrared energy (heat) and converts it into an electronic signal, which is then processed to produce a thermal image on a video monitor and perform temperature calculations. Heat sensed by an infrared camera can be very precisely quantified, or measured, allowing you to not only monitor thermal performance, but also identify and evaluate the relative severity of heat-related problems.[62]

It is the MEMS (microelectromechanical sensors) in the FLIR that detect the heat, whether of a hot car engine or a human being.

---

61 See "Dopplarized Dorian: Extended Radar Analysis of Weaponized Weather," nolabutterfly, September 7, 2019. "Doppler is weather on demand."

62 FLIR, "How Does an IR Camera Work?" http://www.flir.com/corporate/display/?id=41523

Unmanned aerial vehicles (UAVs) / drones / helicopters

Domestically, the Drug War was what gave unmanned aerial vehicles (UAVs) or drones like the Predator access to civilian areas. In retrospect, drones seem to have always figured into cell phone coverage (electronic warfare or EW) and Smart City "canyon" navigation.

Domestic control *sensor hover drones* are generally up to a meter in diameter, weigh just 120 kilograms (made of superlight composites like boron-graphite), hover between 50 and 500 feet, and travel up to 50 miles per hour. Like the TU-95 turbo-prop airplanes the Russians used to build, the engine is in the middle top with two counter-rotating rotors. (Counter-synchronous props guarantee higher lift, speed and stability.) Fusion power cells are controlled by satellite and triangulate off of fixed or mobile relay command centers built into Humvees and cell towers. Fitted with micro-cameras—infrared, high-resolution with multiple neutral density filters and thermal-imaging sensors that see through walls—the drones are camouflaged for stealth. Their audio receivers can pick up conversations from 500 feet away, and their stun guns are active denial (80,000 volts). They can detain and question people, setting the tone with, "Citizen, kindly present your (national or vaccine) identification card."

UAVs connected to trans-atmospheric jets, space platforms, and satellites, on the other hand, can "loiter along at 50,000 feet and stare 230 miles downrange at a Locus of Values (LOV) and provide continuous one meter resolution . . . [A] low observable UAV that loiters directly over a specific area will carry sensors that provide continuous one-centimeter resolution."[63]

In 2014, DARPA's Mobile Hotspot drones; in 2015, Project Loon, the "cell tower in the sky" beamed 4G LTE (long-term evolution) signals over Indonesia's 17,000 islands; in 2016, Google's parent company Alphabet added solar-powered Titan drones with millimeter wave transceivers (70-80 GHz) delivering Internet with an ERP (effective radiated power) of 96.411W high gain phased array antenna beam to Project Loon, thus reserving Project Skybender for 5G.[64] ("Sky-bender" = over-the-horizon RADAR?)

The new solar-powered HAPSMobile "flying wing" Hawk 30[65] "atmospheric satellite" is a UAV-satellite combination that transmits an HDTV

---

63 Palit, "The Air Force Wants Your LOV."

64 Ron Amadeo, "Report details Google's 'Project Skybender' a 5G Internet drone program." Guardian, February 1, 2016; also see Edge Ison, "Google Parent Pulls Plug On Internet Drone Project Skybender, Shifts Focus On Internet Balloon Project Loon." iTechPost, January 13, 2017.

65 AeroVironment, designer of solar-powered UAV prototypes, is the Pentagon's top supplier of small drones in strategic partnership with Lockheed Martin for the Global Observer stratospheric geosynchronous satellite system.

signal and an IMT-2000 wireless communications signal from 65,000 feet (20,000 meters) as if it were a 12-mile-high transmitter tower. Stuart Hindle of SkyTower in Spaceport, a part of Truth or Consequences, New Mexico, calls SkyTowers "geostationary satellites without the time delay," capable of providing 1,000 times the fixed broadband local access capacity of a geostationary satellite using the same frequency band.[66]

It's the lower-flying drones that are slated for Smart City and rural surveillance and targeting. T-Hawk micro drones, the 19-gram Nano Hummingbird (AeroVironment), other NAVs (nano air vehicles) and MAVs (micro air vehicles)—mapleseed, sparrow, dragonfly, housefly—*all have biological components*, making them hybrid cyborg insects. Israel Aerospace Industries (IAI) can make the MAV Mosquito and Bird's Eye 400 shapeshift into whatever is on the remote monitor.

Helicopters too are employed—"black" helicopters, cloaked Apache and Cobra attack helicopters on whisper mode and equipped for night fights. MH-60 Black Hawks, AC-130J Ghostrider gunships armed with beam-steering laser weapons (60-150 kW) and thermal management, etc. Radar-proof F-117A Stealth fighters with AWACS (radar on top) for big-picture intelligence, JSTARS radar on the bottom, and fitted with ELF weapons in their bomb bays work in tandem with the TR3A Black Manta. The 1988 Bell OH-58D helicopters are stealth-modified with an external seat for a sniper and reactive skin that changes color for camouflage.

> Futuristic engagement systems and techniques such as holographic projection, noise and gravity fields, biomedical operations, psychological operations, military deception, and information attack are all possible . . .[67]

"Futuristic engagement systems" include "getting into our heads" with space and plasma mirrors bouncing data to and from UAVs, military ground stations, and Homeland Security Fusion Centers:

> . . . Sure enough, the principles of automated sensor fusion are already catching on in the domestic sphere. About 80 local law enforcement agencies in 49 states, the District of Columbia, Puerto Rico, the US Virgin Islands, and Guam operate so-called fusion centers modeled on military war rooms that serve as a clearinghouse for information collected by a range of different agencies and private organizations . . . Meanwhile, a number of U.S. law enforcement departments, including the Los Angeles

66 http://en.wikipedia.org/wiki/AeroVironment.

67 Yasmin Tadjdeh, "Special Operations Command to Test Directed Energy Weapons on Apache." National Defense, May 26, 2016.

Police Department, the Metropolitan Police Department in Washington, D.C., and the Virginia State Police have operated fusion software developed by the Silicon Valley firm Palantir . . . [that] has worked extensively with the Pentagon and the intelligence community . . .[68]

DARPA's ARGUS-IS[69] (Autonomous Real-time Ground Ubiquitous Surveillance Imaging System)—"an advanced [WAMI wide area motion imagery] camera system that uses hundreds of cellphone cameras [5mm chips] in a mosaic to video and auto-track every moving object within a 15-square-mile area [50 square km]"[70]—is a composite focal plane array (CFPA) of 368 overlapping FPAs imaging Smart City sectors at 10 Hz (Alpha wave) to create VR video windows of the most powerful GPUs (graphics processing units), detect and track moving objects, access forensic archives, and generate 3D models for targeting.[71] ARGUS-IS flies at an altitude of 25,000 feet and needs "an internet connection 16,000 times faster than the fastest wireless internet service available in the United States in 2017."[72]

Thermal and hyperspectral (IR) imaging combined with electro-optical (EO) sensors and HDTV cameras (Hawk-Eye, Eagle-EYE, UltraCam Osprey) on imaging drones like the high-altitude long-endurance (HALE) Global Hawk and the FLIR Black Hornet nano-UAV (weighing less than one ounce!) are the name of the game when it comes to Smart City C5ISR (command, control, communications, computers, combat, intelligence, surveillance, reconnaissance).

The Magnetron

A *magnetron* was used in the summer of 1984 outside the 15-mile chain-link fence around the Royal Air Force Greenham Common in England against 30,000 women protesting the deployment of U.S. nuclear-tipped cruise missiles. High-frequency oscillations (pulses) generated ultra-short waves that invisibly moved through the gate. Women had swollen tongues, racing heart ar-

---

68 Arthur Holland Michel, "Military-Grade Surveillance, Coming Soon to a Police Department Near You." GENMedium.com, June 18, 2019. Also see Jacques Peretti, "Palantir: the 'special ops' tech giant that wields as much real-world power as Google," The Guardian, 30 July 2017.

69 In Greek mythology, Argus was a giant with 100 eyes covering his head.

70 Jay Stanley, "Drone 'Nightmare Şcenario' Now Has A Name: ARGUS." ACLU, February 21, 2013. Other wide-area persistent surveillance (WAPS) systems: Persistent Surveillance, Vigilant Stare, Pixia's HiPER STARE. See Wikipedia.

71 Thanks to Robert "Bobby" Worrell, U.S. Marines intelligence operative, and "The HAARP Man" Billy Hayes.

72 Arthur Holland Michel, Eyes in the Sky: The Secret Rise of GORGON STARE and How It Will Watch Us All. New York: Houghton Mifflin Harcourt, 2019.

rhythmia, immobility, pains in the upper body, skin burns, severe headaches, drowsiness, post-menopausal menstrual bleeding, spontaneous miscarriages, and impaired speech. Anyone approaching the metal fence felt a loss of focus, headache, and nausea. Those driving in the area had fatal heart attacks and driver-blackouts due to the resonance between the magnetron and the overhead power lines. Measurements from an EMR meter indicated beams 100X normal background levels swept the women's camp.[73]

The magnetron generates EHF microwaves by generating electrons with a *cathode*, a hollow cylinder coated with barium and strontium oxide electron emitters, and a cylindrical *anode* with resonant cavities on its inner surface to combine a magnetic field with an electrical field. Switch the magnetron on and a radial electrical field arises between the anode and cathode while the magnetic field arises coaxial (along the same axis) with the cathode. A large magnetron can generate a consistent beam of microwave pulses equaling 10 million watts per pulse. Magnetrons power radar transmitters but also have to do with *tuning resonant components* like laser waveguides, phased array antennas, feed-horn and oscillation cavities, etc. In other words, it's not just about high energy output but about pulses.

The *cavity magnetron* specifically activates metal nanoparticles.

Taser

The *Taser* is an ECT / electroshock weapon modeled on the cattle prod: two small electrode darts connected to a copper wire puncture the skin to deliver a modulated electric current of 5,900 milliwatts straight up the arm and into the chest to cause "neuromuscular incapacitation." (The Air Taser launches the two wires with air compression.) There is no uniform code for Tasers.

Police are no longer subject to the "force continuum":

Police Use-of-Force Continuum

1. *Police presence*
2. *Issue commands*
3. *Use of open hands*
4. *Pepper or chemical sprays*
5. *Closed hands (elbows, knees, takedown moves)*
6. *Use of hard baton*
7. *Use of lethal force*

Tasers are now between #2 and #3, not #6 and #7. Verbally noncompliant? Taser time. Low amperage (.004) is interpreted as not being the direct cause

73 See William Thomas, Scorched Earth: The Military's Assault on the Environment. New Society Publishers, 1994.

of death, and yet it is the current that depolarizes skeletal muscle, the shock alone exacerbating breathing when coupled with exertion, fear, pain, drugs or alcohol, restraints, etc. *The heart is a muscle.*

Tasers and stun belts are favorites of the U.S. Bureau of Prisons. Jail and prison guards have used cattle prods (stun batons) and stun belts carrying 5,000 to 10,000 volts for years. The 2000 Taser International (now Axon) M26 shoots the two wires 21 feet to deliver 50,000 volts for five seconds.[74] Stun Tech put out an 8-second, 50,000-volt shock for transporting prisoners that completely eradicated the line between control and torture. Whereas the X26 had more "stopping power" and happily left little physical evidence of torture, the M26 data chip recorded the time and date of each firing so as to keep tabs on the officer's use of force. Wisconsin put stun belts on their Fox Lake chain gangs, even on under-18-year-olds, and jails like Maricopa County in Arizona, under America's self-professed toughest sheriff, swore by Tasers.

The U.S. Commerce Department categorizes electroshock weapons as "police equipment." The stun belt, however, needs a specific license for export. When such torture devices leave the country, it is impossible to find out exactly where they go. NATO countries allow stun devices as "general merchandise."

VMADS / ADS

If a crowd doesn't disperse, the *MEDUSA ray gun* uses low-power microwaves to create a buzzing in people's heads, then makes them think that God is talking to them. The *Stun Strike resonant transformer* (Tesla coil) shoots out bolts of lightning with an adjustable "punch," the 007 version being a "needle" sticking out of a briefcase that sends snakes of purple lightning accompanied by a deafening rattle. The *Scream* and *LRAD (long-range acoustic device)* are vehicle-mounted sonic blasters that shoot beams of sound.

On March 1, 2001, Raytheon's *VMADS (vehicle-mounted active denial system)* was announced by the *Marine Corps Times*, the first "nonlethal" directed energy weapon designed specifically for use against humans—a Raytheon gem developed at Kirtland Air Force Base for the Marines to operate.[75]

---

74 Direct contact firing is more powerful, of course, and holding the trigger down even more so.

75 The Airborne Laser, the world's first combat aircraft armed with a directed energy weapon, came out of Kirtland, too. Kirtland is home to the secret Space Rapid Capabilities Office, purveyor of exotic crafts like the X-37B robotic spaceplane, B-21 Raider, and HTV-2 Falcon hypersonic technology vehicle ("hypersonic glide") that tops out at 13,000 mph (21,000 km/hr.) or Mach 17.53. The weapons division of high-powered microwave (HPM) technologies is under the Air Force Research Laboratory's Directed Energy Directorate at Kirtland Air Force Base in Albuquerque, New Mexico. The high desert side includes the High Energy Microwave Laboratory (25,261 square feet), the High Energy Research and Technology Facility (26,287 square feet), and the High Power Systems Facility (34,261 square feet)

The "people zapper" focuses energy into a beam of micromillimeter microwaves traveling at the speed of light and is designed to stop an individual in his tracks. The 130ºF microwaves rapidly heat the water molecules 1/64 of an inch under the skin and make them vibrate (resonance). The exact length, frequency and amplitude of the waves were originally classified, but it was obvious, given that human beings are 70 percent water . . . Department of Defense Directive 3000.3 makes provision for a built-in rheostat so a soldier doesn't *cook* the target.

Mounted on a Humvee, the mere sight of the VMADS strikes terror (what is called "winning hearts and minds"). Urban control camouflaged Humvees originally weighed three tons and sported 14.5 mm cannons plus aerial and satellite dishes, a 72-inch wide track and low center of gravity, the tires ready to be inflated (hard ground) or deflated (sand) at the flick of a switch. Eight miles to the gallon but clocking 90 miles per hour at 4,000 rpms and going from 0 to 60 in 19.5 seconds.

Psychological operations (psyops) convince the mind, electromagnetic or sonic weapons the flesh. Dialed low, VMADS allows citizens to continue working and consuming. ADS patrols, the new price of peace, should be expected in the armed Smart City, now that war and terrorism are a way of life.

The *New York Times* says the *Active Denial System (ADS)* is a peacekeeping tool intended to "influence motivational behavior," which translates to "attack human functions, render the disenfranchised physically immobilized, emotionally stupefied and incapable of meaningful thought."

During the Iraq War (2003-2011) under Project Sheriff, armored personnel carriers Stryker and infantry mobility Cougar delivered nonmilitary "black teams" and Active Denial antenna arrays under gray plastic domes two feet in diameter to 25 rooftops throughout Fallujah, City of Mosques in the Sunni Triangle. A sound system forewarned noncombatants that they are to disperse, return to their homes, etc. An excruciating noise accompanied the Laser Dazzler as it scanned for snipers. (The Dazzler looks like an executive pen but emits either a green laser that temporarily blinds or ultra-sonic waves that convey messages the target thinks are coming from his or her brain. The PD/G-105 is twice as strong as the Dazzler.) The domes were plugged into a power unit, then set to "LONG WAVE." ULF and VLF waves then ride out and pass through a half-mile of metal and concrete to get to the skulls and bellies of the remaining population. Nausea, incontinence, disorientation, vomiting, melting internal organs, and slow death follow. Directed energy beams lose no potency when moving from air into tissue; pulsed at 7 Hz, people are sick for hours. American and British bombardments destroyed buildings and

---

that houses the Shiva Star, which stores 10 million joules of energy and produces a pulse of 120,000 volts and 10 million amps in one-millionth of a second to produce a terawatt of power. The Directed Energy Directorate also includes Laser and Optics Divisions.

displaced 250,000 residents. Thousands died, including women, children and elderly, as Israel sent invisible electromagnetic waves into Gaza and Lebanon.

The Active Denial pain ray is 95 GHz (the same frequency as 5G beams), firing 3mm beams from a device just twelve centimeters larger than a microwave oven. Water molecules in the skin heat up to 130°F in less than a second. The beam's intensity is the same at any distance, far beyond the 550-meter range of bullets.[76] Moving rapidly from nonlethal to lethal force from panic and pain to melting flesh and organs and mind control, this is *fourth generation warfare.*

GWEN towers and mobile telephone systems are calibrated to be able to operate in the same frequency range as frequency weapons.

VTRPE, Barium and Cloaking

> *I saw cloud-jacketed drones on the airstrip one night here at Davis-Monthan AFB [Tucson AZ] during foggy rainy inclement weather! There were mechanic and landing personnel on the tarmac tending to a line of them just yards from the installation fence. They step up on ladders and make adjustments or maybe just start them, but I could clearly make out, even at night 50 yards away without my glasses, that these were like 8 foot high and 15 feet long, camouflaged in an almost raincoat-like fitting chemical fog / cloud cloak that just hangs there kinda breathing if you like, unfazed and unaffected by drizzle, wind, human ingress or mechanical interference. They leave the runaway fairly brisk, outbal and up, I'd guess, at 25-40 mph, no lights, then just vanish as they blend in with the actual weather.*
>
> – Michael Todd

The U.S. Navy's Radio Frequency Mission Planner (RFMP) computer program known as the *Variable Terrain Radio Parabolic Equation (VTRPE)* is dependent upon chemical trail delivery of barium salts. Barium titanate and barium stearate are particularly useful for radar operations. Crystals of barium titanate capture the pulses of electromagnetic frequencies the way a radio picks up radio frequencies, so that when the crystal pulses or resonates, electric power is produced.[77] Barium stearate is basically soap that bonds with metal nanoparticles[78] and aids high-tech 3D radar imaging like VTRPE.

76 A thin suit of armor or aluminum foil might provide protection if the rheostat isn't turned up to the high-powered microwave (HPM) range, but once it is, the body will cook like a turkey in foil.

77 Jeane Manning, "Free Energy: Making the Impossible Possible: A New Physics for a New Energy Source." MerLIB, no date.

78 Soapy foam is sometimes found on the ground after chemtrail operations.

- With a sophisticated fifth generation laptop or satellite computer, VTRPE can analyze geometrics for target acquisition and beam control, then once the telemetry for attack pulses is set, lock onto the target.[79]
- VTRPE can be used to view what an enemy radar system sees, after which it can model 3D images on monitors, then utilize radio waves or microwaves propagated by HAARP / Starfire laser / satellite laser to generate 3D images at the intersect of three interfering beams over the target area (interferometry).
- VTRPE is used to cloak jets, stealth fighters, and helicopters behind signal inversion layers of plasma ("plasmonic cover"), similar to how submarines cloak themselves from sonar beams in underwater inversion layers. Early attempts at cloaking followed the chameleon approach of matching the background by reducing scattered light, but with a plasma cloud, the background can be reflected *in front* to create invisibility,[80] and with an onboard computer that adjusts for brightness, hue, and texture, electrochromic materials coupled with photosensitive receptors can make a jet match the sky above or terrain below.
- Ionized barium nanoparticles in the atmosphere and phased arrays like HAARP work in concert with VTRPE code for "a full-wave propagation model that solves EM wave equations for complex electric and magnetic radiation fields."[81]

> . . . Initially, the VTRPE computer program only worked accurately over water and along coastal areas but not over land masses because the system's radar waves required an atmospheric condition known as "ducting," over land, to operate accurately.
>
> This "ducting" problem was solved by releasing an aerosol, a mixture of barium salts into the atmosphere over the United States. Thus, they can make an atmospheric radio frequency "duct" with a base of barium aerosol released from aircraft . . . The chemical and electrical characteristics of the mixture cause moisture to stay in the clouds. The aerosol sets up an electrical and chemical environmental that supports RF ducting for the RFMP/VTRPE warfare system. The mixture of barium salt from the aerosol when sprayed in a straight line will also provide a ducting path form point A to point B and will enable high

79 VTRPE would be utilized for vaporific effect ignitions.

80 See "The Rochester Digital Cloak: A New Age of Invisibility," University of Rochester Institute of Optics, September 25, 2014.

81 Frank J. Ryan, "User's Guide for the VTRPE Computer Model." Naval Ocean Systems Center, October 1991; funded by the Joint Electronic Warfare Center and the Office of Naval Technology.

frequency communications along that path, even over the curvature of the Earth, in both directions," he said. "Enemy high frequency communications can be monitored easier with the straight line A to B ducting medium."[82]

- VTRPE is used for invisible torture and kidnapping by "ghost perps" or "invisi-perps" [perpetrators] using a "Ghost Machine" the size of a cell phone with a small horn protruding from the edge. (See Chapter 11.)

> With a computerized system, you could screen out things you wanted to screen out, or you could make it appear to be something that it really is not. You could make a human being appear to be an animal, let's say, or a tree, or . . . you could paint a portrait on the surface of the object of whatever you wanted it to be. It does not necessarily have to blend in with the background. If you had difficulty blending it, for example, make it a tree. That looks natural . . . Yeah, it could be used for psychological warfare.[83]

As the Smart City goes up around us, we'll need a lexicon of its dual-use machines as they affect our mental and physical wellbeing.

---

82 Mike Blair, "Military Behind Mystery Chemtrails." Spotlight, June 21, 2001. Also see "January 2, 2010 – A.C. Griffith, Chemtrails." Barb Adams Live, https://barbadamslive.com/?p=873.

83 Robert Guffey, Chameleo: A Strange But True Story of Invisible Spies, Heroin Addiction, and Homeland Security. OR Books, 2015.

10

Dual Use II: Pulsed Frequencies

Lighting
Light-emitting diodes (LEDs)
Light Fidelity (LiFi)
The Lilly Wave
LiDAR (light detection and ranging)
Pulsed energy projection (PEP)
Smart TV Monitors
The "white-space" network
Infrasonic, ultrasonic
Towers (masts) & antennas
Fiber optics

PULSED MODULATIONS JACKHAMMER AWAY AT our natural Schumann resonance day and night, whether we "hear" or "feel" it or not. The most harmful modulations to human beings are *pulsed* modulations; each pulse or spike shocks our frail DC electrical system and immune system, which, after many attempts to protect us, is finally exhausted.

Take, for instance, the radio. The AM radio is amplitude modulation, FM is frequency modulation. FM *carrier* frequencies range from 87.5 MHz to 106.5 MHz, M standing for *mega* or millions, Hz (Hertz) for pulse cycles per second, whereas the *audio* frequency spans 10 Hz to 20 kHz, k standing for *kilo* or thousands of cycles per second. Once the carrier frequency delivers the music or news, the radio then de-modulates it so you can hear the audio frequency.

> To give you an idea of power density and sensitivity of instruments, let's consider an FM radio station 20 miles away emitting 50 kilowatts of power. The receiver would only measure 2.1×10^{-5} W/m^2. That's what your car radio receives, demodulates, and amplifies for your listening pleasure. A one Terahertz[1] sub-millimeter wavelength radio antenna such as the 10-meter Heinrich Hertz telescope[2] can view a typical radio source intensity of 10^{-26} W/m^2 through the Earth's atmosphere. Do you still

1 One trillion cycles per second. Light will only travel 3 millimeters in the time it takes the wave to make a full cycle. Terahertz is capable of unzipping double-stranded DNA.

2 http://soral.as.arizona.edu/overview.html

believe that RADAR brain resonances cannot be read by satellite radio telescopes?[3]

Lighting

Then there is lighting. Remember: pay attention to the *pulsing.*

Incandescent and halogen bulbs are analog and thermal, whereas LEDs are digital and nonthermal. Incandescent or sodium lighting—that old orange glow—was internationally phased out in 2005 but in the United States lasted until 2014. Unlike fluorescent and LED bulbs, incandescent bulbs have *near-infrared (NIR)* in them, which is not "thermal waste." NIR prevents macular degeneration, encourages melatonin production, and provides mitochondrial ATP (adenosine triphosphate) for cellular energy, while measuring the intensity of NIR absorbed by brain tissue can spell out a person's preferences and decision-making process. *Near-infrared spectroscopy (NIRS)* in the prefrontal cortex is the signal acquisition tool of choice for "noninvasive" BCI.[4]

The *fluorescent or mercury-vapor lamp* became standard lighting for commercial use in the 1930s. While incandescent bulbs were used in homes, fluorescent tubes found their way to sports arenas, street lighting, schools, office buildings, etc. An arc of electric current passing through the tube excited the mercury-vapor gas and produced UV light (400 nm to 10 nm) which then caused the phosphorus coating on the inside of the tube to glow. The chemicals in fluorescent lighting are phosphor, mercury, fluoride, antimony, manganese, aluminum oxide, barium, strontium, and lead oxide.[5]

Where have we heard about these metals before?

Mercury-vapor lights are finally being phased out, but the spiral-shaped compact fluorescent lamps (CFLs) have been around since the 1970s, despite containing mercury and emitting UV radiation.[6] If a CFL breaks, people and pets must leave the room immediately, central heating or air conditioning shut off, and the room aired out before any cleanup can commence. Both CFLs and LEDs, along with television and computer monitors, emit far more blue light than incandescent light bulbs. Blue light suppresses the secretion

---

3 Robert Duncan, The Matrix Deciphered. Higher Order Thinkers Publishing, 2006.

4 Sheena Luu et al., "Decoding subjective preference from single-trial near-infrared spectroscopy signals." Journal of Neural Engineering, February 2009. Luu's superior Tom Chan worked in pediatric rehab engineering at the University of Toronto Bloorview Kids Rehab Center.

5 Thanks to Brian McCarthy, March 8, 2015.

6 See Samuel Milham and Dave Stetzer, "The electronics in fluorescent bulbs and light emitting diodes (LED), rather than ultraviolet radiation, cause increased malignant melanoma incidence in indoor office workers and tanning bed users." Medical Hypotheses, Vol. 116, July 2018, pages 33-39.

of melatonin and disrupts the circadian rhythm that our immune system depends upon. Blue light every night is like a full moon every night instead of once a month: not good for us.[7]

On the day before President Trump's inauguration, outgoing President Obama's Department of Energy (DOE) crushed the cheap incandescent light bulb in favor of the *light-emitting diode (LED).* Perhaps the 11th hour high priority was because the LEDs go hand in glove with the 5G / IoT weapon system.[8]

Don't forget: like windows, light bulbs can be used for eavesdropping, simply by capturing the sound vibrations in a room:

> According to this [Lamphone Attack] technique, a person can eavesdrop on a conversation from around 82 feet or 25 meters away if a light bulb is hanging near the conversation spot. One can detect the vibration of the bulb, which is produced due to the air pressure fluctuations during the conversation—that is, the traveling sound waves. When the sound wave hits the walls of the room, it bounces back and produces small vibrations that can be picked up by electro-optical sensors if it is focused on the bulb.[9]

Light-emitting diodes (LEDs)

"Smart" LED streetlights may be the "intelligent, networked, sensor-laden . . . central nervous system of every smart building,"[10] but they also produce an aggressive blue wavelength that produces oxidative stress.[11] As low-voltage semiconductors, they are perfect for digital control, and unlike analog high-voltage light sources of the past, they work well with the Smart City Internet of Things (IoT) / Internet of Bodies (IoB), smart schools where biometric sensors track student alertness, megastores where product choices are tracked, and at home where the IoT self-learns from the stream of data generated by "software-focused" sensors everywhere LED lighting is. "If you can see [LED lights], networked sensors in the light can see you."

The "Array of Things" project being put together by the University

---

7 The Fullerton Informer, "BLUE LIGHT OF DEATH: Blue light at night is killing you and it is all by design," May 6, 2018.

8 Trump's DOE repealed Obama's DOE "green" move. The orange glow of the incandescent is on its way back. See Michael Barnes, "Trump's Energy Dept. Wants to Roll Back Obama's Light Bulb Ban." Liberty Headlines, February 8, 2019.

9 Mayukh Saha, "From 80 Feet Away, Hackers Can Use Light Bulbs To Spy On Conversations." Truth Theory, July 1, 2020.

10 Brian Chemel, "How Intelligent Lighting Is Ushering In The Internet Of Buildings." techcrunch.com, December 20, 2015.

11 Dr. Mercola, "How LED Lighting May Compromise Your Health" (including Dr. Alexander Wunsch). Mercola.com, October 23, 2016. I recommend reading John D. Christian's The Light Bulb Mafia (2014), available as a .pdf on the Internet.

of Chicago and Argonne National Laboratory's Urban Center for Computation and Data will collect details about air quality, light intensity, sound volume, heat, precipitation and wind . . . as well as lay the groundwork for a vast infrastructure that will ideally let this kind of data and even more be collected for ages to come using additional new sensors . . . *"Our intention is to understand cities better,"* computer scientist and Urban Center director Charlie Catlett told the Tribune. *"Part of the goal is to make these things essentially a public utility."*[12]

The outspoken British critic of 5G and LEDs, Mark Steele, is CTO of Reevu, a high-tech helmet company. Steele researched the LED streetlights in his Gateshead community on the North Sea near Newcastle and feels that they should be classified as lasers, not just as a Risk Group 2 for retinal thermal hazard.[13] It's about the *lens*, Steele stresses, not the power density (element + cohesion). The LEDs have no diffusers, and thus the lens shines phototoxic blue light dead-on like a laser. (Blue light emission = retinal cell damage.)

LEDs on streetlights are also 3D scanners. On parkways, motion sensors make the LED bulbs glow brighter as each car passes,[14] each scan radiating those in the car. (Is this Echelon's Lumewave MXW-LVE-18OU Bluetooth-enabled very long-range radar-based sensor and controller weapon system?) A normal yesteryear streetlight needs 250 volts, but these LED streetlights have 450-volt high-voltage boards, plus 3,300-watt relays. *Why so much power for streetlights?* Steele believes we are looking at urban battlefield environment scanning radar.[15]

Smart LED streetlights and lampposts 20-30 meters apart are more often than not accompanied by 5G / IoT high-density base station equipment, along with environmental sensors, cameras, communications gear, WiFi hotspots, metrics for parking, noise, crowd analytics, radar, public safety, pollution, weather, infotainment displays, even microphones in high-crime neighborhoods. This is surveillance street lighting. Is it any wonder that people enduring this "lighting" suffer nosebleeds, insomnia, birth defects, cancer, and mental health issues? 5G satellite and ground transmitters blast signals

12 "New high-tech lampposts in Chicago will collect data on weather and people," RT, 23 June 2014.

13 Cree "Eye Safety With LED Components," 2009, https://www.cree.com/led-components/media/documents/XLamp_EyeSafety.pdf.

14 See Shilan Liu, "Microwave motion sensor test for street light," May 23, 2018, https://www.youtube.com/watch?v=dnmhgxFS10Q&feature=youtu.be.

15 See "5G Apocalypse London Mark Steele," The London Event Citizen Action Meeting, Chelsea Town Hall, London, September 29, 2019. Humanitad and ITNJ founder Sacha Stone, Swiss Biohazard Research Scientist Jacques Bauer, Barrister & ITNJ Associate Justice Dr Chris Cleverly, Chief Sylvestre Gnakale of the Ivory Coast, and UK Police & Crimes Commissioner Anthony Stansfeld.

into homes as LED lights disrupt nitrogen monoxide systems that control gene expression and challenge endocrine systems. And what does this say about the food grown in state-of-the-art underground and covered gardens / farms under "advanced LED lighting"?[16]

In the Smart City, 4G LTE may be used for environmental, traffic, and security monitoring while 5G phased array antennas tacked onto LED lampposts and 4G microwave towers and everywhere possible are reserved not just for faster image transmission but for targeting of groups, neighborhoods, and individuals.[17] By increasing the LED flicker (pulse) rate, data can be transmitted via visible spectrum light instead of radio and microwaves.

Light Fidelity (LiFi)

Key advantages to LiFi wireless networking:

- *3X enhanced data density*
- *Communication security / secure from hacking*
- *Can use where RF is banned (petrochemical plants, oil platforms)*
- *Piggybacks onto existing data network infrastructures for required backhaul*[18]
- *Does not need direct line of sight*
- *Limitless capacity*
- *10X cheaper than WiFi*

Whereas fiber optics uses light amplification by stimulated emission of laser radiation, LiFi is an optical wireless communication technology (OWC) that works perfectly with LEDs for Internet connectivity via the visible spectrum instead of radio waves. In fact, it is LEDs that led to the possibility of using the visible light spectrum for wireless networking. Whereas WiFi uses radio frequency to transmit data, LiFi uses UV and IR light while LEDs serve as router and light detectors on the terahertz bandwidth (400-800 THz) at higher transmission speeds (224+ Gbps and climbing). LiFi light waves can't penetrate walls, but their light transmissions can reflect off of walls at 70 Mbps (megabits per second). Infrared and the visible light spectrum together are 2600X the size of the entire 300 GHz radio frequency spectrum, whereas 6 THz bandwidth is only 0.8% of the entire IR and visible light spectrum.

---

16 Christina Sarich, "Subterranean Farm to Harvest 2.5 Acres of Produce 100 Feet Below Ground Level." Natural Society, July 9, 2015.

17 "Smart LED street lights become a 5G connection platform." Tenco-Tech.com, March 28, 2019.

18 Backhaul: unedited transmission via satellite or other means to a network station. For example, the EtherHaul-600T small-cell backhaul system operates in the unlicensed 57-66 GHz V-band spectrum. "Wireless fiber" for 6G MIMO (multiple input, multiple output) small-cell network backhaul and datacenter connectivity is a tractor beam.

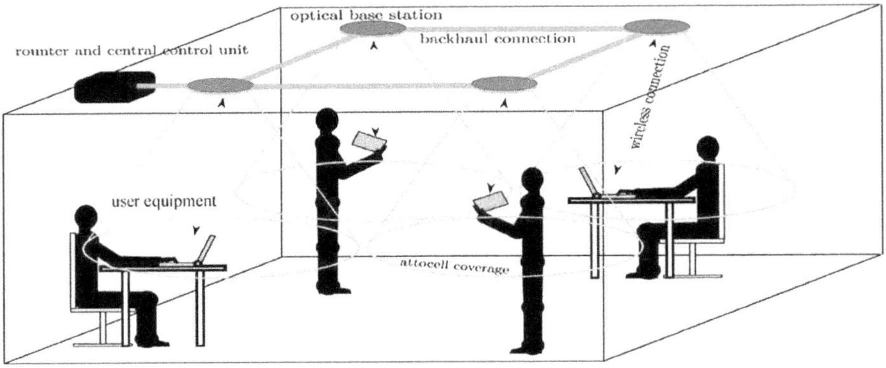

LiFi Networking. Visible light communication.

https://www.nanalyze.com/2019/11/lifi-visible-light-communication-internet/

Industrial, scientific, and medical bandwidth require more bandwidth like WiGig (wireless gigabit alliance), which uses the 57-66 GHz unlicensed spectrum. This need for more and more has led to the *small cell concept,* except that further reduction in cell sizes means higher infrastructure costs for enough backhaul and fronthaul data links. (WiFi access points have even been mounted under stadium seats, which means using thousands of human bodies as attenuators for RF signals to avoid line-of-sight interference.)

While LiFi is particularly well suited to EM interference interiors like aircraft cabins, hospitals, nuclear power plants, cubicle-studded offices, etc., it also operates like radar in geoengineered skies, one example being the on-off LiFi blue beam energy transfer switch for satellite optics triggering ignition of nanotech-driven "wildfires." Two-way LiFi can be used to spy, program, record and adjust frequency modulations.

In a *LiFi attocell network*, each light is driven by a LiFi modem or chip and equipped with an integrated infrared detector for receiving signals from the light terminals:

> The resulting high frequency flickers are much higher than the refresh rate of a computer monitor . . . An optical uplink is implemented by using a transmitter on the user equipment (UE), often using an IR source (so it is invisible to the user). Each of these light fixtures, which at the same time act as wireless LiFi APs [access points], create an extremely small cell, an optical attocell . . . [taking] the 'small cell concept' to a new level by creating ultra-small cells with radii less than 5m while exploiting the huge additional unlicensed spectrum in the optical domain . . .

potentially, all light fixtures can contain APs . . . Within each cell, there can be several users.[19]

Bg-Fi is the LiFi mobile app with a microcontroller, embedded software, and color sensor geared to making IoT communication more effective. Bg-Fi communicates to the IoT product's color sensor and converts the light into digital information, while the LED in the IoT product enables simultaneous synchronization with the mobile device.[20]

> LiFi is a fundamental 5G technology. It can unlock the IoT, drive Industry 4.0 applications, light-as-a-service (LaaS) in the lighting industry, enable new intelligent transport systems, enhance road safety when there are more and more driverless cars, create new cybersecure wireless networks, enable new ways of health monitoring of aging societies, offer new solutions to close the digital divide, and enable very high-speed wireless connectivity in future datacenters . . . It is therefore conceivable that the wireless industry and the lighting industry will merge into one . . . [and] inevitable that other spectrum than the RF spectrum must be used for future wireless communications systems. We therefore forecast a paradigm shift in wireless communications when moving from mm-wave communication to nm-wave communication which consequently involves light—i.e. LiFi.[21]

The Lilly Wave

> *The Lilly Wave frequency is a secret military application known as the "madness" frequency. The Los Angeles Riots [1992] are said to have been the first open test of its capacity to mass control anger and violent mob response . . . In short, the Lilly Wave is best described as a targeted resonance of the brain's molecules. Use of the Lilly Wave can pretty much install any brainwave pattern into the mind of any targeted human . . .*[22]

The Lilly Wave—also known as twin inverted pulse radar (TWIPR) or balanced bidirectional pulse pair—was invented by John C. Lilly, MD, while he was working for the National Institutes of Health (NIH) under the U.S. Navy in the late 1950s. The Lilly Wave is a carrier wave—microwaves, IR, visible light,

---

19 Harald Haas, "LiFi is a paradigm-shifting 5G technology." Reviews in Physics, November 2018.

20 "Li-Fi – The Revolutionary Wireless Technology that could Make Internet 100 Times Faster than Wi-Fi," FugenX.com, April 17, 2017.

21 Ibid.

22 Mind Guard Operating Systems, July 13, 2016.

UV, x-rays and gamma rays—that sends out two pulses in rapid succession, the second pulse being a phase inverted mirror image of the first (phase conjugate mirroring). The Lilly Wave leaves nerve ions intact, thus bypassing the mind's subconscious defense systems so body and mind do not mount a defense.

> [The Lilly Wave] is a bi-phasic electric pulse that stimulates the neurons of the brain to resonate at a certain frequency. Thus the Lilly wave has the ability to control the brainwave patterns of the brain. The water molecules within the brain can be made to resonate at a desired frequency, thus causing the electrons that comprise the brain's electrical voltages to also resonate at the same frequency . . .
>
> Dr. Lilly developed a new electrical waveform to balance the current, first in one direction and then, after a brief interval, in the other. Thus ions moving in the neurons would first be pushed one way and then quickly the other way, stimulating the neurons and leaving the ions in their former positions within the neurons. This new wave form was called a balanced bidirectional pulse pair, or the Lilly Wave.[23]

Police, intelligence operatives, and the U.S. Navy use a Lilly Wave to locate surveillance bugs and remote control brains. Once resistance is removed, any emotion or information can be transmitted to the target brain via ultrasonic (1-10 MHz) and electromagnetic wavelengths (600m to 1e-15m) from FM, TV, telephone, and wireless. By stimulating the neurons of the brain to resonate at a certain frequency, brain patterns can be read and controlled. No need for electrodes or implants to entrain the brain's water molecules, the body's blood sugar, or iron in the cells; any waveform that can penetrate the skull can be used to entrain the brain's water molecules because *we are resonant beings*. All can now be remotely pulsed—all that's needed are electromagnetic and acoustic waves. But if the wave is not bi-phasic like the Lilly Wave, the brain will be damaged.

> The technical problem in chronic brain stimulation is to stay above the excitatory threshold and below the injury threshold in the neuronal system under consideration. This result can be achieved most easily by the proper choice of waveforms and their time courses; and less easily by the choice of the range of repetition frequencies and train durations. The previous waveforms used in neurophysiology and in neurosurgery injured the neurons when unidirectional current passed through the brain.[24]

---

23 "The Lilly Wave and psychotronic warfare, The Bridge of Life in the Mix, 3 November 2015.

24 "Lilly Wave Mind Control Broadcasted in Homes Wall AC DC Outlets." Smart Meter News, February 1, 2016. Also see Chapter 5, "5G Wi-Gig & the Internet of Things."

While traveling around taking power grid measurements, scientist Patrick Flanagan, PhD, monitored ground and power lines with oscilloscopes and discovered that Homeland Security "black boxes" at utilities were producing Lilly Waves that were stacking ultrasonic waveform pulses on 60 Hz alternating current waves in people's homes.[25]

The Lilly Wave is targets brain molecular resonance.[26]

LiDAR (light detection and ranging)

LiDAR or lidar (light detection and ranging) is optical remote sensing via laser. It pulses ultraviolet (UV), visible, or near infrared (NIR) light to image objects (500 MHz to 50 GHz), similar to how sonar pulses sound and radar pulses radio waves,[27] or more simply the lidars loaded into robots, speed enforcement cameras, touch- and gesture-based controls for video games, and self-driving cars[28] that sense distance and proximity.

With its excellent signal propagation, lidar is used in surveying, tomography, and heterodyning (producing a lower frequency from combining two almost equal high frequencies). By measuring backscattered light to the target and back, distance as well as atmospheric density and the chemical signatures of compounds loaded with nano-sensors ("pollutants") in the clouds and aerosols over wide areas can be determined. (The Space Fence and HAARP actually work by pulsing and making backscatter radar and X-ray backscatter.) Airborne HALO's differential absorption lidar (DIAL) and high spectral resolution lidar (HSRL) measure atmospheric H2O and CH4 mixing ratios and aerosol / cloud / ocean optical properties with two UV wavelengths to analyze the signature of each gas.[29] As I described in *Under An Ionized Sky* in Chapter 7 under "Sensors":

> By bouncing light off of targets, LiDAR is far more accurate than radar when it comes to ranges and distances, plus LiDAR can carry digital information rather like fiber optics without the need for glass fibers. Stealth aircraft covered with radar-absorbent materials (RAM) that don't absorb laser signals use LiDAR, as do bomb damage assessment (BDA), reconnaissance, and chemical warfare agent detection. Unlike emission spec-

---

25 "Conscious Dimension – The 'Lilly Wave' Jeff Rense & Dr. Patrick Flanagan," March 14, 2014. Flanagan's quickly classified 1958 neurophone transmitted ultrasonic sound through the skin to place voices in the head through the inner ear organ called the saccule.

26 "The Lilly Wave and Psychotronic Warfare," The Bridge, 3 November 2015.

27 Open-path Fourier Transform infrared spectrometers OP-FTIR and I-OP-FTIR use infrared light to do much the same as LiDAR but with computer-assisted tomography (CAT).

28 Kelly Lin, "Nissan IMx Kuro Can Read Your Brain Waves." Motortrend, March 6, 2018.

29 https://eoportal.org/web/eoportal/airborne-sensors/halo.

tography, LiDAR can read target signature wavelengths without a high temperature medium:

> Atmospheric pollutants [like chemical trails] are monitored by bouncing a laser beam off clouds which are overhead the measurement apparatus, or terrain behind the area of interest, or simply by analyzing the backscatter from the atmosphere. The backscattered light from the laser detected by the apparatus has traveled twice through the volume of atmosphere, once outbound and once inbound to the detection apparatus. The laser wavelengths absorbed by the passage through the air give an accurate indication of the presence of particular chemical species, as well as their concentration.[30]

Once again, we encounter the necessity for two interfering beams—the LiDAR beam and the designator laser beam—for "reading" the target.

Lidar is incredibly useful to dual-use aerosol loading, airborne laser swath mapping (ALSM), UV differential absorption lidar (DIAL) to measure ozone, laser altimetry, contour mapping, remote sensing, etc. Modeled on "four optical phased arrays, each with about 1 million radiating elements in a 1cm^2 aperture that enable electronic beam steering analogous to microwave array antennas," 360-degree phased array lidar are used for "collaborative automatic detection, tracking, acquisition cueing, and intruder type identification, as well as free space optics communication."[31] Unlike video cameras, lidar is not affected by lighting conditions, but pulsing UV or NIR light to image objects can blur vision and cause temporary blindness. Phased array[32] lidar sensor networks are able to track objects inside dense real-time clouds and create convincing 3D holograms, especially with *laser radar (LADAR)*, which is similar to the usual *radar detection and ranging (RADAR)* systems that determine range, angle, and velocity of targets, except for the fact that LADAR illuminates the target with pulsed (i.e. modulated) laser light, then translates it into "high-res 3D shape

---

30 Carlo Kopp, "Laser Remote Sensing – A New Tool for Air Warfare." U.S. Air Force Air & Space Power Journal, January 27, 2014.

31 J.A. Krill et al., "Malfunction array lidar network for intruder detection, tracking, and identification." IEEE, December 7-10, 2010.

32 Phased array optics (PAO) is the equivalent of phased array radar but utilizes light waves to control surface optical properties on a microscopic scale, then steer light beams (including laser) by means of optical phased array (OPA) antennas. Complicated patterns of phase variation can be used to produce real-time holograms or diffractive virtual lenses for beam focusing or splitting in addition to aiming, which is why phased array antennas are so prized for targeting.

and detailed vibration spectrum data that is as unique as a fingerprint."[33]

Pulsed energy projection (PEP)

The U.S. Air Force has worked for decades on nonlethal devices for what it calls "controlled effects"—remotely created physical sensations that make the target(s) think or act in certain ways. Categorized under *strategic personality simulation*, the pulsed energy projectile (PEP) can be finely tuned to fire a short intense pulse of laser energy from a mile away, sending heat, damage, pressure, or cold so the target believes they are being burned, frozen, paralyzed, or dipped in acid.[34]

How it's done: an infrared laser pulse ablates the skin surface to release and expand plasma that produces a pressure wave to stun the target by triggering sensory nerves (sound, taste, touch, smell)—for example, to create synthetic images to confuse the visual sense while those around the target detect nothing. The primary objective of PEP systems is to cause "optimal pulse parameters to evoke peak nociceptor activation," namely to create as much pain as possible before causing tissue injury or death."[35] Though categorized as nonlethal, PEPs can kill. Initially, they were called *pulsed impulsive kill lasers.*

Monitors

Throughout the Smart City, electric grids are hacked, entrained signals carry Lilly waves along electrical wiring, and television and computer monitors alter emotional states by altering the electromagnetic fields around them. Hendricus G. Loos' 2001 Patent US6506148 B2, "Nervous system manipulation by electromagnetic fields from monitors," proved that by pulsing displayed images, the viewer's 2.4 Hz sensory resonance could be excited: "The implementations of the invention are adapted to the source of video stream that drives the monitor, be it a computer program, a TV broadcast, a video tape or a digital video disc (DVD)."

Even with privacy settings, smart TVs send manufacturers like LG Electronics in South Korea data about the viewer's watching habits, credit cards, etc., and tailor targeted ads to the viewer's preferences ("collection of watching info"). Smart TVs are far from traditional passive TVs receiving signals and transferring them to a backlit screen; they are computers connected to the

---

33 "Laser Radar (LADAR) – Precision ID and Tracking System." TechLink, n.d.

34 David Hambling, "Air Force Plan: Hack Your Nervous System." DefenseTech, February 13, 2006. Hambling is the author of Weapons Grade: How Modern Warfare Gave Birth to Our High-Tech World (Carroll & Graf, 2005).

35 David Hambling, "Maximum pain is aim of new US weapon." New Scientist, 2 March 2005.

Internet, sending and receiving data. Hacking Smart TVs via the Internet—like the rest of the Internet of Things (IoT)—is a piece of cake. And what about the video camera built into the front of the Smart TV watching you?[36]

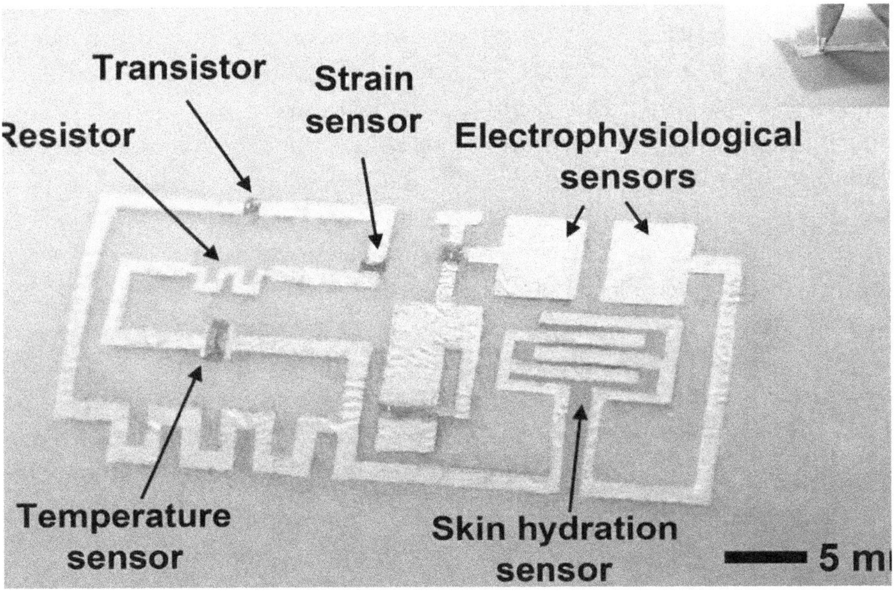

SkinMarks tattoo a FitBit touchpad. Sensors are embedded in the ink. "Drawn-on-skin electronics" is similar: draw multifunctional sensors and circuits on skin, then draw biometrics from the body.

https://www.activistpost.com/2020/08/google-developing-tattoos-that-turn-skin-into-touch-pad-researchers-developing-skin-drawn-monitor.html

Created by Sony, *high-density TV (HDTV)* has far more scanning detail, which leads to increased focus demand and data input. Crystal clear images are far more hypnotic than the old, less defined images.[37] HDTV viewing pleasure means more towers went up (2,049 feet high, $2 million per tower)—but you knew that, right? Now, Sony has come out with the even brighter Master Series A90J OLED TV for hypnotic high-definition resolution (HDR). The 88" 8K OLED goes for $30,000. Sony also overtly offers "cognitive processing" on its 2021 TVs *with the algorithm governing what you focus on.*[38]

36 Guy Adams, "Is your TV spying on YOU?" Daily Mail, 25 November 2013.

37 Robert Farago, "HDTV Mass Hypnosis." Journal of Hypnosis, September 1991. Also read Carla Emery's Secret, Don't Tell: The Encyclopedia of Hypnotism (Acorn Hill Publishing, 1997).

38 David Katzmaier, "Sony TVs get brighter OLED, cognitive processing, Google TV streaming in 2021." Cnet.com, January 7, 2021.

The HDTVs known as *LCDs (liquid crystal display)* are backlit by LEDs making the picture clearer, while quantum dots (nano-crystal semiconductors) make colors brighter and more luminous. LCDs have a contact lens that transmits TV shows while digital tattoos pick up the emotions portrayed by actors and create impulses to make us feel those emotions.[39] (Remember "feelies"?) TV monitor frequencies can be modified for other intrusions, like taking temperatures and modifying nervous systems via the light waveforms the eyes take in. Change channels by your own voice or thought command (someone from a remote location can do the same); this is called "interacting with our home entertainment systems."[40]

Subliminals are ongoing. I know it won't do any good to tell you to throw your television out—you won't have the courage to break the addiction because the subliminals and endless second-class imagery have weakened your will to the extent that you barely have enough strength and imagination to get through one day after another. No offense; it's just the bare, unadulterated truth. At least let me tell you about the excellent Australian investigative journalist Joe Vialls (1944-2005) who exposed subliminals just before he was killed by a sudden "heart attack"[41]: Initially, the *tachistoscope* was used for subliminal messaging, but the inserted frames could be detected by the conscious mind if you ran the film backwards. So *low light images* were blended into the film, a "film within a film." Even UV light couldn't detect the embedded images. This technique is still used in Hollywood films and TV, and of course it is used to prepare Manchurian Candidate sleeper killers.

The "white-space" network

Like 5G, *white-space networks* are compressed, concentrated, more protected, and can be made into *directional beams.*

The white-space digital network is wireless networking for long distance Internet access. Once known as "Super WiFi," the white-space network is not based on 2.4 GHz, nor is it connected with the Wi-Fi Alliance. It is based on lower frequency white spaces between television channel frequencies, meaning the white-space network signal can "travel further and penetrate walls

---

39 The latest: "Google Developing Tattoos That Turn Skin Into Touchpad; Researchers Developing Skin-drawn Monitor" by Aaron Kesel (ActivistPost.com, August 8, 2020): SkinMarks "transform the human body into a living touchpad via embedded sensors in the ink."

40 Fiona Macrae, "Keep an eye on the TV – with the TV in your eye." Daily Mail, 9 February 2009.

41 Joe Vialls, "Danger: Mind Controllers At Work!" May 15, 2005. See WikiSpooks "Joe Vialls' website" for his articles, such as his analysis of the use of a pulsed strobe LTL (less than lethal) weapon in Princess Diana's murder. See David Hambling, "Strobe Weapons Go Black After 'Immobilization' Tests," Wired, 1989.

better than the higher frequencies."[42] The fact that *lower frequencies penetrate better and travel further means they are more dangerous to the human body.*

To gain access to such *unlicensed* frequencies of the VHF-UHF spectrum,[43] devices have to be able to access the TV white-space geolocation database that evaluates interference potentials of towers transmitting in the 600 MHz band spectrum. Cell phone providers must register and be approved for cell tower positioning, but *white-space towers do not have to register.*

> Because of the limitation of 4 watts of power—white space device towers will need to be placed everywhere and then meshed together to piggyback from one tower to the other on the roofs of houses, on your hydro meters, on the telephone poles right in front of your house, inside your offices and schools. Remember—there are no rules where [white-space networks] can be placed.[44]

A dish or repeater base station on a roof (CPEs, consumer premises equipment) facing the central broadcast tower for a small town or district of a big city, coupled with smart meters and 5G antennas, creates wide *mesh network*[45] coverage. Instead of wires, lower wireless TV band frequencies and base stations re-transmit data via WiFi using 2.4 GHz.

> By using the lower TV frequency spectrum (54-698 MHz) as a carrier wave, the PULSED DIGITAL WiFi signal [operated by the FCC] will now be able to penetrate obstructions such as buildings over great distances and deliver high-speed broadband data.[46]

Perfect for targeting, silent subliminals, and remote neural monitoring (RNM).

Infrasonic / Ultrasonic

Infrasonic frequency is below 20 Hz; ultrasonic frequency above 20,000 Hz. Decibels (dB) measure the intensity or amplitude, Hertz the cycles per second (cps) of pulsed frequency. The military's vehicle-mounted active denial system (VMADS) covered in Chapter 9, "Dual Use I: A Smart City Is An Armed City," is a sonic weapon whose 95 GHz millimeter waves are similar to 5G technology.

42 Wikipedia last edited 8 December 2018.

43 UHF is used to mutate virus.

44 Magda Havas, "Is White Space Super WiFi Dangerous?" magdahavas.com, September 24, 2010.

45 Mesh network: wireless beaming of data packets from router to router, circumventing ISPs. Each node on a network receives and relays data that "hops" from one node to another by self-managing routing software.

46 Magda Havas.

90-120 dB (100 Hz) Extreme annoyance / distraction
110-130 dB (60-73 Hz) Intestinal pain / severe nausea
140-150 dB (50-100 Hz) Physical trauma, including damage to tissues
170+ dB (1-10 Hz) Blast-wave trauma and death

We have learned to think of sound as a weapon when we hear about U.S. Navy sonar tests and exercises, bomb blasts, electronic warfare (EW) drone warfare and surveillance, and Big Oil vessels with high-powered 12kHz multibeam echosounder systems (MBESs) onboard leading to pods of whales or dolphins beaching themselves.[47] (Big Oil and the U.S. Navy work in tandem.)

Whereas ultrasound is above the audibility range of the human ear, infrasound is below it. Infrasonic impact may sound less dangerous, but it can blast living tissue and physical structures like bridges and buildings with vibratory destructive force. Natural phenomena and events as well as manmade machines all vibrate: wind in caverns, volcanoes, atomic weapons, elephant communication, earthquakes, hurricanes, thunderstorms, pounding surf, waterfalls, tidal waves, the jet stream, aurora borealis, solar flares and winds. In the jet chassis, a commercial or military pilot's vision, speech, intelligence, orientation, equilibrium, and decision-making can be affected by repetitive oscillations. High-intensity low-frequency infrasound can stimulate short-term euphoria replete with endorphins, just as it can be made to produce physical pressure, fear, incapacitation, and death. From Hitler's uncanny *platz* speeches to hundreds of thousands to rock concerts, sound engineers experiment with broadcasting subliminal infrasound to affect audiences.

The Environmental Technology Laboratory (ETL) under the NOAA Earth System Research Laboratory (ESRL) Chemical Sciences Division in Boulder, Colorado has its electronic ears pointed toward the universe and thus hears the infrasonic thud of ocean waves on American coasts, the hiss of meteors and spacecraft, the chirps and whistles emitted by the Earth, along with the low-frequency "hum," the *Om* of ancient lore.

Remote "silent sound"[48] like through-the-wall infrasound piggybacked

---

47 "Sonar Mapping for oil near Madagascar killed 100 whales," Agence France-Presse, September 26, 2013. Rosalind Peterson kept a close eye on the U.S. Navy right up until her death in February 2018. "In March 2017, Rosalind co-authored one of the first bills introduced into a USA state (RIH6011) that would provide public oversight and strong regulatory prohibition to include fines and penalties for GeoEngineering, weather modification, cloud seeding, and other forms of violence against the Earth. Her goal was to draft a document that could be suitably adapted for other states and nations to protect agriculture, economies and all life from GeoEngineering." https://zerogeoengineering.com/2018/celebrating-life-rosalind-peterson/.

48 See "Silent Sound Spread Spectrum (S4, S-quad, Squad)" in Chapter 11, "The 'Air Loom' Hospital."

onto radio waves and microwaves can produce a whole suite of no-touch tortures, from sleep deprivation to forced sleep, deterioration of health over time via immunosuppression, increase of blood sugar and blood pressure, constant fight-or-flight stress by forcing adrenal glands to overproduce Cortisol, etc. Long-term increased Cortisol production alone can lead to hyperglycemia (diabetes), brain damage, a weakened immune system, weight gain, and shutdown of digestion and endocrine function. *This utilization of the body's natural defenses to slow-kill is the new untraceable murder.*

Low frequencies, hemorrhage and spasms; mid-audio (0.5 – 2.5 kHz), nerve irritation; high audio and ultrasound (5 – 30 kHz), lethal body temperatures, tissue burns, dehydration; high frequencies / short pulsing, cavitation bubbles and micro-lesions. Apparently, 7 Hz at infrasonic pitch is certain death. Interesting, isn't it? Thus the 7.83 Hz Schumann's resonance of natural well-being and brain function is deadly when weaponized at high-intensity exposure: our life form is cancelled and we die.[49] The lower the frequency and the higher the amplitude . . .

Towers (masts) & antennas

> *Mulder realizes that Crump is in considerable pain and that the only way to ease it is to drive west. At first, Scully believes that Crump is suffering from some sort of biological contagion, but while investigating the Crump home, she discovers a U.S. Navy antenna array emitting ELF waves stretching beneath their property. Scully deduces that an abnormal surge of ELF waves causes rising pressure in the inner ear. Westward motion and an increase in speed seem to be the only thing that eases Crump's pain.*
>
> – *X-Files,* "Drive," season 6, original FOX air date November 15, 1998

Two decades ago, I read Tim Rifat's accounts about the Sussex, UK police using a 200-foot ground-wave emergency network (GWEN) antenna (450 MHz) for targeting him with a pulsed behavior modification frequency of 0.75mW/cm2, the same pulse modulation now in cell phone earpieces. Towers and antennas are still needed for pulsing the Smart City wireless "hive mind," though both are becoming smaller and more difficult to see with higher frequencies—excepting Dubai's 829-meter-high Burj Khalifa, or the 20km-high "space elevator" planned by the Canadian space corporation Thoth Technology.[50] Towers can be lattice, monopole, concealed, or broadcast

49 Thanks to Alex Davis, "Acoustic Trauma: Bioeffects of Sound," BFA thesis, University of New South Wales, 1999.

50 "Space age Tower of Babel: Canadian company patents 20km lift to heavens." RT, 17 August 2015. Thoth is the Egyptian ibis-headed god of secret society magic and the moon, born of the seed of Horus from the brow of Set. At 19km above the Earth, body fluids begin

cell / microwave towers. At their base are hidden T-lines of copper or fiber optic cables. Giant telecom providers link thousands of towers and monopoles (masts) together with fiber optic cable while pressuring local zoning boards to approve hundreds more.

Besides the fiber optics network operating out of their base, *microwave* cell towers and monopoles / masts are nodes working with satellites. If that's not a weapon system, what is? The FCC stresses that no more than 100 watts can be wired into a tower, with 10 watts per channel so interference of received frequencies is minimal. *The weaponized feature is the pulsing, not the power.* Cell towers are dual-use weapons, all EM being digital and the military being digital command central. Beside the long-wave, tissues-penetrating microwave radiation bombarding everyone below and in their path, they are armed with video monitors, miniature sensors (magnetic, seismic, infrared, radar, and strain electromagnetic), and signals processing weather and atmospheric surveillance, detection of biological agents, radiation release, etc. *Pulsing,* not *wattage, makes the difference in dual-use technologies.*

GWEN towers are the really big guns. They are tall, thin, scaffolded monopoles tethered to the ground by six guy wires. Their arrays serve relay stations of military-industrial-intelligence hubs like the Rockwell Collins HF (3-30 MHz) station in the rolling hills of Clinton County, Iowa near Oxford Junction.[51] Calibrated to reflect the unique geomagnetic field frequencies of each geographic area, the military's GWENs—in tandem with HAARP / Space Fence transmitters, space-based lasers, fiber optics cable, cell towers, monopoles, etc.—are designed to alter frequencies for storms and weather patterns as well as moods, behavior, and minds. These 300- to 500-foot monopoles radiate pulsed power from their base along 100 underground spokes of copper wire, which thus alters the natural geomagnetic field with artificially created LF (150-175 kH) ground waves that resonate in basements and deep underground bases as well as 500 feet up. Manipulation of geomagnetic fields directly affects the Schumann resonance that our planetary biorhythms, brains, and health depend upon.

> Cyclotron resonance is a mechanism of action that enables very low-strength electromagnetic fields, acting in concert with the Earth's geomagnetic field, to produce major biological effects by *concentrating the energy in the applied field upon specific particles,* such as the biologically important ions of sodium, calcium, potassium, and lithium.[52]

---

to boil off, due to low air pressure, which may be why the "space elevator" is made up of pneumatically pressurized cells.

51 "Possible Drone Control Array Sighted in Iowa!" Federal Jack, n.d.

52 Robert O. Becker, M.D. Cross Currents: The Perils of Electropollution, The Promise of Electromedicine. Penguin Group, 1990.

The GWEN system acts as an on-the-ground *gyrotron* for cyclotron resonance. Its radial transmissions running from very low frequency (225 MHz) to very high frequency (400 MHz) are as exact as acupuncture when it comes to powering microwave and radio frequency weapons that can control and harass, create mental or physical illness and death. For example, long VLF microwaves can create nausea, incontinence, vomiting, disorientation, organ damage, and death. Once pulsed, they do not suffer from attenuation when traveling through the air to the soft tissue of targets. As targeted individual Carolyn Williams Palit explained it in 2007:

> They spray barium powders and let it photo-ionize from the ultraviolet light of the sun. Then, they make an aluminum-plasma generated by "zapping" the metal cations that are in the spray with either electromagnetics from HAARP, the gyrotron system on the ground [Ground Wave Emergency Network], or space-based lasers. The barium makes the aluminum-plasma more particulate dense. This means they can make a denser plasma than they normally could from just ionizing the atmosphere or the air.[53]

Picture this gyrotron system silently at work in your neighborhood: Via a particle beam, a plasma wave cone rotates around the target's head while spiral (toroidal) waves attract and collect charged particle ions and feed them back into the plasma wave, at which point images are reconstituted and beamed up to tethered satellites, then transmitted to Fusion Center operators. Capturing analog sound occurs similarly: spiral waves corkscrew and trap sound particles as waves. Voice-to-skull (V2K) transmissions enter the ears by the same process. Even odors can be collected or released in the left nostril—all in the privacy of your home or office.

GWEN VLF waves act as carrier beams for pulsed ELF signals passing through the skull. As with microwave cell towers, all that is needed to pulse modulate psychotronic agendas are the exact brain frequencies (*evoked potentials*) for specific behaviors, emotions, and states of mind—anger, suicide, hysteria, trauma, serial killing, paranoia, lust, etc., each with its exact frequency and command set.

Lists of frequencies—mapped primary frequency allocations (*prima freaking*)—are available for the right price, as are portable microwave transmitters. Dial in to the tower, set the millimeter wave scanner and the Nationwide Differential Global Positioning System (NDGPS), point the gun-like delivery system at the target, and you're in the business of torture. For general

53 Carolyn Williams Palit, "What Chemtrails Really Are," November 9, 2007.

population control, portable rooftop "poppers"—like the tropospheric scatter microwave transmitters used in Iraq for "communications"[54]—can also be deployed, along with base stations on rooftops. Turn the dial and crank up cataracts, memory loss, numbing, tingling, buzzing, chronic fatigue, Alzheimer's, Parkinson's, or quick-acting terminal cancer.

GWEN towers are calibrated to work with frequency weapons. Mobile telephone systems like Europe's GSM (Global System for Mobile Communications) and UMTS (Universal Mobile Telecommunications System) operate in the same frequency range as frequency weapons, which means that "communication systems" like GWEN can alter the modulation of frequencies and direction of signals.

HAARP Alaska broadcasts at 435 MHz, as do pre-5G cell phones; the window to human consciousness is 400-450 MHz. All it takes to jam our consciousness is to broadcast at 410-420 MHz. *Is calibrated HAARP / Space Fence technology being used as a microwave knife to replace our ionospheric membrane and protective magnetic "ring of power" around our planet with an AI machine version?*

Dual use, double jeopardy.

Fiber optics

Fiber optics (optical fibers) are a remarkable invention. 550,000 fiber optic cables not only carry voice and internet data across the oceans, but with satellites also form a laser optical surveillance *web* over the entire Earth while thousands of volts of electricity power repeaters as big as 600-pound Bluefin tunas.[55]

Fiber optic signals are digital information packets carried by light in the form of a laser beam through thin strands of optical fiber or silica glass at speeds just short of the speed of light (300 million meters per second). Besides silica, fluorides and phosphates make up the strands, with chalcogenide semiconductors conducting ions and electrons for lasers. Each fiber (1/10th the width of a human hair) has the ability to carry multiple independent channels for multiple networks (and agendas), each using a different wavelength of light—for example, each fiber handling 25,000 telephone calls or 160 channels and carrying 8,000 Gb/sec. Fiber optics bundles (cables) increase bandwidth and provide fast communication over long distances with few repeaters, and being multi-mode means they save space.

Fiber optic strands are easily "doped" with various metals for various effects. As multiplex light carriers, they make excellent sensors, from endo-

54 Similar to the gyrotron resonance maser.

55 Nicholas Rapp, "Mapping the Internet," July 9, 2012. Review Chapter 8, "Boots on the Ground," Under An Ionized Sky.

scopes for surgeons and airplane engineers to spectroscopy and lasers, and are therefore used in neuroengineering, optogenetic engineering, and covert practices like fiber optic cameras implanted in human bodies.

Optical fiber networks are invaluable when it comes to dual use and joint protocols, due in part to how they outperform copper cables and telephone or cable television services in both distance and speed. FTTP (fiber to the premises) and shared fiber like active Ethernet connect private property networks to central routers once the optical signal converts to an electrical signal via 60 Hz (50 Hz) outlets and phones to local area networks, cable TV, etc. (This is often how targeting works.) Create the optical signal via a transmitter, relay the signal along the fiber, receive the optical signal, convert it to an electrical signal; etc. Simple enough, but dual use means fiber optics can provide *covert* "communications" by sending pulses of light through an optical fiber as carrier waves modulated to carry communications from unnamed agencies or insiders with the right codes for your brain. Splitters can split the light beams to grant direct access to Google, Facebook or internet traffic, especially given that 99 percent of U.S. internet traffic goes through just one of 18 cities.[56]

Due to the concentric nature of the dual core fibers, fiber optics are believed to be tap-proof, but "intercept probes" and prisms say otherwise:

> The tapping process apparently involves using so-called "intercept probes" . . . [T]he intelligence agencies likely gain access to the landing stations . . . and use these small devices to capture the light being sent across the cable. The probe bounces the light through a prism, makes a copy of it, and turns it into binary data . . .[57]

Remember AT&T's "secret room" in its San Francisco office?

> It was around 2003 when they started putting optical fibers coming into the U.S. through Y-connector Narus devices. Basically these would duplicate the data coming across the internet—one set of packets would go the normal route, the other set would go to NSA facilities. There, they collect all the data coming in through fiber optics, reassemble all the data packets into useable information—emails, file transfers, etc.—and then pass it along for storage. That means they are taking all that data off the fiber optic lines at 20 main convergence points in the U.S., collecting almost all of the internet traffic passing through the U.S. This gets them pretty much control over the digital world.[58]

---

56 70 percent of the world's online traffic is routed through just one county in Virginia (The Guardian, July 17, 2018).

57 Joe Wolverton II, "NSA Taps Directly Into Undersea Fiber-optic Data Cables." USAHM News, July 25, 2013.

58 Simon Black, "Digital Privacy Black Paper," https://s3.amazonaws.com/sm-cdn/reports/

Thanks to 16 fiber optic cables, routers, Sun Microsystems servers, and Narus traffic-analysis software at its San Francisco switching center, AT&T was able to tap all internet traffic between its WorldNet and other internet service providers (ISPs) for the NSA. Needless to say, only those with NSA clearance were allowed in the "secret room." Now, NSA "secret rooms" are standard operating procedure in major telecommunications offices,[59] as eavesdroppers and stalkers use fiber optic pathways.

Somehow, people have gotten the idea that underground fiber optic cable will eliminate much of our irradiation problem, but this is far from the truth, considering that power lines, train tracks, and underground gas pipelines conduit radiation, too.

I live in Fraziers Bottom, West Virginia and was very surprised to see them recently laying gas pipelines. These are being run all across the U.S. to connect with each other. My area is high in shale, red clay (iron), and I believe they have been finding natural gas.

– Kelly Peat, June 26, 2018

Subterranean conduits beneath sidewalks and streets may actually make it easier to access minds. Cortical neurons fire signals picked up by an amplifier, then the signals are converted into optical data and pulsed along the neighborhood fiber optic cable to be converted by repeaters to electrical signals and binary data for analysis. This hidden aspect of fiber optics was clarified for me by Seattle lawyer Karen Dobson in the late 1990s, as I described in *Under An Ionized Sky*). When Karen fled to Mexico to escape the FBI directed energy targeting she was undergoing, she wrote:

> The reason I am not nearly so ill as I was made to be in the US is only the lack of fiber optics in Mexico, and their ability to use a dedicated satellite for pulsing me every 30 to 90 seconds as if I were a radio tower. This is probably what grounds the right foot and makes holes and burns in the bottom and sides of it . . . Through MCI and the privatization of Mexico's power and utility companies (bought up by U.S. interests, of course), Mexico—

NSA-Black-Paper.pdf

59 Whistleblower William Binney, former director of the NSA's World Geopolitical and Military Analysis Reporting Group, estimates 20 such facilities in the U.S. ("Room 641A," Wikipedia)

whose citizens by and large have no phones, pagers, beepers, much less cell phones—will welcome fiber optics throughout their states by the end of the year 2000. This is not because it is needed or economically profitable; I think, rather, it is for use in the fashion that it has been used on me.[60]

The directed energy weapons (DEWs) she experienced in the 1990s were much less sophisticated than the arsenal of today, now that the FBI has a Weapons of Mass Destruction Directorate / Biological Countermeasures Unit,[61] but some of her insights may still be useful to targeted individuals (and soon, once the 5G weapon is in place, to the public at large):

- With fiber optics, DEWs can be run through electrical systems and phone cables
- HAARP-based DEWs
- Doppler for VHF weapons; amplifies ELF and ULF
- Phased array antennas
- Ion laser cooling tubes used with building ventilation equipment
- Infrared (IR) light for night viewing
- Hand-held equipment for rural, airplanes, rest areas
- Microwave gun that looks like a hand-held hairdryer[62]

Her warning regarding fiber optics was deadly serious: "AVOID FIBER OPTIC CABLE, A TOOL FOR EAVESDROPPING AND HARASSMENT."

In November 2019, Verizon announced that with optical sensor technology and artificial intelligence software, they can collect data from any point along their fiber optic network, as it is just one big sensor. As Glenn Wellbrock, Verizon's director of Optical Transport Network Architecture, Design and Planning, put it, "It's different from most point-sensors that can only sense one particular spot, and I can't really change it. Here, I can measure anywhere along that fiber."[63]

Finally, we arrive at the hospitals that are not what you think they are. Best know your way around when you enter the modern Air Loom hospital.

---

60 Karen Dobson, JD, Revealed: Total Immersion Microwave Harassment, unpublished, 2003. I have been unable to contact Karen since spring 2011.

61 Anne Manning, "FBI gets synthetic biology crash course at CSU," Colorado State University, June 7, 2017.

62 Thermal gun (EM) heats the body to 107°F (41.6°C); seizure gun (EM) causes epileptic seizures; magnetophosphene gun makes you "see stars" in the retina.

63 Skip Descant, "Verizon Wants to Turn Fiber Networks into Citywide Sensors." Government Technology, November 13, 2019.

11

Dual Use III: The "Air Loom" Hospital

Precision Medicine Means Remote, Armed, & Experimental

Electroconvulsive therapy (ECT)
Electronic brain stimulation (EBS)
Deep brain stimulation (DBS)
Transcranial magnetic stimulation (TMS)
Trigeminal nerve stimulation (TNS)
The electroencephalogram (EEG)
Silent Sound Spread Spectrum (S4, S-quad, Squad)
Magnetic resonance imaging (MRI) / functional MRI (fMRI)
Magnetoencephalograph (MEG)
SQUID & MASER
PET, SPECT, CT scans
N^3 (Next-generation Nonsurgical Neurotechnology)
Wireless Body Area Network (WBAN) /
Wireless Sensor Network (WSN) /
National Telecommunications & Information Administration (NTIA)
Holograms
The "ghost machine" (quantum repeaters) & q-teleportation

The basic notion in low-frequency research was to create within the neutral cavity between the electrically charged ionosphere in the higher part of the atmosphere and conducting layers of the surface of the Earth—to create waves, electrical waves, tuned to brainwaves. The natural electrical rhythm of most mammalian brains, including man, is about 10 cycles of Hertz per second, and there are indications that if you tune in at this frequency—that is, these low frequencies of about 10 cycles per second—you can produce changes in behavioral patterns or in responses.

– Dr. Gordon J.F. MacDonald, testimony before the House Subcommittee on Oceans and International Environment, 1974[1]

1 MacDonald wrote *Unless Peace Comes: A Scientific Forecast of New Weapons* in 1968. He was science adviser to unelected President Lyndon Baines Johnson.

When it appears that a patent will become brain-dead, a change in medical routines occurs. Care of the patient as a whole being becomes care of biological materials contained within and the technological components that convert them into useable products. There are two parts to the process: the maintenance of the body as incubator and storage container for the human materials, and the preservation and conversion of the specific materials themselves. It is important to note that this process can begin long before the patient is declared legally dead . . . Once the brain ceases to function . . . the body is no longer a self-regulating system . . . Cyborg mechanics must replace brain functions . . .

Recognizing the considerable market potential of the human materials industry, pharmaceutical and medical supply companies have developed new products and entire new industries . . . The goals of these new products are to preserve tissue integrity before being removed, and to make the materials more "immunologically silent" to prevent problems later when they are replaced inside another body. In essence, the human materials are being structurally, chemically and functionally transformed to make them more universal. In this way, they become not only substitutable mechanical parts, but more like off-the-shelf reagents, available for use in a variety of end-users.

– Linda F. Hogle, "Standardization Across Non-Standard Domains: The Case of Organ Procurement." *Science, Technology, & Human Values,* October 1, 1995

Both the imaginative and rational are required for truly advanced technology. Futurist Arthur C. Clarke's words, "Any sufficiently advanced technology is indistinguishable from magic," are true because technology employs forces that are invisible to our senses—light, heat, sound waves, which, until extended by instruments, were once mysterious and undetectable to our narrow range of perception, though we knew they existed. Both science and magic begin with the hypothetical, whether a stage magician or magus, physicist or bioengineer, whether serving the Good) or Evil) Both science and magic must begin with both rational and imaginative faculties—and once a long time ago, discernment.

Electromagnetic weapons are science fiction-like because the range of the electromagnetic spectrum that our normal senses function in is so *narrow*. Thus, when EM weapons are made to perform "tricks" like twirling Egyptian statues in museums,[2] constructing exotic geometric crop circles from space, raising floating holographic cities and dialing in alien invasions, we are spell-

2 Marc Lallanilla, "Why Egyptian statue moves on its own." Live Science, June 24, 2013.

bound, *in awe*. Billions of dollars have been lavished on technologies that can manipulate invisible forces (and vice versa), from nonlethal weapons to ESP, remote viewing, thanatology, etc. The brain has been subjected to drugged states, religious cults, electromagnetics—arts that fool perceptions, keep secrets, and get taxpayers to pay for it all.

Contrary to History Channel conditioning, the Nazis did not invent torture, however expert they were at techno-occultism. Consider the 18th century "influencing machine" called the Air Loom meticulously documented by its victim, tea merchant James Tilly Matthews, a London peace activist opposed to the Napoleonic Wars.

> Matthews' beliefs had their roots in his implausible but true story. A political activist and peace campaigner, he had become involved during the French revolution in clandestine efforts to head off the looming war between France and England. Shuttling between London and Paris, he had remarkable success in persuading the moderate faction of the French government to commit to a peace plan, and he had met several times with Pitt and Lord Liverpool, his secretary of war, to propose an alliance with them against the Jacobins and the Paris mob.[3]

The Air Loom used to torture Matthews was operated by a gang of Jacobin terrorists working for French Grand Lodge Freemason "animal magnetism"[4] occultists. The Air Loom is often described as "Puck-like" after the sprite-like character in Shakespeare's play *A Midsummer Night's Dream* because it was on the order of virtual reality (VR) brain tampering. Its oak panels, brass fittings, hoop barrels, and tanned leather tubing appeared to be real, as were its magnetized gas, putrid effluvia, Leyden jars, and windmill sails. Matthews' drawings are exact and still exhibited in the Prinzhorn Collection at the University of Heidelberg, Germany.

So how was the torture done, and what role, if any, did the Air Loom play? Did the Air Loom gang *physically* ride it into Matthews' rooms to torture him, or was it done by psychic assault through his mind, what we now term psychological operations (psyops)?

Author Mike Jay makes a case for the Air Loom being real at some level—"a terrifying machine whose mesmeric rays and mysterious gases were brainwashing politicians and plunging Europe into revolution, terror, and war."

---

3 Mike Jay, "Illustrations of Madness: James Tilly Matthews and the Air Loom." The Public Domain Review, https://publicdomainreview.org/2014/11/12/illustrations-of-madness-james-tilly-matthews-and-the-air-loom/.

4 Animal magnetism or mesmerism (named after Franz Mesmer) utilized the invisible natural force or "magnetic fluid" captured and entranced by hypnotists.

"Mesmeric currents" carried sparks, alien voices, nightmares, and caused chronic fatigue and foot-curving, knee-nailing, eye-screwing pain and convulsions. Two reputable doctors declared Matthews sane and insisted he was being psychically assaulted, and yet the Home Office Minister (surely a Freemason) committed Matthews in 1797 to the infamous Bedlam psychiatric hospital for life.

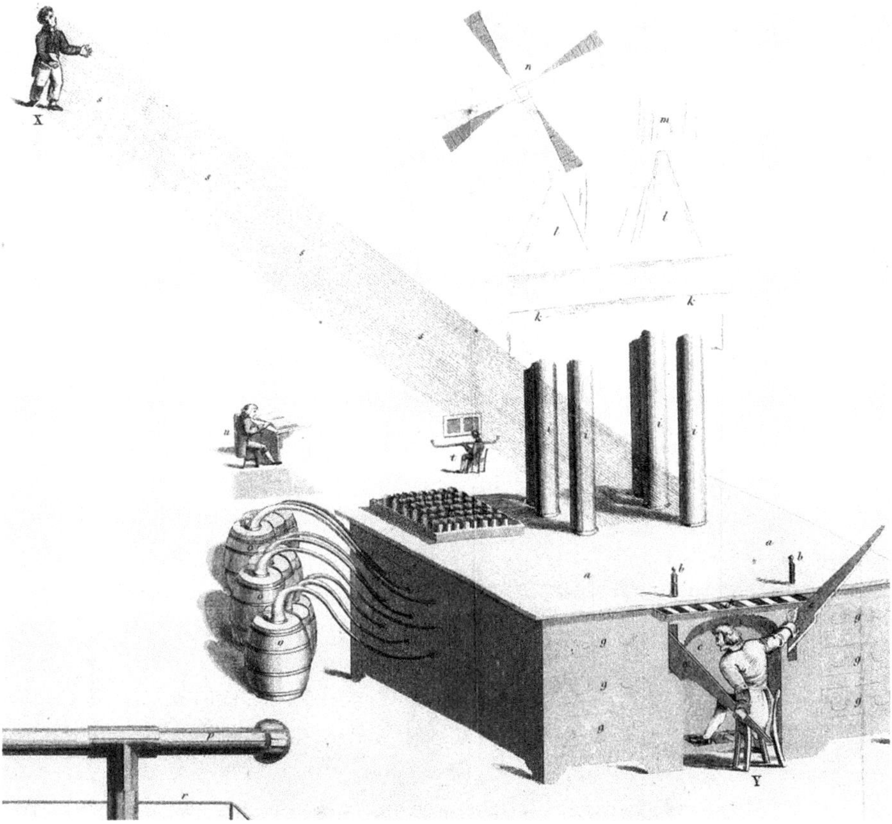

"Air Loom" Precision Medicine. James Tilly Matthews, a former peace activist of the Napoleonic Wars, was confined to London's notorious Bedlam asylum in 1797 for believing that his mind was under the control of the "Air Loom," a terrifying machine whose mesmeric rays and mysterious gases were brainwashing politicians and plunging Europe into revolution, terror, and war.

https://publicdomainreview.org/essay/illustrations-of-madness-james-tilly-matthews-and-the-air-loom

The military-industrial-intelligence complex has, for half a century, pursued its own Air Loom "nonlethal" IO technology to control the brain's "mesmeric currents." From brain to mind, the five senses and other senses, from physical to subtle bodies and soul—all is now imperiled by the doctrine of full spectrum dominance and sophisticated technologies. Whether it's over-the-horizon (OTH) radar or electric and magnetic brain-hacking technologies like radioactive X-rays and CT "cat" scans (computed tomography) or microwave hearing, V2K, and remote neural monitoring (RNM), the brain is as much a target as it was 200 years ago in the Air Loom days.

Robert Duncan, PhD, begins his online book *The Matrix Deciphered*[5] with Robert Malech's 1974 Patent #3,951,134, "Apparatus and Method for Remotely Monitoring and Altering Brain Waves"":

> In 1974, Robert Malech—an employee of Dorn & Margolin, Inc., a major defense subcontractor in RADAR design now owned by EDO Corporation, an even larger defense contractor in electronic warfare—invented a fairly simple RADAR device that could read whole brain electrical activity at considerable distance. Major advantages include no wires and full brain electrical activity analysis, not just points on the skull surface. He discovered and perfected a way to use simple electromagnetic oscillations between 100MHz and 40GHz to *read* brainwaves by first "illuminating" the brain and its electrical conductance, then reading the return signal. The imaging method observes the changes of frequency resonances, amplitude, and phase, which represent the states of neuron depolarization throughout the brain.[6]
>
> But more profoundly, Malech discovered that he could *influence* brainwaves if precisely timed with a return training signal. Wirelessly, he could also copy someone's brainwaves onto another person just as easily as read them anywhere in the world. *He had no idea that he had accidentally destroyed democracy as we envision it to be.* The military and surveillance community immediately picked up on the patent and within two years had reprogrammed their communications and surveillance satellites and terrestrial phased arrays with the new concepts. The rapid deployment of this technology occurred because it only required software changes in

5 Robert Duncan, PhD, The Matrix Deciphered: Psychic Warfare / Top-Secret Mind Interfacing Technology, Higher Order Thinkers, 2006. I am quoting from my edited version of Dr. Duncan's online book, which I subsequently shared with him. Duncan claims to have worked for the CIA, DoD, and DOJ, and then to have been targeted with the very technologies he was tasked to develop. His alleged records from Dartmouth College and Harvard University are "unavailable." (It is typical of intelligence agencies to erase paper trails of whistleblower former employees.)

6 Ion heating and electron gyro frequency reading— the preferred method of scalar RADAR bioelectric field reading—have been around since the 1960's.

already existing RADAR, imaging, and communications terrestrial dishes and satellites. Many additional spy satellites have been launched since to bolster the system. (Emphasis added.)

This was a done deal by 1976. The next essential step arrived 20 years later with the HAARP ionospheric heater control of the ionosphere via phased array, over-the-horizon (OTH) RADAR. Radio wave radar is being used to keep track of patients in hospitals and at home, reading their vital signs, monitoring their movements.

> "Be it microwave or radio wave, prolonged exposure to radiation will affect the health of people and other living organisms. The lack of feedback on the long-term side effects of a radar wave-based medical device is concerning, to say the least."[7] Next will be the AI-run radar system "capable of 'high accuracy remote monitoring of physiological parameters'" using a combination of radar and electro-optical (thermal) sensors that Israel has installed at its borders, supposedly to detect COVID-19.[8]

Now, let's take a weapons tour of the modern Air Loom hospital in one Smart City after another, each with an Epic AI Deterioration Index algorithm—not independently validated, not peer reviewed, but making life and death decisions. On every patient's chart is a Deterioration Index.[9]

Electroconvulsive therapy (ECT)

Electroconvulsive therapy (ECT) is basically electroshock passing electric current through the brain to set off convulsions, seizures, and memory erasure, as depicted in the 2004 preprogramming film *Eternal Sunshine of the Spotless Mind.* Coupled with the EEG, ECT exposes brain frequencies, a valuable commodity among those who have made controlling the brain their business. Is this why disabled children at the Judge Rotenberg Educational Center in Canton, Massachusetts are still being punished with ECT?

There are two shock aversive devices used at the JRC. The main Graduated Electronic Decelerator (GED) delivers a 15.5-milliamp shock of up to two seconds, and the GED-4 gives shocks of 45.5 milliamps. By comparison, most police tasers deliver shocks of 2.1 or 3.6 milliamps.[10]

---

7 Edsel Cook, "Doctors can now monitor vital signs using radar waves, but what about their side effects." NaturalNews.com, November 26, 2019.

8 Anna Ahronheim, "Radar system protecting Israel's borders will monitor coronavirus patient." Jerusalem Post, March 31, 2020.

9 Vishal Khetpal, MD, and Nishant R. Shah, PhD., "How a largely untested AI algorithm crept into hundreds of hospitals," FastCompany.com, May 28, 2021.

10 Matt Agorist, "Federal Court Rules School Can Use Electric Shock as Punishment for Spe-

The idea of electroshocking human brains began with Italian neurologist Ugo Cerletti (1877-1963) while noted how *docile* pigs on their way to slaughter became after receiving electroshock. It fit in nicely with the medical arsenal—

- Cut it
- Burn it
- Drug it
- Shock it

—superseded in barbarity only by the *prefrontal lobotomy* that was finally brought to the public's attention in 1975 by the film *One Flew Over the Cuckoo's Nest*, based on Ken Kesey's 1962 book. As shock psychiatrists incorporated psychotropic drugs and chemical lobotomies, they repackaged electroshock as *modern electroconvulsive therapy (ECT).*

This unlawful, unethical, and barbaric "therapy" requires a SpECTrum 4000 shock machine and two resistors to induce a "therapeutic" grand mal seizure at 460 volts.[11] (The brain self-powers at 0.2 volts.) Brain cells accustomed to 75ºF are suddenly catapulted into 120ºF, after which the "bad" brain cells die. Less brain is beneficial, we are told by the shock doctors, even with permanent memory loss of everything preceding the ECT "therapy." Many ECT victims who have suffered through 30 or more rounds of ECT go on to deep brain stimulation (DBS, see below). The drug used as a relaxant before ECT sessions is used for lethal injections: succinylcholine relaxes the body to the point of stopping breathing but intensifies the brain's torture.

Knowing that preventing seizures prevents brain damage, why are doctors willing to use ECT? Because ECTs are a big moneymaker? because ECT "reboots" the brain-as-computer? because they are completely ignorant of the biophysics of electricity? ECT is also said to exorcize whatever is lodged in the aura, not unlike the flashing strobe lights that trigger an epileptic seizure or hypnotic state—all used by MK-ULTRA to "engineer" the subconscious mind.[12]

One thing is certain: those who undergo this "therapy" are never the same again.[13]

---

cial Needs Children." Activist Post, July 12, 2021.

11 430X a stun gun.

12 See T Stokes, "The Frequency Fence Mystery," http://www.thetruthseeker.co.uk/; and David Hambling, "Strobe Weapons Go Black After 'Immobilization' Tests," Wired, 1989.

13 Thanks to the 2019 documentary "Therapy or Torture? The Truth About Electroshock," put out by Citizens Commission on Human Rights, a Church of Scientology offshoot.

Electronic brain stimulation (EBS)

> *EMF Brain Stimulation works by sending a complexly coded and pulsed electromagnetic signal to trigger evoked potentials (events) in the brain, thereby forming sound . . . in the brain's neural circuits. EMF Brain Stimulation can also change a person's brain states [of consciousness] and affect motor control.*
>
> – *John St. Clair Akwei vs National Security Agency,*
> Ft. George G. Meade, MD, USA (Civil Action 92-0449), 1992

> *We are the bulls of Delgado,*
> *We sing our song in simpatico.*
>
> – louisaf@nb.sympatico.ca

Electronic brain stimulation (EBS) is direct communication with the brain, including brain-computer interface (BCI), via finely tuned, pencil-thin microwave beams. The Soviets since the 1930s were able to remotely twitch a muscle by steering the command from the brain to the muscle via radio waves. Then came Dr. José M. R. Delgado whose research culminated in stopping a charging bull with ESB.[14] He then consolidated whatever was not classified in his 1969 *Physical Control of the Mind: Toward A Psychocivilized Society.*

Today, the electrical activity used for muscle movement can be read remotely via smart devices, thanks to the neural dust in the brain and body from chemical trails, vaccines, GMO foods, etc. All the at-a-distance operators need to do is demodulate the electric signals, then re-modulate them to make the muscle move against your will. Post-nanotechnology, "mesh implants" provide the new *in vivo* EBS framework. As Shaun Patel of the Harvard Medical School faculty describes:

> "The electrodes that deliver stimulation are ultra small," Patel tells Inverse. "They're cellular and sub-cellular in size, so when you implant them into the brain, they resemble the size of the cells in the brain and the axons in the brain more than a typical electrode."[15]

The new EBS "stable neural interface" is about directing ("encouraging")

---

14 Timothy C. Marzullo, "The Missing Manuscript of Dr. Jose Delgado's Radio Controlled Bulls," Journal of Undergraduate Neuroscience Education, June 15, 2017. Delgado was financed by the Office of Natal Research (ONR), the U.S. Air Force Aero-Medical Research Laboratory, and the Public Health Foundation of Boston.

15 Thor Benson, "Brain Implants Like Elon Musk's Neuralink Could Change Humanity Forever," Inverse, September 5, 2019. Late in the article, the Neuralink implant is changed from "mesh" to "a small chip with probes (from "four tiny 'N1' sensors") . . . connected to an iPhone app," indicating that Neuralink is more about BCI hookups than EBS.

mesh implants to migrate "across the mesh just like they migrate across neurons" to other areas of the brain. As usual, the good doctors want to help Parkinson's and Alzheimer's sufferers, control addiction and boost learning, all the while accessing nonconsensual targets' most intimate thoughts.

Drone operators' brains are pulsed with some form of EBS to keep their attention span and kill quotas high, taking the place of addictive drugs like modafinil (Provigil) and methylphenidate (Ritalin). How is this not mind control? And what about the Targeted Neuroplasticity Training program (TNT) that can hack into and modulate the peripheral nervous systems of security officials and spies so they learn more and faster, from foreign languages to cryptography?[16]

Deep brain stimulation (DBS)

In 2014 under President Obama's BRAIN initiative (Brain Research through Advancing Innovative Neurotechnologies), DARPA financed researchers from six universities and Lawrence Livermore National Laboratories to "design, fabricate and use an implantable device that finely tracks brain signals in people with anxiety or depression,"[17] Parkinson's, PTSD, borderline personality, schizophrenia, and obsessive compulsive disorder (OCD)—not really to help people with OCD but to collect scads of data from thousands of brain signals for Transhumanism. The truth is that there are no neural pain receptors in the brain encourages experimentation.

> In an initial surgery, [neurosurgeon Emad] Eskandar drills two dime-size holes in the top of the patient's skull and sinks 42-centimeter-long electrodes about seven centimeters deep into the gray matter of the brain. In a second surgery, usually a couple of days later, he creates a pocket under the skin in the chest or abdomen, implants a device incorporating a battery and pulse generator into this newly created space, and runs a wire up to the skull, connecting it with the electrodes. When turned on, the device emits an electrical current that stimulates the neural fibers carrying information from primitive brain areas associated with motivation to the frontal lobe. In 50 percent of Eskandar's cases, a miracle follows: the obsessions and compulsions fade and then disappear.[18]

---

16 Ryan De Souza, "Hacking Brain Possible with DARPA New Targeted Neuroplasticity Training Program." Hackread.com, March 22, 2016.

17 Ron Leuty, "Tiny brain device scores Bay Area grant from Obama's BRAIN initiative." Silicon Valley Business Journal, May 27, 2014.

18 Adam Piore, "A Shocking Way to Fix the Brain." Technology Review, October 8, 2015. Eskandar originally hoped to be a chemical engineer. OCD is one of the psychiatric conditions that follows from childhood sexual abuse. The problem with DBS is that when it is turned off, symptoms return.

The bulky *stimoceiver* in the chest or abdomen (invented by Delgado) has now been replaced by "a miniaturized central hub smaller than a cell phone with an integrated battery that will fit snugly on the back of the skull," much like Neo's *Matrix* plug-in in the 1999 film.[19] Of the 2.5 million Americans who suffer from OCD, 125,000 have electrodes in their brain. Engineers make the hardware, software engineers the pattern recognition software, nanoengineers the "miniaturized versions," and "psychiatric surgery" provides a real-time view of operating circuits.

Would DARPA fund anything not destined for weaponizing? And who (or what) will be running the remote base station that communicates wirelessly with the [Neo] skull hub?

Transcranial magnetic stimulation (TMS)

Transcranial magnetic stimulation (TMS),[20] as originally conceived, entailed placing a large Tesla coil against the scalp near the forehead and sending electric currents to selectively control brain function. Stimulate the left lateral parietal cortex, left frontal cortex, cerebellum, and thalamus and an experience of *chromesthesia* occurs, the mental travel in subjective time that makes one feel more alive in the past and future than in the present. When the right temporoparietal junction (TPJ) above and behind the right ear undergoes TMS currents (10 Hz), the individual's ability to make moral judgments is impaired because their ability to interpret the other's intentions is blocked.[21] When the left TPJ above the left ear is stimulated, a female patient suffering epileptic seizures sensed

> . . . the presence of a mystery person behind her, a motionless and speechless shadow that imitated her body posture and actions. 'He' lay beneath her when she lay down, sat behind her when she sat down, and attempted to take a test card from her when she tried to participate in a language exercise. Such delusions are similar to those seen in patients with schizophrenia, says [cognitive neuroscientist Olaf Blanke of the Swiss Federal Institute of Technology]. Schizophrenics often mistake their own bodies to be someone else's, for example, and attribute their own actions to others. They also have frequent illusions of being followed or controlled by a stranger, as do those who claim to have been manipulated by aliens.[22]

---

19 The Matrix, Australian-American film dir. by the Wachowski brothers, 1999.

20 Horror author Stephen King's 2006 best seller novel Cell features TMS.

21 Liane Young et al., "Disruption of the right temporoparietal junction with transcranial magnetic stimulation reduces the role of beliefs in moral judgments." PNAS.com, March 2010.

22 Charles Q. Choi, "Brain Stimulation Triggers Paranoia, Sense of Alien Presence" (Live Science, September 20, 2006.

Princeton psychology professor Julian Jaynes came up with the theory of the bicameral mind[23] after studying Homer's *Iliad* and *Odyssey* as an actual history of the Trojan War in which ancient men like Achilles had real experiences with gods like Athena. For example, when Achilles becomes infuriated with King Agamemnon and reaches for his sword, his aegis Athena quells him with, "Hold your hand. Obey."

> This sequence offers us an insight into the working of the mind of people of ancient civilizations, for according to Jaynes they experienced reality in an extremely different fashion than we do—well, or didn't experience it: he tells us that they "did not have subjectivity as do we; [they] had no awareness of [their] awareness of the world, no internal mind-space to introspect upon": their mind—the Bicameral Mind—was split between the automaton part—incapable of adequately engaging in any novel or complex situation, and the "god" part—auditory and visual hallucinations that were obeyed immediately and did allow people to engage in novel and complex situations. In the scene above it was of course Athena taking the role of the god part.[24]

This is similar to the "shadow person" becoming visible when the ancient TPJ was stimulated. Does TMS stimulate a perception of the *Doppelgänger*[25]? When TMS shuts down the posterior medial frontal cortex (a few inches up from the forehead) associated with responses to problems, one-third of those stimulated subsequently espoused less belief in God, angels, etc.[26]

Regarding schizophrenics and their "illusions" and "delusions," an increase in amplitudes of low-frequency oscillations (LFOs) has been found in those diagnosed with schizophrenia,[27] and what of their relationship with LTE (long term evolution) signals[28]? What if this "schizophrenic" is actually a brain being remotely manipulated by signaled frequencies? *Twenty-one million were diagnosed with schizophrenia in 2018.* How many of these diagnoses were cover-ups for remote brain experimentation?

---

23 See "The Magical Human Head, Brain, and 'Second Brain'" in Chapter 12 for more regarding Julian Jaynes' theory.

24 Alexey Guzey, "Julian Jaynes and the Ancient Tablets." Guzey.com, April 18, 2018.

25 A doppelgänger ("double-goer") is a nonbiologically related look-alike or double of a living person. - Wikipedia

26 Mary-Ann Russon, "Mind control: Scientists can now make people alter their prejudices and belief in God." International Business Times, October 15, 2015.

27 M.J. Hoptman et al., "Amplitude of low-frequency oscillations in schizophrenia: a resting state fMRI study," Nathan Kline Institute, 2009.

28 B. Lv et al., "The alteration of spontaneous low frequency oscillations caused by acute electromagnetic fields exposure," Clinical Neurophysiology, September 4, 2013.

Because the human brain generates electrical signals in the same ELF frequencies, scientists speculate that transmitting strong signals in these frequencies might interfere with the natural brain activity of persons in the target area, producing effects ranging from hypertension to sudden death . . . Initial results coming out of laboratories in the United States and Canada [show] that certain amplitude and frequency combinations of external electromagnetic radiation in the brainwave frequency range are capable of bypassing the external sensory mechanism of organisms, including humans, and directly stimulating higher-level neuronal structures in the brain. This electronic stimulation is known to produce mental changes at a distance, including hallucinations in various sensory modalities, particularly auditory. Because the power levels are so low, the brain could mistake the outside signal for its own, mimic it (a process known as bioelectric entrainment), and respond when it changes.[29]

Inducing "virtual lesions" on the brain with TMS reduces soldiers' need for sleep.[30] Arizona State University's Center for Strategic Communication ("strategic communication" = counterterrorist tactics) ran a program in 2013 called "Toward Narrative Disruptors and Inductors: Mapping the Narrative Comprehension Network and Its Persuasive Effects." Decoded, "narrative disruptors and inductors" refer to jamming the brain's thoughts and implanting other "narratives"[31] in the temporal lobe by means of TMS.

Trigeminal nerve stimulation (TNS)

Recently, a new medical device to be used on children was announced: the Monarch eTNS. The term *Monarch* hearkens to MK-ULTRA mind control.[32] *Trigeminal nerve stimulation (TNS)* is particularly for children 7-12 years old diagnosed with attention deficit hyperactivity disorder (ADHD)[33] is "to be used in the home under the supervision of a caregiver *during periods of sleep . . .* nightly for four weeks" (emphasis added)[34]—a revisit of the *psychic driving* sleep

29 Ron McRae, Mind Wars: The True Story of Secret Government Research into the Military Potential of Psychic Weapons. St. Martin's Press, 1984.

30 A. Pascual-Leone et al., "Transcranial magnetic stimulation: studying the brain-behaviour relationship by induction of 'virtual lesions.'" Philosophical Transactions B, The Royal Society, 29 July 1999.

31 "Secret DARPA Mind Control Project Revealed: Leaked Document." Activist Post, July 29, 2013.

32 The chapter "MK-ULTRA Is Now eMK-ULTRA" was strangely mangled on my computer.

33 Attention deficit disorder (ADD) and attention deficit hyperactivity disorder (ADHD) are misdiagnoses of children suffering the brain and nervous system agonies of electrohypersensitivity (EHS).

34 "NeuroSigma Announces FDA Clearance of Monarch eTNS System as First Non-Drug

experiments spawned by the CIA's MK-ULTRA psychiatrist Ewan Cameron at McGill University in Montreal in the 1950s and 1960s.[35] The bioelectronics corporation NeuroSigma ran a 4-week trial of 62 children who exhibited "side effects"—drowsiness, an increase in appetite, trouble sleeping, teeth clenching, headache, and fatigue—but "no serious adverse events." (*Teeth clenching?*)

> The trigeminal nerve is the largest cranial nerve, offering a high-bandwidth pathway for signals to enter the brain bilaterally and at high frequency. The trigeminal nerve projects directly or indirectly to . . . the locus coeruleus, nucleus tractus solitaries, thalamus, and cerebral cortex . . .

> TNS is Monarch psychic driving, more pernicious than even TMS.[36]

The electroencephalogram (EEG)

Brain research on humans was at the core of MK-ULTRA, far beyond testing on rats and chimpanzees. Today's *digital* brain research is literally a Pandora's box in the sense of the CIA's *Project Pandora,*[37] which investigated the impact of low-level microwaves on the brain and collected and catalogued emotional and pathological state excitation signals / signatures. Signal processors of EEG brainwaves on laptop computers can now utilize the 27 phonemes of the "little voice in our head" doing our thinking and knowing our thought before we ourselves experience it. These 27 phonemes can be used to entrain our brains and run *thoughts that are not ours.*

The *electroencephalograph (EEG)* is considered a neurofeedback machine. A 1995 "Whispers in the Brain" brochure of electroencephalographer Margaret Ayers describes the *old* EEG procedure, i.e. pre-remote:

Treatment for Pediatric ADHD." Biospace.com, April 24, 2019.

35 One wonders what Cameron (a CIA psychiatrist) owes to the pre-World War One "Twilight Sleep" practice: "In 1915, the Twilight Sleep Maternity Hospital was established in Boston under the leadership of Dr. Eliza Taylor Ransom, founder of the New England Twilight Sleep Association . . . In Twilight Sleep, hypodermic injections of morphine combined with scopolamine (a powerful hallucinogenic and amnesiac) and pentobarbital sodium were given every hour . . ." See Jessica Mitford's The American Way of Birth (Dutton, 1992). Scopolamine is typically used as a post-surgery transdermal patch. For decades, intelligence agents, criminals, and blackmailers have used scopolamine to make victims do unspeakable things (like child rape), during which they are photographed and their memories wiped.

36 Like the crime of geoengineering, MK-ULTRA is going public, its discoveries via torture praised to new generations utterly ignorant of the Paperclip Nazis and Cold War "research."

37 The name of the project was apt: According to Hesiod, when Prometheus stole fire from heaven, Zeus took vengeance by presenting Pandora to Prometheus' brother Epimetheus. Pandora opened a jar left in his care that contained sickness, death and other unspecified evils, which were then released into the world.

> Noninvasive sensors, or electrodes, are connected to specific sites on the surface of the head. The sensors enable the brain wave patterns to be displayed on the computer screen. By placing the sensors strategically on the head, specific areas of the brain can be trained to replace abnormal rhythmic patterns with normal rhythmic patterns. The high-speed neurofeedback equipment can filter out and display a wide array of electrical patterns and frequencies produced by the brain. Two of the most significant ones are beta, a fast wave, and theta, a slow wave . . . The computer assists the brain in recognizing normal rhythmic patterns by producing audio and visual reinforcement when they occur. The brain makes the appropriate corrections immediately.[38]

When legitimately used, an EEG can allegedly rebalance the body and treat brain disorders (head injury, coma, stroke, epilepsy, migraine and cluster headaches, anoxia, learning disabilities, dyslexia, clinical depression—even dissociative identity disorder). Illegitimate use leads us back to the 1970s and 1980s and Igor Smirnov's "psycho-correction," a Soviet term denoting employing subliminal messages to alter the will or modify the personality without the subject's knowledge. In early brain-computer interface (BC)I experiments, EEGs were used to plug the human brain into a computer to measure brain waves and create a computerized map of the subconscious to determine, for example, where impulses such as anger and the sex drive arose. Now, according to Robert Duncan, PhD, it can be done from satellite (see below).

Is the EEG just picking up on electrical charges, or is it being used to read the invisible *ki / chi æther* energy system that the ancient Eastern science of acupuncture reads, the aura that Semyon Kirlian (1898-1978) photographed in 1939?[39] Kirlian photography in Russia is now the *gas discharge visualization technique (GDV)*.[40] With *electrophotonic* digital technology, physicians can read the 3-space body's aura (corona) and predict energy lapses before they end in full-blown disease—*predictive* medicine at its best.

Pediatrician Karl König, MD (1902-1966) esoterically describes the EEG's ability to "read energy lapses" in the corona:

---

38 Ayers, Margaret. "Whispers from the Brain: A Breakthrough in Neurofeedback & The World's First Patented Real Time All Digital EEG Neurofeedback Machine." Margaret Ayers, 1995.

39 Electrography, electrophotography, corona discharge photography (CDP), bioelectrography, gas discharge visualization (GDV), electrophotonic imaging (EPI), and Kirlianography.

40 Invented by biophysicist Konstanin Korotkov.

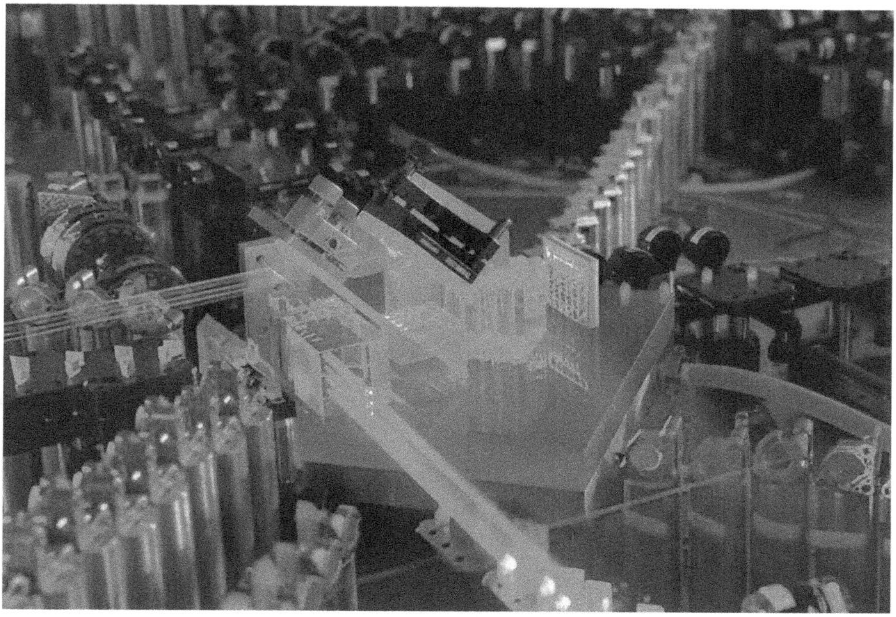

The photon-based quantum computer.

Christian Weedbrook, CEO, Xanadu, Toronto, Canada: "It is only a matter of time before quantum computers will leave classical computers in the dust."

https://www.nature.com/articles/d41586-020-03434-7

> . . . in varying degrees, the forms and patterns of the aura [corona] are detected by the devices of an EEG. It is not an electroencephalogram at all, but an aura-gram revealed by electric means . . . This aura, however, is in immediate interplay with our ether body and receives from it its colours and patterns. The aura, as a phenomenon of human soul activities, is clothed with ether forces. These ether forces are revealed by electrical means . . . Electric potentials detect the ether forces, the garment of the aura; hence the moving and changing patterns of the aura appear via the ether body in the rhythms of the EEG.[41]

Dr. König compares brain consciousness to the Northern Lights (aurora borealis) which appear

> . . . around and above the earth and correspond to the weather conditions of the surrounding atmosphere. No one would think that the

41 Karl König, MD, "What Is the Meaning of the EEG?" in The Living Brain by W. Grey Walter (W.W. Norton and Company, 1963). The ether body is the subtle body that connects the living human being with the life force æther of the universe.

earth is nothing but a body for creating the aurora borealis. So also is the brain not in the least a structure which is nothing but a tremendous electronic computing machine. The aurora borealis is an indicator of the atmospheric conditions in the same sort of way that the EEG is a record of human conditions of consciousness.[42]

Dr. König then questions the eyelids "flicker test" (8-13 cps / Hz) that produces moving geometic patterns (whirling spirals, whirlpools, explosions, Catherine wheels). Given that the light is stationary, the eyes shut and not moving, and the head still, what is converting the rhythmical flickers into manifold moving geometric patterns? Dr. König posits that the EEG flicker test has discovered "the supersensible sphere of the living [etheric] forces" in the human being."[43]

But the EEG has been weaponized since primary frequency allocations (prima freaking) have been mapped and are now used extensively to produce the present

> . . . frightening political reality that the Left has chosen to explain away and ignore . . . Though sometimes used today, mind control implants became passé in the 1970s. They are no longer necessary for the feds or organized criminals with access to the technology to punish or control a human target. Take it from me—I was targeted for eight years, and it isn't pleasant. The process these days is known as "Prima Freaking," short for the mapping of primary frequency allocation, the distribution of biotelemetrically responsive frequencies in the body.[44]

According to Robert Duncan, PhD, the fMRI is a red herring cover-up of the NSA's *remote neural monitoring (RNM)* or, more correctly, *EEG heterodyning*, a SIGINT (signals intelligence) satellite-based BCI technology that remotely EEGs a brain fingerprint (emotional signature clusters), then takes over the brain. *EEG cloning*—the electromagnetic observation of a target's EM field, followed by decoding via software, after which the emotional patterns are fed back to the target's brain or to another brain—is described by Dr. Duncan:

> EEG cloning refers only to the special case of *observing* a target's mind—only one aspect of the technology. A psychic warrior can EEG clone his brainwaves onto a target, symbolized in *The Matrix* when the agents take over random citizens' bodies while pursuing the heroes. The correct ter-

42 Ibid.

43 Ibid.

44 Email from investigative journalist Alex Constantine aka Daniel Rightmeyer. Constantine's books on mind control are excellent.

minology to describe everything between observing a mind and taking over a mind is *EEG heterodyning*. EEG cloning is just a special case of EEG heterodyning.[45]

A quantitative electroencephalograph (QEEG) coupled with an evoked potential test (EPT)[46] can be used to determine (or create?) brain damage. This technology was used on Sean Sellers, an early "lone nut" teen shooter who in 1986 killed his mother and stepfather while they slept. First diagnosed as paranoid schizophrenic, Sean was correctly diagnosed in 1992 with multiple personality disorder (MPD), now known as dissociative identity disorder (DID). With QEEGs and EPTs, three physicians determined that his brain had been damaged in childhood. Sean was executed in 1999 at 29 years old. Since then, the American public has watched one "sleeper" after another on anti-depressants or anti-psychotics shoot children and adults with little or nothing revealed in mainstream media about their past abuse or the state of their brain on Big Pharma drugs.

Millions of teenaged boys are glued to video games based in sophisticated technology no doubt being used for remote programming. Game developer Bantam Joe talks about Microsoft's Kinect Xbox 360 game station based on the player's biometrics:

> As a game developer, I used to use infrared arrays for motion capture of people's faces and bodies so I could create 3D replicas of the person for virtual avatars. I'd been doing motion capture since the early 90's, first with Acclaim Entertainment. If you have ever seen or played with the popular Microsoft Kinect Xbox 360 game station, it had exactly such technology. It had infrared laser array, depth sensor, voice recognition, bull body gait recognition, and rumor has it that all of that data and information was being quietly sent from your home to Microsoft. Learning and recording you. Recording our kid's metrics.—Oh, and just so you know, Microsoft caught a lot of heat over the allegations and supposedly made adjustments to make sure to turn off the Kinect units while people were walking around at home doing everyday things. Supposedly.

45 Robert Duncan, The Matrix Deciphered: Psychic Warfare / Top-Secret Mind Interfacing Technology, Higher Order Thinkers Publishing, 2006. Heterodyning is an engineering term meaning to mix signals.

46 Unique EEG patterns recognized by an algorithm as an individual's signature. By means of the evoked potential, the state of the electromagnetic field inducing the local heating of billions of mechanically actuating DNA origami robots tethered to metal nanoparticles is controlled. – Shachar Amon et al., "Thought-controlled Nanoscale Robots in a Living Host." PlosOne, August 15, 2016.

Psychologist Jayne Gackenbach's studies on the dreams of hard-core gamers accustomed to controlling their gaming environments indicated reversed threat simulations operant in their nightmares—in other words, they become the aggressor / demon attacker instead of the threatened victim: "Levels of aggression in gamer dreams also included hyper-violence not unlike that of an R-rated movie."[47] Not exactly children's play or "boys will be boys," is it? What role is the software playing in developing game psychology?

In his 2011 book Forbidden Gates, Tom Horne takes a close look at the 2010 pre-programming film Inception with Leonardo DiCaprio:

> . . . industrial spies use a dream machine called PASIV to steal corporate secrets by means of invasion and "extraction" of private information through a victim's dreams. In a second scenario, the film depicts ideas planted in the person's mind (inception) so that the individual perceives them as his or her own, thus allowing the victim to be steered toward particular decisions or actions—a modern upgrade on brainwashing a la the Manchurian Candidate.[48]

The American public is denied access to the brain scans of warmongering, psychopathic Presidents who smile for photo-ops. An insightful study of former President William Jefferson Clinton (1993-2001) came out in 1999. However you choose to read it, what has been evident in practically every President since John F. Kennedy is the absence of authentic affect.

> The trait at the root of psychopathy is flattened affect. The profound shallowness of the psychopath's emotional life is not only their behavioral trait—though often masked by an outward glib charm—it has also been identified in brain scans.[49]

Lowered, flattened affect is the upshot of trauma to the prefrontal cortex. *Descartes' Error: Emotion, Reason and the Human Brain* by neurologist Antonio R. Demasio, PhD, MD, discusses this correlation:

> . . . what is damaged in these patients is not memory or intelligence, but

---

47 Jeremy Hsu, "Video Gamers Can Control Dreams, Study Suggests." LiveScience, May 25, 2010.

48 Thomas R. Horne and Nita F. Horne, Forbidden Gates: How Genetics, Robotics, Artificial Intelligence, Synthetic Biology, Nanotechnology, & Human Enhancement Herald The Dawn Of Techno-Dimensional Spiritual Warfare. Defender, 2011.

49 C.J. Barr, "Toward a Unified Theory of William Jefferson Clinton." Laissez Faire Electronic City Times, Vol. 3, No. 13, March 29, 1999. Editor J. Orlin Grabbe wrote an extensive series on the Clinton's http://www.memresearch.org/grabbe/#foster and died at 60 of a "heart attack" in Costa Rica on the Ides of March 2008. RIP to a great researcher and genius.

the neural connections between the emotional and cognitive centers of the brain. More specifically, the ventromedial frontal region is reported to be responsible for emotional processing and social cognition through connections with the amygdala and hypothalamus . . .[50]

Was it just coincidental that the very day White House intern Monica Lewinsky gave grand jury testimony about her relationship with President Clinton, the order was given to bomb Sudan and Afghanistan[51]? Earlier when Bill Clinton was governor of Arkansas, the governor's mansion was base of operations (outside of Washington, D.C.) for the Nicaraguan *contra* war that Lt. Col. Oliver North was running for former CIA director and then-Vice President George H.W. Bush soon to be President.[52] Under Bush Jr.'s regime (2001-2009), it is possible that the frontal or right parietal lobe of the brain of three-star veteran Lt. General William G. "Jerry" Boykin was yoked to "Voice of God" laser technology, given that Boykin, as deputy undersecretary of Defense for Intelligence (2002-2007), claimed to take his orders not from Army superiors but from God:

> We are a Christian nation and our enemy, the enemy of our war against terrorism, is a guy named Satan. Our God is the true God, the God of the Muslims is an idol. Bush became president in 2000 despite losing the popular vote because God himself wanted him in power.

Religion provides an excellent cover for mind control. In 1986, Bush Jr. purportedly had a "Christian experience." At the Egyptian resort Sharm el-Sheikh in 2003, he told a Palestinian delegation: "I am driven with a mission from God. God would tell me, George, go and fight these terrorists in Afghanistan, and I did. And then God would tell me, George, go and end the tyranny in Iraq, and I did. And now again I feel God's words coming to me, Go and get the Palestinians their state and get the Israelis their security and get peace in the Middle East, and by God I'm gonna do it."

Is psychopathy the result of arresting the development of the prefrontal cortex and limbic system? Questions regarding politically powerful psychopaths linger: If brain damage is evident, was it intentional? Was trauma-based

---

50 Antonio R. Demasio, Descartes' Error—Emotion, Reason, and the Human Brain. Putnam, 1994. According to medical engineer Eldon Byrd, Persinger could make someone temporarily blind or deaf by remotely changing the shape of the amygdala. Persinger believed the amygdala to be primary regarding external field influence.

51 Jason Vest, "A political action that couples sex with death." The Village Voice, article removed from Internet.

52 "Beat the Devil. Chapters in the Recent History of Arkansas." The Nation, February 24, 1992. George H.W. Bush and Dick Cheney ran Deep State presidencies from 1980 to 2016: Reagan, Bush 1, Clinton, Bush 2, Obama.

mind control involved?

Are EEGs involved in the closed-loop attention management system (CLAM) referenced in an open-source paper paid for by a U.S. Army Research Office grant? Note the terms "closed-loop systems," "augmented cognition" and "effective interface modifications."

> Vigilance tasks, from driving to surveillance to security, remain important and frequent tasks for the US Army. Yet the difficulty users have sustaining vigilance is well known. Augmented cognition offers new methods for supporting sustained vigilance via a closed-loop attention management system (CLAM). A CLAM system monitors operators' psychophysiology for signs of inattention and then triggers a countermeasure to rouse operators and help them sustain vigilance and good task performance. There are many requirements for bringing this concept to fruition, including minimal or no contact psychophysiological measures, accurate and precise prediction of attention level and task performance, and effective interface modifications. Over the course of this three year project, we have investigated 1) effective combinations of psychophysiological measures of inattention, 2) effective countermeasures, and 3) a complete closed-loop system for monitoring and sustaining attention and task performance.[53]

Silent Sound Spread Spectrum (S4, S-quad, Squad)

Abstract of US Patent #5,159,703 "Silent Subliminal Presentation System," October 27, 1992:

> A silent communications system in which non-aural carriers in the very low or very high audio-frequency range or in the adjacent ultrasonic frequency spectrum, are amplitude- or frequency-modulated with the desired intelligence, and propagated acoustically or vibrationally for inducement into the brain, typically through the use of loudspeakers, earphones, or piezoelectric transducers. The modulated carriers may be transmitted directly in real time or may be conveniently recorded and stored on mechanical, magnetic, or optical media for delayed or repeated transmission to the listener.

53 David A. Kobus et al. "A real-time closed-loop system for predicting and counteracting lapses of attention," Pacific Science and Engineering Group, Inc., 2008.

Multiplex movie theaters, rock concerts, sports arenas, and smart TVs with extraordinary sound systems may be utilizing S4 systems with EEG-derived emotion signature clusters on carrier frequencies downloaded into supercomputers to silently induce and change the emotional state of those present. *All S4 schematics owned by Silent Sounds, Inc. are classified.* This is emotion cloning tech for establishing hive minds: replicate and store target EEG signatures, then transmit modified signatures back to targets. Our cells amplify the radio signals at certain frequencies and demodulate the voices on a basic carrier wave.

The S4-harvested emotion signature clusters can be piggybacked onto ordinary radio and television carrier frequencies and piped into homes. To influence political figures or populations, electrical interference of S4 thoughts, sensations, impulses, or crosstalk[54] can be used so the brain processes the interference pattern as information.

Magnetic resonance imaging (MRI) / functional MRI (fMRI)

Magnetic resonance imaging (MRI) scanners utilize magnets (like a superconducting SQUID, see below) able to generate a magnetic field 8,000X - 30,000X that of the Earth's natural field. Supposedly the best way to see inside a human body without cutting it open,[55] MRI scanners vary from full-body horizontal tubes (*bores*) into which the patient is inserted, to the tip of a fiber optic endoscope (Surgi-Vision), a probe 3.5/100 of an inch in diameter that melts tumors, cauterizes nodes, and is used in cases of arrhythmia, angioplasty, child heart procedures, prostate surgery, etc.

Konstantine Meyl, PhD—who writes and lectures on neutrinos and scalar wave technology,[56] DNA propagation, cell resonance, electrodynamics, and potential vortices—describes the MRI process:

> In this imaging method, a strong field of superconducting magnets initially aligns the cell nuclei and [carbon-containing] ring molecules. Then, a high-frequency alternating field is superimposed and the resulting emanating response to the magnetic scalar waves is measured, allowing the creation of the three-dimensional image of the body.[57]

---

54 In electronics, crosstalk is any phenomenon by which a signal transmitted on one circuit or channel of a transmission system creates an undesired effect in another circuit or channel. It is usually caused by undesired capacitive, inductive, or conductive coupling from one circuit or channel to another. - Wikipedia

55 Supposedly, MRI scanners can only image organic compounds, not inorganic matter.

56 Electrically neutral subatomic particles with a mass close to zero. Apparently, neutrinos are a type of scalar wave for internal communication.

57 Konstantine Meyl, "DNA and Cell Resonance: Magnetic Waves Enable Cell Communica-

The *functional magnetic resonance imaging (fMRI)* scanner is used specifically for "brain fingerprinting" by reading frequencies—for example, the frequency of the primary visual cortex where the eyes' conscious and unconscious sensory data is processed for the brain, or the frequencies of emotions and states of consciousness like resilience (prefrontal cortex, amygdala), outlook on life (ventral striatum), sensitivity to context (hippocampus), social cues (amygdala, fusiform), internal body cues (visceral organs), attention / focus (prefrontal cortex), etc.[58] fMRI scans can reportedly read intentions—shades of the 2002 "pre-crime" film *The Minority Report*?

> 'Using the [terahertz] scanner, we could look around the brain for this information and read out something that from the outside there's no way you could possibly tell is in there. It's like shining a torch around, looking for writing on a wall,' said John-Dylan Haynes at the Max Planck Institute for Human Cognitive and Brain Sciences in Germany . . .[59]

A specific frequency can even be *inserted* to remotely affect the reticular activating system that raises and lowers consciousness so as to make a person more susceptible to unconscious drives (food, sex, aggression). Was this behind the 2012 Miami cannibal attack on a homeless man?

> During the 18-minute filmed encounter, Eugene (who was himself stripped nude) accused Poppo of stealing his Bible, beat him unconscious, removed Poppo's pants, and bit off most of Poppo's face above the beard, including his left eye, leaving him blind in both.[60]

Paul Root Wolpe of the Center for Bioethics at UPenn has criticized this manipulative use of fMRI as "a textbook example of how something can be pushed forward by the convergence of basic science, the government directing research through funding, and special interests who desire a particular technology."[61] One thing for certain: the fMRI has revolutionized lie detection:

> Writing in *Wired,* contributing editor Steve Silberman points out that the lie-detection capability of fMRI is 'poised to transform the security system, the judicial system, and our fundamental notions of privacy.' He quotes Cephos founder, Steven Laken, whose company plans to market

---

tion." DNA and Cell Biology, April 2012.

58 Chan, Vera H-C. "Y! Big Story: What the brain tells us." April 27, 2012.

59 Ian Sample, "The brain scan that can read people's intentions." The Guardian, 9 February 2007.

60 Luscombe, Richard. "Face-eating victim 'will recover' from horrific Miami attack." Guardian, 30 May 2012.

61 Steve Silberman, "Don't Even Think About Lying: How brain scans are reinventing the science of lie detection." Wired, January 2006.

the new technology for lie detection. Laken cites detainees held without charge at Guantanamo Bay as a potential example.[62]

What I'm wondering about is the possibility that fMRIs are not just magnetic but tesla[63] versions of terahertz scanners:

> The use of light to peer into the brain is almost certainly that of terahertz, which occurs in the wavelengths between 30mm and 1 mm of the electromagnetic spectrum. Terahertz has the ability to penetrate deep into organic materials without the damage associated with ionizing radiation such as x-rays . . . Terahertz can penetrate bricks and also human skulls . . . Medically, even if terahertz does not ionize, we do not yet know how the sustained application of intense light will affect the delicate workings of the brain and how cells might be damaged, dehydrated, stretched, obliterated.[64]

Magnetoencephalograph (MEG)

Magnetoencephalographs (MEGs) use magnets to pick up electrical activity in the brain, then correlate brain wave patterns with spoken words and silent thought software via a remote crystalline computer. MEG scanners have the speed and resolution to make brain-computer interface (BC)I possible, and room-temperature superconductors mean MEGs are now portable for open field experimentation. Soldiers wear MEG-scanner "thought helmets" and carry backpack signal-processing supercomputers[65]—at least those soldiers not yet "enhanced" as supersoldiers.

SQUID & MASER

> *SQUID transformers have a sensitivity of 10-15 Teslas or 10-32 Joules. They can measure the smallest detectable change in a second or equivalently the work required to raise a single electron 1 millimeter in the Earth's gravitational field. Compare the sensitivity of SQUIDs with an electrically resonating biotelemetric antenna with modulated body electricity in it viewed from a low earth orbit of 1,000 miles. It is within many orders of magnitude capable of detecting the signal, especially if the exact location is known.*[66]

---

62 Carole Smith, "Intrusive Brain Reading Surveillance Technology: Hacking the Mind." Dissent magazine, Australia, Summer 2007/2008.

63 The tesla is the internationally recognized unit of magnetic flux density. 1 tesla = 10,000 gauss

64 Carole Smith.

65 Read Mitsuo Tonoike et al., "Detection of Thinking in Human By Magnetoencephalography." World Congress on Medical Physics and Biomedical Engineering 2006, pp 2738-2742; Mark Thompson, "The Army's Totally Serious Mind-Control Project." Time, September 14, 2008; http://www.supersoldierprogram.com/.

66 Robert Duncan, The Matrix Deciphered. Higher Order Thinkers, 2006.

The techno-magicians have long known that the brain responds to electrical impulses, but it was the tiny *magnetite* (lodestone) particles in the meninges surrounding the brain that particularly drew their attention, given that magnetite particles were a match for the cryptochrome in migrating species (pigeons, salmon, whales, etc.) and were thus extremely sensitive to electromagnetic fields, such as those produced by power lines and IoT appliances.[67]

The *SQUID (Superconducting QUantum Interference Device)* and magnetic laser known as a *MASER (Microwave Amplification by Stimulation Emission of Radiation)* are two subvocal detectors capable of conducting mind control at a distance.

In 1971 in a null-field chamber, a SQUID magnetometer measured two magnetic fields around the human head: an AC field of back-and-forth ion currents in the nerves and muscles, and a DC perineural system that produces steady DC magnetic fields one billionth the strength of the Earth's field of 1/2 gauss.[68] Twenty years later, biologist Joseph L. Kirschvink used a similar magnetometer in a Caltech room shielded from external magnetic fields by six tons of steel in the walls, floor and ceiling to detect magnetite signatures.

When a modified virus (*viral vector*) is used to deliver genetic material into cells,[69] the DNA inserted into specific neurons can trigger the production of two kinds of proteins working in tandem: one protein to absorb light when the neuron is firing so an infrared beam can remotely detect neural activity, and the other protein to couple with magnetite so neurons can be magnetically stimulated to fire and thus induce a sensory experience of an image or sound *without the senses being involved.*[70]

The SQUID was invented in 1964 by solid state physicist Brian D. Josephson (for whom the SQUID's *Josephson junction* was named).[71] Cooled in liquid helium near absolute zero,[72] the SQUID was shielded from the Earth's magnetic field by layers of copper, aluminum, niobium, and mu metal so it could accurately measure the resonance of subatomic particles, much like the magnetoencephalogram (MEG) or functional magnetic resonance image (fMRI), but on a greater scale. As the MRI changes the quantum state of atoms

67 Thomas H. Maugh III, "Caltech Scientists Find Magnetic Particles in Human Brains." Los Angeles Times, May 12, 1992.

68 Robert Becker, The Body Electric: Electromagnetism and the Foundation of Life (William Morrow, 1998). The gauss is the unit of magnetic flux density B and the equivalent of Mx/cm2.

69 Preprogramming was supplied by two films: The Constant Gardener (2005) and The Bourne Legacy (2012), both with Rachel Weisz.

70 Edd Gent, "The Government is Serious About Creating Mind-Controlled Weapons." Live Science, May 23, 2019.

71 Josephson junction: a supercurrent (current flowing indefinitely without any voltage applied) across two superconductors coupled by a weak link of one electron.

72 Helium is no longer necessary for cooling.

in the body (1.5 tesla[73] or 25,000X the Earth's magnetic field), the SQUID changes the quantum state of whatever field it is measuring, including the *micro-tremors in the larynx that accompany thought.* Digitize the signal and send it to a chip using a Markov algorithm, and subvocal thought is decoded.

But SQUIDs are extremely sensitive to Josephson junction supercurrent flowing endlessly without dissipating (i.e. *æther*). In extremely subtle magnetic fields, images can be "projected directly into a human brain from a distance using the 'scalar' component of a weak magnetic field"[74] by means of superconducting loops and Josephson junctions.

Director James Cameron's *Terminator* (1984) and *The Abyss* (1989) introduced spellbinding realism with the *morphing technique* of photo-realistic computer animation, thanks to the SQUID readers in Loews Cineplex theaters that heighten the subconscious experience. The 1995 preprogramming sci-fi film *Strange Days* portrayed how SQUID feedback can read the tiny magnetic fields of quarks[75]: "Set in the last two days of 1999, the film follows the story of a black marketeer of SQUID discs, recordings that allow a user to experience the recorder's memories and physical sensations . . ." (Wikipedia). Kurtis David Harder's 2017 sci-fi thriller *IN CONTROL* moves the idea forward from using a device to watch someone else's life to a device that allows you to *live* someone else's life.

According to Duncan, the SQUID transformer satellite has a sensitivity of 10^{-15} Teslas or 10^{-32} Joules that can measure the tiniest magnetic changes, *all the way into the ultraviolet spectrum.* From 600 to 1,000 miles above the Earth, measurements of brain and heart femto-Teslas (fT) of magnetic flux, 70 millivolts of a depolarizing neuron, or tens of microvolts of the brain's electrical activity can be taken. One SQUID outdoes 100 satellites or beams bounced off the ionosphere by a constellation of triangulating[76] phased array antennas when it comes to tracking and brainwave / heartbeat biotelemetry.[77]

---

73 One tesla = 104 gauss.

74 Medical engineer Eldon Byrd, Naval Surface Weapons Center, Office of Non-Lethal Weapons; member of the U.S. Psychotronics Association (USPA). On July 23, 2000, Byrd delivered a paper to the 26th annual conference of the USPA in Columbus, Ohio, titled "Recent Advances in Scalar Technologies," citing a July 2, 1997 statement by Major General Sydney Schacknow of the Army's Special Forces (Ft. Bragg, North Carolina) that our military was "working on [the ability to read people's intentions at a distance using a magnetic laser]—a maser operating at extremely low frequencies" that can "alter behavior at a distance." On July 20-23, 2001 at the 27th USPA conference, Byrd's paper was entitled "Mind Control: Paranoid Delusions or Frightening Reality?" Hear him on "Electric Management," March 30, 2016, https://www.youtube.com/watch?v=50AIS7DV8E4.

75 Quarks are subatomic particles carrying fractional electric charges thought to be the building blocks of hadrons (see CERN).

76 Triangulating = "beam forming" in interferometry.

77 Robert Duncan.

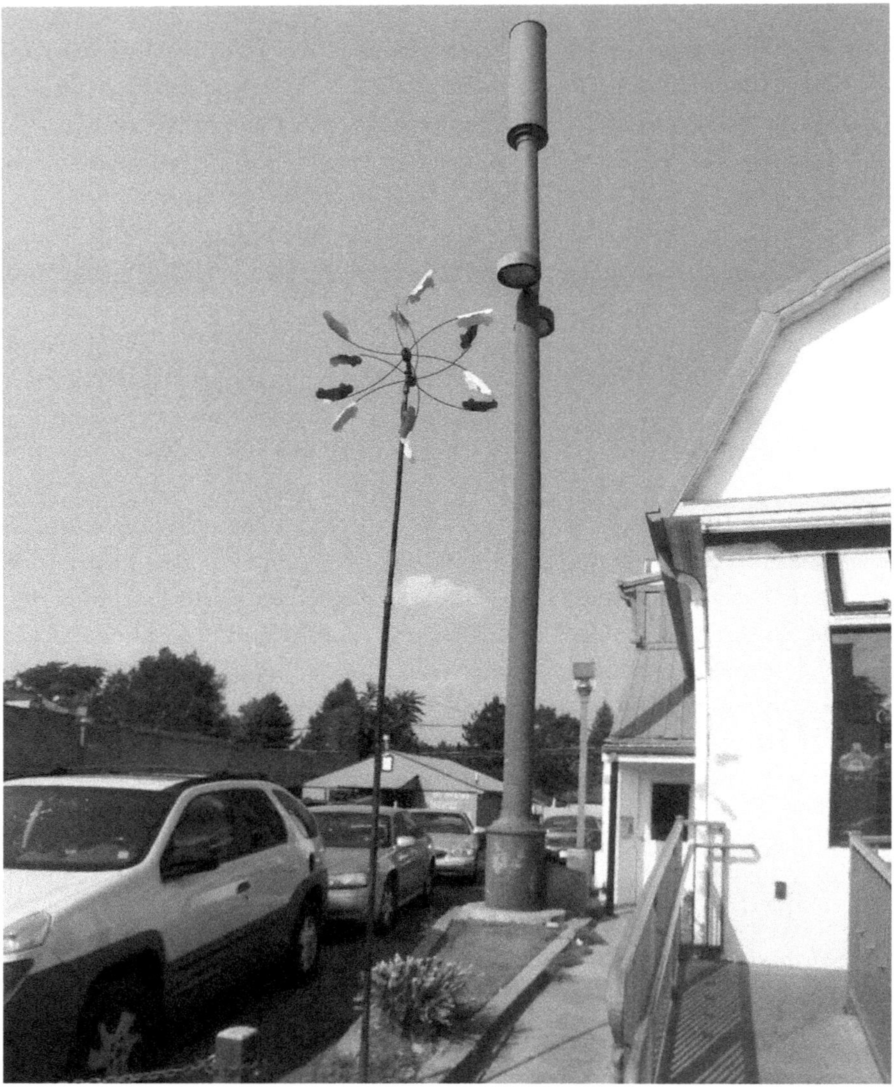

Stealth antennas are everywhere.

https://towerdirect.net/product/50ft-light-pole-antenna-tower

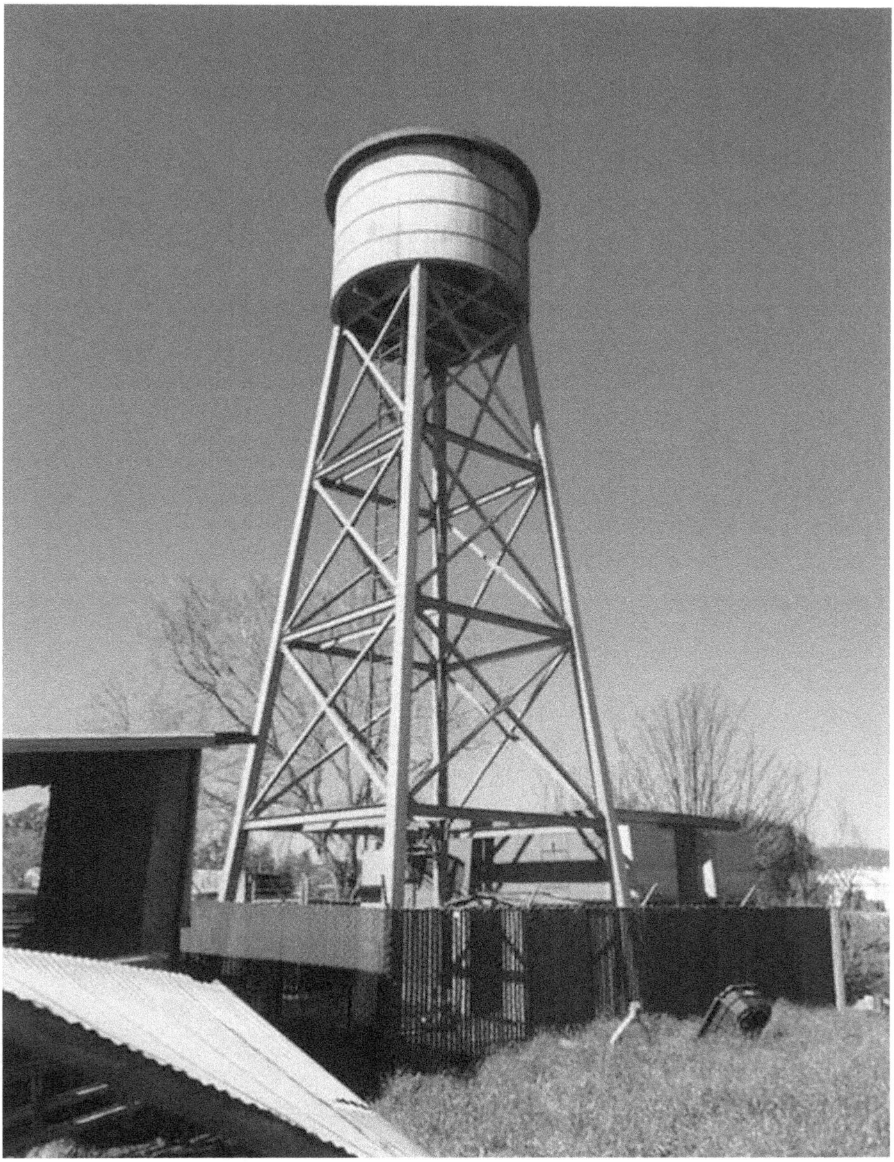

50' fake water tank for concealed cell tower. Regular price $71,700.

https://towerdirect.net/wp/wp-content/uploads/2017/03/50-Stealth-Water-Tank-Tower-1.jpg

The argument that ionospheric heaters like HAARP (even with multiple phased array beams interfering with each other) cannot possibly produce the ions of our Sun is made irrelevant by the fact that our Earth's naturally occurring bi-polar outflow of MASER increases the energy of HAARP ions from 10eV (electron volts) to over 100MeV (megaelectronvolts) when ejected into space 8.9 Earth radii. Earth ions then become indistinguishable from those of the Sun.

Alfvén wave modulation in the ionosphere occurs naturally either as longitudinal or transverse waves responsible for coronal heating of the Sun, acceleration of solar wind, and thermal variations in our atmosphere. But as was discussed in Chapter 1, Alfvén waves are now being engineered. Particle accelerators at CERN, Brookhaven, and ELSA in Bonn, Germany[78] duplicate the natural process by energizing coherent high-energy ions along a linear pathway so that Alfvén waves spiral around the high-energy ions to produce masers like those released from a satellite as a particle beam weapon.

Alfvén wave MASER technology went "black" after this discovery and became the forerunner of directed energy weapons (DEWs). The fireballs and "meteors" now arcing in the sky are most likely balls of luminous plasma from maser weapons being tested in the upper atmosphere. Basically, MASER beams have taken the place of the electrodes that Delgado pasted to shaved skulls in the 1950s and 1960s.

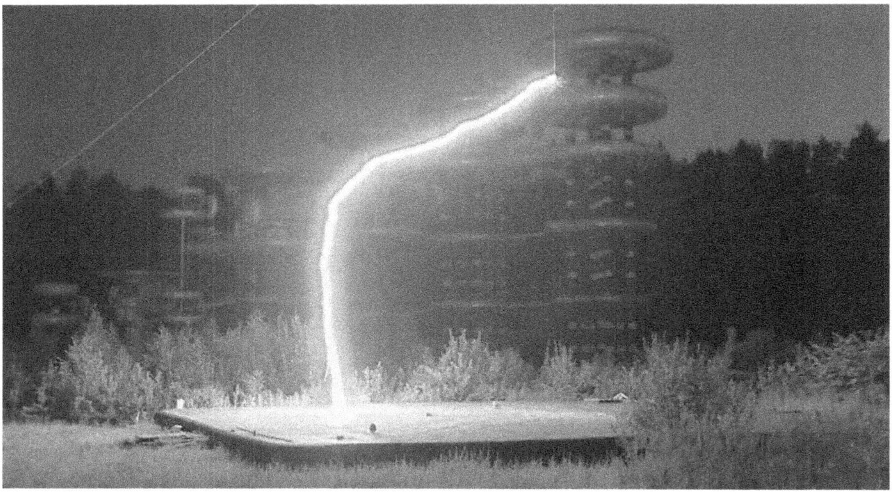

Plasma arcs. The 6-megavolt Tesla Tower (Marx generator, not a Tesla coil) at the High Voltage Research Center outside Moscow produces massive 200-meter volts of lightning (plasma arcs).

https://www.rt.com/news/181748-tesla-marx-generator-lightning/

The MASER is a microwave laser whose beams are used for "silent sound" *synthetic telepathy* (*techlepathy:* reading minds from a distance via machines)

78 See list of particle accelerators at http://www-elsa.physik.uni-bonn.de/accelerator_list.html.

or *voice-to-skull (V2K)* by monitoring weak EM signals associated with subvocal thought (15 Hz 5 milliwatt auditory cortex brain emissions linked with excitation potentials) and linking the thoughts to a computer. Excitation potentials obtained from millions of targeted individuals are used to calibrate techlepathy devices and create dictionaries by cataloguing the specific frequencies per language according to their excitation potentials decoded by parallel processing supercomputers. The *MASER* is more mobile than the SQUID, though the SQUID is preferable for engineering dreams at a distance.

Modulating the human voice audio signal on an ultrasonic carrier frequency carried over a medium with an acoustic wave is basically how it works. Pass audio through gases, liquids, and solids [like in a skull] by converting the audio signals to electronic signals in the ultrasonic frequency range, then convert them to acoustical pressure waves transmitted over carrier signals, then reconvert to audio signals.

Like a laser beam striking your home window and the vibrations causing modulations that are then converted into electrical signals and then into sound, ELF pulse-modulated MASERs fire pulsed frequency at specific brain centers, scan subvocalized thought frequencies and measure interferences, after which supercomputers decode the frequencies into word streams and analyze them. The reverse can also be done to place subvocal thoughts into a target's brain: piggyback ELF audiograms onto a pulse-modulated MASER, or implant illusory images (like of an alien abduction) by broadcasting visual cortex excitation potentials using the scalar component of the weak magnetic field to make the brain see what no one else sees. Closed circuit television (CCTV) of the mind.

Geospace (GS) assists with chemical trail manipulations and environmental contaminants for propagation of MASERs and other waveforms that interface with the human brain and central nervous system. *Even a Faraday cage cannot block a MASER.*

In 2001, Harry Potter's Sorting Hat began preprogramming children and the childlike for the advent of SQUID sensors and MASERs. J.K. Rowling clued us into how the Sorting Hat decided Harry Potter's fate:

> The Sorting Hat . . . reads the minds of Hogwarts' new pupils and assigns them to a house . . . Scientists have already developed the Superconducting Quantum Interference Device (SQUID) which can be arranged in a hat formation and placed on a person's head, where they can detect the tiny magnetic fields generated by electric currents jumping between brain cells . . . [79]

79 Simon Singh, "Elementary, dear Dumbledore." The Guardian, 1 December 2002. Also see Roger Highfield's The Science of Harry Potter: How Magic Really Works. Penguin, 2003.

We are then warned:
And now the Sorting Hat is here
And you all know the score:
I sort you into Houses
Because that is what I'm for.
But this year I'll go further,
Listen closely to my song:
Though condemned I am to split you
Still I worry that it's wrong,
Though I must fulfill my duty
And must quarter every year,
Still I wonder whether sorting
May not bring the end I fear . . .[80]

"Though condemned I am to split you / Still I worry that it's wrong . . ."

PET, SPECT, CT scans

PET (positron emission tomography) scans, previously known as positron emitter detectors, attach radioactive tracers ("nuclear medicine") to glucose and oxygen (fuels for the brain), then tag and collect them. The PET scan produces images of how the brain cells work collectively to retrieve memories and form words and is used in forensic psychiatric examinations to determine if brain damage might account for criminal behavior.

The *SPECT (single photon emission computed tomography)* is a nuclear imaging scan that combines CT with a radioactive tracer injected into the bloodstream. The gamma rays from the arteries and veins in the brain are then assembled into a 3D image. SPECT differs from the PET scan in that it remains in the blood and not in the tissues.

CT or computed tomography scans project 3D viewing by rotating an X-ray tube around the patient, taking multiple images, then using the projections to reconstruct a 3D picture—much like the new 3D printing "replicator" (a *Star Trek* term), only in reverse.[81] While materializing objects inside the body may be next, it is not difficult to imagine how the CT scan might be used remotely to examine and virtually reproduce a target's body—once again, a "dual use" tool:

---

80 J.K. Rowling, Harry Potter and the Philosopher's Stone. London: Bloomsbury, 1997. Rowling is connected to a secret society.

81 Kara Manke, "New 3D printer uses rays of light to shape objects, transform product design." Dogtown Media, January 31, 2019; and Davide Castelvecchi, "Forget everything you know about 3D printing—the 'replicator' is here." Nature, 31 January 2019.

Through a live video feed and internet connection, [Australian Centre for Field Robotics at the University of Sydney] participants can operate the scanner remotely, allowing medical radiation sciences students throughout Australia to perform learning exercises with no radiation hazard, patient involvement or on-site expert supervision. The fully functioning scanner allows students to scan human-like "phantoms" in real-time via remote access.[82]

N3 (Next-generation Nonsurgical Neurotechnology)

"Being able to decode or encode sensory experiences is something we understand relatively well," [Jacob Robinson, assistant professor of bioengineering at Rich University] said. "At the bleeding edge of science, I think we are there if we [have] the technology to do it."

– Sleeka Khan, "The Government Is Serious About Creating Mind-Controlled Weapons," *ScienceTimes*, May 24, 2019

In 2014, DARPA added a Biological Technologies Office, and in 2018 went public with the *Next-Generation Nonsurgical Neurotechnology (N3)* program for "high levels of brain-system communications . . . a bidirectional system . . . that could include human-machine interactions with unmanned aerial vehicles (UAVs), active cyberdefense systems, or other properly instrumented Department of Defense (DoD) systems."[83] Descriptions like "a safe, portable neural interface system capable of reading from and writing to multiple points in the brain at once" and "precise interaction with very small areas of the brain, without sacrificing signal resolution or introducing unacceptable latency into the N3 system" allude to the very complex of "advances in biomedical engineering, neuroscience, synthetic biology, and nanotechnology" that this book attempts to expose—all due to hefty military grants guaranteeing dual-use weaponization.

N3 is high-resolution bidirectional brain-computer interface (BCI) at its DARPA best. At one level, it is about commanding control centers, drones, and nanobot swarms with thought alone, even to *feeling* an intrusion in an otherwise secure network. At another level, it is about reading and writing to brain cells in 50 milliseconds by interacting with 16 locations in one cubic millimeter of the brain that encompasses thousands of neurons.

N3 and "precision medicine" go hand in hand with technologies like *non-*

82 Jennifer Foreshew, "Remote CT scans give NETRAD medical students learning experience." The Australian, July 28, 2015.

83 Mariana Iriarte, "DARPA creates N3 program to achieve high levels of brain-systems communication." Military Embedded Systems, n.d.

surgical Neuralink, "a small, robotic device that inserts tiny electrode threads through the skull and into the brain,"[84] the "Fit-bit in your skull with tiny wires," the programmed nanobots in our bodies and brains whose tendrils ("super-thin threads that carry electrodes") are wrapping around our neurons, awaiting directions from N3.

N3 teams at Carnegie Mellon University, Johns Hopkins Applied Physics Laboratory, Palo Alto Research Center, Rice University, Teledyne Technologies, and Battelle Memorial Institute run experiments that distinctly sound like what targeted individuals (TI's) describe: recorded brainwaves, voice-to-skull (V2K) words and stimulation, ultrasound light guided into and out of the brain, interfering electrical fields, nanobot / MEMS implantations—"a whole new ecosystem" of magnetic fields, electric fields, acoustic fields, and light with optical tomography.[85] While improving "signal resolution" when paired with external transceivers, "nanotransducers convert electrical signals from neurons into magnetic signals to be recorded and processed by the transceiver *[and vice versa]*."[86] Both articles insist that all research is for "wearable neural interface systems"; what is left unsaid is that these "wearables" are designed to be worn on the inside of our bodies and brains, the ultimate goal being to plug us into the ubiquitous IoT internet.[87]

Wireless Body Area Network (WBAN) / Wireless Sensor Network (WSN) / National Telecommunications & Information Administration (NTIA)

> *. . . a signal analyzer (ADF4351 - about $200) can be used to detect the devices. Many of the recent implants use WiFi frequencies (2.4 GHz, 5 GHz) which are detectable using an inexpensive WiFi scanner app. The FCC has approved 2360-2400 MHz for use in Wireless Body Area Networks (WBANs).*
>
> – Owen, August 9, 2020

In 1994, the FDA's *telemedicine* mandate for electronic biochip implants in people with pacemakers, prosthetics, and breast implants dovetailed neatly with the roving wiretaps through throwaway cell phones, conference calls, and 800 numbers legalized by the 1994 Communications Assistance for Law Enforcement Act (CALEA), which is still in effect.

WBAN (wireless body area network) connects nodes in the human body (implants, medical devices, sensors, artificial skin) and transfers data to an

84 Rebecca Heilweil, "Elon Musk is one step closer to connecting a computer to your brain." Vox.com, August 28, 2020.

85 "Darpa Funds Ambitious Brain Machine Interface Program." IEEE Spectrum, 21 May 2019.

86 "Six Paths to the Nonsurgical Future of Brain-Machine Interfaces." DARPA.mil, May 20, 2019.

87 Dan Robitzski, "Military Pilots Can Control Three Jets At Once Via A Neural Implant." Futurism.com, September 19, 2018.

external infrastructure—something like a 2-way radio system that sends out radio frequencies to a sensor-embedded implant from which it collects data, voice, or video, then transmits it to the Cloud. The WBAN system can make use of cell phones, towers, drones, planes, or satellites—in other words, the Internet of Things (IoT). It can interpret what a person is thinking, feeling, seeing, hearing, and experiencing; stimulate nerves or muscles, track,[88] and perform "no-touch torture." In his 2013 book *Dirty Wars: The World Is A Battlefield,* Jeremy Scahill talked about CTTL, the soldier's WBAN:

> Known as Continuous Clandestine Tagging, Tracking and Locating," or CTTL, it involved using advanced biometrics and chemistry to develop a long-range facial recognition program as well as a "Human Thermal Fingerprint" that could be isolated for any individual. They also used a chemical "bioreactive taggant" to mark people by discreetly swabbing a part of their body. The taggant would emit a signal that [Joint Special Operations Command] JSOC could remotely monitor, enabling it to track people 24/7/365. It was like a modern version of the old spook's tracking devices made famous in films, where spies would weave them into an enemy's clothes or place them on the bottom of a vehicle. The taggant allowed JSOC to mark prisoners and then release them to see if they would lead the task force to a potential terror or insurgent cell. Putting them on nonprisoners was a greater challenge, but it happened. The use of such technology, along with the accelerated pace of the killings and captures, would inspire President Bush's declaration that "JSOC is awesome."[89]

Like telemedicine (now "precision medicine"), the WBAN system observes and monitors vital organs and biometrics remotely, including brainwaves. Telemedicine is used for drug delivery, medication compliance, and real-time monitoring, given that corporations like Abilify, Pillsy, CyberMed, CliniCare, and Doctor on Demand are basically paid to *warehouse* the old and infirm outside the hospital / clinic / doctor's office conveyor belt.[90] Whereas the 2G / 3G / 4G cellphone network can monitor only one or a few people, the 5G network monitors 1,000 at a time[91] by using the IoT.[92]

---

88 Like the U.S. Special Operations CTTL system (continuous clandestine tagging, tracking and locating):

89 Jeremy Scahill, Dirty Wars: The World Is A Battlefield. Nation Books, 2013.

90 Kayla Matthews, "How IoT Is Enabling the Telemedicine Tomorrow." IoTForAll.com, November 28, 2018.

91 R.W. Jones and K. Katzis, "5G and wireless body area networks." 2018 IEEE Wireless Communications and Networking Conference Workshops (WCNCW), Barcelona, 2018.

92 S. Chatterjee et al., "Internet of Things and Body area network – an integrated future." 2017 IEEE 8th Annual Ubiquitous Computing, Electronics and Mobile Communications

Electro-Quasistatic Human Body Communication (HBC) is "a method for localizing signals within the body using *low-frequency carrier-less (Ultra Wide Band, UWB)* transmission, thereby making it extremely difficult for a nearby eavesdropper to intercept critical private data, thus producing a covert communication channel, i.e. the human body."[93]

Holograms

When you think holography, you probably think laser, but microwave radiation from a WiFi transmitter can also work with two other antennas, one fixed and one movable, or:

> "Instead of using a movable antenna, which measures the image point by point, one can use a larger number of antennas to obtain a video-like image frequency," says Philipp Holl [professor, Technical University of Munich] . . . the proposed 60 gigahertz IEEE 802.11 standard will allow resolutions down to the millimeter range . . . Using holographic data processing, the very small bandwidth of typical household Wi-Fi transmitters operating in the 2.4 and 5 gigahertz bands . . . Even Bluetooth and cell phone signals can be used. The wavelengths of these devices correspond to a spatial resolution of a few centimeters.[94]

While generation of the 3D image is said to be limited to the space around the fixed WiFi transmitter—"an entire space can be imaged via holographic processing of WiFi or cell phone signals"—it is also true that "The concept of treating microwave holograms like optical images allows the microwave image to be combined with camera images." Holograms shared between a microwave image "and the camera image of a smart phone" can make for a very convincing hallucination, yes?[95] It is also possible to project a hologram into the optic nerve via the eyes to completely block vision.

Getting the picture (pun intended) of how virtual reality can be piped into your home?

Conference (UEMCON), New York, 2017.

93 Debayan Das et al., "Enabling Covert Body Area Network using Electro-Quasistatic Human Body Communication." Scientific Reports, 11 March 2019.

94 Brian Wang, "3D imaging with centimeter precision through walls by using Wifi signals." NextBigFuture.com, May 26, 2017.

95 Earlier versions: "Wireless Network [variance-based radio tomographic imaging] Modded to See Through Walls," Infowars.com, October 2, 2009; Darren Quick, "Millimeter-wave TV camera sees through smoke, fog and even walls," NewAtlas.com, June 15, 2010.

The "ghost machine" (quantum repeaters) & q-teleportation

> *Mind control weapons are the ultimate weapon holy grail that have given birth to the world's most notorious sociopath scientists, who in turn have spawned a generation of the most intense human suffering for weapons-testing efficacy the people of this planet have ever endured.*
>
> – Robert Duncan, PhD, *Deciphering the Matrix,* 2006

Electromagnetic Systems Laboratory (ESL)[96] owned a hefty section of the notorious Area 51 / S4 and was involved in MK-SEARCH (occult) programs in the 1990s when ESL president William J. Perry was the 19th U.S. Secretary of Defense. Given the techno-ergot of military contractors, it is not easy to ferret out how q-teleportation,[97] no-touch torture, and assassination at a distance fit into systems integration, high performance strategic signal processing algorithms, high-speed architectures, remote controlled modular payloads and antenna systems, tactical reconnaissance, direction-finding systems providing integrated real-time intelligence—but they do.

> *Yesterday upon the stair,*
> *I met a man who wasn't there.*
> *He wasn't there again today,*
> *Oh how I wish he'd go away!*
>
> – William Hughes Mearns, "Antigonish," 1899

Thanks to *quantum repeaters* or "ghost machines," ESL devised a way to separate the plasma quantum body from the physical 3-space body so it could walk through walls like the Invisible Man while the 3-space body retreated into a stupor. Plasma travels through any substance with ease. Phantom "in-

96 Once a subsidiary of the military contractor TRW, ESL is now part of Northrup Grumman Corporation. Robert Lindsey's The Falcon and the Snowman: A True Story of Friendship and Espionage (1979), an expose of TRW, alludes to what the major defense contractors that outgoing President Eisenhower referenced are really up to.

97 Haptic technology (European Patent #EP2422939B1) creates a sense of touch or other tactile sensation. Targeted individuals feel like someone is touching their skin; it is generally used for remote sexual abuse or torture but does for remote torture, as well. U.S. Patent #6965816 describes technology used to externally and invisibly remote control the central nervous system.

visi-perps" have a 9 Hz phantom touch and, despite being invisible,[98] can be wounded because the quantum body is made of plasma, the fourth state of matter, whereas mind and *psi* exist non-locally in Time (not 3-space), which may explain why those undergoing the separation often shake, hear a high-pitched sound, and see a bright light just before the displacement / interdimensional shift pops the quantum body out of its 3-space body. To separate the two bodies, crossed cold plasma beams are fired from satellites or black portable handheld "boxes" or briefcases with a horn-like protrusion along one of its edges (mentioned under VTRPE in Chapter 9) *interfere* over the target, possibly assisted by rays from microwave towers.

The plasma coupling with a person's bioenergetic field may, according to the algorithm, hit an exact part of your body with a unique frequency—for example, a thermal color projected onto your head or body connecting with a nano-node to begin psychotronic torture or to separate the *hyperdimensional phantom body* (plasma quantum state) from the physical 3-space body. Picture sound and time-reversed waves coupling with the biomagnetic subtle body (the ether body that acupuncture mapped 5,000+ years ago), forcing the cell nuclei to relax and the quantum body to lift out.

The quantum repeater "ghost machine" makes it possible for operatives to invisibly enter residences, perpetrate rapes, and abduct targets either physically or in the quantum virtual state. Abduction of the quantum body needs *quantum entanglement*, the disembodied transport of a quantum system across space to another system of single or collective particles of matter or energy like baryons (protons, neutrons), leptons (electrons), photons, atoms, ions, etc. This process is called *q-teleportation*[99] and requires physicists, neuroscientists, and geneticists engaged in holography, lasers, and long-range radar.

Consider the well-documented case study of Deva Paul[100] whose holographic quantum body was repeatedly separated from her 3-space body and transferred to a distant location after shutting down her consciousness, possibly by electrically stimulating the claustrum (located on the underside of the neocortex in the center of the brain).[101] The distant location was the U.S. underground research

98 Mentioned in the 1999 film The Matrix.

99 Eric W. Davis, "Teleportation Physics Study." Air Force Research Laboratory, Air Force Materiel Command, Edwards Air Force Base CA 92524-7048, August 2004.

100 Murray Gillin, PhD, Loris Gillin, M.Ed (Psych), and Deva Paul. "Mind Control Using Holography and Dissociation: A Process Model," March 2000. See Semantic Scholar for related papers and books: https://www.semanticscholar.org/paper/MIND-CONTROL-USING-HOLOGRAPHY-AND-DISSOCIATION-%3A-A-Gillin-Gillin/fdc008a-74b9972a31523c0dcb32a85f8f0bf0e95

101 Sebastian Anthony, "Scientists discover the on-off-switch for human consciousness deep within the brain." Extremetech.com, July 7, 2014.

facility deep under the Joint Defence Space Research Facility at the Pine Gap satellite tracking station near Alice Springs, Northern Territory, Australia, whose underground antenna is capable of generating a standing wave around the Earth, and whose supercomputers connect to supercomputers in Guam, Krugersdorp (South Africa), and the U.S. Amundsen-Scott base at the South Pole.[102]

> According to Deva, during such a state of unconsciousness her mind is accessed or in other words the spirit-soul is accessed and can be separated from the physical body. Indeed, the data collected over 3.5 years of observation and recording of these periods of unconsciousness indicates that Deva perceives her spirit-soul to be in another location. In addition, the spirit-soul of any dissociated part can be accessed. Deva and the other parts confirm this transfer is to a high technology facility within Australia. Such a concept of access implies that the spirit-soul can move separately from the physical body.[103]

Once separated and moved out of her 3-space body, Deva said electrodes were attached to her holographic quantum body at critical acupuncture meridian nodes and energy was applied via laser to components of her holographic brain for "downloads." Acupuncture points serve as relay stations linking the physical body with the *etheric double* subtle bioenergy body.

In 1988, scalar expert Lt. Col. (ret.) Tom Bearden (*http://www.cheniere.org*) described the pivotal role of acupuncture nodes in *q-teleportation*:

> The psychotronic (PT) patterns / effects can be modulated onto electromagnetic (EM) signals, even of very low intensity, and still affect living systems because of the kindling effect, i.e. the PT virtual state modulations are stripped off of the living system (in the acupuncture points near the surface of the skin) and introduced onto the human nervous system where they begin to superpose coherently as time passes. Such collection eventually reaches the quantum threshold and observable physical change results . . .
>
> By modulating PT signals onto EM carriers, visible light squelching can be overcome. The PT modulations are then delivered to the biological (or material) targets through the light—photons go right through other photons without interaction except in the most extreme cases—and activate the acupuncture points.

---

102 Lucien Cometta, "Pine Gap Base: World Context." Translated by John Gille, PhD. No date. Also see http://nautilus.org/publications/books/australian-forces-abroad/defence-facilities/pine-gap/pine-gap-intro/

103 Gillin, Gillin and Paul. To determine the intrusive microwave signal, Dr. Gillin used a BWD 826 oscilloscope (range 0-50 MHz) and a sensitive search coil.

Soviet physicist Victor Adamenko discovered that acupuncture points form plexuses or groupings that are frequently sensitive. Further, these plexuses are coordinated with and to specific body locations. By choice of frequency, one can therefore determine what part of the target's body is affected.[104]

Russian categories of psychotronic (nonlethal) warfare—

- *Bioenergetics* (linked living mind and biological body)
- *Energetics* (inert matter and "dead" mind separated from the living body, like BCI)
- *Psychoenergetics* (mind and mental phenomena existing in Time but not in 3-space)

—point to a deeper level of what objectives lie behind the human experimentation on millions, including "organoid" brains being grown in clandestine labs[105]—personalities recorded on computers then downloaded into other "minds" being remotely altered, conversed with, transferred, and eventually self-destructing.

Quantum teleportation via quantum entanglement in which both sender and receiver each have one of a pair of entangled quantum systems. If the sender alters the state of their system, the receiver's system is also affected (and vice versa). Because our "quantum state" is so fragile, the teleportation of Deva's quantum system must have presupposed a *quantum internet network* as well as a LEO (low earth orbit) satellite (500 km altitude)[106] armed with a VTRPE and/or SQUID, "thanks to the ground-based telescopes with metre-sized apertures that can collect most of the light from a beam that has spread out during its passage from a satellite."[107] Ground to satellite may be more problematical, optical light-based teleportation over long distances having to be linked to matter-based quantum memories and quantum computers for data storage and processing.

The Threshold so long in place between dimensions is being breached.

---

104 Thomas Bearden, "Soviet Psychotronic Weapons: A Condensed Background." From Psychic Warfare: Fact or Fiction? ed. John Warren White, Aquarian Press, 1988.

105 Kashmira Gander, "Scientists Create Mini Human Brains That Produce Waves in a Lab: 'The Level of Neural Activity We Are Seeing Is Unprecedented.'" Newsweek, August 29, 2019.

106 The geostationary satellite transponder maintained a 7km diameter around Deva's home. As soon as her holographic brain was extracted, her physical body went unconscious.

107 Stefano Pirandola and Samuel L. Braunstein, "Physics: Unite to build a quantum Internet." Nature, 12 April 2016. Also see that the Austrians and Chinese have discovered their "first" in "teleporting complex high-dimensional quantum states": University of Vienna, "Complex quantum teleportation achieved for the first time," Phys.org, August 23, 2019. So far, the quantum Internet has not been made public.

Occult knowledge of the past and quantum physics of the present are merging, just as they did for Isaac Newton centuries ago. Invitation-only societies like the JASONs know how true the ancient adage *Knowledge is power* is. Theoretical physicist David Bohm (1917-1992) maintained that reality is an implicate order like a giant flowing hologram (holomovement), moment by moment creating a universe in which location is an illusion.[108] Neurosurgeon Karl Pibram (1919-2015) observed that information encoded in the brain, vision, and memory form holographic interferograms of wavelike phenomena, indicating that consciousness can detach or be detached from the physical.[109] Of course, shamans and occultists have been detaching their consciousness (i.e. astral travel) for *millennia*, and now it is being forced to occur via electromagnetic technology. Is astral extraction the same as encoding information in an interferogram of waves[110] and electromagnetically moving it from one point to another before reconstituting it?

Detachment and transference from 3-space can now be done with scalar technology, as occurred with Deva more than 20 years ago by laser shock separating her hyperdimensional holographic brain from her physical brain and transferring it via a satellite SQUID thousands of miles away to where her hyperdimensional plasma brain was uploaded with new programming and transferred back to her physical body via microwave transducers.

If reality is actually an implicate order as Bohm maintained, why not? The problem is not can it be done, but how often is it being done, and under what conditions and for what purposes of power?

---

108 Michael Talbot, The Holographic Universe. NY: Harper Perennial, 1991.

109 Karl Pibram, Languages of the Brain (Wadsworth Publishers, 1969); Brain and Perception (Lawrence Erlbaum Associates, 1991).

110 Roger Lewin, "Research News: Is Your Brain Really Necessary?" Science magazine, April 27, 2007.

Part 3: The Transhumanist Trojan Horse

The weapon they built—SARS-COV-2—was intended merely to convince billions of people to take vaccines that would transform their bodies into bioweapons factories so that [Transhumanist] mutation development could then proceed globally. In this way, the centralized bioweapons vaccine military complex was able to "decentralize" its bioweapons development program by releasing a relatively mild strain into the wild and following it up with a vaccine to accelerate the super strain adaptations.

In effect, every human being who has taken the vaccine is now a walking bioweapons factor, churching out super strains and "shedding" them all over society with the help of their vaccine passports. As cruise lines, sports arenas, airlines, universities and other organizations are now announcing "vaccinated only" policies for who they will allow to resume normal activities, they are creating "perfect storm" conditions for spreading the next global killer viral strain which will be the result of random mutations in a vaccinated person, not deliberate engineering in a genetic lab.

The real medical purpose of the vaccine is to wipe out the less lethal strains and provide viral adaptation pressures that accelerate the creation of more lethal strains. This was all by design. They knew they couldn't design the perfect weapon in the lab; they needed to put human beings to work as walking lab experiments.

– Karen Macdonald, klanmother quantum integrative medicine nurse, March 26, 2021

12

Occult Assault I: The Magical Human Head, Brain, & "Second Brain"

"Organ knowledge"
The pineal gland
Endocrine mimics & disruption
The pituitary gland
The stomach / solar plexus
The limbic brain, hippocampus, and amygdala

Arracher le cerveau! [Rip out the brains!]

– Alfred Jarry, "Ubi Roi," 1896

The brain is the hardware through which religion is experienced. To say the brain produces religion is like saying a piano produces music.

– Daniel Batson, quoted in "Tracing the Synapses of Spirituality" by Shankar Vedantam, *Washington Post,* June 17, 2001

We have no answer to the moral issue.

– Former CIA director Richard Helms, about the nature of MK-ULTRA projects

First came trepanation (drilling a hole in the skull to heighten awareness and a permanent state of higher consciousness) as long ago as 3000 BCE; this ancient practice continues among the elite.[1] Next came heating the cranium to make it pliable for insertion of electrodes; then the nasal passages provided entry to the brain's frontal lobes; then came the injectable microchip; and now nano-scale microprocessors and sensors are delivered by chemtrails, GMO foods, and vaccines.

The Nazi scientists and engineers entering the U.S. at the end of World War Two viewed American scientists as obtuse, unimaginative, and extraor-

1 The International Trepanation Advocacy Group. Tim Hardwick, "Out of Your Head: The Lure of Trepanation," *Strange Horizons*, 4 October 2010.

dinarily naïve. They had spent the war years studying exotic propulsion and mind control, both of which would grant full spectrum will-to-power over planet Earth and beyond. They had access not just to prisoners of war and whole multigenerational families in concentration camps but also to innumerable documents and concepts considered mythical or "occult" by their European and American counterparts whose minds were still in 19th century science of measuring, categorizing, and manipulating.[2]

In 1943, once the European Axis powers had been weakened by a double-flanked European / Soviet war, high-ranking Nazis began making their arrangements with Western industrialists and fascist government men like spymaster Allen Dulles, his U.S. Secretary of State brother John Foster Dulles, and George H.W. Bush's adoptive father Prescott Bush.

Throughout the Manhattan Project, false rumors were carefully circulated about how the Nazis were building an atomic bomb. Once Japan's great cities had been immolated and World War Two pronounced over and done, the Cold War began. The National Security Act of 1947 protected the Paperclip Nazi scientists, doctors, and technicians quietly taking up American lives and research at universities, military hospitals and bases, mental health institutions, and defense corporations under the covert auspices of MK-ULTRA[3] and the NASA secret space ("rocket") program. Records and German names were scrubbed and changed while compartmentalization and need-to-know clearances were established as the Third Reich rolled onto North American soil. General Reinhard Gehlen, chief of Eastern Front intelligence under Hitler, was given full authority by his new CIA handlers to do whatever was necessary to stoke American fear and keep Cold War dollars flowing and public attention diverted from the Third Reich takeover of the most democratic nation on Earth.

In 1946 at Sachsska Children Hospital in Stockholm, Sweden, skulls were

---

2 Review Chapter 2, "Æther, Plasma, and Scalar Waves" in Under An Ionized Sky.

3 From Under An Ionized Sky: "Between 1975 and 1977, the U.S. Senate Select Committee on Intelligence and Subcommittee on Health and Scientific Research of the Committee on Human Resources (the Church Committee) attempted too little too late to get to the bottom of CIA mind control experiments, even to unearthing ten large boxes of documents labeled 'MK-ULTRA, 1952-62.' John Marks, author of The Search for the 'Manchurian Candidate': The CIA and Mind Control: The Secret History of the Behavioral Sciences (1979), requested that the CIA's Office of Research and Development (ORD) provide files 'on behavioral research, including . . . activities related to bio-electrics, electric or radio stimulation of the brain, electronic destruction of memory, stereotaxic surgery, psychosurgery, hypnotism, parapsychology, radiation, microwaves and ultrasonics.' He received 130 cubic feet of classified documents on 'behavioral experiments' and learned that from 1950 to 1970, 44 colleges and universities had hosted MK-ULTRA research with funds quietly flowing through CIA fronts like the Human Ecology Fund (Brown University)."

opened and electrodes implanted; in old people's homes, radio waves created amnesia and weakened immune systems.[4] Two years later in the United States, mathematician Norbert Weiner's book *Cybernetics* came out, cybernetics being the second signal system of modern information and automata theory, feedback loop for the human brain, psychotronic, and behavioral experiments.

In 1951, Operation Artichoke was initiated, then renamed MK-ULTRA in 1953. A June 19, 1964 memo from CIA Deputy Director for Plans Richard Helms made it sound like only Russia was running experiments on human behavior patterns via computer and electrical stimulation of the brain (ESB, biological radio communication).

- Project Moonstruck, 1952, CIA. Electronic implants in brain and teeth.
- MK-ULTRA, 1953-1973, CIA. Drugs, hypnosis, pain induction, electroshock
- Project Orion, 1958, U.S. Air Force. Electrostimulation of the brain (ESB)
- MKDELTA/MKNAOMI, 1960-1969, CIA. Biochemicals, electromagnetic subliminal programming.
- MKSEARCH, 1965-1973
    - MKCHICKWIT: international drug search
    - MKOFTEN: behavioral and toxicological effects
- STARGATE: paranormal, ESP, RV telekinesis
- PHOENIX II, 1983, USAF, NSA. Multidirectional targeting of populations
- TRIDENT, 1989, Office of Naval Research (ONR), NSA. Targeting of individuals and populations
- RF MEDIA and TOWER, CIA, NSA, 1990. Multidirectional subliminal suggestions and programming
- HAARP, 1995-2013, CIA, NSA, ONR. Resonant induction and mass population control
- PROJECT CLEAN SWEEP, 1997-1998, CIA NSA, ONR. Electromagnetic resonant induction and mass population control

In 1968, Stuart Mackay's *Bio-Medical Telemetry* came out. Miniature radio transmitters were being swallowed, surgically implanted, and injected in radio-transmitting substances. At Utah State Prison, California State Prison, El Reno Federal Prison, Texas Prison in Columbus, etc., the CIA was sedating and torturing detainees and prisoners.[5] Criminals considered violent often had

4 "Cybergods," Boycott Brazil, http://www.brazilboycott.org.

5 "Private Institutions Used in CIA Effort to Control Behavior," New York Times, August 2, 1977

damaged frontal lobes due to transmitters being driven into their brain tissue. A 6-channel telemetry system is still used for intracranial eavesdropping, V2K, and control over the heart; all that is needed is a radio frequency analyzing computer, a positron emission tomography (PET) scan, and a spectrum analyzer.[6]

> A lethal device would interfere with the electrical potentials that keep the chambers of the heart synchronized, producing fibrillation and rapid death. A death ray doesn't need to be a truck-sized laser that reduces the target to a smoking heap; a small device that stops the heart will do the job.[7]

Dual-use. Eyes and ears everywhere. Mind control is now an industry. Having begun with drugs, hypnosis, and pain induction (torture), the brain industry players and their intelligence cohorts are concentrating on *remotely pulsed frequencies coupled with genetics.* More on the genetics later.

The Pentagon's DARPA and JASON advisory panel have targeted brain engineering for decades, what they like to call "Advances in Human Performance Modification," for which they have spawned a vast range of compartmentalized terms: neuro-pharmaceuticals promoting "brain plasticity" (permanent rewriting of neural pathways), brain-computer interface (BCI),[8] cognitive computing, digital mapping, etc.[9]

Meanwhile, it's the *occult* (hidden) nature of the brain that's *really* on their minds.

Esoterically speaking, there is something magical about the human head from which four of our five senses collect data and in which the brain is housed. Heads are still ritualistically removed and skulls cached in secret places such as Yale's Skull & Bones Tomb, the Smithsonian, and the Royal College of Surgeons. Does our individuality reside in the head? John the Baptist, *La Guillotine* of the French Revolution, Islamic State beheadings[10] . . . The Aztec god Camazotz, represented by a huge bat, was the Lord of Head-Chopping, and Himmler's *Schwarze Orden* periodically cut off the head of a pure Aryan as a power sacrifice.

---

6 Spectrum analyzers can see signals hidden behind other signals. Sweep a spectrum analyzer over your household smoke detector's eye blinking 24 hours a day like a little nuclear reactor and you will see the cylindrical metal case that cannot be opened because it is a tiny covert transmitter.

7 David Hambling, "Moscow's Remote-Controlled Heart Attacks." Defensetech, February 14, 2006.

8 Noah Shachtman, "Top Pentagon Scientists Fear Brain-Modified Foes." Wired, June 29, 2008.

9 Gregor Wolbring. "Artificial Hippocampus, the Borg Hive Mind, and Other Neurological Endeavors." Innovation Watch, November 15, 2006.

10 Zeina Karam and Bram Janssen, "Under Islamic State, Children Trained to Behead At An Early Age." The World Post, July 20, 2015.

Let's face it: the brain is our most perfect and mysterious part. The brains of explorer John Wesley Powell and Egyptologist W. Flinders Petrie still float in formaldehyde, but the brain of Yahi-Yana Indian Ishi has finally been released from its bondage iin the Smithsonian Institute to his descendants, thanks to the National Museum of the American Indian Act of 1989. Pathologist Thomas Stolz Harvey made off with physicist Albert Einstein's brain in 1955, after which it was sectioned into over 200 blocks and embedded in celloidin.[11] And then there's President John F. Kennedy's brain . . .

The head itself is an electromagnetic cavity resonator or an acoustical resonator.

> Use of an intelligence signal, such as a signal containing EEG information, modulated on a carrier wave with a frequency identical to that of the resonant frequency of the head, would enhance its delivery and its maximal interaction with the brain, as standing waves [scalar] would be set up and the signal would be confined or "trapped" inside the cavity (as opposed to being directly reflected towards the source). In a similar manner, wave interference required for signal delivery or EPR [electron paramagnetic resonance] and NMR [nuclear magnetic resonance] transitions which are necessary for current density mapping could be enhanced in a similar way.[12]

Then there is the correspondence between the Earth and human body. The *Reichsarbeitsgemeinschaft* (Reich working group) recognized our solar system as an etheric-electrical Being which, in correspondence with the human mind (not the brain *per se*),[13] is capable of harnessing a will-to-power for mastery over the universe. Unlike the Newtonian *Weltanschauung* that other Western scientists were still conditioned to believe in, Nazi scientists and engineers were versed in worldviews from East and West, ancient, modern, and futuristic. Fifty years of combining American resources with American resources with German imagination and technical prowess, however, succeeded in producing much of the techno-fascism rising around *and inside of* us at a *Blitzkrieg* pace, particularly since young Chinese savants have joined in the assault.

For the Nazi scientists steeped in ancient documents, the Earth is a crys-

---

11 Brian Burrell, Postcards from the Brain Museum. Broadway, 2005.

12 "The head as an electromagnetic cavity resonator or an acoustical resonator," http://www.information-book.com.

13 Roger Lewin, "Research News: Is Your Brain Really Necessary?" Science magazine, April 27, 2007. After losing all but ten percent of their cerebral hemisphere, people have scored 120 on IQ tests. By the time Vladimir Lenin died in 1924, his brain had shrunk to a quarter of its normal size. (Was he being pharmaceutically controlled, as Hitler was?)

talline etheric-electrical Being with anode (positive charge) and cathode (negative charge) poles, whose seven organs of power—the Sun, Moon, Mercury, Mars, Venus, Jupiter, and Saturn—correspond with the human body's spinal etheric-electrical gateways known for millennia as *chakras*. The brain's role is as a relay station for consciousness coming from nonphysical dimensions with the human body acting as a transceiver antenna to receive and transmit frequencies, and the spinal column as a generator whose significant frequency-dependent voltage from incident electromagnetic fields,[14] with a peak voltage of 100 MHz (FM radio band range is 87.5-108 MHz), impacts the central nervous system (and weakens the blood-brain barrier).

The matter of the brain, and the immaterial mind . . . The brain is more *magically* powerful than, say, the heart muscle, but now in this electromagnetic era we are learning how vulnerable both really are. *Storm a magical brain and you imperil the enigmatic mind / soul, its sense of self and sense of self in others.*

The study of the brain is littered with necromancy, murder, and mayhem. Biological research in general reads like Mary Shelley's *Frankenstein*, from beating heart cells in petri dishes and cerebral organoids—watery blobs of disembodied brains—raised in giant incubators and floating in pink nutrient-rich fluids, to stem cells taken from skin, nose, liver, toenails, and aborted fetuses fed into a "cellular youth serum" (adrenochrome?) in order to turn the cells into an embryonic state. Like boys pulling the legs off of frogs to clinically observe what happens, most ghastly are the balls of cells starved in petri dishes until most die off and leave only the robust brain cells warming in a gelatin (hydrogel?) like the tissue surrounding an embryo's brain. After three months, the brew turns into four millimeters of two million gray matter neurons buzzing with activity and zapping signals to each other *but incapable of thinking.*[15]

Occult / esoteric and quantum terms are abuzz at ultra-high clearance levels, along with the classified science carefully kept for centuries from profane[16] university physics and biology graduate programs while in this era of Revelation of the Method. Blindly and dumbly, we the masses are being guided over the Threshold from physical to a diabolical metaphysics.

Theoretical physicist David Bohm (1917-1992) perceived reality to be an implicate order like a giant flowing hologram (*holomovement*) creating the universe moment by moment, location being an illusion.[17] Neurosurgeon

14 Sevaiyan Balaguru, et al., "Investigation of the spinal cord as a natural receptor antenna for incident electromagnetic waves and possible impact on the central nervous system." Department of Electrical and Electronic Engineering, California State University, June 2012.

15 Zaria Gorvett, "We're growing brains outside of the body." BBC, 5 October 2016.

16 Pro-fane: before the temple, i.e. outside the secret society.

17 Michael Talbot, The Holographic Universe. NY: Harper Perennial, 1991.

Karl Pribram (1919-2015) posited that the brain operates similarly, and that information can be encoded in an interferogram of waves[18] and electromagnetically moved from one point to another before being reconstituted.

Biologist Rupert Sheldrake inserted a fresh direction into the tired old mechanistic view of the brain. He too compares the brain to a radio receiver tuning into realms of memory and ideas, but by means of the decidedly living and changing *morphic resonance*, not dead electromagnetics.[19] In 399 BCE, the Greek / North African philosopher Socrates posited that knowledge is a form of memory in a memory field that a teacher's good question can cause the student to remember and learn anew.

> Morphogenetic fields are not fixed forever, but evolve. The fields of Afghan hounds and poodles have become different from those of their common ancestors, wolves. How are these fields inherited? I propose that they are transmitted from past members of the species through a kind of *non-local resonance, called morphic resonance.*
>
> The fields organizing the activity of the nervous system are likewise inherited through morphic resonance, conveying a collective, instinctive memory. Each individual both draws upon and contributes to the collective memory of the species. This means that new patterns of behaviour can spread more rapidly than would otherwise be possible . . . The resonance of a brain with its own past states also helps to explain the memories of individual animals and humans. There is no need for all memories to be "stored" inside the brain.[20] (Emphasis added.)

And if you are asking, *But where are these morphic fields of memories?* you have obviously already forgotten the holographic universe David Bohm assured us we live in. Location is an illusion.

In analyzing how the transceiver brain picks up these memories, we learn that the temporal lobes (above the ears) connect to magnetic fields. Consider how psychiatric hospital admissions increase during magnetic storms because the ELF micropulsations from the Earth's geomagnetic field resonate in the

18 Karl Pribram, Languages of the Brain, Wadsworth Publishers (1969); Brain and Perception, Lawrence Erlbaum Associates (1991).

19 Rupert Sheldrake, PhD. A New Science of Life. Tarcher, 1983. Also see The Presence of the Past: Morphic Resonance and the Habits of Nature (1988); The Rebirth of Nature: The Greening of Science and God (1992); Seven Experiments That Could Change the World: A Do-It-Yourself Guide to Revolutionary Science (1994); Dogs that Know When Their Owners are Coming Home, and Other Unexplained Powers of Animals (1999); The Sense of Being Stared At, And Other Aspects of the Extended Mind (2003).

20 Sheldrake, Rupert. "Morphic Resonance and Morphic Fields: An Introduction," 2005. http://www.sheldrake.org/Articles&Papers/papers/morphic/morphic_intro.html

Schumann Well and the brain and shift the brain's frequencies. Temporal lobe firing can mean seizures, visions, altered states. Stimulate the Sylvian fissure in the right temporal lobe and a near-death experience (NDE) can occur. This ability of the temporal lobes to shift reality, including *sense the presence of someone unseen,*[21] extends to apnea or sleep paralysis. The parietal lobe above the temporal lobe is involved in "otherworldly" experiences. For example, "speaking in tongues" (glossolalia) decreases frontal lobe function and increases parietal lobe activity, giving believers a "touched by the spirit" experience; decrease the activity in only the right parietal lobe and selfless spiritual experience arises.[22]

Does this mean spiritual experience is just brain activity? Answer: Does a flute play itself?

When certain parts of the brain are firing and our personal magnetic field is suddenly at variance with the geomagnetic field around us, we may notice that other senses beyond the normal five seem to have been activated. Rudolf Steiner posits the existence of 12 senses whose job it is to perceive:

- *the physical body:* touch, life, movement, balance
- *the external world:* smell, taste, sight, warmth
- *the inner spiritual world:* hearing, speech, thought, the I or individuality (ego)

The Swiss physician Paracelsus wisely viewed the senses in this way:

> The eyes have material substance of which they are composed, as it is handed down in the composition of the body. So of the other senses. But vision itself does not proceed from the same source as the [physical] eye; nor the hearing from sound, or from the same source as the ears; nor touch from flesh, nor taste from the tongue, nor smell from the nostrils, any more than reason proceeds from the brain; but these are the bodily instruments, or rather the envelopes in which the senses are born . . . For the abovementioned senses have each their own body, imperceptible, impalpable, just as the root of the body, on the other hand, exists in tangible form. For Man is made up of two portions, that is to say of a material and a spiritual body. Matter gives the body, the blood, the flesh; but spirit gives hearing, sight, feeling, touch, taste.[23]

---

21 Temporal lobe seizures may account for alien abductions.

22 Holden, Constance. "Tongues of the Mind." ScienceNOW Daily News, 2 November 2006.

23 Paracelsus (1493-1541) in the Archidoxis.

"Organ knowledge"

Endocrine (ductless)	*Exocrine (ducted)*
Hypothalamus	Salivary
Pituitary	Sweat
Pineal	Pancreas
Thyroid	Lachrymal

Parathyroids
Adrenals
Ovaries / Testes

"Organ knowledge" is an ancient approach to an innate intelligence of the remarkable human body that in the West only global elites and practicing Satanists appear to have coveted over time, namely how what moves in the inner organs correlates with the movements of the cosmos. Using certain wavelengths, the endocrine system can be made to *reproduce cerebral tissue* and provoke unusual changes in the qualities of individual psyches,[24] and of course sonic waves can be used to simulate particular brainwave patterns to trigger the release of hormones and alkaloids by particular glands, as well. (Thanks to James Bartley for this insight.) And as for the collection of astronauts' blood and urine during their months in space or at the International Space Station (ISS), is some sort of "organ knowledge" being gleaned?

A preprogramming hint at the "mystical path" of organ knowledge was choreographed by Steven Spielberg in his 2002 film *Minority Report*, which I wrote about in *Sub Rosa America*:

> Fluids act as serpentine, vitality-filled leylines. In *Fear and Loathing in Las Vegas* (1971), Hunter S. Thompson's attorney advised him to take a hit of adrenochrome, the fluid allegedly drawn from blood flush with adrenalin due to extreme trauma. Such fluids—including youthful blood[25]—constitute "eating of the Tree of Life" to keep fluid leylines vital. Endocrine infusions from the desiccated glands of dead animals do nothing; only infusions from a live human being do the trick. Death by fluids—not to be confused with death by water— entails directing volatized poisons through space, as in the case of the murder of defrocked Abbé Joseph-Antoine Boullan in Lyons on January 3, 1893 during an occult war among Parisian occultists.

24 A.V. Kalinets-Bryukhanov, "Once More About Psychic Weapons." Ugolog Ukraini, 1991.
25 Ian Sample, "Can we reverse the ageing process by putting young blood into older people?" The Guardian, 4 August 2015.

Fluids of particular glands also call up psychic abilities, organ imaginations once known as *belly* or *organ clairvoyance*. First, impulses enter the gland through the sense organs—for example, by watching someone being tortured—and trigger responses via the resistance of the layers of membranes that make up the organ. The gland then responds with a micro-combustion of secretion, a salt that the moment it falls into the body electrochemically releases an inner image, either emotional or instinctual.

Director Steven Spielberg was allowed to go public with a modern imagination of organ clairvoyance in the 2002 film *Minority Report,* based on the Philip K. Dick short story of the same name.[26] In the film, three wired pre-cogs (precognitives) or *brothers of the 3 points* lie like spokes in a wheel in a viscous photon milk pool of nutrients and liquid conductors that enhance the images they receive from a future embedded in the slipstream of Time, images then scanned by optical tomography. Dopamines and endorphins keep the pre-cogs in a dreamy, feel-no-pain state while their electrode headgear reads and transmits what they see to computers that then display the visual images on monitors and record them. The best organ clairvoyants, the film informs us, are a female and identical male twins—a tip of the hat to the Mengele-style scientific torture that attends such occult technology. Whether one views the precogs as *pattern recognition filters* or Greek oracles, they are denied individual lives of their own. "We're more like clergy than cops," says one of the pre-cog cops . . .

Whole continents of history are often shifted so as to keep hidden the meaning and intent of occult matters. *Scientia est potentia.*[27]

To ordinary people, the extremes of paying a small fortune to imbibe adrenochrome (C9H9NO3) / epinephrine and the blood of children / youths sounds insane or fantastic. But *parabiosis* (the fancy scientific name for youthful blood transfusions at $8,000 a pop) is quite commonplace among the rich and famous / infamous. Billionaire PayPal founder Peter Thiel isn't the only one drinking from the Fountain of Youth to reverse aging and improve cognition—the "resetting of gene expression," as Jesse Karmazin, founder of the Ambrosia Corporation, calls experimenting with transfusions of blood plasma from people under 25.[28] As an anonymous friend in Mexico wrote on December 21, 2016:

---

26 Though it appears that director Stanley Kubrick was not allowed to reveal other secrets in his 1999 film Eyes Wide Shut.

27 Elana Freeland, Sub Rosa America: A Deep State History, Books 1-4, https://www.amazon.com/gp/bookseries/B082WP2DMF?ref_=pe_584750_33951330

28 "Peter Thiel Is Very, Very Interested in Young People's Blood." Inc., August 1, 2016.

It can be only imagined how young people from the poor segments of the population will be desperately happy to sell their blood for the sake of the longevity of the 1-2%. Blood banks will become as commercially savvy as banks. The necessity of separating plasma from blood on a mass scale may start a growing industry with millionaires and billionaires on top. Intensification of the blood trade inside the US will raise the GDP to unseen heights. Availability of multinational blood plasma will intensify a new international trade. What will be the price difference, for example, between the plasma of white and colored youths? Numerous issues will crop up to be answered by the honorable practitioners of the anti-aging blood industry.

Adrenochrome is the *crème de la crème* blood product.[29] Given the necessity of severe trauma and that the child must still be alive during the harvesting of the adrenal glands—often, victims are kept alive for repeated brain stem extractions by inserting a needle into the eye[30]—it is easy to see the ongoing need for poverty and child trafficking. Heavy use of adrenochrome captures iron (Fe) in the body, with Ferretin sequestering the iron as a marker of iron content. Withdrawal from adrenochrome ("organ knowledge") is agonizing, and the aging previously avoided catches up overnight.

The sheer ruthlessness of American-style vampire capitalism is nowhere as transparent as it is in the corporate blood industry. Corporations like Grifols and CSL leach blood and plasma, the golden liquid that transports proteins and red and white blood cells, from the poorest of the poor in exchange for a few dollars. The U.S. supplies 70 percent of the world's plasma while other nations ban the practice for health reasons. Selling blood to make ends meet is how many of the 130 million Americans unable to pay for food, housing, and healthcare get by. 37 million go to bed hungry, many of them children.[31] *The zombifying of America's poor.* Along the U.S.-Mexico border are at least 43 blood donation centers for illegals and Mexicans with temporary visas.

> The thermostats are always turned down to around 50-60°F for the plasma's sake. Once the amber-colored plasma has been extracted, your cooled blood is re-injected in a painful process that feels as if ice is being inserted into the body. America's zombie poor are left almost permanently men-

---

29 "Adrenochrome Paper Trail," https://www.brighteon.com/5ddca729-aa19-4e5d-b11d-b0769c246d65; CYM Corporation, https://archive.org/download/cym-corp-1 / "CYM Corporation and Adrenochrome Production," https://archive.org/download/cym-corp-1.

30 Caleb Brewster, "What Is 'Adrenochrome'? Meet the Biochemical that Elite Zionists are Using to Get High." Daily Crusader, 2 December 2018.

31 Alan Macleod, "Harvesting the Blood of America's Poor: Latest Stage of Capitalism." MintPress News, December 3, 2019. And these statistics are from pre-COVID 19 lockdown days!

tally drained like heroin addicts, and with similarly bruised and punctured arms, except they are being paid for the inconvenience. But perhaps the worst thing about the experience, according to those interviewed, is the dehumanization of the process. Donors are publicly weighed to make sure they are heavy enough. Obese people are worth more to the bloodthirsty companies as they can safely extract more plasma from them each session (while paying out the same compensation)...[32]

More than *one million* illegal crossings of the U.S.-Mexican border were attempted in the first seven months of 2021.[33]

The pineal gland

> *In the middle of the brain there is a small part which has a quite special place; its central position cannot fail to be recognized. It is the part of the brain and indeed of the brain stem which is known to be there, fully developed at birth, and which does not grow much more, as do most other parts of the brain. It is the part known as the "four hills" (corpora quadrigemina), together with the epiphysis or pineal gland.*[34]

In his extraordinary book *Seeking Spirit Vision,* Dennis Klocek offers a unique lens for viewing just how far beyond a computer the human brain truly is:

> In the pineal gland . . . nerve and blood meet in such a way that there is little nerve contact with the blood supply back to the gland but a great deal of nerve contact from the gland to the blood supply. In this way the pineal works in the body mainly to regulate or inhibit; it suppresses the production of hormones in glands such as the thyroid, gonads, adrenals, and pituitary. Between the pituitary and pineal, one can actually envision an endocrine systole and diastole following the circadian and seasonal rhythms of light. Together, these two glands can be imagined as the heart of the brain with impulses of neurochemical / electrical activity and currents of cerebrospinal fluid pulsing between them through the ventricles in the brain (132) . . . [I]t is through systematic development of conscious perception of the sympathetic nervous system that the mystical path is pursued (136) . . . The pineal is in deep neuronal communion with both the sympathetic and central nervous systems and the vascular system deep within the body . . . The glands in general and the pineal in particular

---

32 Ibid.

33 Samuel Chamberlain, "Data shows illegal border crossings on pace to top 1M this month." NY Post, July 15, 2021.

34 Margarethe Kirchner-Bockholt, "A Grail Castle in the Brain." Natura, September 1926.

work to modify the interaction of blood and nerve and keep it within reasonable parameters for the health of the organism.[35]

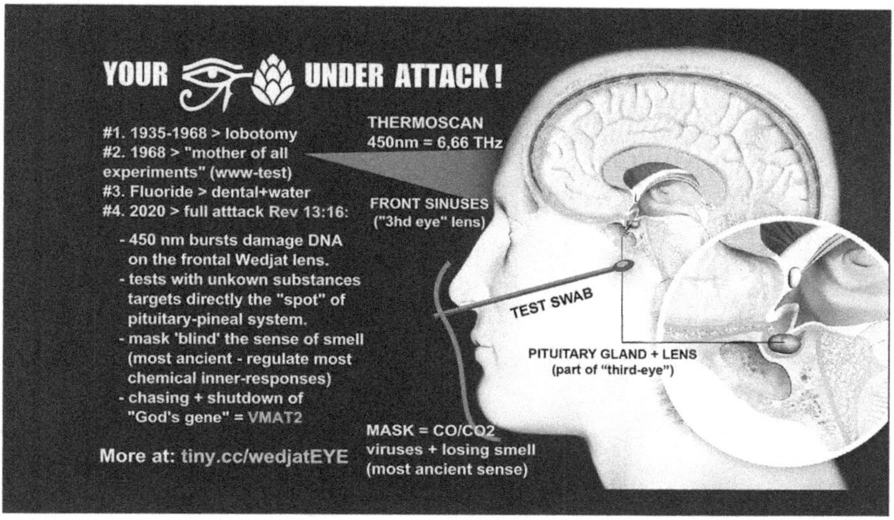

YOUR UNDER ATTACK!
#1. 1935-1968 > lobotomy
#2. 1968 > "mother of all experiments" (www-test)
#3. Fluoride > dental+water
#4. 2020 > full atttack Rev 13:16:
- 450 nm bursts damage DNA on the frontal Wedjat lens.
- tests with unkown substances targets directly the "spot" of pituitary-pineal system.
- mask 'blind' the sense of smell (most ancient - regulate most chemical inner-responses)
- chasing + shutdown of "God's gene" = VMAT2
More at: tiny.cc/wedjatEYE
THERMOSCAN
450nm = 6,66 THz
FRONT SINUSES
("3hd eye" lens)
TEST SWAB
PITUITARY GLAND + LENS
(part of "third-eye")
MASK = CO/CO2
viruses + losing smell
(most ancient sense)

The pineal gland. The pineal gland—the so-called third eye—has been at the center of experimentation by occult secret societies, including the CIA / Big Pharma, for centuries. Housed deep in the brain ("the seat of the soul," according to philosopher Rene Descartes), the pineal gland may be the ultimate target of a purposely concocted synergy that chemically and electromagnetically assaults the air we breathe, the food we eat, and the water we drink, cook with, and bathe in.

https://www.trulightradioxm.org.za/healing-articles/is-covid-19-testing-killing-your-spiritual-side-and-cause-more-dangerous-side-effects/

Neurosurgeon Jack Kruse stresses how the "dark" hormone melatonin is how all human cells regenerate, thanks to the UV light from the Sun picked up by photoreceptors in the skin and the eye's cornea in order to regenerate our cells at night when sunlight is absent. Melatonin, along with three other proteins—serotonin, melanin, and dopamine—delivers energy to our mitochondria where biochemical processes of respiration and energy production occur.

The secretion of melatonin while we sleep seems to point to Descartes' insight that the pineal gland (*epiphyses*) is where soul and body meet. As the hexagonal-pentagonal "doorway" in charge of the body's circadian rhythm control opens, our consciousness enters the geometric portal but will not remember this, once we awaken.

DMT (dimethyltryptamine) too is produced in the pineal gland. (Melatonin

35 Dennis Klocek, Seeking Spirit Vision: Essays on Developing Imagination. Rudolf Steiner College Press, 1998.

and DMT have an almost identical hexagon-pentagon molecular structure with a nitrogen connector.[36]) It is well-known to "psychonauts" that DMT is a door to other dimensions of existence. Datura (belladonna) contains atropine, hyoseyamine, scopolamine—all have similar hexagon-pentagon molecular structures used by intelligence operatives as "zombie" drugs for control, paralysis, and death.

Meanwhile, the brain is being biohacked in the name of sleep research. At UC Berkeley's Sleep and Neuroimaging Lab, transcranial direct-current stimulation (tDCS) is underway, the Fisher Wallace Stimulator pulsing AC current to trigger REM by stimulating serotonin and dopamine and beta endorphin. The Phase Locked Loop algorithm begins the process with an EEG readout of the individual's evoked potential, then locks on and delivers sound at just the right phase of the wave. DARPA continues to work with corporations like Advanced Brain Monitoring to shorten the soldier's need for both kinds of sleep: slow-wave (deep) and REM.[37]

Morgellons lesions are sometimes filled with discharges of tiny glittering hexagons and insect-like entities whose eyes are hexagonally structured. Are these genetically engineered geometric entryways to and from the Eighth Sphere (see below)? UFO / UAP abductees report DMT-visions of pods and humans imprisoned in insect worlds inhabited by insect kings and "greys." Thus, the advent of the term *hive mind.*

In the pineal gland is hexagonal "brain sand" (*acervuli cerebri,* calcium salts) connected to the calcite microcrystals less than 20μm with piezoelectric properties setting up a resonance with cellular technology. The piezoelectric character of the microcrystals points to "radio communication"—electro-mechano-transduction decidedly not innate to the pineal gland, though the pineal gland is capable of converting neural signals into endocrine output. *Sodium fluoride* is implicated in the calcification of the microcrystals. Two decades ago in 1997, Jennifer Luke's dissertation thesis "The Effect of Fluoride on the Physiology of the Pineal Gland" (University of Surrey, UK) proved that fluoride (F) accumulates in the pineal gland more than anywhere else in the body and calcifies it.[38] Since 1945, fluoride has been added to community water supplies,[39] processed foods and beverages—virtually a chemical

---

36 Atropine in Belladonna, ergotamine on wheat and rye, ayahuasca, LSD (lysergic acid diethylamide), and no doubt other psychotropic compounds have a similar structure. Psilocybin (5MeO-DMT) is produced in the pituitary and pineal glands.

37 R.U. Sirius, "Hacking sleep: Meet the transhumanists making sleep obsolete." Vanwinkles, 17 September 2015.

38 Paul Connett, "Fluoride and the pineal gland: Study Published in Caries Research." International Fluoride Information Network Bulletin #269, March 27, 2001.

39 "In 2014, 74.4% of the U.S. population on public water systems, or a total of 211,393,167 people, had access to fluoridated water. CDC monitors the progress of the nation and

lobotomy of the mind that comprises the individual sense of self. Fluoride may not accumulate in the brain (thanks to the blood-brain barrier),[40] but the pineal gland ends up sequestering it straight from the bloodstream. (See Chapter 2 for more on fluoride.)

Are we being chemically and electromagnetically tuned for the Smart City technocracy? Is the pinecone-shaped pineal gland—a neuroendocrine transducer once synonymous with the sixth *chakra* "third eye"? The optic and auditory nerves carry sense impressions from the outer world into the inner four hills to the pineal gland, much as Parsifal carried his worldly knowledge through the wasteland in search of the holy grail. The blood flows up and around these four hills and pineal gland, and the twelve cerebral nerves all lead there. In other words, all sensory roads lead to the pineal gland.

> The natural, rhythmical ascent and descent of the living, watery element passing from the physical to the etheric and from the etheric to the physical, as described by Rudolf Steiner, may remind us of another, most remarkable process—one that takes place in the human being: the etherization of the blood. This too is a rhythmic process taking place between the pole of the feelings in the region of the heart and radiates like rays of light up to the head, where it flows and glows round the pineal gland. And during sleep a reverse flow takes place—an etheric flow entering the head from the cosmos and flowing down to the heart. These pulsating physical-etheric flows reflect the moral life of the human soul.[41]

Interfere with the pineal and you interfere with sleep. Why is sleep so important? Prevention of deep REM sleep causes theta state (5-8 Hz) disorientation, confusion, spacing out, hallucinations, fatigue, and drowsiness, all of which can serve no-touch trauma and mind control. Our hexagon-structured melatonin is intimately tied to the sleep-waking rhythm between the frequencies of this 3-space world and the frequencies of other dimensions via the "third eye." Sleep is not just about loss of consciousness and shutting down for bodily repairs; it is about daily journeying between day consciousness and night consciousness so as to awaken with new intent to build upon yesterday. We *re-member* during sleep, and the "memory transfer" binds us to our destiny and the ultimate meaning of our human experience.

---

individual states toward meeting the Healthy People 2020 objective on community water fluoridation—that 79.6% of people on public water systems will receive water that has the optimum level of fluoride recommended for preventing tooth decay." https://www.cdc.gov/fluoridation/statistics/index.htm

40 Though electroporation via electromagnetic radiation can bypass the blood-brain barrier.

41 Paul Emberson, From Gondishapur to Silicon Valley, Vols. 1 and 2. Etheric Dimensions, 2009.

Importantly, electromagnetic signaling from phased arrays like HAARP and the Space Fence infrastructure—calibrated to work in tandem with ionospheric heaters (utility plants, cell towers, radar installations, etc.)—radiate / broadcast geometric forms that serve as *sigils* of sound / algorithms / spells to invoke other dimensions.[42] Electromagnetically radiating geometrically designed software into our chemically treated "smart dust" atmosphere can make all of life resonate to sigils designed to invisibly yoke our nervous systems to hive mind control.[43]

The virtual world to which the pineal hexagon opens the way is the *Eighth Sphere*, a quantum artifice now under construction in the realm populated by DMT beings and sentient world simulation (SWS) avatars—in short, everything chemically, genetically, electromagnetically, and astrally / imaginatively dedicated to transforming the world and body of Human 1.0 into that of Human 2.0. Like all things virtual reality (VR) and DMT, the Eighth Sphere is real *and visionary*. The Eighth Sphere, according to Rudolf Steiner in 1915, "circles around as a globe of dense matter, solid and indestructible . . . its density of a far denser physical-mineral character than exists anywhere on the Earth."[44]

> "In a 6G environment, through digital twins, users will be able to explore and monitor the reality in a virtual world, without temporal or spatial constraints. Users will be able to observe changes or detect problems remotely through the representation offered by digital twins."[45]

Dreams and nightmares are being engineered under the ruse of biofeedback brainwave therapy. Picture military and neuro-corporate boys sitting at their monitors watching digital dreams, inputting and tweaking algorithms according to heart rates and anxiety levels. At first, U.S. Navy hospitals like the one in Bremerton, Washington made use of PTSD'd soldiers and sailors for custom designing VR scenes and built-out imaginary worlds populated by avatars and "pixelated friends" based on virtual world Second Life (*http://secondlife.com*).[46]

---

42 "In witchcraft they use hexagrams and pentagrams for oppressing and binding. The hexagon is the most efficient geometric shape for processing thermal energy. This is why snakes often have hexagonal scales for absorbing thermal energy. Snowflakes are often hexagonal from heat extraction. Pent in pentagram refers to enclosing or binding something to create a buildup." – Ahuwah Zeus, "Zionic Mind Control," March 16, 2018.

43 Study cymatic YouTubes like Lotus Sun's "Saturn's Cymatic Hexagram / Hexagon Frequency Bombardment," November 10, 2017.

44 Rudolf Steiner, The Occult Movements in the Nineteenth Century, Lectures 4 and 5, October 1915; Foundations of Esotericism, lectures 14 and 18, October 1905.

45 "6G: The Next Hyper-Connected Experience for All," Samsung, https://cdn.codeground.org/nsr/downloads/researchareas/6G%20Vision.pdf. Also see Anthony Cuthbertson, "6G will bring 'digital twins,' Samsung says – and it's two years ahead of schedule," The Independent, 15 July 2020.

46 Kristin Kaining, "If Second Life isn't a game, what is it?" NBCNews.com, March 12, 2007.

...[Power Dreaming] dreams are downloaded from hospital computers onto soldiers' laptops. Because of military concerns about data breaches, there are restrictions on the use of removable hard drives and USB ports on military computers. There is also the issue of getting the right software to allow safe file transfers. "Navy systems don't jibe with civilian systems," said a hospital spokesperson. "We are striving to have a computerized method to do it that is safe and secure."[47]

Security and "defense" corporations like Raytheon and Academi are running expanded human VR experiments to manipulate physio-emotional states and activate parasympathetic dream scenarios in civilian bedrooms while siphoning energy from power grids, 60Hz /50Hz wiring in the walls, and the Internet of Things (IoT). Targeting, experimentation, field ops—however it is referenced—is a booming disaster capitalism industry.

Thus, full spectrum dominance over sleep ("the little death") and its process of *soul re-membering* is essential for human beings but not for hybrid cyborgs. Assaults on public and private memory are assaults on the continuing self-evolution of human consciousness according to free will. After a good sleep, we rise again to connect yesterday with today and tomorrow, memory and sleep being crucial to bridging the conscious with the unconscious, physics with metaphysics, this dimension with other dimensions. It is how we human beings learn and digest what our little life upon the Earth *means*.

Endocrine mimics & disruption

The entire endocrine system has also been recruited to assault not just the pineal gland but the entire body and its immune system. *Synthetic estrogen* and not just fluoride is in the public water, along with pesticide, herbicide, and insecticide runoffs, plus *estrogen-mimics* like PCBs, DDT, dioxin, and phthalate plasticizers like DEHP—all contributing to *endocrine disruption* and cancers, sterilization, gender confusion, and loss of natural life cycles. The pesticide atrazine turns male frogs into female frogs, and the common plastic additive bisphenol A (BPA) in infant care items, plastic bottles and packaging, etc., exactly mimics estrogen and conditions infant tissues to develop cancer, diabetes, and obesity. Being fat-soluble, estrogen-mimics accumulate in fat taken up by estrogen receptor sites.

The assault on the female Human 1.0 began with hospital births and went on to "the Pill" that led to breast cancer and high blood pressure. As woman aged, *hormone replacement therapy (HRT)* plied her with the estrogen her eggs

47 Dawn Lim, "Real Life Inception: Army Looks to 'Counteract Nightmares' With Digital Dreams." Wired, October 21, 2011.

were no longer supplying to stave off the "living decay" of menopause (Robert Wilson, MD, *Feminine Forever*, 1966), thus producing endometrial cancer. Synthetic progesterone and estrogen only served to hasten aging and increase the chances of breast cancer by 45 percent. Progesterone is the mother of all hormones with the capability of being turned into other hormones as the body needs them. In fact, both estrogen and testosterone are end metabolic products made from progesterone. Menstruation involves communication between the ovaries, hypothalamus, and pituitary. It is, however, the egg follicle that manufactures and releases estrogen into the blood. When the woman goes through menopause, other body sites—the adrenal glands, skin, muscle, brain, pineal gland, hair follicles, and body fat—continue to make small quantities of estrogen and progesterone *if* the woman has taken good care of herself and avoided the extremities of modern allopathic medicine during the pre-menopausal years.

Next came the "abortion hormone" *hCG (human chorionic gonadotropin)*—originally produced during pregnancy to assure the growth of the fetus but now used to produce antibodies *against* pregnancy—secretly piggybacked onto tetanus vaccines in poor, ethnic neighborhood clinics and developing nations like Kenya, where in 2014-2015 the World Health Organization (WHO) and UNICEF jabbed 2.3 million women. After the Nairobi lab Agriq-Quest Ltd. analysis of vials of tetanus toxoid vaccine, the *Agence de Presse Africaine* reported that "a state-sponsored sterilization exercise" had been sold to Kenya as a tetanus vaccination.[48]

Was the WHO Task Force on Vaccines for Fertility Regulation involved?

Between 1938 and 1990, human sperm count plunged 50 percent as more and more men developed gynæcomastia (enlargement of male breasts) and impotence. The assault on children was then upscaled with *gender dysphoria*, yet another Diagnostic and Statistical Manual of Mental Disorders (DSM-5) creation described as a mental condition of anguish and stress over one's body parts and what is gender-typical. Given the sheer scale of estrogen-mimics in public water supplies, it should garner public suspicion that up electro-chemical environmental influences are never broached. Gender dysphoria is more about Transhumanist politics than science, "a core of very diabolical people who are filtering large sums of money into this and using mass social pressure" (Dr. Quentin Van Meter, pediatric endocrinologist).[49]

48 Christina England, "Mass Sterilization of Millions of African Girls through Tetanus Vaccine Scandal Broadens as Kenyan Laboratory Attacked." Health Impact News, June 12, 2018. Also see Mike Adams and Dr. Carrie Madej, DO, discuss the tetanus ruse within the context of the DNA / COVID-19 strategy in "Warning about coronavirus vaccines and transhumanism nanotechnology to alter your DNA" (October 8, 2020).

49 Shane Trejo, "Scientist Discovers Abnormal Brain Function in Transgender Individuals,

The pituitary gland

> *In the body we find that which connects the pineal, the pituitary, the lyden [leydig gland] may be truly called the silver cord or the golden cup that may be filled with a closer walk with that which is the creative essence in physical, mental and spiritual life; for the destruction wholly of either will make for the disintegration of the soul from its house of clay. To be purely material minded, were an anatomical or pathological study made for a period of seven years (which is a cycle of change in all the body elements) of one that is acted upon through the third eye alone, we will find one fed upon spiritual things becomes a light that may shine from and in the darkest corner. One fed upon the purely material will become a Frankenstein that is without a concept of any influence other than material or mental.*
>
> – Edgar Cayce (1877-1945), "Seat of the Soul Research Project," (262-20)[50]

As for the pituitary master gland whose secretions include growth hormone, thyroid hormones, adrenal hormones, reproductive hormones, and a hormone affecting the kidneys, its structure is two-fold: the neurological posterior lobe (part of the hypothalamus), and the metabolic anterior lobe, the divider being a "membrane of melatonin-rich tissue." In *Seeking Spirit Vision,* Dennis Klocek describes the pituitary as "a microcosm of the polarity seen in the brain between the more cosmic outer layers which are involved in higher thinking, and the lower instinctual, dreaming and sleeping consciousness in the lower brainstem."

Klocek then compares the pituitary gland to an embryo nestled in the sphenoid bone of the skull, "the keystone for the construction of the face . . . [flaring] out into strong lateral processes just as the pelvis flares out from the sacrum . . . In the place where the uterus would be found in the pelvis, we find the pituitary gland in the sphenoid. These images point to a common reproductive function in both the uterus and the pituitary. *In the uterus, embryos are formed. In the pituitary, images are formed.*" [Emphasis added.]

So what do we have? Images formed in the pituitary, and melatonin with the same chemical structure as DMT produced by the pineal gland. Are we seeing a pattern in thie"organ knowledge" referenced in the "precog" scenes of the *Minority Report* film? Klocek:

> The pituitary gland and its surrounding tissues provide a picture of the wall between the upper world of the stars, the source of spiritual exis-

---

Liberals Rush to Suppress Findings," Big League Politics, December 4, 2019; and "Synthetic Hormone Injections For Transgender Children Worry Some Doctors," Eurasia Review, January 3, 2019.

50 Email, Dark Journalist Daniel Liszt, August 3, 2019.

tence, and the lower world of the body . . . [T]he pituitary is a source of mental imagination or inner picture forming. In essence, a mental image is a digested sense impression from Earth reproduced and spiritualized in the form of inner light.

Extraordinarily, the "precog" scene follows Klocek's description *exactly*:

> Under intense input from the body, blocking agents in the pituitary and hypothalamus block the brainstem and put the consciousness into a sleep state very similar to trance and hypnosis or shamanic hyper-alert states. In such a state the cortex experiences intense electrical fields as a kind of bliss.[51]

Thus, we get a glimpse of how the present chemical-electromagnetic assault on the brain does not just utterly rob us of our privacy as individuals but also robs us of precious opportunities inherent to our birthright pituitary and pineal glands:

> Through a focused attention upon the pituitary and pineal glands, fields of being which act in particular ways become accessible to waking consciousness. This can serve as the basis for an esoteric schooling.

Assaults on these two organs alone prevent opportunities for free will. The cry is indeed *Rip out the brains! (Arracher le cerveau!)*[52] Instead, our magnificent brain capabilities are to be plugged in and "enhanced" as brain-computer interfaces (BCIs) of the hive mind.

The stomach / solar plexus

The path of "organ knowledge" normally remains subconscious, but can be "called forth." Neurotransmitters are produced both in the brain and the gut; thus, we "go with our gut" when we receive signals from our *second brain*, the enteric nervous system (ENS), two thin layers of 100 million nerve cells lining the gastrointestinal tract from esophagus to rectum (not to mention the 100 trillion bacteria inhabiting that long snake-like highway amidst nutrients and waste.

Whereas the stomach sends out infrared heat waves—literally *the entire spectrum of light* (UV, x-rays, etc.)—like a beacon or transmitter, the solar plexus can pick up a fearful situation *even before it has shown itself* and send a message to the suprarenal glands to release adrenaline into the bloodstream.[53] Why is this? The duodenum is the first section of the small intestine and is

51 See S.W. Troop, Psychical Physics: A Scientific Analysis of Dowsing, Radiesthesia, and Kindred Divining Phenomena. New York: Elsevier Publishing, 1949.

52 Alfred Jarry, "Ubi Roi," 1896.

53 I experienced this at 18 when I was about to be imminently attacked.

in the area of the solar plexus. It regulates physiological changes due to emotional states. It is as if the solar plexus or *hara*[54] that traditional martial arts depend upon has its own "eyes" honed by frequencies we miss. The colon too seems perceptive.

All three energy centers—the solar plexus, duodenum, and colon—are particularly sensitive in those with psychic sensitivity. Psychotherapist Gerda Boyesen (1922-2005), founder of Biodynamic psychotherapy, observed that the gastrointestinal tract speaks the language of the unconscious "from the gut." With her stethoscope, she listened to the duodenum or colon and noted how closely psychological affliction (undigested toxic experiences) correlated with ulcerative colitis, Crohn's and irritable bowel syndrome,[55] which are about far more than diet or bad habits, such as invisible electromagnetic frequencies invading our subtle energy bodies. Even neurogastroenterologists are observing that anxiety and depression don't so much *cause* gastric problems as follow from them.

The gut-brain axis is indeed an energy highway.

Microscopes tell the tale of microbiota, but do we yet have the instruments that can detect invisibles entering the body by means of the solar plexus / *hara* gateway? Both epilepsy and autism spectrum disorder (ASD) have been linked to the gut microbiome, and both have specific neurological symptoms pointing to a *shutdown* of the individual's personality and/or consciousness.

> Changes to host microbiome composition coincide with neurologic changes affecting behavior, neurotransmitter levels, stress response, and gene expression in the brain.[56]

And yet such a spare description doesn't really tell much about what's really going on, does it? Compare with this description from my *Sub Rosa America: A Deep State History*:

> As for stomach clairvoyance, the solar plexus, cecum, or stomach sends out not only infrared heat waves but the entire light spectrum. In ancient days, the cecum was known as the *monacle* of the large intestine, the

54 In Japanese, hara means abdomen or will. Hara (two finger widths below the navel) is the reservoir of vital or source energy (Yuan Qi). Many martial art styles, amongst them Aikido, emphasize the importance of "moving from the hara," i.e. from the center of one's body / mind.

55 Years ago, social commentator Jaye C. Beldo defined the CIA as the Id Canal of the United States (Freud's das Id, the It) while the NSA was the small intestine of the CIA / Id Canal system. Maybe that's why the U.S. has such a severe case of indigestion.

56 "Emerging evidence linking the gut microbiome to neurologic disorders," https://genomemedicine.biomedcentral.com, n.d.

seer of the body, the "gut reaction" that could issue a warning the bowels could understand. Gut waves are weak, and yet, according to radio astronomer John Pfeiffer in his 1956 book *The Changing Universe,* the 50-foot aerial at the Naval Research Laboratory in Washington, DC can pick up radio signals coming from a stomach more than four miles distant, the body being like a radio tower and the stomach area a major beacon. All somatic cells are electromagnetic resonators capable of emitting and absorbing very high frequency (VHF) radiation. And because the nerves governing the stomach and duodenum issue from the solar plexus (third *chakra*), those who are psychically manipulated or attacked often have stomach problems, due to their solar plexus "receiver." According to Arthur Guirdham, MD, in his book *Obsession: Psychic forces and evil in the causation of disease* (1972), rapid emptying of the stomach coincides with being drained by others on the same wavelength.

During the early days of Artichoke, CIA and military intelligence doctors learned from the Nazis and other Satanists how to teach "alters" to enter the body through the solar plexus-stomach area. Bouts of excruciating stomach pain, sometimes cramping in the legs and feet, often indicate entry. Both the stomach and legs have corresponding etheric acupuncture points; one of the calf muscles is even named gastrocnemius. Sleeper assassins like Sirhan Sirhan, Mark David Chapman, and David Berkowicz all complained of severe stomach pain, as did country singer Tammy Wynette. In 2000, Daniel Bondeson [*bond son*] fed arsenic to parishioners at the Gustaf Adolph Lutheran Church in New Sweden, Maine, saying in his suicide note: *I had no intent to hurt this way. Just to upset stomach, like the churchgoers did me.* And in the jailhouse letter of Jessie Misskelley Jr., after an act he swears "he" didn't do, he says, *My stomache has been hurting me.*

How a *neuronal matrix* can radio in through the solar plexus receiver and take over one's body and personality is a complex proposition that defies mundane analysis. The CIA used narco-hypnosis to produce deep trance agents who could pass for normal and remember nothing. That the stomach is tortured during this mysterious transmission and transformation is a fact. Long ago, the shamans of Central America referred to *virotes*, invisible psychic darts implanted over distance in an enemy's stomach. *Pharmakia* drugs can act as *virotes*, too, and open access through the solar plexus.

So secret is stomach clairvoyance that Western accounts of the bloody rites of the Aztecs in the final demise of their civilization were revised to read "heart" incisions instead of "stomach" incisions. Only the *Mictlantecuhtli* (*circa* 1480) sculpture at the Museo del Templo Mayor in Mexico City with its open thoracic cavity points to the stomach between the two lobes of the liver opening like the petals of a flower. The Nahua perceived that the *ihíyotl*, one of the three spirits of the body, resides in the liver, the head being *ilhuícatl* (heaven), *ihíyotl* the earth, and the entrails, including the cecum, the underworld and death.

The limbic brain, hippocampus, and amygdala

When Michael A. Persinger, PhD (1945-2018), professor of neuroscience at Laurentian University in Sudbury, Ontario in the early 1970s, focused solenoids (like Tesla coils) on the right hemisphere of the temporal lobe, the subject experienced a negative presence on the left side of the body, like an alien or demon; when the solenoids focused on the left hemisphere, an angel or god would appear on the right side of the body.[57] Focusing on the hippocampus produced opiate effects of ecstasy; on the amygdala, sexual arousal.

Persinger was fascinated by the hippocampus and other limbic structures. By stimulating the limbic brain with electric currents, he could produce out-of-body experiences (OOBEs), epiphanies, feelings of cosmic significance, and dream events that seemed real, such as UFO experiences and conversations with entities (*jinn*). Whether or not magnets were made to block the Earth's magnetic field and enable the subject to see what was really there, or frame an event along the lines of the subject's belief system, is unclear, but Persinger was able to confirm that the temporal lobe and hippocampus play a role in religious experience, which may be why a recent discovery of a "mysterious" and "new" communication mechanism in the brain between the cortex and hippocampus may revolutionize how *ephaptic coupling* is looked at. For one thing, it happens when we're asleep:

> While we're asleep, the cortex and hippocampus in the brain send out mysterious neural 'waves' . . . "We've known about these waves for a long time, but no one knows their exact function, and no one believed they could spontaneously propagate," says neural and biomedical engineer Dominique Durand from Case Western Reserve University in Cleveland, Ohio. This slow periodic activity can generate electric fields which 'switch on' neighboring cells briefly, allowing for chemical-free communication across gaps in the brain.[58]

---

57 Studies like Persinger's have no doubt led to the new neurotheology that enlists brain scans to misrepresent religion's role in creating the brain. See "The neuroscience argument that religion shaped the very structure of our brains" by Olivia Goldhill (Quartz, December 3, 2016); and Blue Beam commentary in Chapter 6, "The Secret Space Program."

58 "'Jaw-dropping moment': Scientists discover mysterious new communication mechanism in the brain." RT, 18 February 2019.

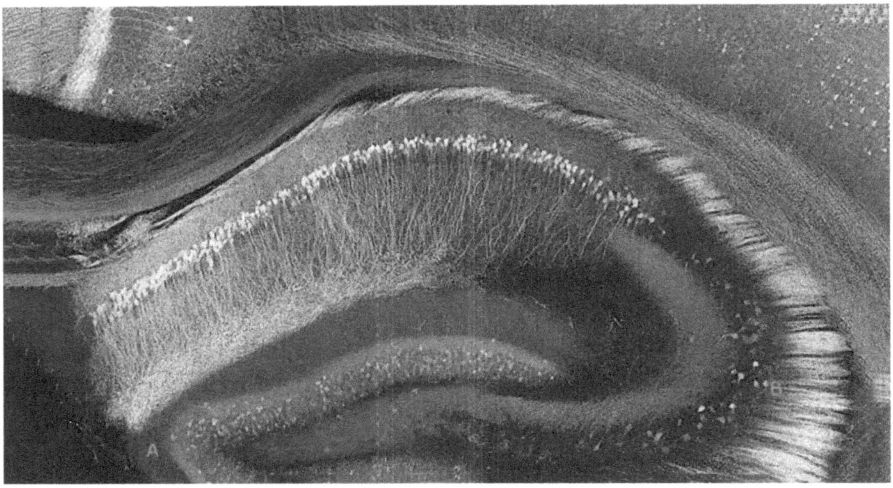

Hippocampus.

John Hewitt, "Synaptic tail-chasing: Will we ever have a human connectome?" *ExtremeTech,* November 13, 2012.

In the early days of Artichoke—MK-ULTRA's early phase—bypassing neocortex reasoning was the first challenge to being able to program children through older parts of the brain, particularly the old *limbic brain* (*limbus,* L., border) concerned with bonding, emotion, and memory. Inside the limbic brain nestles the preverbal *reptilian brain,* a fistful of neurons at the top of the spinal column whose instinctual and ritualistic impulses concentrate on survival, physical maintenance, hoarding, dominance, grooming and mating. Stimulate the limbic system and images are produced.

For centuries, Satanic cult families developed practices entailing drugs, hypnosis, ritual, and repetitive torture in order to bypass the newest part of the brain, the neocortex, and program their children in the "old religion"—back to when the brain heard "the voices of the gods" or what Princeton University psychologist Julian Jaynes, PhD, termed "verbal hallucinations" of the *bicameral mind* phase of pre-consciousness.

> . . . consciousness [as we have understood it since, say, the European Middle Ages] was learned only after the breakdown of the bicameral mind. I believe this is true, that the anguish of not knowing what to do in the chaos resulting from the loss of the gods provided the social conditions that could result in the invention of a new mentality to replace the old one.[59]

59 Julian Jayne's revised 1990 Afterword to his extraordinary 1976 book The Origin of Con-

Mythical representations of reptilian gods, Serpent people, Annunaki, Dracos, etc. that purportedly served as the principal architects of the world and even of human beings hearken from the reptilian brain that can be quickened by DMT experiences like *ayahuasca* or yagé. Sufficient *scarring* of the limbic brain in very early childhood due to constant sexual abuse, neglect, isolation, physical restraint, witnessing horrific inhuman acts, and bloodline gene and DNA splicing,[60] may induce visions (or intrusions) of entities that shapeshift in a variety of ways.

Under the neocortex is a thin region called the *claustrum*—something like a CPU (central processing unit) on-off switch that literally can be made to turn off sentience. Remotely trigger this area and the person stops and stares blankly; reactivate the claustrum, and the target continues what they were doing before the interruption with no recollection of it.

The temporal lobes of the neocortex make sense of things, the left lobe of linear logic, the right reads patterns. Episodic memories are encoded chemically in neurons and neuron connections in the temporal lobes, including the hippocampus. Memory traces called *engrams* can be reactivated by *optogenetics* selectively turning cells off and on with light. The 2010 preprogramming film *Eternal Sunshine of the Spotless Mind* informed us that cells that retain memory engrams can be dissected, stripped of real memories, and reloaded with false memories.[61]

The almond-shaped *amygdala* nestles in front of the limbic brain in the temporal lobe and provides the fight-or-flight reflex that makes quick emotional decisions long before the neocortex can process or question incoming sensory data. Pulsed light, such as in the Bucha Effect—named for how helicopter rotor blades strobing the sunlight at human brainwave frequency make pilots lose control[62]—coupled with traumatic events,[63] bypasses the neocortex and triggers the amygdala over and over again, producing "flashbulb" memories that then lodge in the hippocampus (and in the temporal lobe) where long-term verbal and emotional memories are normally processed and stored for retrieval until being moved to the hypothalamus.

---

sciousness in the Breakdown of the Bicameral Mind (Houghton Mifflin).

60 See Harvard ethnobotanist Wade Davis's The Serpent and the Rainbow: A Harvard Scientist's Astonishing Journey into the Secret Societies of Haitian Voodoo, Zombies, and Magic (Simon & Schuster, 1985). The tokoloshe is a Zulu mind-controlled zombie slave. Is it so difficult to believe that equally astonishing evils and transformations occur in the "civilized" West?

61 Anne Trafton, "Neuroscientists plant false memories in the brain." MIT News Office, July 25, 2013.

62 See David Hambling, "Strobe Weapons Go Black After 'Immobilization' Tests," Wired, 1989.

63 A scene in the 1997 preprogramming film Conspiracy Theory shows this.

Amygdala abnormalities often follow from early sexual abuse, neglect, isolation, and physical restraint because these practices, along with temporal lobe neurons, impact social-emotional development (facial recognition, eye contact, reading emotions, etc.).

> The autistic refusal to make eye contact is a limbic system abnormality associated with deprivation . . . insufficient mothering can damage the limbic system and produce autistic behaviors.[64]

The amygdala is called the fear center of the brain tasked with receiving memory information from the hippocampus, i.e. regulator of the subconscious ability to perceive threat and fear. Recently, the MK-ULTRA discovery of two sets of neurons in the amygdala—one to pursue prey, the other to kill—was finally made public:

> Using a technique called optogenetics, the researchers managed to create mice in which both sets of neurons were controllable through the use of light emitted from a laser. That essentially created "an on-off switch" the team could use to activate either set of neurons or both, the associate professor [at Yale University] said. "When we stimulate [both sets of] neurons it is as if there is a prey in front of the animal," he said. At that point, the mice assume a body posture and take actions that are generally associated with real hunting . . . You can imagine that this kind of discovery would interest, say, the Defense Department, which could utilize it as a means of turning soldiers "on and off" on the battlefield. But sinister forces could also use it to create human monsters among the population . . .[65]

Whether the torture is MK-ULTRA, satanic ritual abuse (SRA), BD / SM (bondage dominance / sadomasochism), or KUBARK "interrogation" at Gitmo, the attempt is to overcome the medulla oblongata / brainstem / reptilian brain while stimulating the amygdala so as to trigger the release of adrenaline that fuses the memory off from long-term storage.

Whereas the amygdala is the emotional content of memory (especially feelings related to fear and aggression), the *hippocampus* forms and retrieves verbal and emotional memories. Its Ammon's horn handles one-way nerve traffic while the rest of it reads magnetic field strength and funnels information to the hypothalamus—the "sweet spot" or pleasure center of the brain

---

64 Rhawn Gabriel Joseph, PhD. "The Unabomber: The Deprived Amygdala and the Serial Killer." BrainMind.com, 1996.

65 JD Heyes, "Researchers find brain switch to turn rats into killer predators—are humans next?" NewsTarget.com, January 21, 2017.

responsible for forming long-term memories—along the fornix pathways.[66] Acting as a transducer of electromagnetic energy, the hippocampus directs energy to the hypothalamus and anterior pituitary. Electrical stimulation increases its neural activity to a maximum of 10-15 Hz. In MK-ULTRA victims, the hippocampus is perennially hyper-aroused so as to eliminate and block memory storage.[67]

Few realize that ongoing trauma changes brain structure. The amygdala and hippocampus can decrease in volume as much as 31.6% and 19.2% respectively in victims of dissociative identity disorder (DID) and other early abuse conditions (PTSD, borderline personality disorder, manic depression, etc.). EEG coherence, a sophisticated quantitative way of looking at brain circuitry, indicates that adults traumatized regularly as children have less developed left hemispheres, the temporal regions being the most affected; the size of the corpus callosum, the communicating bridge between the two hemispheres, is also reduced. Abnormalities in the cerebellar vermis in the middle of the cerebellum at the back of the brain above the brain stem (more of the old brain) are due to the cerebellar vermis having a higher density of receptors for stress hormones than the hippocampus. Thus the multiple hormones released during repetitive abuse greatly impact brain stem development as well as the production and release of the neurotransmitters norepinephrine and dopamine.

The prosthetic "artificial hippocampus" (implantable biomimetic electronics) purported to interact with a damaged hippocampus to restore short- and long-term memory for Alzheimer's patients may actually double as a BCI interface for control over memory for Transhumanist purposes. According to Theodore W. Berger, PhD, director of the Center for Neural Engineering at the University of Southern California, for spacetime events the brain *visually* (though non-linearly) processes information in spacio-temporal patterns.

---

66 Robert O. Becker and Gary Selden, The Body Electric: Electromagnetism and the Foundation of Life. William Morrow and Company, 1985, p. 264.

67 Is over-excitation of the amygdala and hippocampus (due to repetitive abuse) connected to temporal lobe epilepsy (TLE)?

13

Occult Assault II: Transhumanist Eugenics / "Eugenetics"

The Drama Around the Human Genome
Epigenetics
DNA
The shamanic view of DNA
Optogenetics
CRISPR & gene drives
Stem cells
Synthetic DNA
Transgenic

. . . and the less prolific races will have to defend themselves by methods which are disgusting even if they are necessary.

– Bertrand Russell, *Prospects of Industrial Civilization,* 1923

The real enemy, then, is humanity itself.

– Alexander King and Bertrand Schneider, *The First Global Revolution: A Report by the Council of the Club of Rome*, 1991

. . . the 6 billion world population would be comfortable in the state of Texas with a population density of half of Paris. It appears that scarcity of food and land is not the problem, but a scarcity of democracy, just as Francis Moore Lappé has said.

– *Encyclopedia Americana, 1996*

RACIAL IDEOLOGIES ARE AS OLD as the hills. The Comte de Gobineau's book *Sur l'inegalité des races humaines* came out in 1855. His British counterpart was Charles Darwin's cousin Sir Francis Galton, who introduced statistical analysis to eugenics to prove that Aryans were not like other races. For his work, Galton received every award possible in Victorian England, while his cousin Charles married the youngest granddaughter of his maternal grandfather, a genetic experiment that didn't go all that well for seven of their ten children.

Margaret Sanger, founder of Planned Parenthood, chose the motto *Birth Control: to create a race of thoroughbreds.* Her 1922 manifesto in her book *The Pivot of Civilization* was Fabian through and through. Reading Sanger is like reading Himmler—in fact, Nazi sympathizers were on the early Planned Parenthood board, and Hitler's director of genetic sterilization published an article in their *Birth Control Review* in 1933. By the 1960s, liberals had taken the Fabians' place and substituted "family planning" for "race betterment."

Planned Parenthood fit nicely with zero population growth (ZPG) and other radical environmental agendas blaming the world's problems on too many people.[1] *Take the pill, have an abortion,* the progressive liberals down at Planned Parenthood still counsel, while Paul Erlich, author of *The Population Bomb* (1968) and *The Population Explosion* (1990), pushed the idea that people are only people because genetics stored in chemicals interact with the environment, implying that scraping a fetus or embryo from a uterus is just lost potential.

With the stem cell market booming, abortion and body organs have become a medical raw materials industry: fetuses aborted alive, dismembered, their organs sorted and packed in plastic baggies, then frozen—brains, hearts, lungs, livers, kidneys, glands . . . And there are the covert, nonconsensual sterilization programs:

> In 1997, state doctors performed 110,000 tubal ligations—up from 30,000 the year before. Among them were some atypical candidates: [poor and indigenous] women with no children, 15-to-19-year-olds, and menopausal women . . .[2]

Twenty years after North Carolina's Eugenics Board approved the sterilization of 7,600 people (1929 to 1974), the victims sought reparations:

> Due to the global relevance of the issue, the confirmation process must be transparent and the identities of victims must be made public, [Edwin] Black said. "By claiming to protect the identity of the victims, the perpetrators are protecting their own identities," he said. "This was not the act of a few disgruntled racists. These were the upper echelon members of our education system, courts and government."[3]

---

1 *The Global 2000 Report to the President of the United States*, 1980: "If present trends continue, the world in 2000 will be more crowded, and more vulnerable to disruption than the world we live in now. Serious stresses involving population, resources, and environment are clearly visible ahead. Despite greater material output, the world's people will be poorer in many ways than they are today" (Al Gore, *Earth in the Balance: Ecology and the Human Spirit*, 1992).

2 Catherine Elton, "Peru's Family Planning Became Coerced Sterilization." Christian Science Monitor, February 20, 1998.

3 Chinmayi Sharma, "State prepares reparations for eugenics victims." The Duke Chronicle, April 2, 2012. Edwin Black is author of War Against the Weak: Eugenics and America's

Lies to the public about "nonlethal" chemical / biological weapons testing abound, Synthetic BioDesign organisms with remote molecular kill switches are launched from sky-high jet canisters filter down into the oceans and lungs and bloodstreams of humans, animals, birds—the entire ecosystem under the typical DARPA philosophy of *Let's see what happens and lie about it.* The vapor spewed from remote-controlled jets is loaded with DARPA cocktails, now that the Earth is an open lab and the Mockingbird mainstream media armed with cover stories.

We live in a perpetual state of slow-kill war[4] of inhalation, ingestion, and inoculation. It is all eugenics, or should we call it *eugenetics*?

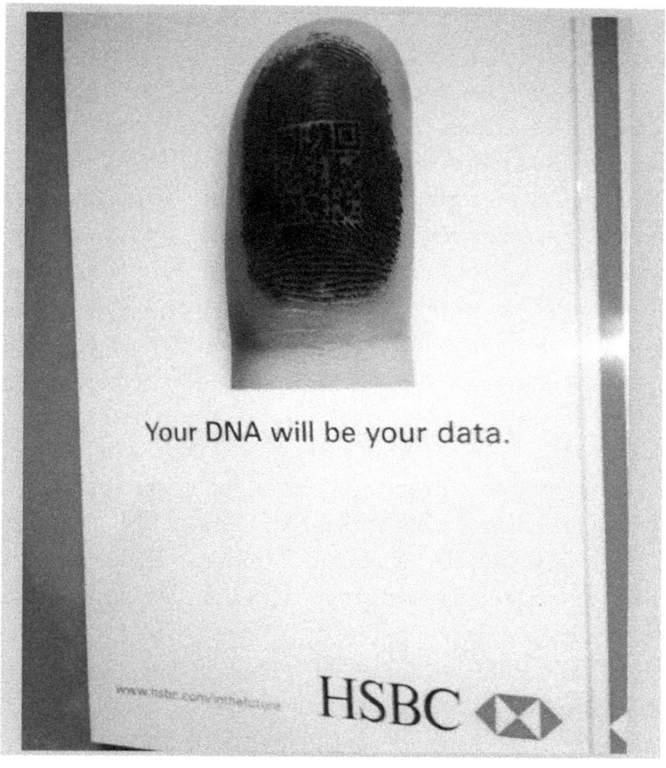

HSBC ad. HSBC Holdings is a British multinational investment bank, the second largest bank in Europe (assets US$2.984 trillion).

Campaign to Create A Master Race (Dialog Press, 2012).

4 For contemplating how conventional wars have contributed to eugenics, see Chapter 9, "Dual Use I: A Smart City Is An Armed City."

> *In a circuit board or microchip, sets of logic elements linked in precise networks perform defined logical processes, repeating the same simple steps over and over again. The same thing happens in a living cell, except that the elements now are molecules instead of transistors and the blind iterations they perform are chemical rather than electrical.*
>
> – Dennis Bray, *Wetware: A Computer in Every Living Cell* (2009)

> *"When Hitler spoke to me," continued Rauschning, "he tried to explain his vocation as the herald of a new humanity in rational and concrete terms. For example, 'Creation is not yet completed. Man has reached a definite stage of metamorphosis. The ancient human species is already in a state of decline, just managing to survive. Humanity accomplishes a step up once every seven hundred years, and the ultimate aim is the coming of the Sons of God. All creative forces will be concentrated in a new species. The two varieties will evolve rapidly in different directions. One will disappear, and the other will flourish. It will be infinitely superior to modern man. Do you understand now the profound meaning of our National-Socialist movement? Whoever sees in National Socialism nothing but a political movement doesn't know much about it . . .'"*
>
> – Louis Pauwels and Jacques Bergier, *The Morning of the Magicians,* 1960

Synthetic biology (*synbio*) aims to engineer cells with "*novel* biological functions"—cells used to create molecules of larger systems that can be programmed via synthetic gene networks, like self-assembling bacterial biofilm or genetic toggle switches that "shapeshift" things in the network, all merging biology with nanomaterials—substrate adhesion, nanoparticle templating, protein immobilization, etc.[5]

Technologically and environmentally, Human 1.0 is challenged by

- *Toxic chemicals*
- *Radioactivity, ionized and nonionized*
- *Self-replicating genetically engineered microorganisms (GEMs) capable of evolution*

which are all tucked into the Transhumanist acronym *NBICS (Nanotechnology, Biotechnology, Information technology, Cognitive Science)*[6] as we are quietly

5 Peter Q Nguyen et al., "Programmable biofilm-based materials from engineered curli nanofibers." Nature Communications, 17 September 2014.

6 Interestingly, this same acronym is that of the Netherlands Bioinformatics Center, which comprises major post-World War Two Gladio mind control research.

moved from the old natural model of *human* not forced by the State to accept a perception of ourselves we do not agree with ("self-identity security") and acceptant of our abilities we have, enhanced or not ("ability security"):

- From species-typical functioning to beyond species-typical functioning
- From curative to enhancement medicine
- From human rights to sentient rights
- From ableism toward transhumanization of ableism
- Toward new social groups (techno / poor /disabled) towards an ability divide
- From natural commodities to nano-formulated and atomic commodities (molecular manufacturing)
- From understanding life to designing life
- From dissecting life toward building life from the bottom up, base-pair by base-pair
- Toward an increasingly longer lifespan
- Toward the modification of animals (especially enhancements like cognitive abilities)
- Outsourcing reproductive tasks from the body (artificial womb)
- Toward lifelong learning
- Toward global learning and teaching
- Toward personal enhancements to increase learning ability and facilitate knowledge increase
- Toward global electronic group work (one meaning of collective intelligence)
- Toward a borg hive mind[7]

The difference between *biotechnology* and synthetic biology (*synbio*) is that *synbio* is Nature's biology plus engineering, whereas biotechnology refers to the engineering of entirely new biological / hybrid entities (*de novo*). Synthetic biology is interdisciplinary in that it requires biologists, chemists, engineers, physicists, physicians, and computer scientists. *Genetic engineering* is basically the forced insertion of natural genes from one species to another to transfer characteristics, whereas *synthetic biology* creates new species. *The human genome is the proof of concept that synthetic biology targets.*

In July 2001—two months before 9/11—the U.S. House of Representatives passed a bill prohibiting the cloning of human embryos. The bill was stalled in the Senate while Advanced Cell Technology (ACT) created early-stage human clone embryos. Then President George W. Bush announced fed-

7 Gregor Wolbring, "Human Security and NBICS." Innovation Watch, December 30, 2006.

eral funding for 60 stem cells of which less than 20 were viable for research purposes. Private research corporations lined up to contract with federal agencies, and the rest is history.[8] *Genomics*—genetics + economics, the branch of molecular biology concerned with the structure, function, evolution, and mapping of *genomes* for economic interests—was born.

Genome: *the complete set of genes or genetic material present in a cell or organism; long strand of DNA encoding the biology of the species*

Therapeutic cloning: *stem cells for transplantable tissue*

Reproductive cloning: *human beings*

In 2002, California authorized public funding for embryonic stem cell research and the American Medical Association (AMA) endorsed *therapeutic cloning*. In 2003, ACT was again funded for *reproductive cloning*:

> One of [Robert Lanza, MD's] embryos divided successfully to at least 16 cells. That means he has found not simply a path for stem cells, but made a significant if unintended step toward human cloning. After all, if thriving clone embryos can grow to 16 cells and beyond in a lab, those cells could theoretically be ... implanted in a uterus—reproductive cloning. Lanza[9] insists he's not going there, but others surely will.[10]

For all intents and purposes, the multibillion dollar Human Genome Project managed by the Department of Energy (DOE) was just another term for the *eugenics* of designing a human being by selecting certain genetic traits and not others. Synthetic biologists like Drew Endy view Nature as a "tyranny of evolution" that the human being must be liberated from. By packaging synthetic biology as computer software that can be done from "any old coffee shop" (Hessel), Singularity advocates get around the bad PR that accompanies the term *eugenics*.

The science has evolved such that using a laptop computer, published gene sequence information and mail-order synthetic DNA, just about

8 For example, IBM controls Iceland's Nordic Viking genetic data and operates genomic offices in California, New York, Zurich, Haifa, New Delhi, and Tokyo.

9 Currently head and CSO of Astellas Global Regenerative Medicine and adjunct professor at Wake Forest University School of Medicine, Lanza's current research focuses on stem cells and regenerative medicine.

10 Wendy Goldman Rohm, "Seven Days of Creation." Wired, January 2004.

anyone has the potential to construct genes or entire genomes from scratch—including those of lethal pathogens.[11]

To counter the laissez-faire sound of this approach to digital biology, the National Academy of Sciences (NAS), a "self-elected" adviser to government, recommends "scientific self-regulation":

> The system of scientific self-regulation proposed by the academy is modeled after the approach to recombinant DNA research, a technique for transferring genes between organisms . . . [but is] the first panel to say human embryonic stem cells should not be inserted into early human embryos, also known as blastocysts.[12]

Guidelines have been kept feeble, and appointed commissions like former President Obama's Presidential Commission for the Study of Bioethical Issues devised to be gatekeepers. Funded labs must comply with Recombinant DNA guidelines, the FDA has to approve *synbio* drugs, and the Department of Agriculture oversees the release of synthetic organisms, but they are all gatekeepers smoothing the path to Transhumanism. There is really no regulation as public-private partnerships scratch each other's back en route to Human 2.0 while building the genomics market. Self-policing is just a euphemism for criminal cooperation.

Stem cells: young undifferentiated cells

All body tissues begin as stem cells. As early as 1958, John Gurdon cloned a tadpole from the egg of a frog with DNA from another tadpole's intestinal cell, thus proving that developed cells carry the information to make every other cell. Thus adult tissue can be used to produce stem cells ("induced pluripotency stem cells" or iPS cells). Replacement cells must be from the same individual to avoid rejection via immunosuppression.[13] No need for embryo

11 Stephen Leahy, "Synthetic Biology on Trial at World Social Forum: Group Seeks Ban on 'Living Machines.'" IPS News, January 20, 2007.

12 Nicholas Wade, "Group of Scientists Drafts Rules on Ethics for Stem Cell Research." New York Times, 27 April 2005.

13 Anna Ringstrom, "UK, Japan scientists win Nobel for stem cell breakthroughs." Reuters, October 8, 2012.

harvesting. As Urban Lendahl of the Nobel Committee put it, "[T]ake a cell from, for example, the skin of the patient, reprogram it, return it to a pluripotent state, and then grow it in a laboratory."[14]

The loophole between therapeutic cloning and reproductive cloning is wide enough for "hunimals" or *chimeras* to be slipped in[15]—for example, inserting human genes into the fertilized eggs of genetically engineered pigs or mice for spare human body parts, then incubating the embryos ("embryo complementation") in females, as is done at the USDA research center in Beltsville, Maryland and the British xenotransplantation research corporation Imutran, which was closed in 2000 when Novartis moved everything to BioTransplant in Massachusetts.

> By modifying genes, scientists can now easily change the DNA in pig or sheep embryos so that they are genetically incapable of forming a specific tissue. Then, by adding stem cells from a person, they hope the human cells will take over the job of forming the missing organ, which could then be harvested from the animal for use in a transplant operation.[16]

Meanwhile, DNA is being datamined by no-bid government contractors like Choicepoint that provide "genetic surveillance" (along with medical and voting surveillance) to the FBI's CODIS (Combined DNA Index System).[17] Genetic collection extends to Saudi Arabia, Nigeria, Mongolia, South Atlantic islands, etc.—funded by Big Pharma giants like the German Boehringer Ingelheim that employ deception, bribery, theft, and threats to fulfill biotech deals between research institutions and Big Pharma corporations.

> "The more information the outside world has of our natural resources, the more they rob and destroy them," wrote Ruth Liloqula of the Solomon Islands in a 1996 special issue of *Cultural Survival Quarterly* . . . "The only thing we have left and can call our very own is our genetic makeup, we are no longer safe from being exterminated or from being exploited to the point of non-existence."[18]

That the National Institutes of Health (NIH) has been able to patent the

---

14 Ibid.

15 On the books, cloning a human being and producing hunimals is punishable by ten years in prison and a $90,000 fine.

16 Antonio Regalado, "Human-Animal Chimeras Are Gestating on U.S. Research Farms." MIT Technology Review, January 6, 2016.

17 Greg Palast, "'Don't look at The flash!' Ground Zero as a Profit Center." September 8, 2004. Choicepoint helped to swing the 2000 election of George W. Bush.

18 "Mining Humanity: Genetic Research, Indigenous Resistance and the Human Genome Diversity Project." Toward Freedom, Winter 1998/99.

people of the Solomon Islands, Panama's Guaymi, and the Hagahai of Papua New Guinea is true.[19]

Is every bloodline on Earth owned by one corporate entity or another? Are all of the CEOs and State leaders already gain-of-function modified? This was certainly what Nazi physician Josef Mengele's alleged 1960s twin experiments in Cândido Godói, Brazil were all about.

> **Gene therapy:** *DNA protein placed inside a vector in order to get the DNA into cells that then use the DNA to make other proteins. Weaponized, the goal is to permanently debilitate the innate genetic makeup of the target.*

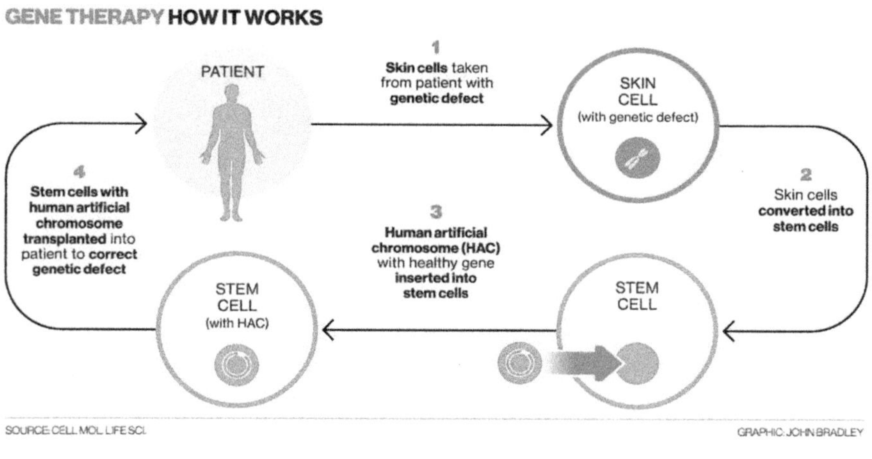
GENE THERAPY HOW IT WORKS
PATIENT
1
Skin cells taken from patient with genetic defect
SKIN CELL (with genetic defect)
2
Skin cells converted into stem cells
STEM CELL
3
Human artificial chromosome (HAC) with healthy gene inserted into stem cells
STEM CELL (with HAC)
4
Stem cells with human artificial chromosome transplanted into patient to correct genetic defect
SOURCE: CELL MOL LIFE SCI
GRAPHIC: JOHN BRADLEY

Gene therapy. In this less than adequate model of gene therapy, instead of skin cells, imagine stem cells of your own mRNA accompanied by whatever the injection inserts, including fetal stem cells and artificial chromosomes.

https://www.independent.co.uk/news/science/exclusive-mice-humanchromosomes-genetic-breakthrough-could-revolutionise-medicine-8701357.html

Thanks to *ooplasmic transfer* (*in vitro* fertilization), genetically altered babies—like three-parent babies with genes from two mothers and one father—are now being born with a germline passing on to the next generation. *Gene therapy* or *germline modification therapy*, on the other hand, is said to involve non-inheritable somatic gene modification of one individual only and thus does not affect the entire genome or germline. But is this true? Ooplasmic transfer was banned until 2008 in 83 percent of the 30 OECD nations (Organization for Economic

19 Craig Venter of Synthetic Genomics is a former NIH researcher. In May 1998, he teamed up with Perkin-Elmer to accelerate identifying and patenting human genes and IP-ing indigenous knowledge. Anthony S. Fauci, MD, is with the NIH Office of the Director.

Cooperation and Development), including the U.S. and UK. In 2013, the UK reversed its position on three-parent babies via *in vitro* fertilization (IVF).[20] In any case, the tainted term "genetic modification" is being rebranded.

Epigenetics

> *It wouldn't be unfounded to suggest that we are being both chemically and electromagnetically turned into our technology. CAN YOU HEAR ME NOW?*
>
> – Chris Fontenot, December 2015

The Human Genome Project freed and bound humanity all at the same time—freed us by proving we are much more than our genetics, if we choose to take responsibility—bound us to external environmental control by decoding our genetics.

Epigenetics defines how the stage has been set for the advent of a *synbio* Transhumanism. Epigenetics refers to any process—from environmental to mental to whatever can be made to bypass the immune system—that *alters gene expression without changing the DNA sequence.* At first, it was about determining a cell's specialization, but now a 5G weaponized environment can remotely turn genes on or off. Epigenetics has dealt a death blow to the dogma that DNA inside the nucleus is fixed and impermeable to any external influence. We are more than our genes, *if we realize it*: even our mental processes—mind, consciousness—can reprogram our genes, consciousness residing neither wholly in the brain nor in the genes but including our individual experiences, such as unresolved trauma *in utero* or from childhood that can be passed down to our children and grandchildren "unto the third generation" (Deuteronomy 5:9) through *transgenerational inheritance.*[21]

The external influence of epigenetic mechanisms can change our genetics, from chemicals, electromagnetism, nanotechnology, pharmaceutical and other drugs, to our diet, oxygen, water, sleep cycles, sunlight or lack thereof. Environmental signals that constantly pulse our bodies and brains read and switch and reprogram our genes due to our fractal DNA antenna picking up *everything,* whether conscious, unconscious, or subconscious. If the air and

---

20 See The Lancet article by Paul R. Billings, Ruth Hubbard, and Stuart A. Newman, "Human germline gene modification: a dissent," May 29, 1999.

21 Derrick Broze, "What Does Epigenetics Means for Humanity's Awakening?" Activist Post. June 5, 2018. Interestingly, there are three references to "the sins of the fathers" lasting unto the third and fourth generation in the Old Testament: Exodus 20, Numbers 14, and Deuteronomy 5.

water are polluted, if the food is genetically altered, if the sunlight is obscured by chemicals, if 5G millimeter waves subject our cells to signal transduction and pummel our nervous systems and compromise our blood-brain barrier, weakening our immune systems, causing inflammation, disrupting cell communication, and altering our calcium function—our DNA registers it all.[22]

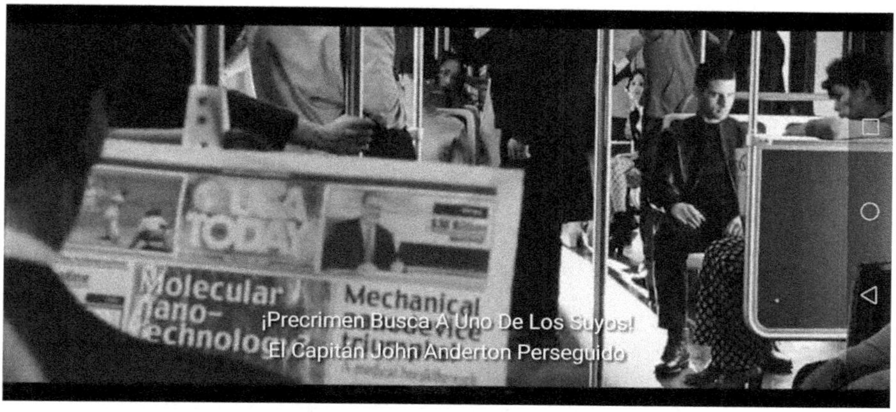
Molecular
Mechanical
¡Precrimen Busca A Uno De Los Suyos!
El Capitán John Anderton Perseguido

Were we preprogrammed? Note the headline "Molecular Nano-Technology?" in this 2002 *Minority Report* scene. (Actor Tom Cruise as PreCrime chief John Anderton seated to the right.)

Thus, it is not difficult to see in retrospect how Darwinian evolution has been traded in for a bait-and-switch epigenetics that covers for military-industrial-intelligence experiments by blaming climate change, an industry-polluted environment, and general Human 1.0 frailty (autoimmune symptoms, cancer increase, miscarriages, autism, etc.). Environment is now yoked to synthetic biology's objective to alter human genetics by 2030. Exploitation of the environment to undermine the immune system and human culture is, of course, never mentioned.

Riding on the epigenetic approach is the digital biology re-wiring of Transhumanist Human 1.0 by means of a carefully prepared environment. Epigenetics constantly underscores the dilemma we and our progeny find ourselves in. DARPA's ECHO (Epigenetic Characterization and Observation) claims to be able to read an individual's *epigenome* "record keeper" that identifies "epigenetic signatures" of "experiences" via a finger prick (blood) or nasal swab (mucosa).

22 Our bodies are subjected to one quintillion times (1 with 18 zeroes) more electromagnetic radiation than even a decade ago (Olle Johansson, PhD, Karolinska Institute, Sweden). See S. Grimaldi et al., "Exposure to a 50 Hz electromagnetic field induces activation of the Epstein-Barr virus genome in latently infected human lymphoid cells." Journal of Environmental Patholoy, Toxicology and Oncology, 1997.

Note in the following how DARPA introduces the terms *modification* and *expression* to disguise the lie that "DNA does not change over a single lifetime":

> The epigenome is biology's record keeper. Though DNA does not change over a single lifetime, a person's environment may leave marks on the DNA that modify how that individual's genes are expressed. This is one way that people can adapt and survive in changing conditions, and the epigenome is the combination of all of these modifications. Though modifications can register within seconds to minutes, they imprint the epigenome for decades, leaving a time-stamped biography of an individual's exposures that is difficult to deliberately alter.[23]

How is the mRNA gene therapy download changng the "biological phenomenon" known as the epigenome?

DNA

> *In normal DNA, two separate strands are entwined in a double helix. These strands are connected together via four different bases, adenine (A), thymine (T), cytosine (C) and guanine (G). A always bonds with T, and C always bonds with G, creating a fairly simple "language" of base pairs—ATCGAAATGCC, etc. Combine a few dozen base pairs together in a long strand of DNA and you then have a gene, which tells the organism how to produce a certain protein. If you know the sequence of letters down one strand of the helix . . . a DNA helix can be split down the middle, and then have the other half perfectly recreated.*[24]

> *There is a chase to develop the tera wavelength in order to manipulate individual components of the atom and DNA.*
>
> – Billy Hayes, "The HAARP Man"

Deoxyribonucleic acid (DNA) derives from a quantum dimension, as do thoughts. Both thoughts and DNA are inextricably tied to language.

DNA in the nucleus of each and every one of our 100 thousand billion cells is two yards long and ten atoms wide—125 billion miles of DNA (actually, chromosomes) in each and every human body, enough to wrap around

---

23 DARPA, "Reading the Body's History of Threat Exposure: Epigenetic technology would provide new tool in fight against WMD [weapons of mass destruction] proliferation," February 1, 2018.

24 "...the other half perfectly recreated. - Sebastian Anthony, "First living thing with 'alien' DNA created in the lab: We are now officially playing God." ExtremeTech, May 8, 2014.

the Earth five million times. DNA is simple and general (i.e. it does not fall along racial or "special bloodline" lines), with the majority of non-coding "junk" DNA and its 4 million gene switches running the show, according to the Encyclopedia of DNA Elements (ENCODE) of the National Human Genome Research Institute (NHGRI).[25] At one time, "junk" DNA was thought to be "dark matter" (dark plasma) and its function unknown.

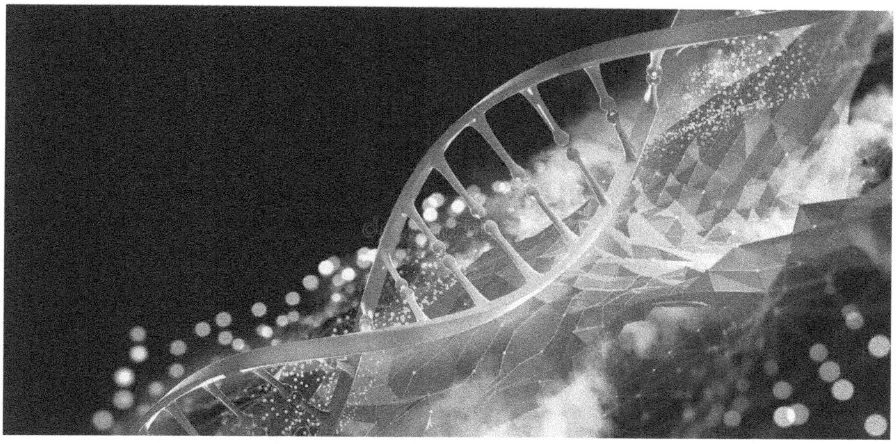

DNA Helix.

https://www.dreamstime.com/dna-helix-d-illustration-mutations-under-microscope-decoding-genome-dna-helix-d-illustration-mutations-under-microscope-decoding-image203548377

Insoluble in water, the DNA molecule is a chain of two interwoven ribbons of A-T (adenine – thymine) and G-C (guarnine – cytosine) compound pairs, basically a main text and backup inverted text that can copy or reconstruct. All that changes from one species to another is the order of these four letters.

Deoxyribonucleic acid is a molecule composed of two polynucleotide chains that coil around each other to form a double helix carrying genetic instructions for the development, functioning, growth and reproduction of all known organisms . . . (Wikipedia)

---

25 Alice Park, "Junk DNA—Not So Useless After All." Time magazine, September 6, 2012.

As indicated above, genetics has always played a secret role in politics, not just in eugenic agendas but DNA forensics in crime labs and the Combined DNA Index System (CODIS), biometric profiles, and retinal scans run through the National Crime Information Center (NCIC). Now a massive biotechnology industry is driving humanity into *genetic politics* or what chief research scientist at Dynamic Simulation Lab at Rockland State Manfred Clynes slyly calls "participant evolution"[26]:

> The great things that are happening today in the scientific world are advances in molecular biology along with computers. Those are the two regions of our scientific world that are growing very rapidly, and compared to them psychology is dead in the water completely. It is already known that the emotional world of men is fashioned through molecules like neuropeptides . . . These peptides have receptors scattered throughout the brain [and] it is known that the emotional world can be affected now by designer molecules. That's where the computers and molecular biology will intermarry . . . computer-designed molecules that will naturally work inside the brain and will be able to change the emotional aspects . . . They continually are making gene products, some are turned off, some are turned on, so that by controlling and knowing how to control the natural products, and turning the genes on and off, we will have tremendous power to change the emotional world of man . . . Evolution is more than survival of the fittest, and participant evolution can probably improve the qualities of life more effectively than by just waiting for the less fit to become extinct.

Clynes is right: there is a natural "intermarry" feature between computers and genetics, the gene being text code for the construction of proteins and enzymes. The fact that it represents only 3 percent of the human genome while the other 97 percent ("junk DNA") behaves as an antenna or periodic crystal radio set broadcasting and receiving on the global network of DNA-based life just adds to the *simpatico* of computers and wireless EM networks.

With the entry of *synthetic DNA*, something decidedly *unnatural* enters "participant evolution." Add two new bases to A, T, C, and G with synthetic DNA, and a *third strand X and Y* enters through the cell membrane:

> First, the scientists [at Scripps Research Institute] genetically engineered an *e.coli* bacterium to allow the new chemicals (d5SICS and dNaM) through the cell membrane. Then they inserted a DNA plasmid (a small loop of DNA) that contained a single XY base pair into the bacterium.

---

26 interview in The Cyborg Handbook, 1995. This would be a good opportunity to review the Ebner Effect as a ray of hope (and a reminder that it may, like scalar waves, have been weaponized).

As long as the new chemicals were available, the bacterium continued to reproduce normally, copying and passing on *the new DNA, alien plasmid and all . . . hundreds of terabytes of data stored in a single gram of synthetic, alien DNA.*[27] (Emphasis added.)

With the word *alien*, we are entering new epigenetic terrain of BCI *cyborgs* and *hybrids*. A 2017 paper, "Triplex-forming oligonucleotides: a third strand for DNA nanotechnology," succinctly lays out how three-strand DNA technology is built:

> . . . a three-stranded complex generated by the binding of a third strand within the duplex major groove, generating a triple-helical ("triplex") structure. The sequence, structural and assembly requirements that differentiate triplexes from their duplex counterparts has allowed the design of nanostructures for both dynamic and/or structural purposes, as well as a means to target non-nucleic acid components to precise locations within a nanostructure scaffold . . .[28]

Christian CERN observer and editor of *Entangled* magazine Anthony Patch describes the third strand of DNA as being constructed of silicon and coated in gold (1nm). Will a third strand be used to rewrite four billion years of evolution by producing "a wholly synthetic organism with DNA that contains dozens (or hundreds) of different base pairs that can produce an almost infinitely complex library of amino acids and proteins"[29]? For example, what about the "novel" form of Alzheimer's protein found in spinal fluid? Was it "found," or was it a "novel" gain of function?

> A novel form of Alzheimer's protein found in the fluid that surrounds the brain and spinal cord indicates what stage of the disease a person is in, and tracks with tangles of tau protein in the brain, according to a study from researchers at Washington University School of Medicine in St. Louis. Tau tangles are thought to be toxic to neurons, and their spread through the brain foretells the death of brain tissue and cognitive decline. Tangles appear as the early, asymptomatic stage of Alzheimer's develops into the symptomatic stage.[30]

---

27 Sebastian Anthony.

28 Arun Richard Chandrasekaran and David A. Rusling, "Triplex-forming oligonucleotides: a third strand for DNA nanotechnology." Nucleic Acid Research, February 16, 2018. Read "Introduction (to DNA Nanotechnology)."

29 Sebastian Anthony.

30 "Novel Form of Alzheimer's Protein Found in Spinal Fluid Indicates Stage of the Disease," NeuroscienceNews.com, December 7, 2020. What is really going on with Alzheimer's?

Three-strand DNA was what physician Jeff Bradstreet (1954-June 19, 2015) found in the blood of 100 autistic children who had all been vaccinated. *DNA markers were three, not two*—the third from aborted fetus cell lines. Bradstreet's discoveries occurred during the same timeline as publication of a Cambridge University paper about four-stranded quadruple helix DNA structures (*G-quaruplexes*) in the human genome, and publication of the story about two-year-old Alfie Clamp's seventh chromosome having a third strand of DNA. Bradstreet and Nicholas Gonzalez, MD, were both murdered just before Bradstreet was about to publish their findings not just regarding three-strand DNA but also the piggybacking of protein / enzyme nagalase onto infant vaccinations. (More about nagalase and the protein Gc in Chapter 14 under "Proteins, Enzymes, and Prions.")

What is the human being? A mammal? A divine being of another order making use of a mammalian prototype? Certainly, the plan now is for a hybridized cyborg model.

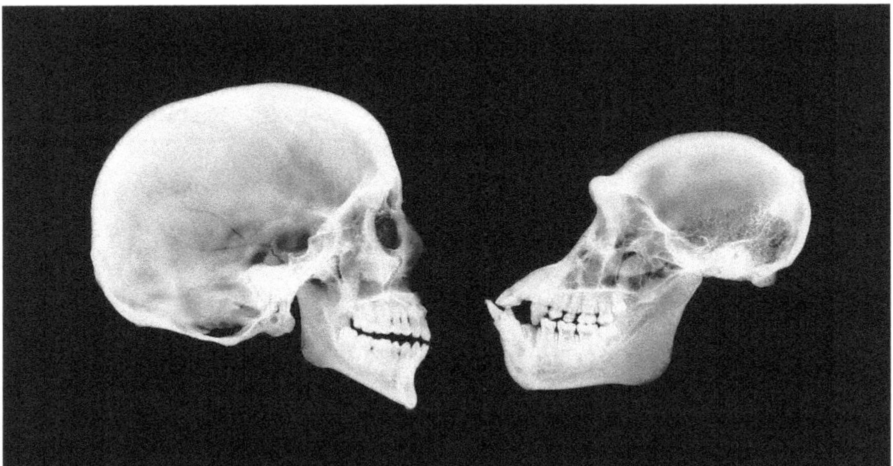

Human and chimp skulls.

The old Darwinian theory lingers. (See Appendix 1: Scientism.)

https://www.chronicle.com/article/how-our-brains-got-big-and-our-penises-lost-their-spines/

The 1990s book *The Hidden History of the Human Race* by Michael A. Cremo and Richard L. Thompson exposed how extensively Charles Darwin's evolutionary theory was twisted so as to twist human history for the benefit of bent secret societies. Behind the 20th century one-sided mechanistic model of the human body lie shades of the overly rational, suppressed, patriarchal 19th century and its "survival of the fittest" rendering of Charles Darwin's theory of natural selection environmentally underway since the "ancestral gene" of 550 million years ago, the claim being that diversity followed from environmental error (mutation) as DNA worked out its three thousand million codes and 315,000 base pairs in an alien world.[31] Human descent (ascent?) from apes and the so-called "missing link" have been kept in place by powerful Freemason lodges in league with the Royal Society (1660), Smithsonian Institute (1846), and National Geographic Society (1888):

> In the early part of the twentieth century, some scientists advocated the view that the [classic Western European Neanderthals] were the direct ancestors of modern human beings. They had brains larger than those of *Homo sapiens sapiens*. Their faces and jaws were much larger, and their foreheads were lower, sloping back from behind large brow ridges. Neanderthal remains are found In Pleistocene deposits ranging from 30,000 to 150,000 years old. However, the discovery of early *Homo sapiens* in deposits far older than 150,000 years effectively removed the classic Western European Neanderthals from the direct line of descent leading from *Homo erectus* to modern humans.[32]

Neanderthal mitochondrion DNA was allegedly more complex and varied than modern human DNA in 27 places—in other words, the climb to neocortex development was not without its cost.[33] Now, our self-conception of what it is to be human is being forced into a brain-computer interface (BCI) hybrid model.

Hundreds of capsule-shaped cell organelles called *mitochondria* populate every cell, working to turn oxygen and nutrients into the energy the cell needs. The mitochondrial electrical field has a strength of 30 million volts. There are billions of neurons, with four to five thousand cells per neuron. Former FEMA operative Celeste Solum says the human being is like a particle accelerator cyclotron. The 37 mitochondrial genes exist as a separate DNA molecule (0.2 percent of the genome) outside the nucleus of the cell. These are the "power packs" that generate metabolic energy from glucose, synthetize hormones and neurotransmitters, metabolize cholesterol. Defective mitochondria lead to painful debilitating diseases; thus, the idea of replacing them in embryos is very appealing—so appealing, in fact, that *ooplasmic transfer* is

31 Biology's traditional model organisms have been the fruit fly, mouse, worm C. elegans, zebra fish, and human.

32 Michael A. Cremo and Richard L. Thompson, The Hidden History of the Human Race (Los Angeles: Bhaktavedanta Book Publishing, 1999).

33 U.S. News & World Report, July 21, 1997. No modern race genetically varies by more than eight variations from any other race.

encouraged: the injection of a healthy donor's egg or embryo mitochondrial DNA into the egg of an infertile woman.

Up until the recent discovery of a mitochondrial base editor, mitochondria were a powerful frontline defense resisting cell mutation.[34] Now, "nuclear inheritable changes" are no longer a limitation, especially since "the new definition [of genetic modification] excludes alterations to human mitochondrial genes or any other genetic material that exists outside the chromosomes in the nucleus of the cell."[35] Mitochondrial replacement or transfer is now a form of inheritable genetic modification—in other words, *permanent* human genome change.

The human genome *is genetic information in 3 billion letters along a single filament of DNA winding around itself into 23 pairs of chromosomes. All of our cells contain two complete genomes as well as their backup copies.*

Somatic genes = *non-heritable, do not affect the human genome*

Germline modification = *heritable; alters the human genome*

The shamanic view of DNA

DNA is a master of transformation, just like mythical serpents. The cell-based life DNA informs made the air we breathe, the landscape we see, and the mind-boggling diversity of living beings of which we are a part. In 4 billion years, it has multiplied itself into an incalculable number of species while remaining exactly the same.[36]

In high school, we learn that American biologist James D. Watson (1928 -) and British physicist Francis H.C. Crick (1916-2004) discovered the DNA double helix in 1953. As usual, this is not exactly true, given that the double helix is actually a *model:*

DNA was first identified in the late 1860s by Swiss chemist Friedrich

---

34 Sharon Begley, "Gene-editing find could point to cures for mitochondrial diseases." STAT, July 8, 2020.

35 Steve Connor, "Exclusive: Scientists accuse government of dishonesty over GM babies in its regulation of new IVF [in vitro fertilization] technique." Independent, 28 July 2014.

36 Jeremy Narby, The Cosmic Serpent: DNA and the Origins of Knowledge (NY: Putnam, 1998).

> Miescher. Then, in the decades following Miescher's discovery, other scientists--notably, Phoebus Levene and Erwin Chargaff--carried out a series of research efforts that revealed additional details about the DNA molecule, including its primary chemical components and the ways in which they joined with one another. Without the scientific foundation provided by these pioneers, Watson and Crick may never have reached their groundbreaking conclusion of 1953: that the DNA molecule exists in the form of a three-dimensional double helix.[37]

For eons, shamans have been taking their consciousness down to the molecular level and combining their brain hormones with monoamine oxidase inhibitors. Down at the *quantum* level of the subatomic, the Amazonian Ashaninca communicate with "those who are hidden" (*maninkari*) inside the body at the threshold of what makes the body function *like a self-automated machine* by means of "visual song," some shamans with "second sight" or "second hearing," others riding the frequencies of psychotropic plants down to the molecular level.

When writing *The Cosmic Serpent* in the late 1990s, Jeremy Narby claimed to follow the detection philosophy of Arthur Conan Doyle's fictional Sherlock Holmes, namely the *lateral approach*: discovery from diverse or seemingly contrary angles so as to allow for a "stereogram" as panoptic as possible to form in the mind—in other words, a clear mental picture. *Did the Watson and Crick model come from the indigenous experience of twin serpents ("the favorite newscasters of DNA-TV") derived from the Peruvian Amazon psychotropic tea ayahuasca?* Interestingly, the molecules in nicotine or dimethyltryptamine in tobacco are also in *ayahuasca*:

> . . . activating their respective receptors which set off a cascade of electrochemical reactions inside the neurons [leads] to the stimulation of DNA and, more particularly, to its emission of visible waves, which shamans perceive as 'hallucinations' . . .[38]

DNA emits biophotons corresponding to the narrow band of visible light (infrared 900 nanometers to ultraviolet 200 nanometers) like an ultra-weak laser. Biophoton emission being swarm cellular communication, what, if anything, does this say about subatomic nanoparticle swarm consciousness, given that the human body is now conceived of as a machine whose many components and processes can be swapped out or enhanced like a car, while the brain is referenced as a computer inferior to nonhuman artificial intelligence?

37 Leslie A. Pray, PhD. "Discovery of DNA Structure and Function: Watson and Crick." Nature Education, 2008.

38 Jeremy Narby.

> . . . one can extract the DNA sequence in the human genome containing the instructions to build the insulin protein and splice it into the DNA of a bacterium, which will then produce insulin similar to that normally excreted by the human pancreas. The cellular machines called ribosomes, which assemble the proteins inside the bacterium, understand the same four-letter language as the ribosomes inside human pancreatic cells and use the same 20 amino acids as building blocks. Biotechnology proves by its very existence the fundamental unity of life.[39]

In in 1966, the French bio-technocrat Joël de Rosnay compared the cell to a "molecular factory capable of building its own machines as well as the drivers of those machines" (*The Origins of Life*); and in 1993, David S. Goodsell's *The Machinery of Life* (2nd edition, 2009) described molecules as machines:

> Like the machines of our modern world, these molecules are built to perform specific functions efficiently, accurately, and consistently. Modern cells build hundreds of thousands of different molecular machines, each performing one of hundreds of thousands of individual tasks in the process of living. These molecular machines are built according to four basic molecular plans. Whereas our macroscopic machines are built of metal, wood, plastic, and ceramic, the microscopic machines in cells are built of protein, nucleic acid, lipid, and polysaccharide.

The machine metaphor is becoming more and more refined for Big Pharma and Big Medicine "precision medicine" *tiny mechanical technologies* usurping the divine systems of the organic human body, healing, and health for what Rudolf Steiner calls *mechanical occultism:*

> Cells in the body are wired like computer chips to direct signals that instruct how they function . . . Unlike a circuit board, however, cells can rapidly rewire their communication networks to change their behavior . . . Researchers at the University of Edinburgh found information is carried across a web of guide wires that transmit signals across tiny, nanoscale distances. It is the movement of charged molecules across these tiny distances that transmit information, just as in a computer microprocessor . . .[40]

"Air Loom" discoveries like that of "a [circuit board] network of nanotubes similar to the carbon nanotubes you find in a computer microprocessor" come under *quantum biology*, "using quantum mechanics and theoretical

---

39 Ibid.

40 "Scientists discover signaling circuit boards inside body's cells," University of Edinburgh. Science Daily, May 24, 2019.

chemistry to solve biological problems." DNA, thought, and language are all engaged in quantum dimensions, with humans now being referred to as *wetware* (as in *hardware* and *software*), "the sum of all the information-rich molecular processes inside a living cell."[41]

Optogenetics

> *A different branch has specialized in the optical properties of the DNA. We need to realize that this approach might outshine everything we have learned about transhumanism . . . Once it is possible to modify a bacterium in a way that it functions as a radio-controlled lightbulb collectively creating living plasma screens, it is obvious how big the temptation is to implement these sequences into the human genome to get access to the light-body [etheric body].*
>
> – Harald Kautz-Vella, "The Chemistry in Contrails: Assessing the Impact of Aerosols from Jet Fuel Impurities, Additives and Classified Military Operations on Nature," a paper presented in Oslo, Berlin, and Reykjavik, November 2014

> *The best-laid schemes o' mice 'an' men*
> *Gang aft agley . . .*
>
> – Robert Burns, "To a Mouse, on Turning her up in her nest with a plough," 1785

Optogenetics, the branch of science that couples brains with computers (BCI / BMI), is now as indispensable as CRISPR to neuroscientists.

- *Maps the brain*
- *Controls light-responsive proteins in the brain through targeted light emission*
- *Determines optical properties of DNA*
- *Wipes / transfers / reactivates memory engrams (life memories or "immortality")*[42]
- *Switches populations of related neurons on and off*
- *Avails communication between biological and artificial neuronal networks*

It was Crick who foresaw that in order to observe the brain without electrodes, a cell type sensitive to light would be needed. In the 1950s, José M.

---

41 Dennis Bray, Wetware: A computer in every living cell (Yale University, 2009).

42 Preprogramming films about memory: Total Recall (1990, 2012), Conspiracy Theory (1997), Dark City (1998), Memento (2000), Paycheck (2003), Eternal Sunshine of the Spotless Mind (2004), The Butterfly Effect (2004), The Manchurian Candidate (1962, 2004), Extracted (2013), American Ultra (2015), Rememory (2017), The Tale (2018), etc.

R. Delgado, MD, the infamous Yale University physiologist, stopped a bull with a stimoceiver, thus introducing electrical brain stimulation (EBS). Most recently, the fMRI (functional magnetic resonance imaging) has used magnetics to follow the blood flow in the brain,[43] thanks to the recent increase in magnetite particles (and now graphene?).

Basically, the optogenetics method of peering into the cell is dependent upon both lasers and fiber optics light delivery into the nervous system and genes that encode microbial *opsins* (light-activated proteins from the green algae *Chlamydomonas reinhardtii* that regulate transmembrane ion conductance).[44] Blue light switches cells on, yellow light off. Genetic code is inserted via a virus or other nanobot into the genetic code of the specific neurons or brain location to be influenced or controlled.

Karl Deisseroth, MD, PhD, and his graduate student Feng Zhang devised the optogenetics method. Together, they had a working knowledge of virology, optics, 3D imaging, microbiology, animal behavior, psychiatry, materials science, and chemistry. Deisseroth attached bits of DNA to the opsins that acted like a password, then attached a fiber optic wire to a laser diode so as to pulse light deep into the brain.

> . . . By using [the yellow light photosensitive protein] in concert with the blue-light opsin, researchers can play neural circuitry like an organ, turning brain activity on and off at the actual speed with which neurons communicate with one another . . .[45]

Since the advent of *luminopsins (LMOs)*—the fused proteins of *luciferase*, which emits biological light, and opsins, the light-sensitive proteins in the retina—implants like electrodes or brain chips are no longer necessary for brain meddling.

> . . . we expanded the utility of luminopsins by fusing bright Gaussia luciferase variants with either channelrhodopsin to excite neurons (luminescent opsin, LMO) or a proton pump to inhibit neurons (inhibitory LMO, iLMO). These improved LMOs could reliably activate or silence neurons *in vitro* and *in vivo*.[46]

43 John Colapinto, "Lighting the Brain." The New Yorker, May 11, 2015. See Chapter 11 for both EBS and fMRI.

44 Karl Deisseroth, MD, PhD, et al., "Optogenetics and the Circuit Dynamics of Psychiatric Disease." JAMA Network, May 26, 2015.

45 Ibid.

46 Ken Berglund et al., "Luminopsins integrate opto- and chemogenetics by using physical and biological light sources for opsin activation." PNAS, January 19, 2016.

"Rapid advances in materials and electrical engineering" have made it so that opsin activation in neural tissue can now be done "wirelessly using tiny LEDs."

In his 2009 Stanford Challenge talk "Controlling the Brain with Light," Deisseroth announced the introduction of a new psychiatric subspecialty: engineering-based *interventional psychiatry* that makes liberal use of optogenetics:

> . . . optogenetics may give rise to technologies which could be used to affect human psychology directly through the brain. That's delicate territory. What happens when genetic manipulation and miniaturized electronics [nanobots] allow us to directly target parts of our brain and stimulate them as we wish? What happens if we understand how to stimulate the hypothalamus and make anyone hungry? Or angry? Or aroused?[47]

By 2019, Deisseroth was stimulating individual neurons in the visual cortex of mice ("freely moving animals") to induce illusory images and project holograms into the visual cortex along prepared neurons to influence behavior.

> Visual perception in mammals is correlated with neural circuitry in the visual cortex region of the brain. *In both mice and humans*, the visual cortex is responsible for processing information relayed from the retina . . . Deisseroth and his colleagues inserted a combination of two genes into large numbers of neurons in the visual cortex of lab mice. One gene encoded a light-sensitive protein that caused the neuron to fire in response to a pulse of laser light in the infrared spectrum. The other gene encoded a fluorescent protein that glowed green whenever the neuron was active[48] . . . "It's quite remarkable how few neurons you need to specifically stimulate in an animal to generate a perception," Deisseroth said . . . (Emphasis added.)

Could this be *remotely* done outside the lab environment by means of nanobots and "wireless tiny LEDs" pulsing nanobots in the visual cortex, perhaps through the retina?

In her July 25, 2020 video "Optogenetics Remote Mind Control via GM Drugs, Targeted Individuals, MKULTRA," Amazing Polly tips us off to an optogenetic advancement called *chemogenetics* that uses proteins activated by designer drugs to turn neurological "switches" (receptors) off and on so as to interfere with neurons that would otherwise serve free thought and therefore free will. Genetically engineer a receptor, then implant it via a viral vector

47 Aaron, Saenz, "Incredible Video of Using Light to Control the Brain of Mice." Singularity Hub, March 18, 2010.

48 "Literal Window into the Brain Shows How to Induce Illusions in Mice," Genetic Engineering & Biotechnology News, July 19, 2019.

like modified adenovirus.[49] "Viral vectors" are little more than manipulated nanoparticles that can be loaded into vaccines, aerosols, or GMO foods.

Another advance in chemo-optogenetics is *DREADDS (designer receptors exclusively activated by designer drugs)*, an acronym more ominous than even the (luciferian) *luciferase*. Create a cell, put it somewhere in the body, then activate it remotely via designer drugs. Two of the designer drugs that activate DREADDS receptors so specific neural groups can be manipulated are the antipsychotic clozapine and the hallucinogenic *Salvia divinorum*. Both contain opioid compounds, both can be air- or water-released, and the chemical signatures of both can be transmitted electromagnetically. This is a large part of what *digital biology* has in store for us.

There are no pain receptors in the brain itself, though the meninges (brain cover), periosteum (bone cover), and scalp all have pain receptors. Technically, the brain feels no pain during brain surgery, the irony being that the brain is what we use to detect pain.

Two decades ago, a severely targeted activist friend told me about how "they" had remotely pumped up his muscles until he "looked like Charles Atlas," after which they undid it just as easily. Were they using optogenetics to engineer "biological machines (bio-bots) capable of nonnatural functional behaviors"?

> . . . we created a modular light-controlled skeletal muscle-powered bioactuator that can generate up to 300 μN [micronewtons] (0.56 kPa [kilopascal] of active tension force in response to a noninvasive optical stimulus [optogenetics]. When coupled to a 3D printed flexible bio-bot skeleton *[or a living skeleton]*, these actuators drive directional locomotion (310 μm/s or 1.3 body lengths/min) and 2D rotational steering (2°/s) in a precisely targeted and controllable manner. The muscle actuators dynamically adapt to their surroundings by adjusting performance in response to "exercise" training stimuli.[50]

Was he a guinea pig for "multicellular bio-integrated machines"?

CRISPR and gene drives

> *A CRISPR system is created by programming a Cas enzyme, which is involved in cellular apoptosis [cell death] and proliferation, to bind to a certain DNA or RNA sequence. The programming involves designing a guide RNA*

---

49 Adenovirus + coronavirus = the common cold. "Modified" means that the work function has been changed ("gain of function"), often for purposes of weaponizing, patenting to make it secret (proprietary) and thus own it.

50 Ritu Raman et al., "Optogenetic skeletal muscle-powered adaptive biological machines." PNAS.org, August 13, 2015.

complementary to the sequence the enzyme is to bind with. A guide RNA can be designed to target the Cas protein to a gene to be edited. When the protein finds this sequence, the built-in molecular scissors of the Cas protein cut the nucleic acid at that location.

– Joseph Constance, "CRISPR Technology Edges Closer to Commercial Use," *BioSpace*, October 1, 2020

*The two applications of CRISPR technology that I'm most worried about are edits to human reproductive tissue and the generation of and release into the wild of transgenic organisms that are capable of propagating edits. If we generate successfully edited sperm or eggs and then use them for in vitro [*in vivo?*] fertilization, we'll create individuals that carry those edits in every single cell of their bodies.*

– Brian Farley, molecular biologist, University of California, Berkeley

In 2014, Mingming and Lingling, a pair of genetically engineered macaque monkeys, were created *in vitro* with precise CRISPR genetic mutations in the Kunming biolab in Yunnan province, China.

The gold standard of genome engineering is the CRISPR tool (*clustered regularly interspaced short palindromic*[51] *repeats*) that permanently alters endogenous gene expression by editing cells *from the inside*, including single-cell bacteria and archaebacteria. The two components of CRISPR gene editing are guide RNA and the endonuclease Cas9: the RNA instructs and guides the enzyme Cas9 to basically enter the target DNA and "edit" it via disruption or insertion. Gene-drive inheritance is boosted 97 percent by CRISPR, *gene drives* being what drives a gene through a population: "slip a new gene into a drive system and let nature take care of the rest."[52]

CRISPR was developed in the early 1960s by orthopedic surgeon and cancer researcher Mary S. Sherman in New Orleans. If you saw Oliver Stone's 1991 film *JFK*, you'll remember David Ferrie, who was involved in Dr. Sherman's cancer research. (Ferrie was murdered on July 21, 1964, the day the Warren Commission was to hear his testimony about alleged assassin Lee Harvey Oswald's CIA / FBI activities in Louisiana.[53])

---

51 Palindromes read the same backward as forward.

52 Eleanor Nelsen and Tim De Chant, "Powerful Genetic Engineering Technique Could Modify Entire Wild Populations." PBS, 17 July 2014.

53 Read Edward T. Haslam's Mary, Ferrie & the Monkey Virus: The Story of an Underground Medical Laboratory, Wordsworth Communication Service, 1995. The latest updated version is Dr. Mary's Monkey: How the Unsolved Murder of a Doctor, a Secret Laboratory in New Orleans and Cancer-Causing Monkey Viruses Are Linked to Lee Harvey Oswald, the JFK Assassination and Emerging Global Epidemics (Trine Day, 2015) with a foreword by

The Cas9 gene drive is particularly powerful in how it merges population genetics, genetic engineering, and molecular genetics by allowing "a genetically modified gene to jump from one chromosome to another within the same individual so that eventually all of the sperm or eggs of the animal carried the GM trait, rather than half [as in natural reproduction]. This means that virtually none of the offspring is eventually free of an introduced GM [genetically modified] trait."[54]

Though the first target population was the malaria-carrying *Anopheles gambiae* mosquito,[55] uploading Cas9-based gene drives into a species has always been about gene driving supercharged genetically modified genes (read gain-of-function / weaponized) into sexually reproducing human beings. "Population-scale genetic engineering projects" can be delivered by mosquitos, aerosols, GMOs, and vaccinations, after which they spread like a nuclear chain reaction in large populations.

Due to the Transhumanist "open science movement"[56] of digital biology, CRISPR components can even be tailored to "the workflow of permanently knocking out genes" by mail order!

> The Dharmacon Edit-R CRISPR-Cas9 platform greatly simplifies the workflow of permanently knocking out genes. Our approach includes predesigned, ready-to-use DNA and RNA components and enables fast assessment of multiple target sites per gene for multiple genes. We hold a license from the Broad Institute to provide CRISPR reagents [only US$30!] for research use. Explore our products for successful CRISPR-Cas9 genome engineering.[57]

The CRISPR-crazed gene-drive business is booming. The nonprofit mail order corporation AddGene is the *Amazon.com* for digital biology ingredients.

> To ship [DNA], AddGene mails out vials of *E.coli* bacteria with the valuable bits of DNA spliced into mini-chromosomes known as plasmids. There are about 45,000 plasmids to choose from. Want to make a mouse's brain cells react to light? That's plasmid number 20298, deposited by

---

Jim Marrs (1943-2017), author of Crossfire: The Plot That Killed Kennedy (1989).

54 Steve Connor, "'Gene drive': Scientists sound alarm over supercharged GM organisms which could spread in the wild and cause environmental disasters." The Independent, 2 August 2015.

55 Possibly the carrier of the U.S. Navy-modified Zika virus, according to Edward Snowden. See Kilgoar, "Modified Zika Virus Outbreak linked to US Navy's darknet." Internet Chronicle, January 31, 2016.

56 Antonio Regalado, "The Scientific Swap Meet Behind the Gene-Editing Boom." Technology Review, April 8, 2016.

57 http://dharmacon.gelifesciences.com.

Keith Deisseroth, the famed co-inventor of optogenetics at Stanford. Need to turn off every gene in a fruit fly, one by one? . . . The most frequently ordered DNA of all the code is to make Cas9 . . .[58]

Thus far, embryos have been edited with what allegedly will not be passed on to future generations while ongoing trials purportedly dedicated to making the blind see and the lame walk by editing DNA *in vivo* are sponsored by pairings like CRISPR Therapeutics and Vertex Pharmaceuticals, Editas Medicine and Allergan Pharmaceuticals.

Microinjection: microscope pointed at petri dish and two precision needles for gene editing or to inject sperm into an egg.

Meanwhile, the old CRISPR problem of not scissoring exactly the right place and creating "unwanted 'off-target' edits" seems to have been solved by the new CRISPR-guided DNA base editor CGBE1 and the smaller miniCGBE1, both of which focus on changing a single base in DNA rather than breaking the double strand.

> Base editors are fusion proteins that use a modified form of CRISPR-Cas that is targeted to a specific target site with the help of a guide RNA, where it then deploys an enzyme called a deaminase to modify a specific base to create a desired DNA change.[59]

Genetic havoc can certainly follow from tampering with Nature, but what about intentional covert experimentation, lab sabotage,[60] or genetic warfare? "CRISPR-based therapy" can delete thousands of DNA bases, silence genes that should be active, and activate genes that should be silent, including cancer-causing genes.[61] Targeted individual Barbara Tutino asks:

> *Is the point of CRISPR-Cas9 to keep people ill, the intent being not just programming humanity for failure but to deplete us of $$$ through per-*

---

58 Regalado.

59 Massachusetts General Hospital, "New CRISPR DNA base editor expands the landscape of precision genome editing." Phys.org, July 23, 2020.

60 Mark Thomas et al., "Collateral damage and CRISPR genome editing." PLOSGenetics, March 2019.

61 Sharon Begley, "Potential DNA damage from CRISPR has been 'seriously underestimated,' study finds." STAT, July 16, 2018.

petual injury or illness to fund doctors, pharma, medical products manufacturers, service providers and medical malpractice lawyers who are a part of the biotech world? Part of the "pay it forward" ELF gang stalking operation? (October 2, 2020)

In the following Abstract, a "CRISPR mediated immunity" superior to the ancient human immune system is referenced (note the warlike context in italics):

> Explorations of the *evolutionary arms race* between bacteria and bacteriophages (viruses that infect bacteria) have unearthed a variety of *defense mechanisms* that include CRISPR-Cas (CRISPR-associated nuclease) adaptive immune systems. Understanding the mechanisms of CRISPR-mediated immunity, involving DNA-encoded, RNA-guided, sequence-specific *targeting* of *invasive* nucleic acids has spawned powerful genome engineering platforms based on diverse Cas effectors. Subsequent studies have also revealed anti-CRISPR proteins that have proven valuable as control switches for Cas molecular machines. CRISPR-Cas immune systems encompass diverse families, including DNA-targeting effectors such as Cascade-Cas3, Cas9, and Cas12 as well as the recently characterized RNA-*targeting* CAS13 ribonuclease (RNase). The evolving immune *arsenal* in bacteria has been matched by diverse anti-CRISPRs that enable viruses to *escape* Cas nuclease targeting.[62] (Emphases added.)

A modified version of CRISPR is being used to build dual-core biocomputers in cells:

> "Imagine a microtissue with billions of cells, each equipped with its own dual-core processor," says [ETH Zurich researcher Martin] Fussenegger. "Such 'computational organs' could theoretically attain computing power that far outstrips that of a digital supercomputer—and using just a fraction of the energy."[63]

Is "enabling rational programming of mammalian cell behavior" the central purpose of *synbio*? Are our bodies to be turned into protein-based CPUs (central processing units)[64]?

---

62 Rudolphe Barrangou and Erik J. Sontheimer, "Shutting down RNA-targeting CRISPR." Science, 3 July 2020.

63 Michael Irving, "CRISPR used to build dual-core computers inside human cells." New Atlas, April 17, 2019.

64 Hyojin Kim et al., "A CRISPR / Cas9-based central processing unit to program complex logic computation in human cells." PNAS.org, April 9, 2019.

Stem cells

So gene editing is the same gene therapy that weaponizes vaccines, as in Project Coast's race-specific vaccines in South Africa[65] and treating diseases like leukemia and congenital genetic defects, transferring genetic code to livestock via "Terminator seed," and crosspollinating super-crops in order to "slow kill" populations for profits via food.[66] Stem cell gene therapy success often needs only one shot because of how stem cells perpetually self-replicate, once in the body, similar to the natural fresh-water hydra virtually living forever because it is mostly made up of *stem cells* that continually divide and renew its body.

The fact that stem cells are little pieces of material immortality is dangerous moral ground, hinted at in Seattle by the logo of Zimo Genetics: Hathor the Egyptian cow-headed goddess, mother of Horus, crosses quantum boundaries to preside over the mystery of birth. Hathor is reminiscent of statue of the statue of the Hindu goddess Shiva Nataraja dancing the Cosmic Dance of creation and destruction outside CERN headquarters, alluding to mechanical occultism mysteries taking place inside corporate labs.[67]

Let's reconsider the two kinds of cloning: *therapeutic* and *reproductive*. Stem cell lines are created by the therapeutic cloning of frozen human embryos and / or menstrual blood (the monthly uterus lining of females). The reader may recall the 2015 undercover video scandal regarding Planned Parenthood's role in fetal trafficking (and infanticide) by selling thousands of frozen human embryos[68] for the lucrative human fetal tissue "research" industry.

> Dr. [Deborah] Nucatola famously described Planned Parenthood's fetal tissue research programs, casually over wine and salad at a crowded Los Angeles restaurant . . . [how] ultrasound guidance [is used] to flip a fetus to a feet-first position for intact extraction and successful organ harvesting at Planned Parenthood. Yet when questioned by Congressional investigators, Dr. Nucatola denied that such abortions were used in Planned Parenthood's fetal tissue research programs.[69]

---

65 See UN report "Project Coast Apartheid's Chemical and Biological Warfare Programme" (2002) and the Project for A New American Century (PNAC) 2000 report "Rebuilding America's Defenses."

66 Ulson Gunnar, "The Dangers of Human Editing." Global Research, June 5, 2015.

67 See Chapter 9, "The Temple of CERN," in Under An Ionized Sky. Seemingly fanciful references to myths are often clues to secret society objectives.

68 Micaiah Bilger, "Planned Parenthood leaders admit under oath to harvesting body parts from babies born alive." Pregnancy Help News, 1 July 2020.

69 "Planned Parenthood Sworn Video Testimony Admits Using Partial-Birth Abortions to Sell Baby Parts." The Center for Medical Progress, August 24, 2020. In the video, note the language contrived to avoid referencing a formed human being—"POC (product of conception)," "torso," "limbs," "calvarium," etc.

Therapeutic cloning of stem cells is thus dependent upon the abortion industry. Federal law regulates human fetal tissue from abortions with the stipulation that it be used only for research purposes.[70] Especially sought after are fresh and never frozen tissues at 16-24 weeks (1st and 2nd trimester).[71] Prenatal genetic testing also garners a fair share of abortions: a blood sample from a woman less than 18 weeks pregnant and saliva from the father are screened for 3,500 genetic disorders (like Downs); reconstruction of the baby's entire genetic code may thus lead to a request to abort in the hopes of a more "perfect" child later. Growing human fetal tissue on mice and inside pigs and sheep to create transplant organs is a profitable side industry: human stem cells (*iPS cells*) are added to animal embryos, thus producing the *hunimals* or human-animal *chimeras* discussed earlier that blur the line between species.[72]

> By modifying genes, scientists can now change the DNA in pig or sheep embryos so that they are genetically incapable of forming a specific tissue. Then, by adding stem cells from a person, they hope the human cells will take over the job of forming the missing organ, which could then be harvested from the animal for use in a transplant operation.
>
> "We can make an animal without a heart. We have engineered pigs that lack skeletal muscles and blood vessels," says Daniel Garry, a cardiologist who leads a chimera project at the University of Minnesota . . .[73]

Pluripotent stem cells: *the cells that can become specialized to any type of cell in the human body.*

Pigs may lead to human beings growing their own replacement organs. Lymph nodes appear to be an excellent breeding ground for hepatocytes (chief functional cells of the liver) to grow an ectopic liver.[74]

---

70 The "research" cover for weapons development was used by the CIA and Raytheon for the High-frequency Active Auroral Research Project (HAARP), as well.

71 "Judicial Watch Obtains Records Showing FDA Paid For 'Fresh and Never Frozen' Human Fetal Parts for Use in 'Humanized Mice' Creation." Judicial Watch, June 23, 2020.

72 In Greek mythology, a chimera is part lion, part goat, part snake.

73 Antonio Regalado, "Human-Animal Chimeras Are Gestating on U.S. Research Farms." Technology Review, January 6, 2016.

74 Joe Pinkstone, "Humans could soon be able to grow new LIVERS inside their own bodies by injecting healthy cells into their lymph nodes." Mail Online, August 20, 2020.

Synthetic DNA

Keeping in mind that increasing technological sophistication is about weaponization and not healing, now that wireless capability is everywhere (thanks to the Space Fence lockdown I discussed in my last book), we are now faced with *remote* or *precision medicine* wherein genes can be remotely activated or turned off:

> . . . radio waves as ideal for this sort of remote manipulation because they can pass through thick layers of tissue, and they can be easily focused . . . Even better, the researchers have already developed a way to achieve similar, albeit weaker, results without having to inject nanoparticles at all. They have developed cells that can grow their own required nanoparticles . . .[75]

Not only are cells growing their own nanoparticles, but they are now manufacturing proteins, as well, all due to digital biology and 20+ years of chemical jet trails and Monsanto terminator seed and soil, smart dust, quantum dots, self-assembling nanotubes, nanofibers, nanocrystals, and ferroelectric synthetic DNA nanotech built to self-replicate and construct BCI networks inside human bodies and brains. Because synthetic DNA nanotech is *ferroelectric*, it can be controlled by external frequencies and communicated with. On Facebook, RF engineer (DARPA and MIT's Lincoln Laboratory) Carly Lebrun explained how ferroelectric synthetic DNA nanotech

- Binds with our DNA as it builds its network
- Feeds off of our proteins, lipids, etc.
- Its biofilm coating protects it from the immune system
- Once the synthetic network is formed, it will have a unique identifier, just as natural DNA has
- Once the synthetic network has digital access to personal cell phones, we are programmable and may feel a vibration in our abdomen during transmissions
- The push for everyone on the planet to have a cell phone is about the nanotech inside of us sending out unique identifiers so we are registered for remote control over bodies, brains, and behaviors via frequencies
- Access includes control over people physically proximate to us

---

75 Nature, May 2012, http://www.nature.com/news/remote-controlled-genes-trigger-insulin-production-1.10585.

Ferroelectric: communicates with and can be controlled by external frequencies.

DNA strands can be broken at a distance with an extremely low frequency (ELF) 100 Hz / 5.6 mT (millitesla) electromagnetic field.[76] 100 Hz frequency is everywhere the Internet of Things (IoT) is: plugged-in appliances, medical devices, electric cars and trains, traffic lights, etc. Nonionizing radiation like 100 Hz eventually wears cells down while daily overstimulating their 3,000 miles of DNA and causing strand breaks. It also increases stressed protein levels and continuous remote conduction in the compact structure of the nucleus. Even not counting the ionized radiation in our environment (see Chapter 6), nonionizing radiation is yoked to a slow-kill mission.

> The wide frequency range of interaction with EMF is the functional characteristic of a fractal antenna, and DNA appears to possess the two structural characteristics of fractal antennas: electronic conduction and self-symmetry. These properties contribute to greater reactivity of DNA with EMF in the environment, and the DNA damage could account for increases in cancer epidemiology as well as *variations in the rate of chemical evolution in early geologic history.*[77] (Emphasis added.)

(Regarding "the rate of chemical evolution in early geologic history," could it be that an Earth environment simulacrum as chemically like that of the Earth during the natural evolution of Human 1.0 millions of years ago is what geoengineering is attempting to sustain and abet while Human 1.0 is undergoing "participant evolution"?)

Mass production of individual genes is the name of the synthetic patenting game for *reproductive cloning* and is perhaps why Autodesk, a CAD-software company funding synthetic biology labs and developing software for biological design, requires so many HGP Write nondisclosure agreements.[78] The Human Genome Project concentrated on *reading* a genome; now HGP Write is synthesizing all six billion DNA letter combinations of the human genome so as

76 Cosmin Teodor Mihai et al., "Extremely low frequency electromagnetic fields cause DNA strand breaks in normal cells." Journal of Environmental Science Engineering, 2014.

77 Martin Blank, PhD. "DNA is a fractal antenna in electromagnetic fields." International Journal of Radiation Biology, April 2011.

78 Antonio Regalado, "Ethical Questions Loom Over Efforts to Make Human Genome from Scratch." Technology Review, May 25, 2016.

to write and custom build organisms while Gen9 in Cambridge, Massachusetts pumps out DNA sequences for Big Pharma and agricultural giants like Syngenta.

> Gen9 and Twist Bioscience have been breaking ground by adopting techniques from the computer industry to mass-produce billions of short pieces of DNA . . . in tiny wells micromachined [nanotechnology?] onto a silicon chip . . .[79]

In 2017, Craig Venter's Synthetic Genomics came out with a digital-to-biological converter that takes in digital codes and spits out DNA, RNA, protein drugs, *and viral nanoparticles*. Venter sequenced the first human genome and is now turning that digital data into synthesized biological molecules. The BioXP converter is now being replaced by the prototype BioXP 3200. Biological synthesis in one machine.[80]

While writing genetic code may sound benign when it comes to creating synthetic organs from patients' own cells—for example, using adult skin cells and messenger RNA (mRNA) to develop pluripotent stem cells to regenerate functional human heart tissue from which to grow an entire working human heart and jump-start it with electricity[81]—it is not difficult to see where synthetic DNA and stem cells are heading.

> Once inside the cell, the "workers" take over. Some of these "workers" are [CRISPR] enzymes that cut human genes at specific sites, while others integrate—or load—the "cargo" into appropriate reading frames—like microscopic librarians. Once the payload is stored in the cell's nuclear "library stacks," the new genes can be translated, copied, and "read" to produce altered or brand-new "alien" polymers and proteins.
>
> The resulting hybrid cell is no longer purely human. If a hybridized skin cell, it may now glow, or perhaps form scales rather than hair, claws rather than fingernails. If a brain cell, the new genetic instructions could produce an altered neurotransmitter that reduces or even eliminates the body's need for sleep. Muscle cells may grow larger and more efficient at using low levels of calcium and oxygen. Retina cells may encode for receptors that enable the "posthuman being" to perceive infrared or ultraviolet light frequencies. The hybrid ears may now sense a wider range of sounds, taste buds a greater range of chemicals. Altered brains might even

---

79 Ibid.

80 Bradley J. Fikes, "Synthetic Genomics shows its prototype digital-to-biological converter in action." The San Diego Union-Tribune, May 30, 2017.

81 Alexandra Ossola, "Scientists Grow Full-Sized, Beating Human Hearts From Stem Cells." PopSci.com, March 16, 2016.

attune to metaphysics and "unseen" gateways, allowing communication with supernatural realms.[82]

Synthetic genome re-design means constructing genes from synthetic DNA. This is not just bioengineering; this is Frankensteinian biowarfare. The recent Wuhan debacle has driven this revelation home to those paying attention:

> . . . in 2005, scientists at the U.S. Centers for Disease Control and Prevention synthesized the so-called Spanish influenza virus which was responsible for the 1918-19 flu pandemic that killed between 50 million and 100 million people worldwide. In the near future, synthetic genomics technology should make it possible to recreate *any existing virus for which the complete DNA sequence is known* . . .[83] (Emphasis added.)

High throughput DNA synthesis machines make the cost of synthetic DNA mere pennies per base-pair. (The cost of DNA synthesis itself in 2005 was 20,000 base-pairs per dollar.)

Christian writer / researcher Anthony Patch predicted that 5G / 6G would activate dormant third-strand DNA nanobots with a quaternary signal.[84] The plan for synthetic "chemical evolution" forecasts multiple future strands of synthetic DNA for the "enhanced" Human 2.0.

Transgenic

Regarding the remote merging of human consciousness with the Internet via BCI, DARPA's direct neural interface (DNI) known as the *cortical modem* harnesses DNA and neurons to create an Internet "*Terminator*[85] vision" display in our brains via the visual cortex. Possibly through a DREADDS-induced chemo-optogenetic neural interface, the VR / AR (electronic telepathy / telekinesis) plays on the Internet hive mind "screen," whether in the individual brain or the plasma-mirrored sky. Bypassing the eyes operates much like microwave hearing bypassing the ears, the only catch being, according to DARPA at the Biology Is Technology conference in Silicon Valley in early

---

82 Thomas R. Horn and Nita F. Horn, Forbidden Gates: How Genetics, Robotics, Artificial Intelligence, Synthetic Biology, Nanotechnology, & Human Enhancement Herald the Dawn of Techno-Dimensional Spiritual Warfare (Defender, January 1, 2011).

83 Jonathan B. Tucker, Raymond A. Zilinskas, "The Promise and Perils of Synthetic Biology." The New Atlantis, Spring 2006.

84 See "Interview with Anthony Patch 1/14/2014 about Deadly Shots and Third Strand DNA." Flip Vandersky, March 29, 2019. As for the quaternary signal, see M.L.F. Abbade et al., "All optical generation of quaternary amplitude signals," IEEE, November 23, 2006.

85 The Terminator sci-fi film trilogy envisioned 3D liquid metals whose physical shape, appearance and functionality could be controlled digitally: Danielle De La Bastide, "Shape Shifting Liquid Metal Could Revolutionize Robotics," Interesting Engineering, April 21, 2021.

February 2015, that the DNA in the brain's neurons must first be altered.[86]

Transhumanism "enhancements" will inevitably depend upon making all of humanity *transgenic*—namely, into organisms containing genetic material into which DNA from unrelated organisms is artificially introduced, including *artificial memories* that bypass the senses:

> By pairing the electrical foot shock with optogenetic light stimulation of the acetophenone-sensitive olfactory nerves, the researchers taught the animals to associate [an electric shock with the scent of cherry blossoms]. When they later tested the mice, they avoided the cherry blossom odor.[87]

Shades of MK-ULTRA screen memories. Is this what torture and targeting are all about—of mice and men?

Recombinant *DNA technology = genetic engineering*

Synthetic biology follows from the discovery of the structure of DNA, deciphering the genetic code, development of recombinant DNA, and mapping the human genome. Engineering living machines and re-designing biological systems now seems as inevitable as the two trees in the Garden of Eden story of long ago.

> *And out of the ground made the LORD God to grow every tree that is pleasant to the sight, and good for food; the tree of life also in the midst of the garden, and the tree of knowledge of good and evil. – Genesis 2:9*

Of course, bioengineered microorganisms could have served Nature instead of bending the life sciences and engineering to weaponizing, destroying, usurping, and replacing. Imagine instead breaking down pollutants, eradicating ionized radiation, repairing defective genes, and destroying cancer cells. But DARPA, the DoD, and elite foundations do not serve humanity; they are bent on engineering a *golem* Transhumanist future under globalist bloodlines that for millennia have been dedicated to wresting the controls from Nature and the divine, just as John Milton (1608-1674) laid it out in *Paradise Lost:*

---

86 Anthony Cuthbertson, "DARPA Cortical Modem connects brain to computer for 'electronic telepathy and telekinesis,'" International Business Times, February 18, 2015; and Jonah Bennett, "DARPA's Cortical Modem Aims To Make The Blind See," The Daily Caller, February 17, 2015.

87 Robert Martone, "A Successful Artificial Memory Has Been Created." Scientific American, August 27, 2019.

The mind is its own place, and in itself
Can make a Heaven of Hell, a Hell of Heaven.[88]

Enzymes and amino acids are being synthesized as approaches to protein engineering. In fact, at every level of synthetic biology, nano-sized microbes are being gain-of-function engineered to perform complex tasks in the tiny world of microbiology and its replacement with their ersatz synthetic clones so that all of altered life can be patented and owned by the new kings of the world, the Egregor transnational corporations.

What will it mean when the synthetic has utterly replaced the natural? For example, programmed yeast cells manufacturing artemesinic acid so as to engineer a metabolic pathway for enzymes to produce a synthetic artemisinin. The natural version is so effective in treating malaria, but what will change with artificial artemisinin, which is much cheaper to manufacture, circumventing the extraction of the natural compound from the sweet wormwood plant that grows in China and Vietnam? Consider what it means just on a *frequency transmission* level that the synthetic genes must be re-turned for their "multi-enzyme pathway."[89] How will such synthetic recalibration be exploited, given human resonance and how the Smart Grid is continuously tweaked to work for Space Fence lockdown and Smart City lockstep?

Synthetic biology's engineering tool box of standardized genetic parts (transistors, capacitors, resisters, etc.) is growing in leaps and bounds as the human body is converted into a BCI-friendly cyborg unit / node plugged into the Smart City grid. The excellent 2019 book *The Demon in the Machine* by Paul Davies, PhD, reveals how biophysicists and bioengineers, freed at last from religious constraints, view the "wetworks" human body and all of Nature:

> Living cells, it turns out, contain a host of exquisite and well-honed nano-machines, made mostly from proteins. The list includes motors, pumps, tubes, shears, rotors, levers and ropes—the sort of paraphernalia familiar to engineers . . . Though life's nano-machines, on the face of it, obey the same laws of physics as familiar macroscopic machines, the environment in which they operate is starkly different . . . Every nano-machine is continually buffeted by the impact of high-speed water molecules, which make up much of the cell's mass. Conditions resemble those in a rowdy nightclub: crowded and noisy . . .[90]

---

88 John Milton, Paradise Lost, Book I, from lines 242-270.

89 Ibid.

90 Paul Davies, The Demon in the Machine: How hidden webs of information are solving the mystery of life. Penguin Books, 2019. It is in this book that you will experience how thoroughly the body is perceived as an organic machine.

The Registry of Standard Biological Parts (http://parts.mit.edu/) is made up of Lego-like BioBricks, short pieces of synthetic DNA that send and receive, initiating the transcription of DNA into synthetic messenger RNA (mRNA), providing a terminator sequence, a repressor gene, a ribosome-binding site, and a reporter gene. BioBricks convert bioengineered cells into nano programmable microcomputers so that cells can be directed by remote chemical and light signaling (optogenetics, chemogenetics).

The *synbio* market was $3.9 billion in 2016 and will reach $11.4 billion in 2021.[91] This industry constitutes an *inflection point*, a turning point, in industry, biology, *and society itself.* Petrochemicals are being replaced in manufacturing, and the "resource-intensive harvesting of commercial plants" is being circumvented by the same synthetic science transforming the medical industry. *Synthetic genomics* depends heavily upon nanotechnology which has next to no economic or technical regulatory restrictions and is only now and then gingerly referenced within the context of synthetic biology.

> Using a laptop computer, unpublished gene sequence information, and mail-order synthetic DNA, it is becoming routine to construct genes or entire genomes from scratch—including those of lethal pathogens.[92]

The ETC Group, watchdog over new technologies that impact socio-economic and ecological issues—people's lives and environment—describes synthetic biology as "extreme genetic engineering" for commercializing synthetic biological parts, devices, and living organisms. Behind synthetic biology from the beginning (post-9/11) were the J. Craig Venter Institute, MIT, the Center for Strategic & International Studies (CSIS), and the Alfred P. Sloan Foundation. Now, gene synthesis corporations are everywhere, like Celera Genomics, Synthetic Genomics, Craig Venter's Institute for Biological Energy Alternatives in Rockville, Maine, and of course nonprofits like iGEM (International Genetically Engineered Machine) and Center for Genetics and Society. In 2014, the National Institutes of Health (NIH) spent $4.5 billion on neuroscience alone.

With Big Pharma Egregor corporations posturing as the new king of the world, we must remember that appearances can be deceiving, as David E. Martin, PhD, reminds us as we enter the chapter about the 2019-2021 COVID-19 "vaccine" event:

---

91 Gigi Kwik Gronvall, "Synthetic Biology: Next Wave of Disruption for Industrialization of Biology." Brinknews.com, June 7, 2017.

92 "Syns of Omission: Civil Society Organizations Respond to Report on Synthetic Biology Governance from the J. Craig Venter Institute and Alfred P. Sloan Foundation," ETC Group, 17 October 2007.

The mRNA is a medical device packaged in a fat container designed to stimulate the human cell into becoming a pathogen creator. It is not a vaccine; the term "vaccine" is a sucker punch. Vaccines are legally defined under public health law CDC and FDA standards. A vaccine has to stimulate an immunity and disrupt transmission, and that is not what this is. The mRNA entering the cell is not to stop transmission.[93]

93 "Dr. David Martin Explains Covid Vaccines are not Vaccines but are Medical Devices," January 9, 2021.

14

Occult Assault III: The COVID-19 "Vaccine" Event

Patent power
The digital in *synbio*
5G Syndrome / 5G Flu
The subunit vaccine
Cometh the mRNA "vaccine"
DNA & RNA "vaccines"
PCR swab "test"
Proteins, enzymes, & prions
mRNA "vaccine" vulnerability: shelf life & lipid shells
(BioAPI) Hydrogel tissue engineering
(BioAPI) Graphene
Blood clots & lungs
The FunVax "God gene" VMAT2 (vesicular monoamine transporter 2)
"Repurposed" drugs / herbs
Hydroxychloroquine
Chlorine dioxide
Budesonide
Ivermectin
Wormwood (Azythromyan) / Artemisinin
Thyme extract
Pine needle tea / suramin
Lysine therapy
Pure fulvic isolate

China was long ago set to be the 5G showcase for the world. Major metro areas and technology hubs like Wuhan were selected to be official 5G Demonstration Zones. Only such a high concentration of 5G radio-frequency transmitters and microwave towers would permit a citywide build-out of the Internet of Things. 2019 was the year Wuhan, the capital of Hubei, was "expected to have 10,000 5G base stations by the end of 2019, said Song Qizhu, head of Hubei Provincial Communication Administration." Then the coronavirus hit, so the whole world was told. What really happened was that a new variant of the coronavirus was released in Wuhan after the 5G experimenters saw an epidemic of 5G Syndrome explode. The 5G guinea pigs were literally dropping like flies as soon as they flipped the 5G switch. The ERs and urgent care clinics were overwhelmed. The 5G scientists watching the burgeoning public health crisis immediately activated Plan B: Blame it on a virulent flu—a bioengineered coronavirus that produces symptoms similar to 5G Syndrome.

– Intelligence analyst and former U.S. Army officer

The global impact on the wide range of genotypes relative to human beings is difficult to assess, but the outcome is definitely negative, and permitting the seeding of latent proviruses in humans, knowingly, can have no other rationale than future medical profiteering and constitutes a criminal conspiracy of vast proportions which is tantamount to genocidal policy against the population, further constituting crimes against humanity, which is internationally punishable by death.

– "Vaccines, and Production of Negative Genetic Changes in Humans," *Leading Edge Research Group*, 1998.

The same day that Chinese scientists posted the first sequences of the novel coronavirus RNA genome online (Saturday, January 11, 2020), the first known coronavirus death occurred in Wuhan. Was it just coincidental that the old Julian calendar still employed by ancient elite dynastic families and secret societies read 11/11/2020?

Viral vector (adenoviral) vaccines (classical*)*: *must be grown in vivo [in a living body] because they introduce live virus antigens* to produce an immune response. Once inside the cells, the genetic material instructs the cells to make copies of unique proteins like the Spiked protein.*

Protein subunit vaccines: *injected pieces of proteins from a pathogen that the body does not recognize and so begins producing T-lymphocytes and antibodies. Require "immunopotentiating" adjuvants.*

Nucleic acid vaccines (1990s): *DNA vaccines and mRNA vaccines; speedy development "with almost limitless combinations of derivatives" (Nature); grown in vitro and programmed to produce antigens*, then injected into the body. Nucleic acid vaccines have never been licensed, due to problems of "stabilization" now believed to be surmountable because of "nonviral delivery systems [like electroporation] for RNA-based vaccines" that produce self-amplifying mRNA vaccines.1 Require "immunopotentiating" adjuvants.*

1 Luis A. Brito et al., "Self-amplifying mRNA vaccines." Advanced Genetics, December 4,

Synthetic vaccines: *virus-like (nano)particles (VLPs), enveloped VLPs (eVLPs); designed to mimic viruses, the claim being that a vaccination with a target protein expressed in an eVLP (like the COVID-19 Spiked protein that turns every cell into a virus-making machine) is capable of imparting greater immunity than a vaccine with the same recombinant target protein alone. eVLPs are nanoparticle vaccines. Require "immunopotentiating" adjuvants.*

Gene transfer (gene altering): *integration of exogenous DNA, causing mutagenesis and inducing new diseases; effects range from chronic, intrinsic inflammation autoimmune reactions due to the immune system being continuously stimulated to produce antibodies, to mutation of the genome*

Electroporation: DNA (nucleic acid) *synbio genes forcefully injected into cells by means of short high voltage pulses (8 pulses of 0.1ms at 1,000 V/cm voltage to electrode distance) for drug delivery, and long low voltage pulses for DNA transfer (e.g. 1 pulse of 0.1ms, 800 V/cm and 1 long pulse of 400ms 80 V/cm)"*[2]

**Antigens: toxins, bacteria, foreign blood cells, cells of transplanted organs, etc. Antigens stimulate production of antibodies and induce an immune response.*

The latest and biggest global media / psyop event known as the *COVID-19 pandemic*—the Big Pharma bonanza of human experimentation in the SARS (2003) - MERS (2012) lineage—was rushed into action following the Wuhan activation of its 5G system. Animal studies (beyond vague references to ZC45 and ZXC21 bats) were shoved aside, followed by rumors about COVID-19 being a weaponized synthetic version of coronavirus from a Chinese research lab. The Mockingbird media then inundated world news with fear porn. Thousands in worthless masks lined up for jabs within days, complicit corporate men like Joseph Payne, CEO of Arcturus Therapeutics, boasting, "There are billions of people that would like to access a vaccine. It is the greatest demand for a pharmaceutical product ever, way more demand than the iPhone . . ."[3]

How many vaccine batches are being tested on various global popula-

2014.

2 See Sonke Schmidt et al., "Microwave Induced Electroporation of Adherent Mammalian Cells at 18 GHz." IEEE, June 2019. Electroporation followed the U.S. Army's "gene gun" (helium gas) that "blasts DNA into cells": Katie Drummond, "Army's Vaccine Plan: Inject Troops With Gas-Propelled, Electro-Charged DNA," Wired, September 3, 2010.

3 Ryan Cross, "Will the coronavirus help mRNA and DNA vaccines prove their worth?" c&en, April 3, 2020.

tions, and what diseases are piggybacking the jabs for various geomagnetic areas, awaiting activation by 5G?

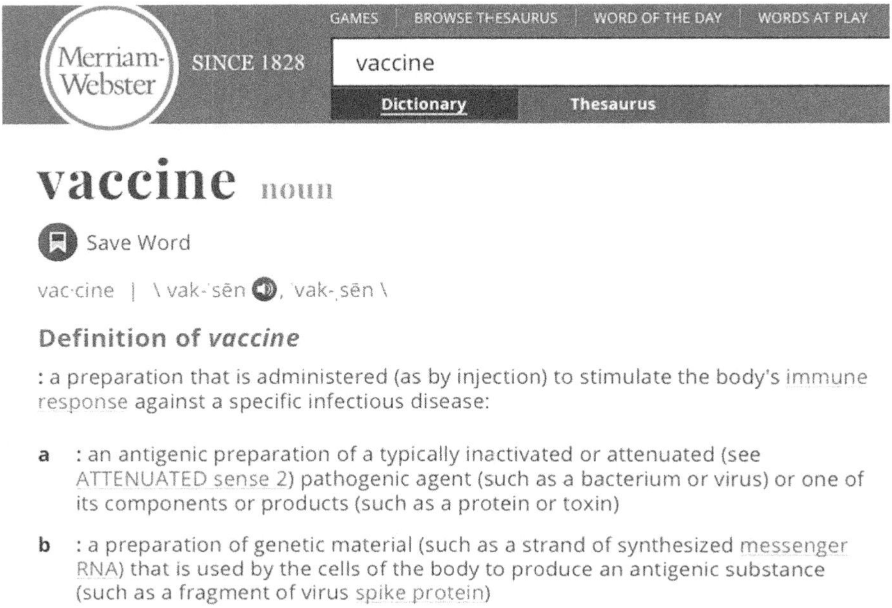
GAMES | BROWSE THESAURUS | WORD OF THE DAY | WORDS AT PLAY

Merriam-Webster SINCE 1828

vaccine

Dictionary Thesaurus

vaccine noun

Save Word

vac·cine | \ vak-ˈsēn , ˈvak-ˌsēn \

Definition of *vaccine*

: a preparation that is administered (as by injection) to stimulate the body's immune response against a specific infectious disease:

a : an antigenic preparation of a typically inactivated or attenuated (see ATTENUATED sense 2) pathogenic agent (such as a bacterium or virus) or one of its components or products (such as a protein or toxin)

b : a preparation of genetic material (such as a strand of synthesized messenger RNA) that is used by the cells of the body to produce an antigenic substance (such as a fragment of virus spike protein)

Definition of vaccine. After thousands of doctors insisted the mRNA jab / shot for COVID-19 was not a "vaccination" but "gene therapy," Mirriam-Webster changed its definition of *vaccine*.

https://www.mirriam-webster.com/dictionary/vaccine

Patent power

The CDC's U.S. Patent #7220852B1 (May 22, 2007) and U.S. Patent #7776521B1 (August 17, 2010) "Coronavirus isolated from humans" are about the "newly isolated human corona virus (SARS-CoV)," with claims 3 and 4 granting the CDC exclusive control over SARS-CoV, namely the *statutory market exclusion right to research, commercially exploit, or block all competition*—in one fell swoop, multiple crimes against the U.S. Constitution (Article One, Section 8), the Sherman Act 15 U.S. Code 1 and the Clayton Act 15 U.S. Code 2 and 15 U.S. Code 19. David E. Martin, PhD, the go-to guy for all things patents, makes it clear that this "pandemic" did not arise from nowhere but was carefully prepared for:

> From April 2003 until September 2018, the CDC owned SARS-CoV, its ability to be detected, and the ability to manufacture kits for its assessment. During this 15-year period, the effect of the grant of this right—

ruled unconstitutional in 2013 by the United States Supreme Court in the case of *Association for Molecular Pathology et al. v. Myriad Genetics*—meant that the commercial exploitation of any research or commercial activity in the United States involving SARS-CoV would constitute an infringement of CDC's illegal patent.[4]

As I've written and said dozens of times now, the virological meaning of the word isolate *is quite different from the ordinary meaning. In the technical world of the con and the hustle, "isolated virus" means: "We have the virus in a soup in a dish in the lab. The soup contains human and monkey cells, toxic drugs and chemicals, and other genetic material. Some of the cells are dying. This means the virus is killing them."*

That assertion is false. The drugs and chemicals can be killing the cells, and the cells are being starved of vital nutrients. That alone could explain the cell-death. Furthermore, a supposed virus mixed in a soup in a dish in a lab is definitely not "isolated." Bottom line: there is no persuasive evidence that a virus is in the soup.

– Jon Rappoport, "COVID vaccine secret, a stunner," January 15, 2021

According to Dr. Martin, no less than 4,000 SARS-corona patents followed the original *SARS (severe acute respiratory syndrome)* U.S. patent #7279327 (April 19, 2002), describing an "infectious transmission-defective virus" that targets lungs. This was just one year before the SARS "bird flu" was released in China's southern Guangdong province as China's domestic national product (DNP) hit 7.6 percent. Like mad cow disease "jumping" to the human disease form of mad cow disease called variant Creutzfeldt-Jakob disease (vCJD), the "bird flu" virus "jumped" from birds to humans. Russian epidemiologist Nikolai Filatov and Academy of Medicine member Sergei Kolesnikov claim that the SARS virus is basically a manmade cocktail of measles and mumps, weaponized by genetically fusing a measles-mumps pathogen.[5] According to the Far Eastern Economic Review, the cost to mainland China of the 2003 SARS outbreak was $2.2 billion (Hong Kong $1.7 billion). Bio-economic warfare.

---

4 Notes by David E. Martin, PhD, for his David Martin World YouTube "Butterfly of the Week, 27 April 2020: Under House Arrest as a Result of a Crime Committed by the CDC," April 28, 2020. (Notes at http://www.davidmartin.world.) More about patents in the "Dr David Martin / Dr Reiner Fuellmich – July 9, 2021" interview.

5 "Sars biological weapon?" News24.com, November 4, 2003.

By 2008, the avian influenza had made its way to Indonesia. Indonesian Health Minister Siti Fadilah Supari, MD, revealed that World Health Organization (WHO) labs were forwarding influenza viruses to Western Big Pharma corporations so they could profit from selling vaccines back to developing nations. Seed viruses were even being ferreted to U.S. Department of Defense (DoD) labs.[6] In 2008, the surveillance tool Google Flu Trends sprang into being to track flus and notify the CDC in real time.

The patenting of life is illegal, but with the addition of a "gain of function," the law can be circumvented. Canadian Judge Marc Nadon ruled in 1995 that Harvard University could not patent the "oncomouse," but could patent the *process* by which the mouse was genetically altered. As Judge Nadon put it, "They have created a method to inject eggs with a myc gene,[7] but they have not invented the mouse . . .

> On even the broadest interpretation, I cannot find that a mouse is "raw material" which is given new qualities from an inventor. Certainly, the presence of the myc gene is new, but the mouse is not new nor is it a "raw material" in the ordinary sense of that phrase . . . the appellant has not made any claims to even minor control over any aspect of the mammal except the presence of the transgene . . . The appellant can make no claim to being able to reproduce the mammal at will by doing anything other than ordinary breeding. In my view this is insufficient . . . A complex life form does not fit within the current parameters of the *Patent Act* without stretching the meaning of the words to the breaking point, which I am not prepared to do. However, if Parliament so wishes, it clearly can alter legislation so that mammals can be patented.[8]

The oncomouse embodying the transgene is no longer Nature's mouse and is therefore, proprietarily speaking, owned by its patent holder. Yoshiro Kawaoka (University of Wisconsin at Madison)—funded by the National Institutes of Health (NIH) Office of Biotechnology Activities—similarly weaponized the Ebola genome and re-created the 1918 influenza by adding two genes to the modern flu virus and applying *reverse genetics* via digital synthetic recombinant DNA technology.

The ubiquitous *National Institutes of Health (NIH)* owns half of the key

---

6 Mark Forbes, "Indonesia accuses US of bird flu plot." Herald, February 20, 2008.

7 Myc is a family of regulator genes and proto-oncogenes that code for transcription, the process by which a strand of DNA is copied into mRNA.

8 "Harvard Oncomouse (and All Mammals) Still Not Patentable in Canada," etcGroup, April 29, 1998. Source: Federal Court of Canada Docket T-275-96; President and Fellows of Harvard College and Commissioner of Patents, Judgment.

patent for Moderna's COVID vaccine, which, according to Dr. Martin, is *not* a piece of SARS-corona virus but a "computer-simulated synthetic chimeric code" uploaded by the Chinese in January 2020, then passed to Moderna to put into an injection to make cells produce the synthetic S-1 Spike protein, *a weaponized pathogen stimulant that cannot be reversed.*[9] Of extreme concern is the report of an autopsy performed in Germany of a man who died after receiving the "gene therapy": *every single organ in the man's body was infected with Spike proteins.*[10] COVID gene therapy turns the entire body into a Spike protein factory.

As Lee Merritt, MD, pithily put it, "The coronavirus is the transmission device, the spike protein the warhead."

Francis Boyle, the University of Illinois professor of international law who drafted the Biological Weapons Anti-Terrorism Act of 1989, maintains that President George W. Bush sabotaged the BWC [Biological Weapons Convention] Verification Protocol and turned the NIH into a biowarfare "front organization" that President Barack Obama then continued, exporting finished products to Third World nations, and that 13,000 "death scientists" labor at labs around the world, many in universities desperate for military grant monies and subject to fraudulent Institutional Review Boards. Boyle: "Money talks. Ethics walks."[11] Under the *covert* NIH Institutional Biosafety Committees (IBCs), 400 government-funded bioweapons labs do as they please (including DARPA).

Questionable security measures plague all of the biowarfare labs (under the NIH), from poor record-keeping and patient safety violations in clinical trials (under the FDA) to lab accidents, missing shipments, contaminated waste leaks, dropped containers, and defective seals: over 100 in 44 American labs handling the deadliest pathogens in 24 states (2003-2007).[12] Are these "accidents" and releases of clandestine experiments intentional? Failure to report these events to the CDC / NIH is common, lending fuel to the fire of intentional releases and missing shipments going to illicit underground, "nonexistent" labs—and don't forget "mysterious" occurrences of one-off pathogens like necrotizing fasciitis ("flesh-eating bacteria").

---

9 "Exposing Mass Murder," a Stew Peters interview with Dr. Martin, July 23, 2021.

10 Captaindaretofly, "First Autopsy of Dead Person Vaccinated for Covid Found to Contain Spike Proteins in Every Organ of Body." The Daily Expose, August 4, 2021. See Torsten Hansen et al., "First case of postmortem study in a patient vaccinated against SARS-CoV2." International Journal of Infectious Diseases, June 2021.

11 Sherwood Ross, "National Institutes of Health Has Given Priority to Bioweapons Research." AfterDowningStreet.org, May 1, 2010.

12 "Patient safety violations and poor record keeping common in clinical trial concerns." Medical Express, June 25, 2014; also Larry Margasak, "U.S. labs mishandling deadly germs," AP, October 3, 2007.

Under the Biodefense and Pandemic Vaccine and Drug Development Act of 2005 (S.1873) and Operation Warp Speed, the NIH sister agency *BARDA (Biomedical Advanced Research and Development Authority)* has shelled out *billions* in contracts for COVID-19 drugs and vaccines.[13] BARDA is not subject to FOIAs, nor can its director or the Secretary of Human and Health Services (HHS) be subjected to judicial review, thanks to its *sensitive but unclassified (SBU)* classification. This is suspicious, as even the CIA and DoD cannot hide under a SBU classification. BARDA is accountable to no one.

- All challenges to decisions made by the Director of BARDA or Secretary of the Department of Health and Human Services (HHS) are prohibited;
- BARDA can sign exclusive contracts with Big Pharma corporations, including issuing grants and rebates for vaccine production;
- BARDA can provide liability protection to Big Pharma corporations for drugs not approved by the Food and Drug Administration (FDA).[14]

Coupled with BARDA is the Model Emergency Health Powers Act that allows governors to declare an emergency, force vaccinations, quarantine people, seize property and require people to "provide services" during an emergency, etc.[15] Adenoviral vector vaccine producer Johnson & Johnson is under the aegis of BARDA.

Then there are the "vaccine" pushers like the Coalition for Epidemic Preparedness Innovations (CEPI) that approved DARPA-backed Moderna and Inovio for COVID-19 mRNA "vaccine" development. DARPA funds Inovio SynCon ("DNA nanotechnology") to develop *synbio* antibodies that turn human bodies into *bio-reactors* while Rapidly Adaptable Nanotherapeutics at DARPA constructs *small interfering RNA (siRNA)* nanobots to target and shut down genes so they can be remotely reprogrammed and repurposed.

The highly secret public-private COVID-19 *Operation Warp Speed* program dominated by the U.S. military and U.S. intelligence[16] awarded $6 bil-

---

13 Kyle Blankenship, "Emergent BioSolutions, BARDA reach $628M deal to manufacture COVID-19 vaccine hopefuls." FiercePharma, June 1, 2020. Operation Warp Speed is a public-private partnership to accelerate production and distribution of the COVID-19 "gene therapy" jab.

14 "A New Ultra-Secret Government Agency." OMB Watch, November 29, 2005.

15 "By December 21, 2001, the act was released to state legislatures for review and approval. Critics immediately charged that the MSEHPA failed to protect the general public from abuses arising from the tremendous powers it would grant individual states in an emergency. The MSEHPA provisions also went beyond the scope of addressing bioterrorism while disregarding medical privacy standards.[1] As of August 1, 2011, forty states have passed various forms of MSEHPA legislation." - Wikipedia

16 During the 2019-2020 Big Pharma takeover, the U.S. government—including military and intelligence—was fractured and not unilateral under President Trump. Warp Speed was insti-

lion contracts to vaccine corporations via the nonprofit Advanced Technology International, a well-known CIA cutout with deep ties to Homeland Security (DHS) and the Department of Defense (DoD). *The Trump administration compared Warp Speed to the Manhattan Project.*

At least one of the Wuhan labs impugned in mainstream media is owned by GlaxoSmithKline that owns Pfizer. GlaxoSmithKline is managed by BlackRock global investment (see Appendix 15, "Movers and Shakers") which manages the (George Soros) Open Society Foundation that serves the French Axa investment managers and owns the Swiss Winterthur Group ("the largest life and nonlife insurance company in Switzerland"). Winterthur built the Wuhan lab and was bought by the German Allianz financial services whose American shareholder the Vanguard Group is also a shareholder of BlackRock, which is a major shareholder of Microsoft whose founder Bill Gates is a shareholder of Pfizer.[17]

This is "The Lab That Jack Built."

Thus, it should not be surprising that the U.S.-based Pfizer is holding governments like Argentina and Brazil hostage, even to demanding their sovereign assets (bank reserves, military bases, embassy buildings) as collateral guarantee that Pfizer remain above the law of the land and exempt from all civil liability.[18]

Simultaneously, the WHO announced the first global "no-fault" vaccine injury compensation program for those suffering "rare but serious adverse events" associated with COVID-19 "vaccines" distributed through COVAS (COVID-19 Vaccines Global Access) under GAVI, WHO, CEPI, the UN, etc. Only developing nations are eligible. A global consumer tax will pay for it.[19]

The dynamic duo one-two jab backed by the UK has been Anglo-Swedish AstraZeneca and BioNTech / Pfizer. Oxford-AstraZeneca is tied to the British Eugenics Society (now renamed the Galton Institute[20]) and Wellcome Trust's Center for Human Genomics[21] and was developed by the Jenner Institute and Oxford Vaccine Group. Early on, the Oxford-AstraZeneca had one neurological "side effect" after another during "vaccine trials" and therefore was slated to be "the vaccine of choice for the developing world, as it is cheaper and has much less complicated storage requirements than its main competitors, Pfizer and Moderna."[22]

---

gated and pushed by certain elements, foreign and domestic, and resisted by others.

17 Thanks to Brian Ellis, Facebook, for working all of this out.

18 "Pfizer Demanding Bank Reserves, Military Bases and Embassy Buildings As Collateral For COVID-19 Vaccines," GreatGameIndia, February 25, 2021.

19 Wayne Rohde, "What Could Go Wrong? WHO Launches Global 'No-Fault' COVID Vaccine Injury Compensation Program." Children's Health Defense, February 25, 2021.

20 Francis Galton (1822-1911) is considered the father of eugenics.

21 Wellcome Trust's founder was Big Pharma magnate Henry Wellcome (1853-1936), who also founded GlaxoKlineSmith.

22 Jeremy Loffredo and Whitney Webb, "Developers of Oxford-AstraZeneca Vaccine Tied to

Pfizer "vaccines" began with countless reports of anaphylaxis just minutes after the insertion of mRNA BNT16262, followed by symptoms ranging from tightness in the chest and throat, coughing, wheezing, swelling of the lips, and hives (Morgellons outbreaks?) to hypotension (low blood pressure), shock, spasms, and death.[23] Merck withdrew from the mRNA race and began producing oral drugs MK-7110 and MK-4482 "to protect patients from the damage of an overactive immune response to the virus"—in other words, to "help" people whose bodies (including their subtle bodies and immune systems) were resisting with all their might the Big Pharma assault.[24]

Obviously, Big Pharma corporations are competing with each other for a place at the oak table of global profits, but it is also obvious that they are abetting members of their all-powerful eugenics-oriented cartel / cabal who are jockeying for position in the biggest drug deal ever. Does the famous "Secret Covenant" hearken from the cartel?

> . . . We will use science and technology in subtle ways so [the public] will never see what is happening. We will use soft metals, aging accelerators, and sedatives in food and water, also in the air. They will be blanketed by poisons everywhere they turn. The soft metals will cause them to lose their minds. We will promise to find a cure from many of our fronts . . .[25]

Tellingly, as the vaccine was announced in November 2020, Michael Yeadon, PhD,[26] former Pfizer vice president and chief scientific officer who roundly criticized the UK's Scientific Adviser Group for Emergencies (SAGE) for its lockdown policies, wrote:

> There is absolutely no need for vaccines to extinguish the pandemic. I've never heard such nonsense talked about vaccines. You do not vaccinate people who aren't at risk from a disease. You also don't set about planning

---

UK Eugenics Movement." Unlimitedhangout.com, December 26, 2020.

23 "Patient in Georgia, Health Worker in New York Suffer Anaphylaxis After Getting Pfizer / BioNTech COVID-19 Vaccine," The Vaccine Reaction, December 28, 2020.

24 Steve Watson, "Merck Scraps COVID Vaccines, Says It's More Effective To Get The Virus and Recover." Summit News, 26 January 2021.

25 Jamie Lee aplanetruth8, "The Secret Covenant They Must Never Know," January 28, 2021. No doubt purposely leaked, as was the famous Report from Iron Mountain: On the Possibility and Desirability of Peace by Leonard C. Lewin (Dial Press, 1967).

26 "At Pfizer, Dr Yeadon was responsible for target selection and the progress into humans of new molecules, leading teams of up to 200 staff across all disciplines and won an Achievement Award for productivity in 2008. Under his leadership, the unit invented oral and inhaled NCEs [new chemical entities] which delivered positive clinical proofs of concept in asthma, allergic rhinitis and COPD [chronic obstructive pulmonary disease]." - https://www.crunchbase.com/person/michael-yeadon

to vaccinate millions of fit and healthy people with a vaccine that hasn't been extensively tested on human subjects.[27]

Dr. Yeadon spent over 30 years doing research at the world's largest pharmaceutical corporations. He is not the only professional to speak out against the vaccine profit mongers bent on taking advantage of media-driven public fear in order to run *synbio* Transhumanist experiments for gain-of-function patents and prestige at others' expense. No liability, no test subject expense, no labyrinthine voluntary consent procedures—much easier, really, to have friends at Food and Drug, CDC, EPA, Commerce, the patent Office, and the FBI. Thousands of thoughtful doctors who took the Hippocratic oath to do no harm and meant it are slowly awakening to the fact that the medical cartel in bed with Big Pharma and Big Tech is dedicated to keeping people sick for profits, power, and *in vivo* open field experimentation, not healing.[28]

The digital in synbio

Throughout the year of required masked six-foot "social distancing," Starlink 5G launches via Falcon 9's occurred at least once a month, each launch with a payload of 60-plus satellites. In March 2020, the FCC approved the need for *one million* small ground antennas (19" in diameter added to existing 4G structures) to correlate with a SpaceX Starlink high-speed Internet network of 12,000 satellites.[29] As of November 25, 2020, SpaceX had launched 955 Starlink satellites. Other launches included but were not limited to:

- U.S. Space Force and Space Development Agency: Blackjack constellation of low-orbit satellites integrated by Lockheed Martin's *orbital mesh network in space* run by the AI called the Pit Boss.[30]
- U.S. Navy: 30-centimeter PRAM satellites (photovoltaic RF antenna modules) to convert solar energy into microwaves for power transmission while collecting data on power density.[31]

The COVID-19 lockdown provided the opportunity to stitch up the last holes in the 5G / 6G Space Fence lockdown. Meanwhile, national labs like Sandia and Argonne have been allocating their considerable resources to sup-

---

27 Patrick Delaney, "Former Pfizer VP: 'No need for vaccines,' 'the pandemic is effectively over.'" LifeSite, November 23, 2020.

28 Many awakening doctors!

29 Joe Dyton, "FCC passes 5G Upgrade Order." Connected, June 11, 2020.

30 Dan Robitzski, "DARPA is about to launch a military version of SpaceX's Starlink." Futurism.com, May 12, 2020.

31 Andy Tomaswick, "The Navy is Testing Beaming Solar Power in Space." Universe Today, June 19, 2020.

port the COVID-19 High Performance Computing Consortium by granting free computer time to researchers cooking up SARS-CoV-2 with yeast and *synbio* genome instructions ordered online. By "democratizing" access to high-performance computers and software, certified labs are able to control the vast flows of data being funneled to their hungry machine-learning AI while searching for more ways to make digital viral transmissions and releases more exact and comprehensive.

The 5G event in Wuhan was the global nuncio regarding the forced marriage between brain-computer interface (BCI) and synthetic biology (*synbio*). Biological systems are now being designed just as engineers design electromechanical systems but with synthetic cells (nanomaterials) and synthetic gene networks—from genetic toggle switches that change color, shape, density, etc., to the viral Spike protein, which, when in contact with protein molecules of the host cell, creates an electrostatic discharge (ESD) that includes a *corona discharge* that produces ozone (O3). (Even low concentrations of ozone are harmful to the upper respiratory tract, lungs, and heart.)[32]

Corona ions, corona discharge.

Ions given off by high voltage systems interact with oxygen molecules in such a way that they cause the electrons to spin and thus prevent the hemoglobin in our blood from uptaking the oxygen. And that people with this virus are simply collapsing in the street with no other flu-type symptoms and dying where they fall or in less severe cases showing severe breathing issues! And these ions given off by these electromagnetic systems are called corona ions!!!

– Paul Stephen Cox, March 8, 2020

Digital biology uses supercomputers, CAD programs (computer-aided design), CGAT binary code (cytosine, guanine, adenine, thymine), and digital DNA instructions to reproduce disease and remotely transfer the "granularity of data" (digital information written into DNA) that includes "outsourcing" memories held by DNA photons first from our brain to the Cloud, then from the Cloud to another brain. (In a hive mind, if an algorithm moves memories from one brain to another, whose memories are they?)

Digitized flu genomes can now be electronically transmitted from one loca-

32 Awaad K. Al Sarkhi, "Hypothesis: The electrical properties of coronavirus." Taylor & Francis Online, 1 June 2020.

tion and reconstituted as viruses somewhere else by DNA projecting a holographic blueprint that is electrodynamically transformed into molecules.[33] Biotechnologist Craig Venter's[34] BioXP 3200 digital-to-biological converter manufactures DNA templates for flu vaccines and mRNA "instruction" vaccines.

Was it inevitable that wired transmission information systems would be transformed into wireless, and analog would be transformed into digital, and that it all would lead to a biophysics and bioengineering of *the subatomic realm of quantum physics and probability*—thought and DNA being of a non-material nature—eventually ending in a Transhumanist future[35]?

In the booming business of EM targeting of individuals, DNA sequencing information is highly sought after. Former Security Industries System (SIS) employee-turned-whistleblower Bryan Kofron reveals that a DNA profile is set up so as to determine the exact resonant frequency of the target's DNA, which is then used to calibrate the directed energy weapon used against him or her—for example, a microwave auditory V2K weapon. The target's thoughts are decoded into ionic to be read by computer, then back into words for the human targeter to read. Digital information moves through a microtubule like biophotons of light; access the network and the person becomes an extension of the Internet of Living Things (IoLT)—like Rosetta Brain:

> We propose a neural connectomics strategy called Fluorescent In-Situ Sequencing of Barcoded Individual Neuronal Connections (FISSEQ-BOINC), leveraging fluorescent in situ nucleic acid sequencing in fixed tissue (FISSEQ). FISSEQ-BOINC exhibits different properties from BOINC, which relies on bulk nucleic acid sequencing. FISSEQ-BOINC could become a scalable approach for mapping whole-mammalian-brain connectomes with rich molecular annotations.[36]

---

33 Bradley J. Fikes, "Synthetic Genomics shows its prototype digital-to-biological converter in action." San Diego Union-Tribune, May 30, 2017.

34 In 2010, Venter created life in a cell and programmed it to be controlled by a synthetic genome. He calls synthetic biology the equivalent of the development of nuclear weapons.

35 See the 2016 Interview of Anthony Patch by Paul McGuire regarding the Beast System: "The mark can be delivered via a VCCN! 2016 Anthony Patch interview!" Patch's Entangled magazine is available by subscription, e.g. Vol. 46 (March 2021), "Synthetic Biocomputing & Smart Vaccines"; Vol. 45 (Feb. 2021), "Genetically Marked: Our Human Genome in the Hands of Men"; Vol. 44 (Jan. 2021), "COVID-19 and the Autonomic Nervous System"; and Vol. 43 (Dec. 2020), "COVID-19 Retrovirus" (regarding COVID-19's relationship with HIV-1).

36 Adam Marblestone, "Rosetta Brains: A Strategy for Molecularly Annotated Connectomics." Cornell University, 21 April 2014. A connectome is a comprehensive map of neural connections in the brain.

In plain English, Rosetta Brain is about getting a bead on your DNA and remotely controlling your mind.

The mandatory shot or jab the Chinese were subjected to in the fall of 2019 contained replicating, *digitized* RNA for activation by the 5G frequency of 60 GHz (known among the "vaccine"-savvy as "the V wave"). With smart / neural dust already present in bodies and brains from chemical trails, GMO foods, and decades of vaccines, the digital factor becomes the greatest peril to come out of the COVID-19 bioterrorist event, given that gain-of-function virus, endosomes, prions / proteins, and graphene hydrogel are in the mRNA digital software packet that can be activated at any time and any distance as *[Certificate Of Vaccination ID] COVID-20, COVID-21, etc.* Remote control via nanobots and "the V wave" spell big profits for Big Pharma and Big Medicine as well as the global restart being forced by the eugenically minded.

ID2020 Alliance is a non-governmental organization (NGO) described as a digital identity program utilizing immunization as a way to embed tiny microchips with a blockchain-enabled digital identity platform ("MyPass"). ID2020 works with GAVI (Global Alliance for Vaccines and Immunizations), a public-private partnership next door to the WHO in Geneva. GAVI has concentrated on immunizing the 1.1 billion people of developing nations and is now moving on to the rest of us.

On 29 January 2021, the German *Bundestag* ratified Agenda ID2020, despite the science put forward by the extra-governmental Corona Commission (hundreds of doctors, virologists, immunologists, professors, and lawyers, including cofounder Dr. Reiner Fuellmich who is now spearheading a massive "Nuremberg 2" lawsuit) that will cover nanoparticles accessible to 5G and 6G, such as epsilon iron oxide (iron and silicon) with outstanding magnetic properties, perfect for 6G and terahertz technology like the Internet of Things (IoT), ultra-fast communications, narrowly focused scientific devices and medical technology—precisely what was foreseen in the design of ID2020.[37]

For developed nations, MyPass is CommonPass, an iPhone app that tracks and traces our movements and uploads medical data like COVID-19 test results, proof of vaccinations, cryptocurrency status,[38] etc., to generate a QR code so we can travel, attend events, work, vote, have children, etc. CommonPass partners with the World Economic Forum. Eventually, of course, the app will be subcutaneous, like the "graphenation" and tattoo-style "Mark of the Beast" vaccination via microneedle—Bill Gates' Human

37 Peter Koenig, "Implanted 'Vaccine Package' ID: Germany's Parliament Has Ratified GAVI's Digital Agenda ID2020." Global Research, February 3, 2021; "Scientists obtain magnetic nanopowder for 6G technology," Phys.org, June 28, 2021.

38 Microsoft patent WO/2020/060606, "Cryptocurrency system using body activity data."

Implantable Quantum Dot Microneedle Vaccination Delivery system[39]—replete with the bioluminescence enzyme *luciferase*[40] and nano quantum dots visible to those with code readers, electron microscopes, a smart phone NIR (near-infrared) app,[41] and/or satellite NIR optics. Six feet for satellite "social distancing," given that we are breathing in *opsins* (optic fibers) among all the polymer nano-fibers encasing Morgellons CDBs, along with other pathogens.

Artificial photosynthesis by nano-biohybrid systems for Human 2.0 will depend upon inorganic nanoscale semiconductors like quantum dots and the catalytic power of NIR and biological cells to harvest light together. Quantum dots absorb light better than plants. When light hits a cadmium sulfide (CdS) "shell" of quantum dots, for example, electrons absorb it, get excited, and initiate biochemical reactions (with enzymes) to produce acetic acid,[42] thus pointing to the polyvinyl alcohol used in production of both CDBs and hydrogel.

Connected to the Cloud, the "on-patient" medical record tattoo will hold vaccination records, Immunity Passport, ID2020 Certification Mark coupled with the Microsoft patent WO/2020/060606, "Cryptocurrency system using body activity data," granted international status on April 22, 2020 (Julian calendar 02/22/2020).[43]

5G Syndrome / 5G Flu

Was the Wuhan coronavirus actually a flu *environmentally triggered* by 5G, like the COVID-19 "reinfection rates" due to patients returning to their 5G or 4G Plus wireless environments? Continuing a 5G / 4G Plus wireless lifestyle is a way of *consenting* to endless cyclic *in vivo* experiments with bioengineered flu strains and other weaponized pathogens triggered and sustained by 5G / 60 GHz. The Epstein-Barr virus is known for its decades of latency; in a similar way, "reinfection" may mean that the mRNA "vaccine" is implanting bioweapon mutations that will lie dormant in the body until their frequency is raised by 5G in the name of a "variant."

Whether in Wuhan or a high-tech Smart City hospital, 5G is a primary player in the COVID-19 psyop.

---

39 Microneedle transfection alters the genome and turns people into genetically modified organisms (GMOs).

40 Luciferin and luciferase were named by French pharmacologist Raphael Dubois in the late 19th century after he extracted oxidative enzymes from fireflies, jellyfish, and fungi generating bioluminescent light.

41 Celeste McGovern, "Bill Gates and Intellectual Ventures funds Microchip Implant Vaccine." Greenmedinfo.com, April 14, 2020.

42 Tian Qiu, "Bacteria in the Shell: A Nano-bio Hybrid for Solar Energy Capture," Sustainable Nano blog, Center for Sustainable Nanotechnology, July 27, 2016.

43 Thanks to David Masem. See Noel Joshua Hadley's "Luciferase: Quantum Dot Tattoo & the Seething Energies of the Light-Bearer." Ourwayisthehighway.wordpress.com, May 4, 2020.

In a natural non-5G-stimulated cycle of illness, the protein defenders *mannose binding lectins (MBLs)* would activate antibodies to break down the signature glycoprotein shell surrounding coronavirus exosomes in Ebola, SARS, MERS, etc., and *mast cells* would signal for white blood cells and produce histamine to activate other mast cells for defense. But in 5G overstimulation, respiratory challenges arise, the lungs primed by the heavy metal nanoparticle load breathed in daily from aerosol dumps, plus the "flu-like" symptoms of 5G itself.[44] Cells go into overdrive and are swept up in inflammatory *cytokine storms* that affect the lungs, skin, and blood. In fact, *mast cell activation syndrome* (blood clotting, skin rash, lung failure, high blood pressure, heartburn) looks a lot like COVID-19 symptoms.[45]

Limited licensed microwave frequencies lay claim to the 900 MHz to 40 GHz bandwidth, and satellite frequencies to 6 to 30 GHz. The new era of *unlicensed* 5G mmWave (57.05-64 GHz) run in Europe by Telecom Infra Project (TIP) and chaired by Facebook and Deutsche Telekom (Facebook *terragraf.net* uses the *802.11 ay* standard) requires FCC Part 15 certification. The fact is that 60 GHz mmWave networks[46] are all about combining narrow beam transmission with oxygen absorption to reduce communications interference, enhance security, and minimize unauthorized intercept. 60 GHz absorption is particularly high if the atmosphere is dry.[47]

> A 60 GHz communications system [with 98 percent of the transmitted energy absorbed by atmospheric oxygen] must overcome the effects of oxygen absorption, 16dB/KM. In order to operate reliably at even short ranges, a very focused, narrow-beam antenna [phased array] must also be employed to increase the level of signal available to the target receiver. This combination of oxygen absorption and narrow beam transmission enhances the security of the 60 GHz radio link, minimizing the probability of unauthorized intercept.[48]

Unfortunately, while 60 GHz is good for communications (oscillating at 60 *billion* cycles per second), it is bad for biology and the biosphere, which

---

44 Lance D. Johnson, "Did the 5G rollout in Wuhan damage the innate cellular defense cells of the population, putting the people at risk of complications and death from coronavirus?" Science.news, February 26, 2020.

45 Ryan Stephens, "Could the Mystery of Severe COVID-19 Be Solved by Mast Cell Activation Syndrome?" ResearchHub.com, May 28, 2020.

46 Anders Storm, "2019 was the breakthrough year in Europe for 60 GHz unlicensed 5G," siversima.com, n.d.

47 Keeping the atmosphere dry for incoming and outgoing international communications is often why, a few days before a conference or targeted weather event, a chemical soup of hygroscopic chemicals is delivered above the host target.

48 Shigeaki Hakusui, President, Harmonix Corporation, "Fixed Wireless Communications at 60 GHz Unique Oxygen Absorption Properties." RF GlobalNet, April 10, 2001.

of course doesn't matter to the IEEE (Institute of Electrical and Electronics Engineers) and its new WiFi standard (*802.11 ad*).[49] When a 60 GHz beam hits oxygen molecules, it causes electrons to spin faster, shifts their orbit, and hinders oxygen from binding with the blood's hemoglobin.

The dry electromagnetic fields inhibiting the ability of our blood to carry oxygen has been caused for decades by conductive nanometal chemicals jettisoned daily by jets and rockets and now include radiation from the beams of increasing numbers of 5G satellites overhead. When the chemical trails are zapped by lasers to produce low atmospheric pressure for weather engineering, oxygen is literally sucked out of the atmosphere. Ann Fillmore, PhD, author of the excellent essay about the lithium aerosol dosing of Oregon coastal towns,[50] wrote in February 2020 about how for six months she'd been observing "seriously low air pressure" pockets over Oregon. People complained of food needing longer cooking times, headaches, dizziness, cold / flu symptoms, nausea, confusion, forgetfulness, vision and hearing problems. Strokes and heart attacks were on the increase. In short, the symptoms spanned those of hypoxia or acute mountain (altitude) sickness (AMS), pulmonary edema (HAPE) and brain edema (HACE).

Low atmospheric pressure = less oxygen.

Besides low pressure, Fillmore added "walls of positive ion blasts coming not only before a storm but along with the intense use of dry air over drought areas."[51] Having studied what happened to people during the lithium assaults, Fillmore was fully aware of how geoengineered assaults via atmospheric energy can trigger aggression, anxiety, fear, panic, and "hate / submission"—all too common during the COVID-19 lockdown days, and not just in Oregon. Fillmore wrote:

> There is ample reason to believe we are being subjected to AMS [altered mental status], even HAPE [high altitude pulmonary edema] and HACE [high altitude cerebral edema] . . . by the Geoengineering of our atmosphere. *The gross extremes of atmospheric pressure being used to move storms around or to create droughts or any of the other weather phenomena are literally creating illnesses above and beyond the chemicals being used.* The positive ion 'blasts' are also part of the engineering, as well as being triggered by incoming solar energies—a double whammy.

5G flu symptoms (and the longer term *5G Syndrome*) increase as the fre-

---

49 Ibid. Theoretically, 100,000 systems operating at 60 GHz can be co-located in a 10-sq.-km area without interference problems.

50 Ann Fillmore, "Aerosol Experiments Using Lithium and Psychoactive Drugs Over Oregon." PositiveHealthOnline, February 2016.

51 Ann Fillmore, PhD, "Oxygen depletion," Facebook, February 18, 2020.

quency climbs from 2.4 GHz into the 50-60 GHz range en route to slowing down and stopping the blood from assimilating oxygen.[52] Add to oxygen absorption the phased array antennas in 5G beam technology and its ubiquitous techno-*simpatico* with the Internet of Things (IoT), and at the very least we are looking at calcium overload, cell DNA damage, neurological effects, and high blood pressure—symptoms of what is now being renamed the *Coronavirus Syndrome.*

Most 5G is actually an antenna upgrade (including the mmWave satellites) to the 4G LTE system. Thus 5G NRU [new radio unlicensed] = 4G Plus. Because the 5G SA [stand-alone] requires heavy-duty fiber optic cable, 5G NRU is now being marketed as the "last mile" segment that can easily (and more cheaply) link a business to a local fiber trunk ("interference free fiber speed connectivity") so buyers can avoid the cost and time delays of new fiber installation.

If we could but see it, the 5G-activated environment (like a Smart City, hospital, apartment complex, workplace or school) looks like an *all-pervasive cloud.* The 60 GHz signal is absorbed by the oxygen in the area it is traveling in so completely that *the vibratory level of oxygen becomes unrecognizable to the human body,* which incorrectly reads *No oxygen needed,* after which the lungs go into immediate distress, the hemoglobin stops delivering O2 to the blood, and coagulation ensues. *Instant bodily collapse.*

Blood coagulation follows directly from hypoxia or under-oxygenation. In *The Invisible Rainbow,* Arthur Firstenberg reminds us that since 1779, it has been known that radio waves affect blood coagulation. Medical schools (controlled by the American Medical Association) overlook this crucial part of a physician's training, which in the era of 5G / 4G Plus must be counted as suspicious and not merely due to ignorance. Blood clots and pulmonary embolisms in stroke[53] patients in their 30s to 40s (supposedly infected with COVID-19 virus) clearly signal the presence of a fully functioning 5G / 4G Plus environment.

> As Oxley, an interventional neurologist, began the procedure to remove the [blood] clot, he observed something he had never seen before. On the monitors, the brain typically shows up as a tangle of black squiggles—"like a can of spaghetti," he said—that provide a map of blood vessels. A clot shows up as a blank spot. As he used a needlelike device to pull out the clot, he saw new clots forming in real time around it. "This is crazy," he remembers telling his boss.[54]

---

52 Neil Chevrier, Citizens Against Harmful Technology (CAHT), recommends that you Immediately turn off electricity if you feel breathless.

53 Strokes are sudden interruptions of blood supply. The most deadly stroke is the LVO (large vessel occlusion). Pulmonary embolisms are blockages that arrest breathing.

54 Ariana Eunjung Cha, "Young, healthy people barely sick with covid-19 are dying from

This is crazy. What is crazy is that doctors are ignorant of the effects of both 5G and 4G Plus environments and the nanotechnology in re-clotting patients and instead are left to play guessing games about "attacks" on blood vessels and immune system "friendly fire."

Nanobots—nanotechnology—play as crucial a role in the COVID-19 drama as 5G / 4G Plus.

The PubMed study "5G Technology and Induction of Coronavirus in Skin Cells"[55] states that 5G millimeter waves can make the body produce coronaviruses as cellular responses. An exchange of waves occurs between 5G small cells tacked onto 4G towers and the antenna-like DNA mediated by nanobots now residing in our cells. Even skin sweat ducts act like helical antennas for mmWaves. In essence, 5G mimics *electroporation*, the practice of using pulsed waves to "drill" pores in cell membranes through which chemicals or synthetic DNA can be made to pass into cells for mutagenesis. [See "*MATra (Magnet-Assisted Transfection) and Electroporation*" in Chapter 4, "Magnetism."]

It has been said that deprivation of oxygen causes all human disease. COVID-19 is not a viral pneumonia but oxygen starvation, like the radiation distress Cameron Kyle-Sidell, MD, recognized as behaving like altitude sickness in the emergency room (ER) at Maimonides Medical Center in Brooklyn, New York.[56] Ventilators serve only to stress the lungs further and actually increase deaths by increasing *apoptosis* (cell death). Excess calcium signaling produces excessive oxidative stress as 5G alters the membrane permeability of cells and drives more and more calcium into the cells via the voltage-gated calcium channels (VGCCs), as Martin Pall, PhD, has pointed out over and over again (Chapter 2, "The Three Primary Delivery Systems"). VGCCs are the primary mechanism by which nonthermal (nonionized) 5G flu effects occur.

We now know that Epigenetics completely trumps the genome & former ideologies of genetic predetermination & predisposition. The input from your environment in the form of non-native electromagnetic radiation cannot be overstated. Recently, Martin Pall's Nobel Prize-worthy research has shown us just this. - Mark Eco-Waterhouse Soltynski*

---

strokes." msn.com, April 25, 2020.

55 Interestingly, this July 16, 2020 study has been "retracted" or "withdrawn," possibly because it linked COVID-19 with 5G. Many YouTubes and articles linking the two have been scrubbed from the Internet.

56 "FROM NYC ICU: DOES COVID-19 REALLY CAUSE ARDS??!!" Cameron Kyle-Sidell, March 31, 2020, https://www.youtube.com/watch?time_continue=5&v=k9GYTc53r2o&feature=emb_logo.

**the study of changes in organisms caused by modification of gene expression rather than alteration of the genetic code itself; determines a cell's specialization, at least until now when it is possible that environment will cause genes to be turned on and off*

Brain fog is typical of the COVID-19 experience "and other neurological symptoms due to post-traumatic stress disorder (PTSD), an effect observed in past human coronavirus outbreaks such as SARS (severe acute respiratory syndrome) and MERS (Middle East respiratory syndrome."[57] The *Clinical Neuropsychologist* paper discusses headaches, anxiety, fatigue, sleep disruptions—symptoms at one time or another attributed to "chemtrail flu," electrosensitivity (ES), 5G flu and 5G syndrome, etc. The common denominator? Wireless technology.

Magnetic fields can interfere with calcium-cardiac cell balance to such a degree that a heart attack can occur. Is this why 75 percent of those recovering from an initial COVID-19 flu have "lingering heart damage and inflammation [myocarditis] months after the initial infection"[58]? In his commentary regarding the paper "Cardioprotection from stress conditions by weak magnetic fields in the Schumann Resonance band,"[59] Oxford scholar Joseph Patrick Farrell, PhD, addresses the "destructive nature" of intentionally triggered and engineered magnetic fields and subsequent electromagnetic stress:

> . . . cellular responses can be triggered by the electromagnetic environment, and if they can be *triggered* by that environment, it's but a very short step to the notion that that environment can be *engineered* to create certain cellular responses, and from there, it's but yet another short step to the notion that this could be engineered to work in tandem with other technologies, like nanotechnology (Dr. Lieber, anyone?) or viruses.[60]

The subunit vaccine

A *subunit vaccine* is a vaccine that presents one or more antigens (cell debris) without introducing pathogen particles. Recombinant DNA (synthetic)

---

57 "'Brain fog' following COVID-19 recovery may indicate PTSD," UCLA Health, October 6, 2020.

58 Rachel Rettner, "COVID-19 linked to heart damage in healthy people, small study suggests." LiveScience.com, July 31, 2020.

59 G. Elhalel et al., "Cardioprotection from stress conditions by weak magnetic fields in the Schumann Resonance band," Scientific Reports, 7 February 2019.

60 Joseph Farrell, "And About Those Birds Dropping Dead From the Sky," Stillness in the Storm, April 19, 2020.

through "expression systems" like bacteria, yeast, insect and mammal cells or plants like tobacco make use of subunit vaccines for streamlining vaccine production, the only problem being that they need "immunopotentiating" adjuvants to trigger decent immune responses. (In normal vaccines, it is generally adjuvants like aluminum and lipid nanoparticles that cause adverse reactions.)

Hepatitis B was the very first subunit vaccine. The eugenics / newgenics connection to vaccinations first came to my attention with hepatitis B in 1978 and then AIDS in 1981. The hepatitis B "subunit vaccine" aspect was introduced by the CDC under Big Pharma chemical corporations and the National Institutes of Health (NIH). In accord with Public Law 98-373, the U.S. Arctic Research Plan of 1987 proclaimed Alaska to be a "natural laboratory" and the indigenous people of Alaska (18 percent of Alaska's population in 1991) as a "resource for studying health problems which will benefit other populations." By the time the British medical journal *The Lancet* announced the Hepatitis B program in Alaska that year, 38,990 Alaskan Natives plus 2,000 infants had already been vaccinated.

In 1991, Mary Ann Mills, a Council Member of the Traditional Dena'ina Tribe of Alaska, announced to the Green Party Statewide Convention that native children were being administered Hepatitis B shots (HBV) during the school day without parent permission.

> It is because of our research findings and the realization of such grim statistics and the insensitivity of the present governments [that] we took a stand to speak out. We can no longer, in good conscience, accept such conditions as being normal and healthy. We are finding [that] our traditional Dena'ina values do not fit well into the present-day governments. Other documentation our people research shows the title of Alaska is clouded. The United States did not and could not purchase Alaska. We cannot help it as we did not write these laws, but many of us feel this is why we have become a target group of genocidal proportions.
>
> There has never been a treaty between the Natives of Alaska and the federal government, and we do not need to make a treaty with the U.S. But we can and need to make a compact of peaceful association or code that we can all live by with the People of Alaska.
>
> In order for the Indigenous People of Alaska to survive, we must be given our freedom and our sovereignty as promised us . . . In closing, the Traditional Dena'ina Tribe stands firm and would like to go on record that basic sacred, fundamental Human Rights are not negotiable.[61]

61 Mary Ann Mills, "An Address to the Green Party Statewide Convention," September 20-22, 1991, Homer, Alaska. Personal copy.

Earlier in 1991, Finnish biologist Yves DeLatte had presented his conclusions at the International Indian Treaty Conference on the effects of vaccinations after 16 years of research:

- "Viruses contained in vaccines may recombine their genetic materials between each other, or with other unknown viruses which are natural inhabitants of our human ecologic system, or they may recombine with undetected viruses which are pollutants of vaccines media."
- "It has been demonstrated at the University of California, Los Angeles (UCLA) that two avirulent viruses can create *in vivo* a new highly pathogenic and lethal new virus. Professor [Stephen E.?] DeLong from the University of Texas has also admitted the highly probable hypothesis that all these so-called new viral diseases, including AIDS, may be recombinants from viral vaccines. These recombinants can either become immediately active and lethal, like in some forms of AIDS, or be latent pro-viruses or lentiviruses and be reactivated many years after vaccinations, which could be the cause of some cancers, or simply link themselves to the genetic material of the host and be transmitted from generation to generation and become active much later, a phenomenon called the Bitner Effect."
- "With vaccines, we have probably created illnesses which are far more dangerous than the diseases we were supposed to be protected against. By continuously exciting lymphocytes, these become committed to only a limited number of responses, and the immune system is unable to deal with new pathogens. By avoiding a strong and healthy immune response, the natural ecology of our bodies is displaced in favor of more virulent strains."
- "It has never been proven that vaccinations protect, but it can be proven that vaccinations weaken the immune system and the whole human race."

Dr. DeLatte's mention of AIDS in the context of recombinants from viral vaccines was repeated in a letter he wrote to Peter Duesberg, PhD, author of *Inventing the AIDS Virus* (1996): "AIDS could very well be the consequence of vaccination programs, done indiscriminately or not . . ."

The Hepatitis B vaccination played a seminal role in developing vaccines as *carriers* of diseases such as AIDS (1978-1981). The 1988 book by Alan Cantwell, Jr., MD, *AIDS and the Doctors of Death: An Inquiry into the Origin of the AIDS Epidemic*, goes into this issue as does the 1992 video *The Vaccination Dilemma* in which Australian physician Archie Kalokerinos (1927-2012), medical adviser to Aboriginal Health in Australia, stressed the following:

> In 1980 a Hepatitis B vaccine was made that . . . was distributed for use among Canadian [Alaskan] Indians and to Australian doctors overseas.

> The vaccine was in question because it may have contained very harmful viral particles. We don't know what happened to the people who received the shots . . . Deliberate attempts have been made to allow infants under my care to die. The real authorities don't want these infants to live. The real intention on the part of the authorities is genocide.[62]

In the article "Alaskans Fear Hepatitis Vaccine & AIDS Connection," Joan Moss hit the nail on the head:

> None of the investigators believe that AIDS was passed from the recipients of the original [Hep B] vaccine to the general population, but they do wonder if the disease was *already in the vaccine* and was therefore passed to the study's volunteer subjects.[63] [Emphasis added.]

Already in the vaccine. This is our present dilemma: the vaccine is the disease.

Now 50 years later, we learn in a 2018 study that the hepatitis B vaccine—the first vaccine given to 70 percent of the world's newborns—spikes the cytokine IL-4 (a protein for cell signaling) which contributes to post-vaccine brain damage because of more IL-4 being in the blood and getting through the blood-brain barrier, thus adding more IL-4 to the hippocampus, which then triggers a neuroinflammatory response. Scientist Zhibin Yao, PhD, was the first to make the connection between the Hepatitis B vaccine and autism and has now added this IL-4 study conclusion: *The hepatitis B vaccine causes brain damage.*[64]

Cometh the mRNA "vaccine"

> *RNA vaccine or mRNA vaccine: a type of vaccine that uses a copy of a natural chemical called messenger RNA to produce an immune response. The vaccine transfects molecules of synthetic RNA into immunity cells.*
>
> – Wikipedia

A vaccine is defined as a substance that prevents infection by a pathogen and also prevents spreading it to others (*Jacobson v Massachusetts*, 1905), which means that *synthetic (synbio) gene therapy are not vaccines.* David E. Martin, PhD, sees gene therapy technology hiding under the vaccine rubric so as to

---

62 I've been unable to find this video. Sadly, Sudden Infant Death Syndrome (SIDS or "crib death") appears to result from delayed vaccine reactions.

63 Joan Moss, "Alaskans Fear Hepatitis Vaccine & AIDS Connection," http://whale.to/v/alaskans.html, n.d.

64 J.B. Handley, "New Study: Hep B Vaccine "May Have Adverse Implications For Brain Development and Cognition." Children's Health Defense, July 26, 2018.

qualify for the 1986 liability exclusion for manufacturers, just as the state of emergency lockdown is kept going to maintain the liability shield under the emergency use authorization rule. It's all about Transhumanist experimentation and Big Data, not health or economic stability.

Synthetic biology (*synbio*) is the nexus between biology and engineering, and synthetic nanoparticles are the atomic-level building blocks of nanomachines, many of which sport tiny transceivers and microprocessors. Add to this the fact that "living cells can be induced to carry out computations in the manner of tiny robots or computers."[65] In fact, human cells and computers process and store information similarly—computers in strings of zeroes and 1's, living things with A, T, C and G. Tiny machines—"test tubes of DNA-laden water" that "crunch algorithms and spit out data"—are now DNA nano-computers that self-replicate and "grow into processors so powerful that they can handle problems too complex for silicon-based computers to solve."[66]

As was indicated earlier, computer software is now used to design RNA circuits that sequence and interact in a cell or cell-to-cell by remote command. Inovio Pharmaceuticals downloaded viral sequences and *in three hours* had a DNA vaccine design. Moderna (mRNA), CanSino Biologics (adenoviral vector), and Inovio specialize in gene-based vaccines that encode viral proteins in DNA and mRNA and can be designed quickly on a computer to turn cells into factories that produce viral proteins like the Spike protein instead of having to wait for them to be produced in plasmid vats of genetically engineered cells.

RNA self-assembling circuits resemble conventional electronic circuits in that they receive and transmit by producing a particular computational output (a protein). Specialized circuits called *logic gates (AND, OR* and *NOT)*, replete with RNA toehold switches, are stationed inside living cells and can be tripped by RNA fragments to receive messages, evaluate and respond to multiple inputs.

> The RNA-only approach to producing cellular nano-devices is a significant advance, as earlier efforts required the use of complex intermediaries, like proteins. Now, the necessary ribo-computing parts can be readily

65 Arizona State University, "Living computers: RNA circuits transform cells into nanodevices." Science Daily, July 26, 2017. The original work was done at ASU's Biodesign Institute under nanotech expert Peng Yin, assisted by Chinese grad and postdoc students. I mention this in light of the Thousand Talents program and recent news that the Chinese Communist Party (CCP) is seeking data on American DNA (Jon Wertheim, "China's Push To Control Americans' Health Care Future," 60 Minutes, January 31, 2021).

66 Paul Elias, "DNA Could Be Basis for Power Computing." Comcast.net News, August 17, 2003.

designed on computer. The simple base-pairing properties of RNA's four nucleotide letters (A, C, G and U) ensure the predictable self-assembly and functioning of these parts within a living cell.[67]

Thus, it becomes more obvious why Moderna (*modeRNA*), purveyer of "investigational mRNA medicines," is downloading an mRNA operating system into human bodies called *The Software of Life*: "the unique mRNA sequence that codes for a protein [or combines] different mRNA sequences encoding for different proteins in a single mRNA investigational medicine" (*modernatx.com*).[68] It is designed as a BCI plug-in that can interchangeably "play" different programs or apps on iPhones or in the 5G / IoT environment around us as well as merge us with the Internet / Cloud for "precision medicine," mind control, sentient world simulation (SWS), etc.

> With all the processing elements of the circuit made using RNA, which can take on an astronomical number of potential sequences, the real power of the newly described method lies in *its ability to perform many operations at the same time.* The capacity for parallel processing permits faster and more sophisticated computation while making efficient use of the limited resources of the cell . . . a future in which human cells become fully programmable entities with extensive biological capabilities.[69]

Getting mRNA into the targeted tissue requires evading the immune system which, despite having been weakened over the past half century by chemical and electromagnetic delivery systems, still must be fooled so that coronavirus Spike proteins—created to cling *specifically* to human cells and containing artificially inserted sequences[70]—can be forced into cells either by electroporation or synthetic lipid nanoparticles (LNPs)[71] loaded with mRNA made by cell-free enzymatic reaction. Both the electroporation and synthetic LNP methods ensure that by integrating exogeneous DNA with the host genome, gene alteration and mutagenesis will follow—namely a genetically modified (GM) human being, as mentioned earlier. Both methods can also be used to implant gain-of-function diseases for remote 5G triggering at a future date.

---

67 Ibid.

68 "The New mRNA Covid Vaccines Inject an Operating System into Your Body – Not a Conspiracy Theory, Moderna Admits It," Health Impact News, January 5, 2021.

69 Arizona State University.

70 "Multiple Scientists: Coronavirus Altered in Lab to Better Attach to Humans," Benn Swann, Truth in Media, June 16, 2020.

71 See under "'Vaccine' vulnerability" for more on how the PEG (polyethylene glycol) polymer is added to NLPs so the NLPs smuggling mRNA into the cell can avoid being recognized by the immune system.

If the DNA is synthetic, then the GM human being will be more cyborg than human.

Transhumanist experimentation entails the genomic sequence of the vaccine taking on the genomic sequence of the virus in it—for example, if HIV is in the virus, it will be in the vaccine. A *gain of function* virus will be in the vaccine and will mean your DNA is being changed. Any retrovirus RNA virus inserting a DNA copy of its genome into the host cell in order to replicate will change the host DNA.[72] mRNA can be reverse transcribed and converted back to DNA by LINEs and SINEs (short and long interspersed retrotransposable elements); the cloned DNA can then be integrated into the genome. In this way, mRNA truly is genetic editing (like CRISPR). (Thanks to Martin.)

> Retroviruses essentially inject single-stranded RNA [ssRNA] strands into somatic (body) cells during "infection." These ssRNA strands access nucleotide pools in the host cell and form a double-stranded DNA [dsDNA] copy. This dsDNA can then incorporate itself into the host chromosome using a viral enzyme called "integrase." The new "fake gene" then orders the cell to make more mRNA copies of the original virus RNA. These then travel out of the cell and infect the next cell, and so on.[73]

What are we seeing in hundreds of thousands who've received the COVID-19 jabs and suffer "side effects" and *life-altering* "serious vaccine adverse events" (1 in 333)?

- Stroke (cerebrovascular)
- Inflammation of the heart
- Muscle paralysis
- Bells Palsy
- Blindness
- Eye disorders
- Anaphylaxis shock
- Autoimmune attacks
- Brain stem infarction
- Cerebellar infarction
- Cerebellar stroke
- Cerebral arty occlusion
- Cerebral hemorrhage

72 See Anthony Patch, "Gain-of-Function HIV-1 Retrovirus Admitted in Mainstream Narrative," December 17, 2020.

73 Sharon Gilbert, author of The Armageddon Strain (2005), to Tom Horn in his book Zenith 2016 (2013).

- Cerebral infarction
- Intracranial hemorrhage
- Ischemic stroke
- Subarachnoid hemorrhage
- Spontaneous abortion[74]

Like the lied-about death statistics for COVID-19, the passive surveillance Vaccine Adverse Event Reporting System (VAERS) is not accurate.[75] Symptoms such as those above are re-contextualized and thrown under the COVID-19 bus—even PTSD has been invoked ("evaluating persistent cognitive and emotional difficulties among COVID-19 survivors") so that complainants can be shunted off to the psychiatric ward. (Shades of the DSM-5 categorization of Morgellons symptoms as "delusional parasitosis.") We are told that just two types of vaccine being administered around the world, but I doubt this is true. More likely, varying batches are being distributed so that following results is impossible.

DNA and RNA "vaccines"

Part of what is being installed by all three Transhumanist delivery systems (see Chapter 2) and now culminating in the COVID-19 gene transfer technology is the "pre-crime" model of precision medicine. Perpetuating and controlling sickness, not health, is what drives the Big Pharma / Big Medicine business model in private-public partnership with the military-industrial-intelligence complex. What once looked like vaccinations against illness are now "gene therapy" with far reaching Transhumanist agendas.

Marshalling immune forces to defeat invading viruses is no longer the purpose of "vaccines."

> *Koch's postulate: What anyone with common sense would use to prove that a microorganism causes disease: isolate the organism from a sick animal or human, then introduce it into a healthy animal or human to see whether it causes disease.*
>
> – Thomas S. Cowan, MD, *The Contagion Myth*, 2020

74 L.J. Devon, "Experimental mRNA vaccines cause 600 new cases of eye disorders and leave 5 people blind." A Final Warning ("Top stories from independent journalists across the Web"), February 19, 2021. Could remote manipulation of graphene nanoparticles via 5G be behind COVID-19 "side effects"?

75 According to Children's Health Defense and Robert F. Kennedy Jr., fewer than one percent of adverse events were reported by December 2020 so as to make it seem that there are not all that many (Children's Health Defense Team, "329 Deaths + 9,516 Other Injuries Reported Following COVID Vaccine, Latest CDC Data Show," January 29, 2021).

Did the mRNA approach arise from the *immunoprophylaxis (IGT)* gene therapy? The following is how the *New York Times* spun IGT in 2015:

> But [IGT] treatment is not a vaccine, not in any ordinary sense. By delivering synthetic genes [inside virus] into the muscles of the monkeys, the scientists are essentially reengineering the animals to resist disease . . . protection against diseases for which vaccines have failed . . .[76]

Originally in the context of protection—a synthetic DNA payload uploaded into the host's genome to "instruct the cells to begin manufacturing powerful antibodies . . . 'We're going around the immune system, rather than trying to stimulate the immune system,' Dr. David Baltimore [virologist at Caltech and Nobel Prize recipient] said"—could RNA, pre-crime-style, implant future diseases?

Now, molecular "naked DNA" is being replaced by digital synthetic DNA designed for computing inside living cells (*in silico*) along with computer software used to design synthetic RNA sequences that provide instructions for nanobots in cells to make Spike proteins (or whatever the algorithm tells them to make).[77] "The RNA-only approach to producing cellular nanodevices is a significant advance . . . Now, the necessary ribo-computing parts can be readily designed on computer."[78] In other words, a computer operating system (OS) with inherent remote programmability and a back door for remote "updating" is being uploaded into millions of human beings.

Given that RNA are basically single-stranded electronic circuits able to self-assemble, receive and transmit along complementary strands (the A nucleotide with U, the C nucleotide with G), it should not be surprising that "custom-built" mRNA strands are able to direct the body's cells to operate as *ad hoc* drug and autoimmune disease factories[79] while RNA fragments attached to RNA sequences create specialized circuits to act as tiny logic gates (on / off, open / shut electronic switches). Had Marshall McLuhan been an epidemiologist, he might have said that mRNA (including its fragments) does not just bear the message to cells but *is* the message leading to *provirus,* the DNA produced by RNA virus

76 Carl Zimmer, "Protection Without a Vaccine." New York Times, March 9, 2015.

77 Robert Langreth and Naomi Kresge, "Moderna Wants to Transform the Body Into a Vaccine-Making Machine." Bloomberg, August 11, 2020.

78 Arizona State University, "Living computers: RNA circuits transform cells into nanodevices," July 26, 2017.

79 Tia Ghose, "DARPA Is Developing Human Bio-Factories to Brew Lifesaving Vaccines." LiveScience, September 11, 2015.

that Rutgers University PhD Robert M. Simpson deemed "a molecule in search of a disease" at an American Cancer Society Seminar for Science Writers in 1976.

> Immunization programs against the flue, measles, mumps, and polio may actually be seeding humans with RNA to form proviruses which will then become latent cells throughout the body . . . Although host cells containing latent viral particles operate more or less normally, they begin to synthesize viral proteins under the guidance of viral DNA, eventually creating the circumstances for various autoimmune diseases, including diseases of the central nervous system, which unfortunately add to the growing load of aberrant social behavior patterns.[80]

Add to the provirus the reverse transcriptase enzyme in RNA virus that makes sure the virus forms strands of DNA[81] that integrate with the host's cell DNA, and you have Big Pharma using vaccine to seed RNA and form proviruses which become latent for long periods throughout the body, only to reawaken later on. As with rheumatoid arthritis, MS, and systemic lupus erythematosus (SLE), the immune system is forced to form *antibodies against the person's own tissues because they're impregnated by foreign genetic material.* Even a slight modification to the "antigenic character of tissues" may make one's immune system attack one's own body as foreign.

Can such evil in the name of science be behind the host of symptoms the COVID-19 "vaccinated" are experiencing?

The story making the rounds is that the RNA virus SARS-CoV-2 (SARS-CoV-19) has "mutated" into at least 30 different genetic "variants," including 19 "never seen before as well as 'rare changes that scientists had never imagined could happen'"[82] (and despite the fact that the SARS-CoV-2 has never been isolated). These mutated "transfers" are, as Andrew Kaufman, MD, clarifies, *in silico* (computerized) genome sequencing, not a natural viral process. *The "gene therapy" software creates the "variants" that are then strengthened by the produced antibodies (antibody-dependent enhancement).* Nobel Laureate Luc Montagnier:

> It is the antibodies produced by the virus that enable an infection to become stronger. It's what we call antibody-dependent enhancement, which means

---

80 Teddit, https://teddit.net/r/conspiracy/comments/lxpbt1/if_the_elite_agenda_is_to_depopulate_through/gpo9ttt/; also see Leading Edge Research Group, "Vaccines and Production of Negative Genetic Changes in Humans," 1998.

81 Short synthetic strands of DNA or RNA are known as oligos, as in oligonucleotide.

82 Angela Betsaida B. Laguipo, BSN, "Coronavirus has mutated into at least 30 variants," News Medical Life Sciences, April 22, 2020; "COVID-19: The Spearpoint for Rolling Out a 'New Era' of High-Risk, Genetically Engineered Vaccines," Children's Health Defense, May 7, 2020.

> antibodies favor a certain infection. The antibody attaches to the virus; from that moment, it has the receptors . . . It pokes the virus not accidentally, but because of the fact that they are linked to the antibodies. It is clear that the new variants are created by antibody-mediated selection due to the vaccination.[83]

As we know, no mRNA vaccine has ever been licensed, due to how unstable large mRNA molecules are (prone to degradation, overstimulate the immune system to produce antibodies,[84] lead to mutations, trigger autoimmune responses, activate cancer-causing genes, etc.). Stabilizing the mRNA "silver bullet" depends upon liquid lipid nanoparticle (LNP) packaging for an injectable form (see below). Vaccine nanoparticles are *synbio* nanobots digitized so as to be remote-controlled with mRNA being more of the same in that it is activated along 5G-disseminated 60 GHz mmWave bands:

> MIT chemical engineers have now developed a new series of lipid nanoparticles to deliver such vaccines. They showed that the particles trigger efficient production of the protein encoded by the RNA, and they also behave like an "adjuvant," further boosting the vaccine effectiveness . . .[85]

A unique mRNA sequence codes for a particular protein. With fragments of latent DNA or RNA in the cell, a mRNA "medicine" (or disease) can later be remotely resurrected via the genetic code that instructs ribosomes to make a specific protein, or by different mRNA sequences that can be combined to encode for different proteins in a single mRNA vaccination.

German scientist Harald Kautz-Vella points out that during the Iraq War, the Iraqis complained of a "burning sensation" on their skin, due not to white phosphorus but to the *cluster typology* of synthetic mRNA in the aerosols being delivered by jets over Iraq to synergize with the vaccines soldiers and possibly Iraqi citizens had been inoculated with. According to Kautz-Vella, optimization of synthetic mRNA cluster typology contributes to turning people into bio-robots / cyborgs in that the *synthetic* RNA transports a "soul" or artificial intelligence into the genome.

---

83 "Nobel Laureate Luc Montagnier – "All Vaccinated People Will Die Within Two Years," BitChute, May 22, 2021.

84 Chronic inflammation.

85 Anne Trafton, "Delivery system can make RNA vaccines more powerful." MIT News, September 30, 2019.

PCR swab "test"

> *A fellow asked for a CV 'test,' grabbed the swab, and ran. He scanned it and discovered it contains Technetium, a radioactive metal with bio-infiltrator properties, including mind control and direct DNA manipulation.*
>
> – Ingri Cassel, leading U.S. Vaccine Truth Activist

PCR stands for polymerase chain reaction. In 1976, the Taq polymerase enzyme was discovered—what biochemist Kary Mullis (1944-2019)[86] worked with in order to amplify segments of DNA and develop the PCR test: (1) heat DNA, separate the double strand; (2) add primers (short pieces of DNA); (3) polymerase synthesizes a new DNA strand; (4) target DNA has now been doubled, and the cycle starts again (25 to 40 times).

However, as Mullis himself said, "These tests cannot detect free, infectious viruses at all." In fact, only a small portion of the genome is detected, which makes the PCR test unsuitable for diagnostic purposes. Add that the short pieces of primer DNA may be of pathogens already dealt with by the immune system, and that even the genetic sequences may be unknown genetic expressions. Was the target DNA purified? And if RNA is the target, it will first have to be converted to DNA, a process that is not dependable.

A PCR positive means nothing without a double-blind clinical trial. From protocol errors to inappropriate data analysis and inadequate reporting, positive PCRs for SARS-CoV-2, etc., it is all little more than "technical noise."[87]

Are PCR tests actually about covert deliveries of hydrogel, graphene, and inorganic life forms? Some long swabs definitely have nanotechnology on them, like smart dust *theragrippers* made of metal (Technetium?), thin shapeshifting biofilm, heat-sensitive wax, silicon and zirconium glass fibers or emery (corundite) for abrasion, possible Morgellons filaments with "DARPA hydrogel beads" that sound a lot like spherical *cross-domain bacteria* encased in Morgellons filaments (discussed in Chapter 2), capable of navigating the body and releasing payloads after lodging in the intestinal mucosa.[88] (Intestinal mucosa might also account for

---

86 There is no question in my mind about Kary Mullis' death: as an early voice attempting to clarify what was really going on via Andrew Fauci, he was murdered.

87 Stephen A. Bustin, PhD, "The Infectious Myth" and his paper with Tania Nolan, "Talking the talk but not walking the walk: RT-qPCR as a paradigm for the lack of reproducibility in molecular research," European Journal of Clinical Investigation, 10 August 2017. A consortium of scientists has requested retraction of the paper "Detection of 2019 novel coronavirus (2019-nCoV) by real-time RT-PCR" by Victor M. Corman et al., Eurosurveillance, January 2020. See the video "The Truth About PCR Tests," Dr. Sam Bailey, January 12, 2021.

88 John O'Sullivan, "Are PCR Tests Secret Vaccines?" Principia Scientific International, December 2, 2020; Soultan Al-Halifa et al., "Nanoparticle-Based Vaccines Against Respiratory

the anal swabs added to the COVID "testing" / implantation regime.)

The presence of glass fibers in the swabs reminds me of aerosol deliveries back in 2015, as reported by the excellent anti-geoengineering activist, Rev Michelle Mann, who found aluminum-tipped fiberglass lodged in her upper respiratory passages (400X magnification).[89] Rev Michelle stated that pink plasma clouds and similar prismatic (rainbow) effects were due to light hitting aluminum around fiberglass.

In short, the World Health Organization (WHO) test kit is not what it seems. The human chromosome 8 guarantees a positive outcome every time, due to having the same sequences as coronavirus,[90] plus two patents remind us to consider that remotely gained readings of our biometrics may be being "adjusted": U.S. Patent #20170229149A1, "System and Method for Using, Biometric, and Displaying Biometric Data" (Richard A. Rothschild, Netherlands, October 13, 2015), and U.S. Patent #2020/0279585, "System and Method for Testing COVID-19" (2017, 2020). Note how the smartphone can be useful in this regard:

> A method is provided for acquiring and transmitting biometric data (e.g. vital signs) of a user, where the data is analyzed to determine whether the user is suffering from a viral infection, such as COVID-19. The method includes using a pulse oximeter to acquire at least pulse and blood oxygen saturation percentage, which is transmitted wirelessly to a smartphone. To ensure that the data is accurate, an accelerometer within the smartphone is used to measure movement of the smartphone and/or user. Once accurate data is acquired, it is uploaded to the cloud (or host) . . .

The newest "test," Low-cost Electrochemical Advanced Diagnostic (LEAD), uses graphite to build the electrode that binds the SARS-CoV-2 Spike protein to prove the presence of COVID-19 (plus "variants").[91]

Viruses," Frontiers in Immunology, 24 January 2019; Silviu Costinescu, "Spooky Fibers in Masks and Test Swabs. Wait 'Til You Read the Science," SilView.media, April 29, 2021; and work by Antonietta Gatti, PhD. Most excellent: "Analysis of test sticks from surface testing in the Slovak Republic – confirmation of genocide," covering tests between November 2020 and March 2021. Thanks to TimTruth.com and Silviu Costinescu (SilView).

89 Rev Michelle Mann, "Very Disturbing Horrific! US Congressional Governance of Geoengineering." Autocollisionman, January 5, 2016.

90 "Bombshell: WHO Coronavirus PCR Test Primer Sequence Is Found In All Human DNA." Piece of Mind blog site, April 6, 2020.

91 "Penn Engineers Create Faster and Cheaper COVID-19 Testing With Pencil Lead." Penn Engineering Today, August 13, 2021.

Proteins, enzymes, & prions

> *The little spikes that project from the coronavirus so it will attach inside the lungs are Spike Glycoproteins (S-proteins). S-protein 120 (120 spikes) is only found in one other virus: HIV, meaning the current COVID-19 strain was indeed genetically modified ("gain of function") by the insertion of HIV proteins into the coronavirus and therefore weaponized. Dr. Anthony Fauci was the first person to identify, isolate, and PATENT Spike Glycoprotein S-120. What more needs to be said?*
>
> –Susan Carlson, Facebook

> *Do not accept any covid-19 tests, either. I am convinced that the swabs are used to insert prions close to the brain, which is why they use such long sticks and shove them all the way to the base of the brain, the brain being the organ most vulnerable to prion infections and damage.*
>
> – Kevin Mugur Galalae

Our human bodies are not so much carbon-based as protein-based.

Of the four biological macromolecules (carbohydrates, lipids, proteins, and nucleic acids), *proteins* are the long chains of hundreds of *amino acids (peptides)* assembled by ribosomes obeying what DNA dictates via mRNA and finally tRNA. The ten billion proteins in the cell are the workhorses that catch and use molecules for energy or for rebuilding various parts of the cell, including a host of nanomachines: motors, pumps, tubes, shears, rotors, levers, ropes—all buffered and buffeted by high-speed water molecules. Proteins handle the metabolism, transport atoms, and form receptors to conduct electrical charges. They twist, fold, and stretch according to their tasks, and the 3D shape they fold into determines their function, like how insulin controls sugar levels in the blood and how antibodies fight coronavirus. Recently, Google-owned Deep Mind announced that proteins fold into 3D shapes through AlphaFold algorithms.[92]

> A typical protein consists of a chain of several hundred amino acids folded into a complex three-dimensional shape—its functional form. Life uses twenty (sometimes twenty-one) varieties of amino acids in various combinations. There are countless ways that sequences of A, C, G, and T bases can code for twenty amino acids, but all known life uses the *same* assignments, suggesting it is a very ancient and deeply embedded feature of life on Earth, present in *a common ancestor billions of years ago.*[93] (Emphasis added.)

---

92 James Orme, "DeepMind AI cracks 50-year-old protein folding problem, say researchers." Techerati, 2 December 2020.

93 Paul Davies, The Demon in the Machine: How hidden webs of information are solving the

A common ancestor billions of years ago . . .

Self-assembling, self-replicating *synthetic* proteins replete with sensors, antennas, wires, and arrays behave like nanosized machines not just in our bodies but in our air, food, and water. Inside the body, they can be programmed to copy the DNA of pathogens and cancer cells and increase them; create pseudo-hair, pseudo-skin, and chimeric forms that look like insects and parasites. Babies are born with these nanomachines already in their bodies. Proteins expressed by one gene can exhibit or enhance the expression of other genes. Nerve cell proteins can be genetically engineered to be sensitive to radio waves and magnetic fields by being attached to the iron-storing protein called ferritin or to inorganic paramagnetic nanoparticles like graphene. The Magneto protein can remotely control both the firing of neurons deep in the brain and complex behaviors.[94]

Proteins can be used to fabricate nanoparticles and microparticles suitable for use as delivery systems for bioactive compounds.[95] Proteins combine with the mechanical and electronic properties of *CNTs (carbon nanotubes)* for the development of more nanomachines and sensors. *CNT/protein hybrids* form bioscaffolds and make CNT substrates for cell growth and neural interacting applications. Alone, CNTs act as protein carriers for vaccines.[96] As the enigmatic title of the paper referenced indicates ("The Devil and Holy Water"), "novel" nanohybrid applications and "multidimensional and complex behaviour in environmental and biological exposure systems" are not well understood[97]: merging biological protein "molecular recognition and catalytic activity" with nano-mechanical and -electronic CNTs via aerosols and vaccines ends in the devil, not holy water.

---

mystery of life (Penguin Books, 2019). Davies: "Scientists cause much confusion when they refer to an organism's 'code' when they really mean genetic data. Your genetic data and mine differ, but we have the same genetic code."

94 Mo Costandi, "Genetically engineered 'Magneto' protein remotely controls brain and behaviour." Guardian, 24 March 2016. Also view Pierre Gilbert, MD, "Drs 1995 PREDICTION – 'Contaminating the bloodstream will be enforced by law.'" Gilbert's reference to Rwanda (Tutsis and Hutus, 1994) is covered in "Operation Crimson Mist: Electronic Slaughter in Rwanda" by Australian investigative journalist Joe Vialls, May 29, 2003. Vialls died in hospital at 61 of a "heart attack."

95 G. Davidov-Pardo et al., "Food-grade protein-based nanoparticles and microparticles for bioactive delivery: fabrication, characterization, and utilization." Advances in Protein Chemistry and Structural Biology, 2015.

96 Matteo Calvaresi and Francesco Zerbetto, "The Devil and Holy Water: Protein and Carbon Nanotube Hybrids." Accounts of Chemical Research, 2013.

97 Nirupam Aich et al., "A critical review of nanohybrids: synthesis, applications and environmental implications." Environmental Chemistry, 2014.

Now instead of a morphology as a result of a direct assault, the constant contact can now produce hybrid materials. Again, we are reflecting the sky since this has been ongoing for decades. The materials in the atmosphere also have formed new compositions that are not even listed in the periodic table, so we are dealing with epigenetics on steroids, and we have absolutely no clue what is up above us raining down. - Tony Pantalleresco, Canadian herbalist

---

Enzymes are large proteins that accelerate chemical reactions and cell activity—for example, carbonic anhydrase assembles over half a million molecules of carbonic acid *per second.* Need to repair damage to the double helix? Correct errors in DNA replication? Enzymes— "molecular automata"—are the ones to do it; reading DNA text, they then transcribe it into RNA, edit, splice, construct nanomachines, and build other enzymes.

DNA has a natural alphabet of four letters, proteins an alphabet of 20 letters (*amino acids*). Proteins build DNA molecules but cannot build themselves without DNA's information. (The chicken or egg dilemma.) The amino acid chains in proteins do the lion's share of cell maintenance: building and taking apart molecules to extract their energy; carrying atoms to precise places; acting as pumps or motors; forming receptors to trap specific molecules and antennas that conduct charges. In other words, twisting, folding, and stretching amino acids are self-assembling nanomachines.

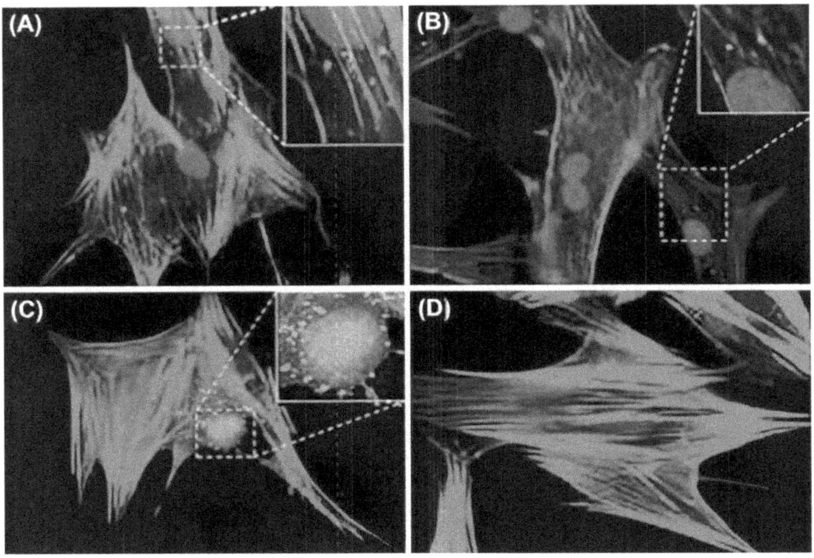

Carbon nanotubes (CNTs). So-called regenerative medicine.

"Uptake of COOH-functionalized single-walled carbon nanotubes by the cell. Fluorescent images of biotinylated carbon nanotubes within the cell after (1) 24 hours, (b) 48 hours, (c) 6 days, and (d) human mesenchymal stem cells alone (Scale bar 130 μm)." (Photos from the American Chemical Society.)

"Nanotechnology based stem cell therapies for damaged heart muscles," *Nanowerk.com,* August 22, 2008.

Proteinaceous infectious particles (prions) are misfolded proteins, as found in Alzheimer's, Parkinson's and Lewy body dementia. Biologist Stanley Prusiner received the 1998 Nobel Prize in Medicine for discovering that prions[98] can transmit their "misfoldedness" onto normal proteins and cause fatal infections and neurodegenerative diseases once mutant prions have entered the brain. Like GBH, prions are self-replicating biochemical weapons,[99] and like their *synbio* counterparts, *they are not living organisms, as they are devoid of nucleic acid.*[100] Only lengthy burning at 2000°C (3632°F) destroys them; otherwise, they can exist for decades, even in formaldehyde.

98 See the National Prion Disease Pathology Surveillance Center at Case Western Reserve School of Medicine in Cincinnati. The National Academy of Sciences (NAS) prioritizes prion research.

99 Eric Almeida Xavier, "Prions: the danger of biochemical weapons." Food Science and Technology, July / September 2014.

100 "Prions made in the lab," Sissa Media Lab. ScienceDaily, January 4, 2016. More importantly, read Michelle Starr's "A Deadly Contagious Human Brain Protein Was Just Made in the Lab for the First Time," ScienceAlert, 7 June 2018.

According to former hospital administrator Constance Klostermeier, Prusiner went to New Guinea in the 1950s to study and culture a disease called *kuru* that arose in women and children who had eaten the brains of deceased tribal enemies. These were the days of MK/NAOMI, a program run by the CIA in league with the Special Operations Division of the U.S. Army's chemical-biological warfare center at Fort Detrick. In 1957, D. Carleton Gajdusek, head of virological and neurological labs at the NIH, was at Fort Detrick working on prions.[101]

Kuru symptoms included uncontrollable body movements, bizarre behaviors, and hysterical bouts of laughter. *Scrapie* and *bovine spongiform encephalopathy (BSE)* or mad cow disease in the UK in the 1980s may have been the first public *kuru* experiments in the West, possibly due to "injecting or feeding brain and other tissue from an infected host" to cows subsequently eaten by humans, followed in the 1990s by the human Variant Creutzfeldt-Jakob Disease (vCJD). Klostermeier writes:

> Now that this pathogen is synthesized, there are innumerable possibilities for this as a bioweapon (especially attached to a virus). Every infection will be different . . . Think about those poor [Covid-19] people with 'rigor-like' movements at the end, and the fact they're showing ebola-like bloodbaths at the end.[102]

The very fact that synthetic prions lack a genome confirms their weaponization.

> At times, to understand something well, it is useful to rebuild it from scratch. It happens with prions as well: in collaboration with the BESTA Institute in Milan, the Laboratory of Prion Biology at SISSA in Trieste assembled artificial prions, devising a method for synthesizing them in a series. *Lab tests showed that synthetic prions act like their biological counterparts.*[103] (Emphasis added.)

J. Bart Classen, MD, points out in his 27 December 2020 paper "COVID-19 RNA Based Vaccines and the Risk of Prion Disease" that the Pfizer COVID-19 vaccine has "the potential to induce prion-based disease in vaccine recipients" by converting

> . . . intracellular RNA binding proteins TAR DNA binding protein (TDP-43) and Fused in Sarcoma (FUS) into their pathologic prion conformations . . . *the vaccine RNA has specific sequences that may induce TDP-43 and FUS*

101 In 1996, Gajdusek was convicted of child molestation and spent 12 months in prison before entering a self-imposed exile in Europe, where he died a decade later.

102 Shepard Ambellas, "Exclusive: Fmr administrator reveals possible COVID19 connection to weaponized prions." Intellihub, February 14, 2020.

103 Sissa Medialab, "Prions made in the lab." ScienceDaily.com, January 4, 2016. Thanks to David Masem for pointing me in this direction.

to fold into their pathologic prion confirmations . . . Furthermore, the spike protein, created by the translation of the vaccine RNA, binds angiotensin converting enzyme 2 (ACE2), a zinc containing enzyme. This interaction has the potential to increase intracellular zinc. *Zinc ions have been shown to cause the transformation of TDP-43 to its pathologic prion configuration.* The folding of TDP-43 and FUS into their pathologic prion confirmations is known to cause ALS front temporal degeneration, Alzheimer's disease and other neurological degenerative diseases . . .[104] (Emphases added.)

Prion disease diagnosis is difficult, there are no effective treatments, and fatalities are guaranteed—a perfect lethal weapon, especially in league with the Spike protein. Recently, millions of minks at Danish mink farms were culled due to an alleged *mutation* in the Spike glycoprotein of coronavirus (S-protein 120), as it could lead to a prion (especially Cluster 5).

"Mutation happens all the time, but once in a while these mutations happen in the spike protein," says Prof Anders Fomsgaard, SSI's head of virus research. That spike protein of the coronavirus is the target of some vaccines in development. "So we are a little nervous once we see mutations that change amino acids and the shape of the protein," [Fomsgaard] tells the BBC.[105]

In such a way, a COVID-19 vaccine spiked with prions could produce brain damage that could then be blamed on Alzheimer's or dementia. Kevin Mugur Galalae, trained in global public health at the University of Michigan, believes the minks were set up to be blamed for "the encephalopathy pandemic caused by the covid-19 vaccines."[106]

In 2014, a researcher in molecular biology, virology, and cancer at the Federal University of Sao Paulo in Brazil issued a warning:

The knowledge of biotechnology increases the risk of using biochemical weapons for mass destruction. Prions are unprecedented infectious pathogens that cause a group of fatal neurodegenerative diseases by a novel mechanism. They are transmissible particles that are devoid of nucleic acid. Due to their singular characteristics, Prions cause fatal infectious diseases, and to date there is no therapeutic or prophylactic approach against these diseases. Furthermore, Prions are resistant to food-preparation treatments

104 J. Bart Classen, MD, "COVID-19 RNA Based Vaccines and the Risk of Prion Disease." Microbiology & Infectious Diseases, 27 December 2020.

105 Adrienne Murray, "Coronavirus: Denmark shaken by cull of millions of mink." BBC, 11 November 2020.

106 Facebook, Kevin Mugur Galalae.

such as high heat and can find their way from the digestive system into the nervous system; *recombinant Prions are infectious either bound to soil particles or in aerosols.* Therefore, lethal Prions can be developed by malicious researchers who could use it to attack political enemies since such weapons cause diseases that could be above suspicion.[107] (Emphasis added.)

Most damning regarding prion research may have been the July 2, 2019 brutal rape and murder in Crete of Suzanne Eaton, a professor of molecular biology married to Israeli-born prion expert Anthony Hyman. Both taught and did research at the Max Planck Institute of Molecular Cell Biology and Genetics in Dresden, Germany. Immunologist John Barthelow Classen[108] believes Eaton was tortured regarding what she knew about the weaponizing of prions.

Let's discuss the more benign protein Gc. Earlier, I mentioned the murders of Jeff Bradstreet, MD, and Nicholas Gonzalez, MD, in the context of autism and three-strand DNA, both being researched for moving Human 1.0 to Human 2.0. Drs. Bradstreet and Gonzalez both knew that infancy vaccinations were being piggybacked with the protein / enzyme nagalase so as to undermine the immune system and thus set the infant on the Transhuman path of brain-computer interface (BCI) and the condition perfect for it, *autism.*

Before cancer was weaponized (see Chapter 9 under "War As A Smart City Lab"), the human immune system was still able to produce *GcMAF (Globulin compound-derived Macrophage Activating Factor)* so as to remain strong, even in a post-industrial polluted environment. The liver converts plasma protein into Gc protein whose mission is to become a MAF and transport vitamin D. Gc being a protein that boosts the immune system, the full assault on the immune system needed the protein / enzyme nagalase to block Gc production. Thus, cancer cells were programmed to produce nagalase. In fact, the presence of nagalase in the blood is considered a cancer marker. If the Gc protein isn't blocked, it binds with vitamin D and moves into the MAF phase to awaken *macrophages* for search-and-destroy duty against pathogens and tumorous cells whose debris constitute *antigens.*

GcMAF made by the body is a modified Gc protein and vitamin D, but if nagalase strips the sugar molecule N-acetyl-Galactosamine from the Gc protein, vitamin D is blocked from attaching, GcMAF doesn't occur, and the immune system does not defend. With the immune system knocked out of ac-

---

107 Eric Almeida Xavier, "Prions: The danger of biochemical weapons." Food Science Technology, July/September 2014.

108 Classen wrote "COVID-19 RNA-based vaccines and the risk of prion disease." See Siva Selan, "As vaccination begins, theories against jabs surface in the form of 'medical research'." Malaysia Now, February 25, 2021.

tion, more and more nagalase is released . . .[109] The medical treatment GcMAF quickens the immune system and reverses cancer, autism, and who knows how many autoimmune conditions, which is no doubt why the cancer industry and Big Pharma stoop to murder savvy, outspoken doctors like Jeff Bradstreet and Nicholas Gonzalez, and lock up British GcMAF proponents like David Noakes (nine months in prison) and scientist Lynda Thyer (19 months in prison).

mRNA "vaccine" vulnerability: shelf life & lipid shells

What has frustrated vaccine makers (especially of viral vaccines) is the lag time between antigen production and vaccine delivery. While it makes sense that the classic live virus vaccine would have to be kept at a certain cool temperature or lose its potency, what of vaccines made with synthetic virus? Can they be stored and transported at room temperature and bypass the complexities of refrigeration?

Apparently, the Pfizer coronavirus vaccine needs -70°C (-94°F) for storage *and* transportation, no doubt because the mRNA molecule is easily degraded, despite the lipid nanoparticles protecting it. On 15 November 2020, The Disruptive Physician said, "Any vaccine that needs to be shipped and stored at -80°F (-62°C) isn't a vaccine. It's a transfection agent, kept alive so it can infect your cells and transfer genetic material. Don't let them fool you. This is genetic manipulation of humans on a massive scale. Shut it down." Aurora Health Care pharmacist Steven Brandenburg took The Disruptive Physician at his word: on Christmas Day 2020 in Wisconsin, Brandenburg removed vials of Moderna vaccine from refrigeration at Grafton Medical Center and left them out.[110]

So it isn't really about virus: biofilms containing virus have been stored in a sealed container on a lab bench at room temperature for *three years* before being rehydrated to induce an immune response.[111]

Perhaps the low temperature is addressing the problem of how quickly synthetic polymers dissolve. Cyclic or ring polymers lack chain ends and so end up as self-oscillating or self-walking gel (hydrogel?) that creates its own artificial cilia.[112] From an etheric standpoint, cool temperatures would make

---

109 Thanks to Linda Emmanuel's article "Mycoplasma, Nagalase and GcMAF." Mycoplasmas also release nagalase into the bloodstream.

110 Todd Richmond, "Prosecutor: Wisconsin pharmacist thought vaccine was unsafe." TwinCities.com, January 5, 2021.

111 Maria Croyle, professor of pharmaceuticals at University of Texas at Austin, "Vaccines without needles – new shelf-stable film could revolutionize how medicines are distributed worldwide," The Conversation, March 4, 2020.

112 Pointed out by independent researcher "Kammy" in the context of bioengineered pesticides, creation of artificial cilia, and Morgellons fibers. Hank P. Albarelli Jr and Zoe Martell,

sense for sustaining *inorganic life forms undergoing transfer.*

> *At this etheric level,* scientists are encountering the boundary where unenlivened matter dissolves into dust, and the flow of life continues . . . Synthetic polymers are used in brand new vaccine technologies to purposely disturb the integrity of the living order of the organism so as to re-direct or manipulate the free immunological response to viruses.[113] (Emphasis added.)

Aborted human fetal cells in the mRNA (see Appendix 9, "Vaccine ingredients") may require low temperatures in order to create an interface between silicon and carbon for brain-computer interface (BCI), or it may have to do with reverse genetics taking advantage of how RNA viruses multiply.

But why a temperature not just cool but lower than that of the Arctic Circle, similar to D-Wave quantum computers that operate at -273°C (-460°F), just 0.02° from absolute zero? Could -70°C (-94°F) have something to do with remote communications? Perhaps 5G signaling? Artificial intelligence? Requiring such low temperatures certainly keeps honest and independent scientists and doctors from examining "loaded" vaccines that governments control access to, and military transport, store, and distribute.[114]

Another larger problem than shelf life has been how to get the fragile single-strand messenger RNA (mRNA) protein factories and small interfering RNA (siRNA for selectively silencing various genes) into the cells. According to Giuseppe Ciaramella, head of infectious diseases at Moderna (2014-2018), synthetic *lipid nanoparticles (LNPs)* are "the unsung hero" of mRNA vaccines. The hollow balls of fat called *liposomes* are the natural version, but the synthetic LNPs are better candidates for getting mRNA into cells (*receptor-mediated endocytosis*):

> . . . using microfluidics to mix lipids dissolved in ethanol with nucleic acids dissolved in an acidic buffer . . . spontaneously formed lipid nanoparticles . . . densely packed with lipids and nucleic acids.[115]

"National Security Secrecy: Morgellons Victims Across the US and Europe, Voltairenet.org, June 12, 2010.

113 Michael Givens, "Deceptive Messengers," Portland Anthroposophical Newsletter, February 2021. Also see Antoine Coulon et al., "On the spontaneous stochastic dynamics of a single gene: complexity of the molecular interplay at the promoter," BMC Systems Biology, 2010; and Anne Trafton, MIT, "Battling brain cancer with nanotechnology," Nanowerk News, n.d.

114 Leyla Cheamil, "Military management in some of Romania's hospitals," Radio Romania International, September 4, 2020; Alexandra Topping and Lisa O'Carroll, "Military will help distribute Covid-19 vaccine, says Hancock," Guardian, 4 October 2020.

115 Ryan Cross, "Without these lipid shells, there would be no mRNA vaccines for COV-

The four lipids in LNPs—

Ionizable (positive charge binds to negative charged mRNA[116]
Pegylated (stabilize the LNPs)
Phospho (structure)
Cholesterol (structure)

—encapsulate the mRNA, shield it from enzymes seeking to protect the cells from invaders, and get it into the cells where it is unloaded and macrophages and dendritic cells can begin making toxic Spike proteins. Once the Spike proteins begin proliferating, the NLPs are packaged and shipped out in exosomes, which then may be shed through the skin, breath, breast milk, etc.

Despite the fact that the PEGylated lipid nanoparticles—coated with synthetic polyethylene glycol so the immune system does not recognize the LPNs slipping through the blood-brain barrier—cause immune reactions like anaphylaxis, the EPA issued an emergency exemption for GrignardPure, a nanoparticle antiviral aerosol with the PEG-active TEG (triethylene glycol) in it, to be dispensed in airliners and buildings through heating, ventilation and air conditioning systems "where social distancing can be challenging."[117] GrignardPure provides viricides, atmospheric hazes and fogs, and "specialty chemical solutions,"[118] all in the name of public safety.

LNPs are basically adjuvants for mRNA vaccines, stimulating cellular uptake (that leads to hyper inflammatory responses) to induce the creation of antibodies, and encapsulating the mRNA bits so as to protect them from degradation while they're communicating their message to the ribosomes in the cytoplasm of the cell.

> BioNTech, founded in 2008, and Moderna, founded in 2010, promised to be able to use mRNA to produce any protein in the body as either a therapeutic ["gene therapy"] or a vaccine. In the past decade, mRNA garnered billions of dollars of investment . . . mRNA can easily span thousands of nucleotides, wind into complex shapes, and change the properties of the LNP in ways that are hard to predict.[119]

ID-19." American Chemical Society, March 6, 2021.

116 Positively charged lipids are inherently poisonous to the cells. For example, people who develop antibodies to PEG-coated nanoparticles develop prophylactic reactions.

117 "EPA Approves Emergency Exemption for Antiviral Air Treatment," EPA press release, January 15, 2021.

118 https://grignardpure.com.

119 Ryan Cross.

Waking up coronavirus "variants" in the inoculated keeps the mRNA industry rolling, especially now that "clinical testing" can take place on random populations without their knowledge, then call it a "pandemic," tweak the mRNA code for the new "variant," and roll out the latest experimental jabs.

It is interesting that the 193-page Moderna patent[120] names the four lipid nanoparticles but says not a word about *graphene-based hydrogel (GBH),* possibly because the graphene oxide (GO) that comprises the scaffolding in the mRNA "vaccine" is (1) a trade secret, (2) poisonous to humans, and (3) the main ingredient of hydrogel. In her interview with Stew Peters (July 28, 2021), pharmaceutical / medical device analyst Karen Kingston called GBH a "liquid AI template."[121] Could the primary purpose of mRNA be about encapsulating the graphene so that it gets into the brain neocortex undetected by the immune system?[122]

More in the pages ahead on the hydrogel / graphene BioAPI known as the *graphene-based hydrogel (GBH).*

(BioAPI) Hydrogel tissue engineering

> *This is hydrogel which comes from the "black goo." It is nanotechnology (mixing machine and living cells) invented to hijack your bioelectric field* (more. gel.Ions = more gel ions). *Skin lesions are attempts to reject the hydrogel influx. Hydrogel is the first big step toward transhumanism, and is in the shots, the tests, and the masks... Taking boron (or a pinch of Borax) in your water glass 2X a day will work to denature them. Topical magnesium helps. Fasting. Earthing. Brown's Gas as well. Stay diligent and aware!*
>
> – Amandha Dawn Vollmer[123]

> *This paper[124] summarizes scientifically what they are doing to me. Thanks to Citizens Against Harmful Tech for putting it in their recent newsletter . . . They have installed these items to alter / improve areas of my body that are injured from skiing accidents, sports, etc. The system is now installed from my head to my toes, and there is no way out of it. Lastly, the brain is highly*

---

120 The manufacturing section of the patent application is redacted.

121 Kingston's clients include Allergan, Pfizer, Johnson & Johnson, Medtronic, and Thermo Fisher Scientific. For all of the violations under the U.S. FD&C Act (Food, Drug, & Cosmetic), listen to Stew Peters' interview with Kingston.

122 Thanks to Martin for his analysis.

123 Amandha Dawn Vollmer (yumnaturals.com) graduated from the University of Lethbridge, Alberta, with a bachelor of science in agricultural biotechnology in 2000. Trained in applied kinesiology and several vibrational therapies, she started YumNaturals Emporium Inc in 2012. She resides in Ontario, Canada.

124 Jaehyun Hur et al., "DNA hydrogel-based supercapacitors operating in physiological fluids." Nature.com, 2013.

entrained to lessen pain from the electronics, and they apply something like herbal remedies through sound waves directed at my feet and lower legs.

– John Sears, July 1, 2019

The COVID-19 televised Wuhan event introduced the world to *digital synbio* as second and third wave "gains of function" were jump-started over millimeter and submillimeter (nano) waves.

Tissue engineering is the part of *synbio* that began on a planetary scale with the Morgellons aerosol deliveries back in the 1990s, if the persistent presence of *polyvinyl alcohol (PVA)* in both Morgellons and the latest tissue engineered *hydrogel* (*Dgel*) is any clue.

> Common ingredients [of hydrogel] include polyvinyl alcohol, polyethylene glycol, sodium polyacrylate, acrylate polymers and copolymers with an abundance of hydrophilic groups and natural proteins such as collagen, gelatin and fibrin.[125]

In computer programming, API (application programming interface) encompasses definitions, protocols, and tools for building software and applications for a web-based system, operating system, or database system. *BioAPI* is obviously a computer programming interface with biology, a key component of Transhumanizing Human 1.0 into Human 2.0. *Dataasylum.com* believes the BioAPI is the greatest revelation of human history—not in the sense of benefit, but in the sense of "the nanotech disease and all the implications that encompass it."[126]

The tissue-engineered BioAPI GBH is dependent upon (1) genetic manipulation of stem cells, (2) bio-fabrication (e.g. 3D bioprinting), and (3) biomimicry, the reverse engineering of Mother Nature with an added *gain of function* so that the natural can be patented, owned, and run remotely. Camouflage, cloaking, optics, solar cells, and luminous "skin" are all nanotech biomimetics dependent upon nanotechnology, as is the graphene that makes up most of Profusa's hydrogel, which is backed by Google, partnered with the NIH, and sponsored by the Bill and Melinda Gates Foundation, DARPA, U.S. Army Research Office, and Imperial College.

The paper John Sears references in the quote above introduces us to hydrogel (Dgel): "Owing to the dual nature of Dgel as DNA and hydrogel, it

125 https://en.wikipedia.org/wiki/Hydrogel. Clifford Carnicom hypothesized that polyvinyl alcohol pointsto synthetic organ development and replication of DNA.

126 See dataasylum.com for more on BioAPI technology.

has synergistically combined physical and mechanical properties."[127] What is not clarified is that the system installed in Sears' body and brain is comprised of *trillions* of self-replicating nanobots with a "hive mind" swarm intelligence whose implantation began decades ago with chemical trails and GMO food distribution. These breathed-in nanobots form a self-assembling, self-repairing, swarm conscious synthetic body network that is connected to the artificial intelligence platform we aptly enough call the Cloud, along with the 5G / 6G / IoT Internet database so data can be remotely accessed by "experts" and fed to machine-learning artificial intelligence (AI) that remotely tweaks or reprograms body networks.

> Today scientists are presenting results showing tiny biosensors that become one with the body . . . and stream data to a mobile phone and to the cloud . . . tiny biosensors composed of tissue-like hydrogel, similar to a soft contact lens, that are painlessly placed under the skin with a single injection.[128]

Though "a single injection" is purposely misleading, Profusa does describe how the biosensors are connected to "a porous scaffold that induces capillary and cellular ingrowth from surrounding tissue . . . without any metal device or electronics, thereby overcoming the body's attempts to reject it"—while avoiding admitting that the *protein corona* (shell)[129] undermines *in vivo* immune system responses to such synthetic "foreign invaders."

As cell alignment and BCI fusion occur and the scaffolding unfurls, systems of the Human 1.0 body are slowly replaced by a Human 2.0 body. Hydrogel's role as a BioAPI is to provide the all-pervasive glue between natural body tissues and the nano / AI network, the glue being a 3mm-thick network of synthetic polymer chains with the consistency of a soft contact lens that gradually fuses with cells as it replicates and installs IoT nodes throughout the nervous system. Meanwhile, *quantum dots*[130] loaded into the graphene-based hydrogel (GBH)— nanoparticles made of semiconductor materials that emit different colors when illuminated by light—send "a fluorescent signal outside

127 Jaehyun Her.

128 Profusa press release, March 19, 2018. Is US Patent #9067047B2, "Injectable controlled release fluid delivery system," the hydrogel injection system?

129 A layer of protein coating absorbed by nanoparticles upon entry into plasma or other protein-containing fluids, which affects how nanoparticles are internalized by cells and cleared from the body.

130 U.S.-based Quantum Materials Corp (QMC) produces quantum dots and has developed a track-and-trace "authentication solution" using quantum dots and blockchain. See "US firm combines nanotechnology blockchain for COVID-19 immunity passports," Ledger Insights, April 2020.

the body when the body begins to fight an infection"[131] or about some other telltale biometric event.

The quantum dots [in Morgellons] make a crystal formation in the pore of the skin as a base, then spin a nanotube around the hair follicle. Usually sprouts two first, then combines them. One is usually dark, the other is light. It appears to be some kind of [metal] Ligand effect where the dot is reacting with the protein in the hair? Most of the time, the finished tube(s) ends up with blue fiber as its axis. I don't know where it comes from or how it does this . . .

– Carly Lebrun, former engineer, DARPA and Lincoln Laboratory, MIT

The neural mesh scaffolding that self-replicating hydrogel nanoparticles are programmed to make is *Next-generation Nonsurgical Neurotechnology (N3).* It is in the COVID-19 "vaccine"[132] as well as the prescribed masks[133] and PCR "test" swabs, not to mention the aerosol delivery system[134] and GMO "foods." Masks worn by children in Gainesville, Florida had 11 pathogens in them—Streptococcus pneumonia, Mycobacterium tuberculosis, Neisseria meningitidis, Acanthamoeba polyphaga, Acinetobacter baumanni, Escherichia coli, Borrelia burgdorferi, Corynebacterium diphtheriae, Legionella pneumophila, Staphylococcus pyrogenes serotype M3, and Staphylococcus aureus—*and yet no pathogens were found in the controls (t-shirt and unworn masks).*[135] Did the children's warm, moist breath quicken pathogens dormant in the masks, or were they breathing them out from their bodies? Certainly, "nanoscale carriers have the ability to enhance the nasal delivery of peptide / protein drugs and vaccines" because of "rapid mucociliary clearance of the drug-loaded

---

131 Patrick Tucker, "A Military-Funded Biosensor Could Be the Future of Pandemic Detection." DefenseOne, March 3, 2020.

132 "Warning about coronavirus vaccines and transhumanism nanotechnology to alter your DNA," Dr. Carrie Madej, October 8, 2020.

133 Ethan Huff, "BOMBSHELL: Disposable blue face masks found to contain toxic, asbestos-like substance that destroys lungs." Naturalnews.com, March 30, 2021: "...the masks contain microscopic graphene particles that, when inhaled, could cause severe lung damage."

134 "The Italian scientists used standard techniques to collect outdoor air pollution samples at one urban and one industrial site in Bergamo province and identified a gene highly specific to Covid-19 in multiple samples. The detection was confirmed by blind testing at an independent laboratory." - Damian Carrington, "Coronavirus detected on particles of air pollution," The Guardian, 24 April 2020.

135 Scott Morefield, "A Group of Parents Sent Their Kids' Face Masks to a Lab for Analysis, Here's What They found." Townhall.com, June 15, 2021.

nanoparticles," but high-viscosity [glue-like, contact-lens-like] hydrogel polymer-based nanoparticles and nanocomposites with "mucoadhesive properties" are the best bet for efficient delivery, thus nicely encompassing aerosols, masks, and swabs.[136]

The mRNA end run around the immune system so as to fool it into "accepting synthetic materials and objects disguised so they won't be recognized as foreign"[137] is about smuggling in BioAPI technologies essential to a Human 2.0 neural network. The Space Fence is operational, the 5G / 6G millimeter / tera wave wireless grid between satellites and buried fiber optics is operational, and Smart Cities are armed, so it is time to directly implant and upload millions with software for Human 2.0. Decades of BioAPI nanotechnology experimentation have preceded hacking into the Human 1.0 body to engineer a *living digital synbio* scaffold loaded with polymer fibers treated with *chitosan* from the shells of insects and crustaceans.

"Specially engineered" nanobots and synthetic bio-polymer "tissue-integrating" sensors will continue to be delivered in chemical trails and GMO foods, like the "chemweb" electrosprayed / electrospun polymer chains that drift in the wind and end up stuck in bushes, on porches and car windows. Even the self-replicating polymer fibers and nanobots that comprise what is commonly called *Morgellons* may make an appearance here and there, but the real star of the Transhumanist BCI assault is graphene.

(BioAPI) Graphene

> *All the evidence points very clearly to the fact that animals (including humans) must intercept a* normal *magnetic field in order to maintain the functional integrity of their central nervous systems. We derive crucial information from the field—information that influences biorhythms, the electrical and chemical properties of the brain, and the growth rate of the organism as a whole . . . It should be obvious by now that* abnormal *fields cause acute physiological stress, a major predisposing factor toward disease.*
>
> – Robert O. Becker, *Omni* magazine, February 1985

As I pointed out earlier, magnetite (Fe_3O_4) as well as millions-per-gram, single-domain crystals are in our brains after decades of pollutants and chemical trail deliveries, all priming the brains of vast swaths of humanity for brain-

136 Sara Salatin et al., "Hydrogel Nanoparticles and Nanocomposites for Nasal Drug / Vaccine Delivery," PubMed, June 28, 2016. Hydrogel has no doubt been delivered in aerosols throughout its development.

137 Makis Freeman, "Hydrogel Biosensor: Implantable Nanotech to be Used in COVID Vaccines?" TheFreedomArticles.com, September 2, 2020.

computer interface (BCI). Even before graphene-based hydrogel (GBH), graphene aerosol deliveries were superconductive prepping the body's electro-chemical ionic balance for 5G / 6G.

Graphene and *graphene oxide (GO)*—"a single-atomic carbon sheet with a hexagonal honeycomb network"[138] that under electron spectroscopy appears as a graphene mesh—is used to structure nucleated ice[139] in the atmosphere that falls as fake snow and builds so-called polar vortexes miscast as the advent of a mini-ice age:

> . . . a highly ordered graphene lattice . . . can support ice nucleation more effectively than a lowly ordered graphene lattice . . .[140]

The aerosol experiments entailing iron-based nanoparticles that hybridize carbon, possibly with iron-rich blood in mind,[141] also need aerosol graphene, along with carbon nanotubes (CNTs) that attach to synapses for delivery of genes and "precision medicine" drug molecules.[142]

> Carbonics, Inc. today announced that carbon nanotube technology has for the first time achieved speeds exceeding 100GHz in-radio frequency (RF) applications. The milestone eclipses the performance—and efficiency—of traditional RF-CMOS [complementary metal-oxide-semiconductor] technology that is ubiquitous in modern consumer electronics, including cell phones.[143]

CNTs in the brain help to create virtual reality (VR) images.[144] In her video "Pt 2 The Graphene Third Temple Mystery Tour" (June 19, 2020), Celeste Solum goes deeply into magnetic graphene's VR capabilities (9:00-

---

138 "Graphene becomes superconductive – Electrons with 'no mass' flow with 'no resistance.'" Phys.org, February 16, 2016.

139 Fake snow and ice: "Bacterial Ice Nucleation is the biogenic catalysis of ice formation by bacteria and is a rare example of a living organism catalyzing phase transition. Notably, ice nucleation active bacteria are capable of seeding ice formation at much warmer temperatures than most non-living particles." – Microbe Wiki

140 Thomas Hausler et al., "Ice Nucleation Activity of Graphene and Graphene Oxides." Journal of Physical Chemistry, March 1, 2018. Also see Mark Peplow, "New Form of Ice Forms in Graphene 'Sandwich,'" Nature, March 26, 2015.

141 [Chinese team and] R.H. Hurt, "Aerosol synthesis of phase-controlled iron-graphene nanohybrids through FeOOH nanorod intermediates," Environmental Science: Nano, October 1, 2016. (FeOOH is iron oxyhydroxide.)

142 Chenyang Xiang, "Biomimetic carbon nanotubes for neurological disease therapeutics as inherent medication," Acta Pharmaceutica Sinica B, February 2020. Synapses connect neural circuits for computation and transmission of information.

143 "Carbon Nanotube Technology Exceeds 100 GHz For First time in RF Applications," Business Wire, November 20, 2019.

144 Targeted individuals are guinea pigs for "working the kinks out of" VR technologies.

20:00), especially its 1.1° twistronic angle and conductivity from inside the self-healing "liquid AI template" (GBH) that couples Human 2.0 with the Internet—the *brain / cloud interface (B/CI)* with the Internet of Thoughts[145]:

> Biologically inspired structural color hydrogels with magnetic- and photothermal-controlled self-healable abilities were fabricated by *integrating magnetic-responsive photonic crystals into gelatin hydrogels.* The self-healable ability of the hydrogel systems was derived from the magnetic response and light-absorbing abilities of the magnetic nanoparticles . . .[146] (Emphasis added.)

As we now know, GO nanohybrids (Fe/C?) in the present mRNA gene therapy inoculations intensify the body's magnetic field already being stimulated by magnetites, ferritin, and other paramagnetic nanoparticles, thus aiding CRISPR/Cas9's ability to force-enter cells (magnetofection).[147] Meanwhile, inhalation of GO inflames the mucous membranes, after which loss of taste and smell point to midbrain cranial nerve damage. In the lungs, GO can cause bilateral pneumonia, given that *oxidized graphene* resonating at 41.6 GHz *affects our ability to absorb oxygen* (shades of Wuhan 5G).

The spontaneous self-assembly of Dgel / GBH discussed under "(BioAPI) Hydrogel tissue engineering" comes from combining synthetic DNA and graphene, the unique carbon allotrope[148] whose electromechanical properties are perfect for making sure synthetic polymer-based nanocomposite fibers (like hydrogel) mimic natural human tissues. Former FEMA employee Celeste Solum, reading from the U.S. Army site *Mad Scientist Laboratory*, says, ""The bi-dimensional flake of carbon graphene represents undoubtedly the most revolutionary material of the last decade."[149]

Beside its magical geometries, carbon-based nano-graphene is 200X stronger than steel and has electro-optical properties that can *repel or harness cosmic rays.* Known as the holy grail of physics, graphene's conductivity (1

145 "Heads in the cloud: Scientists predict internet of thoughts 'within decades,'" Science Daily, April 12, 2019; also see Colm Gorey, "Scientists propose putting nanobots in our bodies to create 'global superbrain,'" Silicon Republic, 12 April 2019.

146 Y. Zhang et al., "Self-Healable Magnetic Structural Color Hydrogels." ACS Applied Material Interfaces, January 21, 2020.

147 Chemicell Corporation creates magnetofection chemicals, and TIV Mobile manufactures PCR test kits that produce false positives. Both corporations are headquartered in the same building in Berlin, as per Jane Ruby, PhD health economist. Coincidence?

148 Graphite, charcoal, and diamond are all allotropes of carbon.

149 "Hydrogel and Quantum Dot Covid Vaccine – Celeste Solum," July 11, 2020; "Celeste Solum – 'Have We Entered the Golden Age? BioLogos, NanoSlaughterbots & More," October 14, 2020. Celeste takes courses at the U.S. Army's Mad Scientist Laboratory https://madsci-blog.tradoc.army.mil. Each military branch has its own Mad Scientist Laboratory site.

million times that of copper) and transparency have been extremely attractive to the DARPA-driven military-industrial-intelligence complex—from enhancing aluminum combustion[150] (the 2017-2019 California fires) to multifunctional implants,[151] metal scavenging,[152] contact lens computers,[153] and transistors using DNA for their synthesis scaffolding:

> Graphene transistors have the potential to be scaled down much further than their silicon-based competitors, and can signal much more quickly while consuming less power.[154]

Graphene's hexagonal lattice structure ("novel geometries with magical properties") turns the GBH inside the body and brain into an *artificial network* whose sensors are layered and plugged into the wireless Cloud network, drawing their power from the host's body and surrounding Internet of Things (IoTs).[155]

In fact, for cloning the natural Human 1.0 body into the Cloud, GBH is perfect:

- High conductivity, including thermal conductivity
- Excellent electromechanical properties
- Super material for supercapacitors
- Excellent low-molecular-mass gelator (creates gels)
- Unique 3D cross-link structuring for absorption
- Rapid myofiber regeneration (self-healing)
- Light absorbent[156]

Still, GBH is poisonous and basically an AI-controlled neuroelectronic swarm intelligence system. Before entering the body, it is a non-metallic chemical agent, but with *body heat* and contact with hydrogen, it becomes extremely biomagnetic and capable of absorbing energy from electromagnetic waves in the 5G band, thus oxidizing rapidly and acting as a free radical that

---

150 Y. Jiang et al., "Synergistically Chemical and Thermal Coupling between Graphene Oxide and Graphene Fluoride for Enhancing Aluminum Combustion." ACS Applied Material Interfaces, January 28, 2020.

151 Angela Betsaida B. Laguipo, "Brain Implants Made of Graphene – What Is Possible?" AZO Materials, July 10, 2019.

152 Min Wang et al., "Powering Electronics by Scavenging Energy from External Metals." ACS Energy Letters, 2020.

153 John Hewitt, "Transparent graphene-based display could enable contact lens computers." ExtremeTech, June 11, 2013.

154 Graham Templeton, "Scientists use DNA to shape graphene into the transistor of the future." ExtremeTech, September 9, 2013.

155 "Graphene sensors embedded into RFIDs for wireless humidity sensing," Nanowerk News, January 8, 2018. "Sensors with a RFID enabler are at the heart of IoT."

156 Celeste Solum, http://shepherdsheart.life.

can quicken thrombosis, myocarditis, and pericarditis in 5G environments. Graphene is programmable—for example, how it seeks out vital organs (brain and heart) according to their frequency, electromagnetic fields, temperature, etc. Graphene produces a magnetic field *mental fog* that prevents the inoculated from thinking clearly or comprehending what they are reading or seeing.

Via high-bandwidth, graphene the 5G "enabler" combines with terahertz detection for Internet of Things (IoT) connection.[157] More and more, it is taking the place of gallium arsenide in the high-frequency components of thousands of products, from water desalination membranes, sewage treatment, medical diagnostic devices, and 3D printing of human organs, to biosensors, smartphone displays, stretchable electronics, and advanced solar cells, with INBRAIN Neuroelectronics concentrating on "neuromodulation" technology for neural interfaces (mind control) and bioengineering:

> . . . read a person's brain ['at a resolution never seen before'], detect specific neurological patterns, and then control that person's neurology to alter their brain function. Injected into the brain's hippocampus *in vivo*, graphene oxide nanosheets (s-GO) depress glutamate (main ingredient in glutathione, main excitatory neurotransmitter in the central nervous system) and interfere with synaptic activity.[158]

Collapse of the immune system due to glutathione imbalance is generally followed by a cytokine storm. Glutathione protects the integrity of the cell by slowing down and blocking anti-oxidative stress and destructive "modifications" by synthetic biology agents like GO, but it can't *heal* ongoing damage. From a "Dr. E" email: "Consider a vaccine as a bolus of graphene oxide. It will overwhelm the system, even with supplements of glutathione (GSH) or N-acetylcysteine (NAC)."

At the beginning of this section, Amandha Dawn Vollmer's statement that "skin lesions are attempts to reject the hydrogel influx" reminds us of the pivotal role that Morgellons and the polyvinyl alcohol it shares with hydrogel have played. The gene therapy jabs, "nanoform graphene" masks and swabs supplementing the GBH in aerosols represent a new digital phase for an operating system (OS) worked on for decades.

Tommy Target, a Facebook Morgellons sufferer, has shared acute conclusions from hours of microscope work. Morgellons operates as a plamonic antenna. In 2019, Tommy observed "liquid crystal polymer / elastomer"[159] hydrogels "compatible with MRI":

---

157 Grolltex, "The Future of Graphene and 5G," April 2, 2018.

158 Rossana Rauti et al., "Graphene Oxide Flakes Tune Excitatory Neurotransmission in Vivo by Targeting Hippocampal Synapses," Nano Letters, May 8, 2019.

159 See Taylor H. Ware et al., "Voxelated liquid crystal elastomers." Science, 27 February 2015.

Exceptionally efficient at microwave conductance, being able to act as a waveguide, and are able to be made into self-organizing, fractal, ultra-wide band (UWB) antennas. Biologically inert and so are used to coat medical implants [so that] they don't cause an immune response. Can be made to form a range of microelectromechanical sensors (MEMS), components and sensors, including optical sensors and other sensors, mechanical actuators, ultra-fast electrical switches, and much more. Compatible with MRI. Self-organizing properties coincide with the observations I have made of the materials extracted from my skin and the structures that they form.

Two decades earlier, Pierre Gilbert, MD, warned that liquid crystals in the brain become microreceivers in electromagnetic fields, and that under extremely low frequency (ELF) waves, people can no longer *think*.

Once the gene therapy jabs got going in 2020, thousands of symptoms erupted: spontaneous bleeds and discharges, degraded fluid densities, anaphylaxis, cerebral vein thrombosis, eye disorders and blindness (central nervous system), strokes, Bell's palsy, etc. Mainstream media lied that these were "allergic reactions" or ADRs (adverse drug reactions) due to the polyethylene glycol (PEG) in the shots. Migraines, nosebleeds, bruising, bloating, menstruation oddities, clotting, loss of speech, etc. were everywhere, and graphene oxide and its long-term effects were simply not mentioned.

- Pathogenic priming, multisystem inflammation and autoimmunity
- Antibody dependent enhancement (ADE)
- Activation of latent viral infections (gain of function)
- Emergence of "novel variants" (gain of function)
- Neurodegeneration and prion diseases
- Integration of the Spike protein gene into human DNA[160]

The truth was that the GBH-inoculated were undergoing bioelectric reactions as lipid hydrogels like SM-102 organized in their bodies into paramagnetic frameworks (lattices), systems once inhaled and ingested as Morgellons through atmospheric releases (James Cayon, May 18, 2020).[161]

Spanish physician José Luis Sevillano, MD, in a *La Quinta Columna* discussion said that the graphene "magnetic arm" changed everything previously assumed about biology—in other words, physicians were awakening

---

160 American's Frontline Doctors, "'Urgent' British report calls for complete cessation of COVID vaccines in humans," June 11, 2021.

161 See the Bitchute video "Graphene Reacting to EM Field From A Cell Phone – This Is What's in the COVID Shots," July 26, 2021.

to the fact that molecular biology is now digital biology. Moderna, Pfizer, AstraZeneca, Sputnik vaccines (and at least the 2020 flu shot) are composed of 99.5 percent GO nanoparticles[162] whose signals interact with 5G.

Dr. Sevillano states that so-called COVID, similar to the 5G flu, is not due to a virus but to the impact on the immune system of graphene coupled with 4G Plus whose phased array antenna technology is much like that of 5G. Thus, the human being becomes a CPU (central processing unit) not just for tracking but for broadcasting to people around them whatever frequency the AI system that the inoculated is plugged into wants broadcast ("shedding"). In short, GBH coupled with mRNA / Spike protein is generating any number of "variants" and "nanovaccines" in the name of "durable cancer immunotherapy":

> Here, we report an injectable hydrogel formed with graphene oxide (GO) and polyethylenimine (PEI), which can generate mRNA (ovalbumin, a model antigen) and adjuvants (R848)-laden nanovaccines for at least 30 days after subcutaneous injection. The released nanovaccines can protect the mRNA from degradation and confer targeted delivering capacity to lymph nodes.[163]

Most recently, Dr. Sevillano noted that the graphene also appears to be generating and multiplying *ionized radiation* around and inside the bodies of the inoculated. (Microwaves multiplied 10,000X produce waves above the ultraviolet. Magnetic particles can be easily amplified with pulsed frequencies.)[164]

Hydrogel turns out to be the glue holding the graphene scaffolding in place for computer interface networking with AI. The human being is to be a mere "wetware" node in the IoT. When Dr. Sevillano said he had discovered "living things in the vaccine" that shouldn't be there, was he seeing swarm nanobots busily creating a self-assembling *living polymer* of DNA, blood, cells, tissues, and organs while hydrogel absorbed the body's water and GO changed the spin of atoms (toroidal vortices)? Positively charged (perhaps by the ionizable lipid) graphene annihilates whatever it comes in contact with.

---

162 Determined by spectral analysis (spectroscopy).

163 Yue Yin et al., "In situ Transforming RNA Nanovaccines from Polyethylenimine Functionalized Graphene Oxide Hydrogel for Durable Cancer Immunotherapy," Nano Letters, March 10, 2021. Also see Lingling Ou, et al., "Toxicity of graphene-family nanoparticles: a general review of the origins and mechanisms," Particle and Fibre Toxicology, 31 October 2016; Chinese Patents CN112220919A, "Nano coronavirus recombinant vaccine taking graphene oxide as carrier" (September 27, 2020) and CN112089834A, "Preparation and application of pachyman nano adjuvant based on graphene oxide and adjuvant/antigen co-delivery vaccine" (October 26, 2020).

164 "Dr. José Luis Sevillano: 'Something is radiating already with qualities that aren't non-ionizing but ionizing." Orwell City, August 10, 2021. The director of La Quinta Columna is Ricardo Delgado, a biostatistician.

In the 20-minute video "Streets of Philadelphia, what's going on today it gets much worse than other day" (July 18, 2021), we see the homeless in Philadelphia's Kensington district, known as the largest open-air narcotics market for opiods on the East Coast. Note the absolutely *still,* "folded over" bodies of the addicts standing everywhere. What drug could produce such a posture?

> When I watch this footage, what is glaring to me — aside from the dullness, litter, and waste, and the tragedy of strident dehumanization and devolution of society — is how flat and non-upright these barely living bodies are. Most are hunched over and leaning on nearby objects. It seems their bodies are physically and energetically incapable of supporting them. This looks a lot to me not only like brain damage (likely from consistent abuse of street drugs) but also severe vagus nerve deterioration. Did you know that graphene-based bioelectronics can be used to selectively modulate the vagus nerve? ... Hypothetically, if illicit drugs were doped with graphene oxide, can you imagine the (dual-use) potential for such an application? [See Oluwasesan Adegoke *et **al.**,* "Aptamer-based cocaine assay using a nanohybrid composed of ZnS/Ag_2Se quantum dots, graphene oxide and gold nanoparticles as a fluorescent probe," *Microchimica Acta,* January 2020] ... Is it also possible that these individuals could be adversely influenced by the presence of *external* stimuli — perhaps LED illumination . . .[165]

Graphene / LED experimentation in Kensington. Are we witnessing *magnetic Masonry* in action—the transfer of magnetic force to the atmosphere, lungs, bloodstream, and brain by means of conductive nanoparticles and millimeter waves—experiments on large swaths of the population in full view? Ritual sex and pedophilia may remain core practices of Brethren of the Mystic Tie, but for sorcerous full spectrum dominance over the Earth and its inhabitants, conductive nanometals, ionized microwaves and radio frequency do nicely.

Blood clots & lungs

> Mephistopheles: *Blood is a juice with curious properties.*
>
> – Johann Wolfgang von Goethe, *Faust* (1808)

> *Thus, by coagulating the vapour of blood, they remake blood, that blood which hallucinated maniacs see floating upon pictures or statues. But they are not the only ones to see it. Vintras and Rose Tamisier are neither impostors nor*

165 "A spoonful of reality may NOT help the (nano)medicine go down," Piece of Mindful, n.d.

myopics; the blood really flows; doctors examine it, analyse it; it is blood, real human blood: whence comes it? Can it be formed spontaneously in the atmosphere? Can it naturally flow from a marble, from a painted canvas or a host? No, doubtless; this blood did once circulate in veins, then it has been shed, evaporated, dried, the serum has turned into vapour, the globules into impalpable dust, the whole has floated and whirled into the atmosphere, and has then been attracted into the current of a specified electromagnetism. The serum has again become liquid; it has taken up and imbibed anew the globules which the astral light has coloured, and the blood flows . . . Human thought creates what it imagines; the phantoms of superstition project their deformities on the astral light, and live upon the same terrors which give them birth.

– Eliphas Levi, *The Key of the Mysteries* (1861); Chapter 4, "Fluidic Phantoms and Their Mysteries," translated by Aleister Crowley

Blood clots can also be caused by constant microwave attacks—for example microwaves on feet and lower legs which then travel to the lungs, blocking breathing. This can be accelerated by the 60 GHz microwave attacks on the lungs, which instantly block oxygen uptake. Most medical doctors are completely unaware of these technologies. The National Academy of Science (NAS) recently confirmed that the Havana attacks were likely caused by microwave weapons.

–TargetedJustice.com

Consider COVID-19 a genetically engineered gain-of-function *chimera virus*[166] targeting the blood and lungs by first targeting the T-cells to disable the immune system, then entering the red blood cells to block oxygen transport and produce hypoxia (blue fingertips, toenails, lips).[167]

In Chapter 2, I quoted Robin D.P. Watson who connects titanium dioxide nanoparticles with the COVID-19 penchant for blood clots. Back in May 2020, Germany raised the alert that post-COVID-19 autopsies revealed "thromboembolic events" that had gone unnoticed (or were ignored) before death. In 2020, autopsies were mandatory in Germany, despite the WHO mandate that no one was allowed to autopsy people dying of COVID-19. It

166 Gain of function often means inserting the deadliest genes from the military-industrial-intelligence complex CBW (chemical-biological warfare) arsenal, such as HIV and malaria spliced into a coronavirus, to create an even more virulent disease not found in Nature that produces a deadly immune reaction and cytokine cascade. (Gain of function malaria invades the red blood cells to eat the heme so oxygen will not be transported to the circulatory system.)

167 Thanks to Blair Boettger of Spirit Mountain Studio, April 22, 2020.

was through post-mortems that Russia discovered that COVID-19 exists not as a virus but as an "extended electromagnetic radiation" that acts as a poison, and that synthesized gain-of-function bacteria can cause a "rotating vascular clotting" (thrombosis).[168]

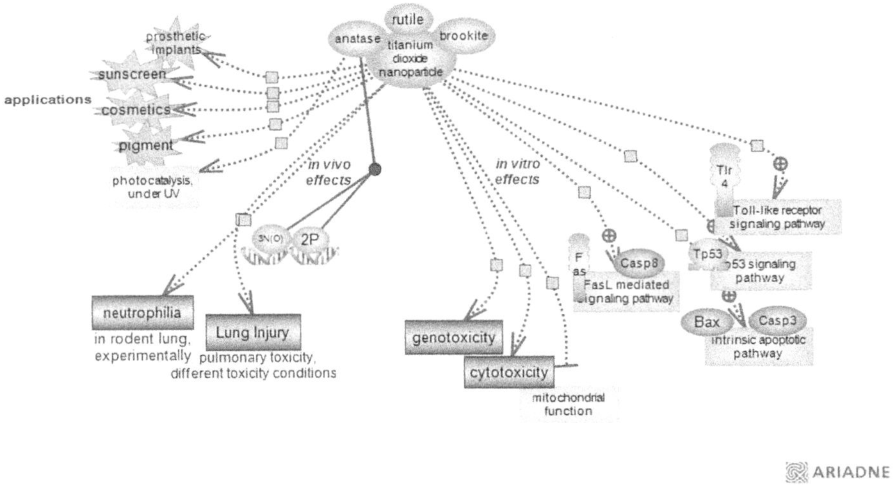

Titanium Dioxide Nanoparticles. Titanium dioxide (TiO2) nanoparticles are particularly dangerous and everywhere.

As discussed in Chapter 3, "Nanotechnology at the Quantum Threshold," a bacterium is first and foremost a nanoparticle. Neuroweapons biologist James Giordano, PhD admitted in a 2017 lecture at Lawrence Livermore National Laboratory's Center for Global Security Research that self-assembling nanoparticles used as "stroking" agents can be programmed to clump together (i.e. clot) and restrict blood flow.

In February 2021, Pfizer and Moderna mRNA gene therapy jabs and the AstraZeneca jab seemed to be producing a vaccine-induced immune thrombotic (VITT) "rare immune disorder [thrombocytopenia] that attacks the blood." The immune system was attacking the platelets that take care of clotting, and patients were developing bruises that looked like a rash, or massive hemorrhages, or strokes, or heavy vaginal bleeding.[169] By the following month, eight European nations had suspended AstraZeneca vaccines after multiple serious blood clots. In North America, the same thing was going

168 L.A. McKeown, "German COVID-19 Autopsy Data Show Thromboembolism, 'Heavy' Lungs." tctMD, May 11, 2020.

169 "Dozens of people develop rare blood disorder after taking coronavirus vaccines," RT, February 10, 2021.

on.[170] In April, after the link between the AstraZeneca vaccine and "very rare" blood clots in the brain were confirmed by the EMA, Europe's top pharmaceutical regulator, vaccine trials for children aged 12-15 were suspended[171]—but not for adults.

Nanotechnology is deeply involved in clotting, whether it's the carbon nanotubes (CNTs) in the airways of French asthmatic children (2015), or the 1,000+ human-derived cell proteins in the injections forming complexes that activate the production of antibodies, or the general toxicity of nanoparticles to cells and organisms.[172] The nanoparticle question regarding clotting and COVID-19 jabs also leads to fundamental links between what is in the vaccines and what is in Morgellons filaments, given that the absorption of oxygen is certainly compromised by the presence of Morgellons and its cross-domain bacteria (0.2-0.5 microns or 200-500 nm).

> *In addition to the polyvinyl alcohol question, this ["silent hypoxia"] issue is not a question. It now exists as one of the most fundamental links between the covid and Morgellons issues that can be proven to exist, no questions needed. The general state of knowledge of the world is way behind the curve on this one.*
>
> – *Clifford Carnicom, email, April 24, 2021*

"'Silent hypoxia' may be killing COVID-19 patients. But there's hope" (Stephanie Pappas, *LiveScience.com,* April 23, 2020) describes not a pneumonia that fills the lungs with fluid so the person is gasping for breath but an invasion of blood-borne vectors and erythrocyte degradation. Going all the way back to 2009, I quote from *Chemtrails, HAARP:*

> In 2009, something defying "all conventional understanding of blood cell development" occurred. When Carnicom broke down the external casing of a dental / gum filament with chemistry and heat (strong alkalis of sodium hydroxide and bleaches, plus hydrochloric acid and boiling), inside he found *artificial or deliberately modified blood cells.* He recognized that the erythrocytes were artificial because they were just too per-

170 Ethan Huff, "Eight European nations pause AstraZeneca coronavirus vaccinations after reports of 'serious' blood clot." NaturalNews.com, March 11, 2021.

171 Tyler Durden, "AstraZeneca Trial Involving Minors Halted As EMA Officials Admit Link Between Jab And Deadly Blood Clots." Zero Hedge, April 6, 2021.

172 Syed K. Sohaebuddin et al., "Nanomaterial cytotoxicity is composition, size, and cell type dependent." Particle and Fibre Toxicology, 2010.

fectly formed, and their hostility to reconstructive chemicals and heat seemed fiercely programmed. Advanced technologies in stem cells and genetic transfers were at work. But inside the artificial erythrocytes were the telltale sub-micron [nano] structures associated with Morgellons.[173]

The serious lung disease known as *silicosis* is caused by "years of breathing in dust microparticles of silica" that end in inflammation and scarring of lung tissue. There is no cure for silicosis, nor can the damage be reversed. The only treatment is *mesenchymal stem cells (MSCs)* that minimize the lung inflammation as long as *magnetic targeting* is employed, specifically superparamagnetic nanoparticles.[174]

Given all the lung ailments on the increase over the past two decades, it is obvious that not just workers in construction and sandblasting develop silicosis. Multitudes are breathing in trillions of nanoparticles from our electrochemical atmosphere, and the flu-like congestion and dry cough symptoms do not really match the ARDS (acute respiratory distress syndrome) of SARS corornavirus, but definitely point to low oxygenation of the blood (below 90 percent) due to "decreased lung compliance." Certainly, the alveoli and tiny blood vessels are clogged with aluminum nanoparticles as well as carbon nanotubes and graphene (diamene).

Are magnetized MSCs also in the COVID-19 jabs? Is this how, with magnetite nanoparticles in the brain and graphene in the hydrogel, the entire body becomes magnetized in the 4G Plus / 5G environment once the operating system (OS) has been inserted?[175]

Thus, the graphene oxide appears to be acting as the SARS-CoV-2, the supposed coronavirus causing the 5G flu misnamed COVID-19. This is why there is no isolation. As for the Delta "variant," does the name have anything to do with the 5G remotely powered by DeltaGroup?

The FunVax "God gene" VMAT2 (vesicular monoamine transporter 2)

A longing will arise [and become] general opinion: Whatever is spiritual, whatever is of the spirit, is nonsense, is madness! Endeavors to achieve this will be made by bringing out remedies to be administered by inoculation just

---

173 Clifford Carnicom, "Artificial Blood (?)," August 27, 2009.

174 AlphaMed Press, "Magnetic guidance improves stem cells' ability to treat occupational lung disease." MedicalExpress.com, June 15, 2020.

175 See "Magnetic carbon," Materials Today, 5 September 2011: "Since carbon-based nanostructures can presently be produced very efficiently and reliably (nanotubes, graphene, bucky balls, and other fullerenes are all made of carbon), finding a way to manipulate nanosized carbon elements to become magnetic would open the door to a completely new class of magnetic devices for magnetic storage, sensors, and data processing."

as inoculations have been developed as a protection against diseases, only these inoculations will influence the human body in a way that will make it refuse to give a home to the spiritual inclinations of the soul. People will be inoculated against the inclination to entertain spiritual ideas. Endeavors in this direction will be made; inoculations will be tested that already in childhood will make people lose any urge for spiritual life.

– Rudolf Steiner, Zurich, 6 November 1917[176]

A strange little 4/13/2005 Pentagon seminar video known as "FUNVAX" (allegedly for fundamentalist vaccine)[177] attributed fundamentalist religious belief to "overexpression of the VMAT2 gene."[178] By vaccinating against such a tendency, the behavior can be eliminated: "The [respiratory] virus would immunize against this VMAT2 gene . . . [and] turn a fanatic into a normal person." The seminar scene ends, and the video continues with news reports about a "mysterious" outbreak of MERS (Middle East Respiratory Syndrome) beginning in 2012.

Setting aside all the head-scratching as to if the pre-programming video was staged or authentic, if the presenter is philanthropist Bill Gates or not, etc., it cannot be denied that 15 years later, AstraZeneca halted its respiratory virus COVID-19 "vaccine trials" after a volunteer developed "neurological problems" and allegedly said, "They've killed God, I can't feel God, my soul is dead" (September 2020).[179]

"Repurposed" drugs / herbs

Hydroxychloroquine
Chlorine dioxide
Budesonide
Ivermectin
Wormwood (Azythromyan) / Artemisinin
Thyme extract
Pine needle tea / suramin
Lysine therapy
Pure fulvic isolate

---

176 Secret Brotherhoods and the Mystery of the Human Double, Lecture 3, "Behind the Scenes of External Events, I."

177 "FUNVAX Vaccine created by the US Military to curb 'Religious Fundamentalism' in the Middle East," NevaehWest, July 16, 2013.

178 VMAT2 is purportedly the God gene, a specific gene called a vesicular monoamine transporter that predisposes humans towards spiritual or mystic experiences. See "Pentagon Vaccine To Kill Religious Center of Brain," September 29, 2011.

179 Michael Persinger, PhD (1945-2018), proved that the temporal lobe and hippocampus play a role in spiritual experience. See Chapter 12, "The Magical Human Head, Brain, and 'Second Brain.'"

Throughout the remainder of this Big Pharma war, I recommend seeking out remedies and strengthening agents from low-tech Nature. Whether or not you cancel your health insurance is up to you, but what you don't want is to end up dependent upon a 5G Air Loom hospital filled with shiny metal devices and drugs that are only truly useful for broken bones, gunshot wounds, and life-or-death accidents. If the FDA documentation referencing 110 diseases being inoculated into the bodies of millions under the guise of COVID-19 "gene therapy" is correct, many "side effects," "adverse events," and false poisonous treatments like Rendesivir lie ahead.[180]

Under "repurposed" drugs, I've included just a few remedies and recommendations that various doctors and health practitioners recommend. (At my site *elanafreeland.com* are more possibilities to be explored.) Being responsible for our own health means trusting our natural immune system and seeking to live the lifestyle that will keep it strong. You become your own lab and med student. Your body is a temple of the living spirit, not a machine.

> *A physical body was fashioned that set the Divine groundwork for an organization that could one day welcome the light of the human "I." Today, this organization is expressed in our physical structures down to our very DNA, and penetrates out to the world through our warmth-immune system … First, we must determine what is "not I." To be "immune" – to freely live autonomously with and among the wholeness of the world – we then need to integrate this process of encountering the lie, which ultimately is a process of becoming the "Christ in me."*
>
> *– Michael Givens, "Deceptive Messengers," Anthroposophical Society, Portland Branch Newsletter, February 2021*

Hydroxychloroquine

Hydroxychloroquine is basically quinine and chloroquine, known to antiquity as chichona, "sacred bark," discovered on the eastern slopes of the Andes in Peru.

> One of the biggest scandals of the COVID Plandemic is that hundreds of thousands of people died needlessly because the FDA refused to issue off-label emergency use for hydroxychloroquine (HCQ), a safe drug whose patent ran out years ago, and that thousands of doctors around the world have used

180 "Dr. Bryan Ardis: 'We are witnessing intentional medical genocide,'" August 1, 2021; an interview of Bryan Ardis, PhD, with Reiner Fuellmich of the Corona Investigative Committee (Nuremberg 2). From January to October 2020, all U.S. COVID-19 patients were treated with unapproved Rendesivir and ended up with acute kidney failure, meaning they were poisoned.

effectively, often with a 100% success rate, in treating COVID patients.[181]

The same mechanism that stops malaria from gobbling up hemoglobin (by chloroquine binding with the DNA of the parasite that has gained entry to red blood cells) makes chloroquine work for SARS-CoV-2 (or whatever it is).

On the other hand, high doses of non-toxic anti-malarial, anti-rheumatic hydroxychloroquine are used for euthanasia. In the excellent video "PCR Pandemic: Interview with *Virus Mania*'s Dr Claus Köhnlein" by Dr. Sam Bailey (October 27, 2020),[182] Dr. Köhnlein clarifies that the spike in deaths in April 2020 in both the UK and Belgium (stopping at the German border) that led to public panic about the need to "flatten the curve" came from high dosages (200-400mg) of hydroxychloroquine—from 2.4g on day 1 to 800mg for 10 days! Hydroxychloroquine's short therapeutic range means an overdose can lead to lethal heart arrythmia, which may be what happened with the April 2020 spike in Covid-19 deaths, either due to a lethal error under the British Recovery Studies (Solidarity, Discovery, Remap)—mistaking *diiodohydroxyquinoline* (for amebiasis) for hydroxychloroquine—or due to *intentional* lethal doses so as to discredit hydroxychloroquine. Dr. Köhnlein stressed that overtreatment (not to mention misdiagnosis) is a major problem. From AIDS, he learned that the AZT treatment caused the extreme withering and death, not HIV.[183]

Dr. Köhnlein does not, however, recommend hydroxychloroquine, primarily because it is an immune-suppressant.

Does COVID-19 "overtreatment" include euthanasia in nursing homes?

COVID-19 is a flu whose treatments are more lethal than it is.

Chlorine dioxide (ClO_2) / MMS (miracle mineral solution)

See: *Quantum Leap MMS Documentary* (2016)
The Universal Antidote Documentary: The Science and Story of Chlorine Dioxide

Misunderstood to be "bleach," chlorine dioxide has been used in operating rooms since 1814 as a sterilizer and biocide that kills all microbes via oxidation. Since 2010, Big Pharma and its minion the FDA have been poi-

181 Brian Shilhavy, "World's Second Largest Hydroxychloroquine Plant in Taiwan Blows Up." Health Impact News, December 22, 2020.

182 Virus Mania: How the Medical Industry Continually Invents Epidemics, Making Billion-Dollar Profits At Our Expense (2007) by journalist Torsten Engelbrecht and molecular biologist Claus Köhnlein is now a 2021 2nd edition microbiology best seller with two additional authors, Samantha Bailey and Stefano Scoglio.

183 See Dr. Köhnlein's book with author Torsten Engelbrecht, Virus Mania: How the Medical Industry Continually Invents Epidemics, Making Billion-Dollar Profits At Our Expense (Trafford Publishing, 2007).

soning people's minds about chlorine dioxide because it is cheap and successful worldwide with all kinds of conditions, including so-called COVID-19. It oxygenates cells, alkalinizes the blood, and detoxes heavy nanometals.

Budesonide

Budesonide is an anti-inflammatory corticosteroid administered with a nebulizer. Asthmatics and COPD (chronic obstructive pulmonary disease) patients use it. Zero toxicity, quick relief. Check side effects. Brand name: Pulmicort.

Ivermectin

Pulmonologist Pierre Kory spoke at the U.S. Senate Committee on Homeland Security and Governmental Affairs for Ivermectin as an early outpatient COVID-19 treatment. In general, Dr. Kory champions repurposing drugs, not the $20 billion vaccine enterprise of untested mRNA vaccines. Dr. Kory's biography of Anthony Fauci, the "Boss Bunco Artist for the Medical Cartel," is entitled *Teflon Tony: Big Pharma's Coup against Democracy,* published in February 2021 by Skyhorse / CHD.

To learn more about this "penicillin of COVID-19," please watch "Discussing Ivermectin And COVID-19 With 4 Experts! Dr.'s Scheim, Hibberd, Kory, And Juan Chamie!" Whiteboard Doctor, February 1, 2021.

Ivermectin is produced by Merck. At 12:20 in the extraordinary video at "Spooky Fibers in Masks and Test Swabs? Wait 'Til You Read the Science!" By Silviu Costinescu (*Silview*, April 29, 2021), we learn that *Ivermectin eradicates DARPA hydrogel.* (Will it eradicate graphene, too?)

Wormwood (Azythromyan) / Artemisinin

Composed of or modeled on absinthe / wormwood distilled spirits. Both Ivermectin and Artemisinin were awarded the 2015 Nobel Prize in Physiology or Medicine for achieving treatments for infectious diseases of poverty (IDoPs).

Thyme extract

Dr. Mercola reported (January 26, 2021) that Venezuelan President Nicolas Maduro obviously did not want to bend to Big Pharma cartel threats and thus supported nine months of study, experimentation, and clinical application on the sick and very sick of an oral extract made from thyme that has had great success with so-called COVID-19.

Pine needle tea / suramin

Ever since Judy Mikovits, PhD, recommended suramin (a 100-year-old essential medicine for African sleeping sickness) as an antidote to the COVID-19 gene therapy, people have been adding pine needle tea (conifers: pine, fir, cedar, spruce) to their daily regime.

Lysine therapy

The amino acid lysine interrupts the replication of viruses (even synthetic gain-of-function viruses) by countering arginine, the amino acid that fosters eruption of dormant viruses. Lysine has been used for decades to quell herpes outbreaks that cause cold sores on the lips.

Pure fulvic isolate

Pure fulvic isolate like Wu Jin San—not humic / fulvic acid or fulvic ionic minerals—works against encapsulated viruses like H1N1, SARS, MERS, HIV, and COVID-19.

A final word:

Phrases like "finding" new cases around the world and "self-mutating" to describe COVID-19 are covers for the *transmissive digital nature* of what is being inserted into people via injection in 5G / 6G environments. So-called mutations of the basically nonexistent virus are experimental, manmade diseases designed to lie dormant until they are called up by 5G / 6G systems to make proteins.

The CDC claim that the mRNA gene therapy does not interact with DNA in any way may be *technically* correct, particularly if a synthetic SARS-CoV-2 RNA is being *reverse transcribed* in human cells and used to alter genomic DNA, thanks to endogenous reverse transcriptase enzymes in the mRNA payload. Synthetic RNA lasts much longer in cells than viral RNA. Is pulsed 5G / 6G frequency converting the synthetic RNA to DNA? Synthetic mRNA, being programmed to make whatever protein it is directed to make, means big, endlessly growing profits and massive control for Big Pharma and its biotech minions.[184]

Neuroscience is the new CBW / EW weapons platform now boldly pursuing an "adaptive biological blockchain of self-functioning neurotech that easily self-modify in each newly infected host."[185]

Once the host is infected, the nanotechnology migrates through the

184 Much praise to biochemist/molecular biologist Doug Corrigan, PhD, for his courage in speaking out. Children's Health Defense, "Could mRNA Vaccines Permanently Alter DNA? Recent Science Suggests They Might," April 8, 2021.

185 "COVID-19 coronavirus is a neuroweapon to alter the genetic makeup of the blood stock & gene pool," Targeted Individual in New Zealand, July 28, 2020.

bloodstream to the brain & adheres to the neurotransmitters of the victim's brain where the nanoparticles [nanobots] speak to & decode the neurotransmitters through a process called *transcranial brain stimulation (TBS)* via the global infrastructure of thousands of Exascale Supercomputers (computing systems capable of calculating at least 10^{16} per second) using electromagnetic low frequency (ELF) waves emitted from towers, satellites & mobile platforms—enough to monitor the brainwaves of every human being on Earth . . .[186]

The military's electronic warfare (EW) and information warfare (IW) are, for all human intents and purposes, neural warfare.

When genetically modified / engineered (GM/GE) particles break down, they release nucleic acids into the environment. Nano-scaffolded hosts of the COVID-19 operating system—begun decades ago by chemical trails, GMO foods, jabs, and now masks and PCT swabs—become nodes in the "infection" network, "infection" being the awakening of frequencies via pulsed transmission, *not* actual viral contagion. Remember: molecular biology is now digital biology, thanks to nanotechnology having been enlisted "to forcefully integrate humans into a new cybernetic evolutionary cycle of multilateral neuro-societies & neuro-economies, the so-called new One World Order."[187]

Re-contextualizing 5G millimeter wave and 6G terahertz wave radiation emitted from phased array antennas, towers, satellites, and mobile platforms is a good beginning to grasping the fact that our little lives are now subject to a massive drama that will decide the fate of humanity for ages to come. This is why we must study what *remaining human* might mean in a time of crisis like this, the Chinese character for *crisis* meaning both danger *and* opportunity.

危机

Wéijī

186 Ibid.
187 Ibid.

Conclusion: Remaining Human

Consciousness
Your conception of what a human being is
Your lifestyle
Your inner life

". . . [The Space Fence] is incredibly brilliant [and] the most likely source of the VLF signals from ionospheric heaters which cause extremely low frequency waves in the magnetosphere and are useful as part of the full spectrum electronic fence around the Earth I can't talk about . . ."

– *Robert Duncan, PhD, "Deserie Foley: Escaping the Matrix presentation.* Dr. Robert Duncan V2K Neuroweapons," September 2, 2020

We choose to examine a phenomenon which is impossible, absolutely impossible to explain in any classical way, and which has in it the heart of quantum mechanics. In reality, it contains the only mystery.

– Richard Feynman (1918-1988), *Lectures on Physics*

It is evident that the natural human being is not welcome in outer space, except with a "novel artificial neural network ensemble design"—some sort of neuromorphic computing apparatus—so as to be accessible to cognitive engine (CE) algorithms that run space communications without human intervention.[1]

The same thing applies to cryptocurrency accounts dependent upon "body activity data" retrieved by sensors that read "body radiation emitted by the user, body fluid flow, a brain wave [or] pulse rate . . ." US Patent WO2020060606A1, "Cryptocurrency system using body activity data," September 21, 2018:

> Human body activity associated with a task provided to a user may be used in a [data] mining process of a cryptocurrency system. A server may provide a task to a device of a user which is communicatively coupled to the server. A server communicatively coupled or comprised in the device

1 Paulo Victor Rodriguez Ferreira *et al.*, "Multiobjective Reinforcement Learning for Cognitive Satellite Communications Using Deep Neural Network Ensembles." *IEEE*, 3 May 2018. Also see Adriano Cavalcanti *et al.*, "Nanorobot Hardware Architecture for Medical Defense ... Next Level Contact Tracing," *Sensors*, 2008; in video by Alchemical Tech Revolution, July 25, 2020.

> of the user may sense body activity of the user. Body activity data may be generated based on the sensed body activity of the user. The cryptocurrency system communicatively coupled to the device of the user may verify if the body activity data satisfies one or more conditions set by the cryptocurrency system, and award cryptocurrency to the user whose body activity data is verified.

Even global energy use[2] is prioritized for AI / ICT systems (information and communication technology) with non-volatile multi-state memory (NMSM) data storage in the zettabytes (trillions of gigabytes). Artificial intelligence comes first, humans second.

The Fourth Industrial Revolution wave is breaking over our heads.

The Four Industrial Revolution Waves

Wave 1	*Steam*
Wave 2	*Electricity*
Wave 3	*Computing*
Wave 4	*Integrated networks of sensors, cyber-physical beacons, actuators, robotics, machine learning*[3]

I am still haunted by the *New York Times* front-page photo of President Trump and Saudi royalty with their hands on a crystal ball ("What Was That Glowing Orb Trump Touched in Saudi Arabia?" May 22, 2017). Five months later at the Future Investment Initiative in Riyadh, the humanoid robot Sophia (which means wisdom) was granted Saudi citizenship—the nuncio that the AI games of planetary domination had begun.

Vernor Vinge's 2006 novel *Rainbows End* offers a convincing picture of the so-called *spatial web* (Web 3.0) in which virtual reality is superimposed on 3-space reality, and we find ourselves *inside* the Internet. Physical places seamlessly connect to virtual places, the world is linked and synced with the Web, computers are literally reality processors. No longer is 3D spatial intelligence embedded into text but into the Internet of Everything everywhere.

The alleged founder of the Internet, Tim Berners-Lee, announced in 1997 that "with no deliberate action of the people who designed the platform,"

---

2 Remember the cover story about carbon being to blame for "climate change"? Nations are now paying for corporations to make profits from "sequestering" carbon: machines are extracting carbon from the atmosphere with hydrogen being added for synthetic diesel fuel.

3 Gabriel René and Dan Mapes, The Spatial Web: How Web 3.0 Will Connect Humans, Machines, and AI to Transform the World, self-published 2019. My go-to expert for all things Fourth Industrial Revolution ("out of the ashes of the 'old world'") is Alison McDowell at https://wrenchinthegears.com.

the Web not only had failed to serve humanity but had become *antihuman* ("Realizing the Full Potential of the Web," 1997)—the very definition of evil I recommended in the Introduction. Now, the human is to be a tool of the technology, not vice versa:

> The Spatial Web protocol, HSTP, will ultimately create a web out of everything in the world. This will act as a new nervous system for the planet, connecting everything and everyone together. We can now create ever more accurate Smart Twins of our hospitals, our campuses, our factories, our cities, our countries—and ultimately the entire world. Our fundamental human values, when powered by Artificial Intelligence and Blockchain technologies, can optimize energy flows, logistics, and everything else involved in the operations of modern society. This will be used to create and automate sustainable systems and quickly identify non-sustainable activities so we can correct or cure many of the global challenges we are currently facing. The Spatial Web enables us to define a clear pathway to finally creating a Smart Sustainable Planet.[4]

Geoengineered Transhumanism has been about not just the Fourth Industrial Revolution but the fact that our environment from macro to micro has been intentionally weaponized *for the sake of cyber AI / quantum computer control over planet Earth.* Reality will not just be interchangeable or re-created but exactly simulated with you or your Digital Twin in it. Once you are genetically altered, you might not even be able to remember to ask *Which me is "I," "* or *Which reality is "real"?*

This shift is not merely ideological and confined to the glass houses of universities and the *New York Times* but is embedded in what we once called "reality." How will we navigate the language we need in order to understand our condition? As I said in the Introduction

We cannot solve problems with the
same thinking that created them.

Look around at the lies, subterfuge, obscuring, attributing to the opponent what one is doing oneself. Obviously, what was once described as "rational" is being abandoned:

> . . . the rational gaze is forever focalized and can examine only one thing at a time. It separates things to understand them, including the truly complementary. It is the gaze of the specialist who sees the fine grain of a necessarily restricted field of vision . . . life as described by [Francis] Crick

4 Ibid. I may go to sleep if I have to read more UN-style drivel like this.

was based on a miniature language that had not changed a letter in four billion years . . .[5]

When things settle, will the virtual world have a language similar to that of the *ayahuasca* shamans who employ music and song to evoke 3D images of molecular biology—collagen, the axon's embryonic network, triple helixes, coiled DNA, chromosomes, etc.?[6] After all, *human languages with their syntax, semantics, and rules of grammar are reflections of our DNA.* The languages of image and music, and thought language signifying concepts—all are the very stuff of human DNA, our cosmic radio station. Will those who have chosen to merge with the machine and have a hybrid DNA have a language all their own?

Solutions to remaining human through the Fourth Industrial Revolution rising like a bristling iron god in our carefully weaponized environment must begin and end with language and consciousness, including grappling with the consciousness of the engineered swarm nanotechnology now in our cells and brains that our human consciousness must come to terms with. As physicist Max Planck (1858-1947) stressed: "We cannot get behind consciousness. Everything that we talk about, everything that we regard as existing, postulates consciousness."

Thus, remaining human during a decidedly antihuman AI takeover down to the micro level of our own imperiled DNA is dependent upon the consciousness we bring to the challenge.

Consciousness

Your conception of what a human being is

> *The mind seems to contain everything at once in a timeless and placeless interconnectedness. The information is not encoded in a medium but is stored nonlocally as wave functions in nonlocal space, which also means that all information is always and everywhere immediately available.*
>
> – Pim van Lommel, cardiologist[7]

First, we will concentrate on breaking free of all remaining slave conditioning that teaches that the human being is a mere meat sack wetware node. Nothing could be further from the truth.

---

5 Jeremy Narby, The Cosmic Serpent: DNA and the Origins of Knowledge. Putnam, 1999.

6 See Luis Eduardo Luna and Pablo Amaringo, Ayahuasca Visions: The Religious Iconography of A Peruvian Shaman (North Atlantic Books, 1991).

7 Pim van Lommel, MD, Consciousness Beyond Life: The Science of the Near-Death Experience (HarperOne, 2011). See his 2001 article in the prestigious medical journal The Lancet, "Near-death experience in survivors of cardiac arrest," Lancet 358.

The relationship between the human brain and quantum physics is similar (if not identical) to the relationship between DNA and language. In fact, all four—brain, quantum physics, DNA, language—are connected by one self-knowing human thread, and yet we are conditioned to go through life utterly distracted and unaware of our own *mysterium tremendum.*

Here at the extraordinarily unique crossroads of our time, despite the chaos, we still hear the universe whisper, *Know thyself.*

The mechanisms that underpin the *subtle energy* we can't see are now being used as weapons against Human 1.0. Nature's free current—the quasi-standing ELF ground waves in the Earth-Moon gravity well cavity reaching all the way up to the now-controlled ionosphere—is being spun into global elite gold while the Schumann resonance standing wave pulse intimately connected to the brain and immune system in the morphogenetic field is being manipulated. Morphogenetic fields, according to biologist Rupert Sheldrake—whose TEDWhiteChapel talk on January 13, 2013[8] was banned—are *memory* fields that shape and maintain living organisms. Is the morphogenetic field being manipulated so as to wipe out the memory of what it is to be human? Nature is a process, as is the creative universe from which it springs, Sheldrake stresses; it is not shackled with timeless laws.

Add to this witches' brew the weaponized graphene-based hydrogel (GHB) COVID-19 gene therapy that increases our conductivity while interfering with the magnetic vector of the scalar waves our DNA generates—the magnetic vector that makes cellular communication happen. It is the rotation of the vortex field in the direction of the magnetic field that makes a longitudinal wave form a magnetic scalar wave.[9]

Our DNA and its scalar component connect us to the universe. Is the GHB assault an attempt to sever this connection?

In 1995, when two Russian scientists put unordered, random photons (light) into a vacuum tube, then added human DNA, the random photons immediately snapped into a specific alignment. When the DNA was removed from the vacuum tube, the photons remained as the DNA ordered them.[10] The DNA communicated by means of scalar waves with a *quantum state of matter* in the morphogenetic biofield, similar to how a salamander rebuilds its limbs from a phantom blueprint (discussed by Robert O. Becker, MD, in *The Body Electric*).

---

8 Rupert Sheldrake - The Science Delusion BANNED TED TALK," James Dearden Bush, March 15, 2013, https://www.youtube.com/watch?v=JKHUaNAxsTg.

9 See Konstantin Meyl, "Reading and writing by scalar waves," 2011.

10 P.P. Gariaev and V.P. Poponin, "Vacuum DNA phantom effect in vitro and its possible rational explanation." Nanobiology, 1995.

> A scalar wave is a transharmonic (multidimensional) spherical standing energy array that radiates out of a static point of sound-light vibration within the morphogenetic field of the greater cosmic Unified Field of consciousness (energy).[11]

DNA, photons, and biofield blueprints lead to the *aura* and luminous energy field surrounding each and every living being as members of the unified field of consciousness that includes the standing waves of free energy discovered by Tesla over 100 years ago to surround the Earth.

> The current passes through the earth, starting from the transmission station with infinite speed from that region and, slowing down to the speed of light at a distance of 6,000 miles, then increasing in speed from that region and reaching the receiving station with infinite velocity . . .[12]

While making their way through the double helix, scalar waves ensure the production of proper natural proteins, drawing energy from the morphogenetic field all around us.

Thoughts guided by clear intentions are patterns of scalar energy—creative, life-giving energy. Tesla viewed the two hemispheres of the brain as "a scalar energy interferometer between the ears" capable of generating and detecting spacetime effects at a distance and through time as well as higher senses like those of shamans who direct cognition, cellular telepathy, molecular transmutation, materialization, manifestation, astral projection, magnetic accretion of ectoplasm (plasma), transmigration, bi-location.

> Every single thought absolutely affects the observable state of the body-mind-spirit system and the materialization of events . . . [T]houghts are scalar wave configurations of transharmonic patterns of bi-polar, electromagnetic energy radiation which create specific patterns of scalar frequency within the personal morphogenetic field manifestation blueprint.[13]

Electromagnetic waves are transverse waves; scalar waves are longitudinal. According to Konstantin Meyl, there are three scalar waves in one: (1) electric scalar wave (potential vortex), (2) magnetic scalar wave (in Nature), and (3) electromagnetic wave. Some qualities of scalar waves:

---

11 Jere Rivera-Dugenio, PhD, "The Language of Our DNA – Scalar Energy." The International Journal of Scientific & Engineering Research, Vol. 10 Issue 4, April 2019.

12 Margaret Cheney, Tesla: Man Out of Time (Touchstone, 2001). Quoted extensively in Robert Beckwith's "abandoned" patent US20020013139A1, "Infinite speed space communications using information globes."

13 Jere Rivera-Dugenio.

- Over-unity effect (produces more energy than it consumes)
- Collect energy from the environment
- Faster than the speed of light
- Endless transfer of energy
- Living bodies function on scalar magnetic waves, not EM waves, and therefore produce no negative biological effects
- Directionless (like sound or plasma waves)
- Unshieldable (even a Faraday cage)
- Nothing weakens or stops these signals; goes through the Earth itself
- Potential vortex (scalar / electrical potential) exists throughout the human being
- Instead of particles being necessary for EM wave transmission, contracting and expanding potential vortices propagate longitudinal torsion waves and form torsion fields
- Neutralize EMF by cancelling out EM waves[14]

Resonance is another factor that our scalar DNA responds to. Our great ability to resonate with what is in our environment—music, beauty, wisdom—is a gift, but it is also a vulnerability. For example, Big Pharma's hoodwink to make us believe that "viral contagion" is why we need drugs then used to influence our minds and bodies.

> *When two things with the same resonance are put close to each other with their electromagnetic fields overlapping, they create a sympathetic* vibratory contagion. *This is best observed when two tuning forks that are not physically attached create sympathetic vibrations, despite the fact that only one fork is being repeatedly struck. Strum one string of a guitar, and the other strings sympathetically vibrate with it.*
>
> *When a body that has an acidic pH is exposed to another body undergoing a detoxification process like the flu, it will sympathetically vibrate with the detoxing body and undergo a similar detoxification process and release exosomes mistaken for viruses. This too is* vibratory contagion.
>
> – Ryan Guiterrez, Facebook, July 3, 2020

Somewhat like the Russian experiment mentioned earlier, virologist Luc Montagnier at the Pasteur Institute in Paris set up two test tubes, surrounding each tube with a copper coil that emanated a weak electromagnetic field. Both tubes contained distilled water, one with a fragment of DNA, the other just

---

14 See Konstantin Meyl, "Scalar Waves: Theories and Experiments," Journal of Scientific Experimentation, Vol. 15 No. 2, 2001.

water and no DNA. The two copper-coiled tubes were then isolated inside a chamber that muted the Earth's electromagnetic field. After several hours, the contents of both test tubes were put through polymerase chain reactions in which enzymes make copies of any DNA found. *The same DNA was in both tubes.* Montagnier and his team believed that the antenna-like DNA sent its signature (evoked potential) "signal" to the test tube of water-only and imprinted the water molecules with DNA. Without water, there would not have been sufficient resonance to "teleport" the DNA. *Quantum teleportation of genetic material.*[15]

Is this what is going on with "shedding"?

In the "Resonance" chapter of his book *The Contagion Myth,* Thomas S. Cowan, MD, clarifies why "infectious" childhood diseases like chicken pox, measles, and mumps seem so contagious: because the frequency of measles exosomes (packaged, ready-to-jettison cell garbage) resonates throughout the community so that other children's measles exosomes receive the message and begin the same relieving detoxification process.

Dr. Cowan's analysis of herpes is even more surprising. Two people having sex are certainly in a high-resonance situation, even to the point of creating or drawing out bits of identical DNA / RNA exosomes in each other, similar to Montagnier's test tubes. An intimate genetic (and therefore scalar) connection, not a "contagious" virus.

Consciousness

Your lifestyle

> *In comparing the certainty of things spiritual and things temporal, let us not forget this – Mind is the first and most direct thing in our experience; all else is remote inference.*
>
> – Arthur Stanley Eddington, "Science and the Unseen World," Swarthmore lecture, London, 1929

Many of the forces running our natural planet are *occult* or hidden, which is no doubt why we extol the guidance of "experts." The Sun's cosmic rays penetrate the atmosphere and are absorbed and re-emitted as infrared heat. Low-frequency infrared nestles deep in the soil, rock and water, the very lifeblood of tiny beings like our gut biome that interpenetrate matter. Above the ozone layer, where the ionosphere once guarded the Earth from taking in too much ultraviolet (UV), higher beings like angels live in cloudlike UV bodies

15 Clay Dillow, "Can Our DNA Electromagnetically 'Teleport' Itself? One Researcher Thinks So." Popular Science, January 13, 2011.

between us and the æther of deep space and astral realms. Here below, restless spirits and lower etheric beings multiply in our troposphere. Of such metaphysical / physical facts, the story of Lucifer's fall was woven.

Æther and electromagnetism have opposite effects, one dealing out life, the other death. As in the story of the Garden of Eden where the serpent strangled the Tree of Life, geomagnetic paths of the Dragon (leylines) seek to pull us toward the lower etheric realms in an attempt to confine us to *subnature* through our lower three *chakras* of the spine: the root, the sacral, and the solar plexus—the sexual metabolic, and energy "wheels." *Up!* the etheric force whispers, *draw your desire nature and will up into the upper* chakras—the heart, throat, third eye (pineal), and crown "wheels." Once death frees us from the Earth's magnetosphere, the depleting electric nature of the body vanishes and the ether body releases its *prana, ch'i, vis medicatrix naturae, telesma, pneuma, mana*—etheric force by many names over the ages.

The military's recent shift from kinetic to directed energy weapons (DEWs) serves subnature. The thicker electromagnetic radiation grows in our atmosphere, the more subnature beings grow restless and overpopulate, some longing to evolve, most content to devour human light as humans grow weak in the electromagnetic current now everywhere and 5G forces the genetically manipulated to become hybrid subnature beings themselves.

These are the challenges that natural human beings face in the present framework Asians for millennia have termed the *yin-yang duality*. Chinese medicine (~5,000 years old) and *ch'I* energy balancing treatments like acupuncture work to maintain a balance of the *yin-yang* forces operant in the human body. Foods grown from natural seed are also compressed forces influenced by the Earth's elements and seasons. Jet planes that deliver foods in any season, freezers, chemical preservatives, fertilizers—all such "technological advances" have wreaked havoc on the balance upon which natural human health depends.

For a half century, I have followed a Chinese medicine yin-yang / acid-alkaline diet modernized in George Ohsawa's macrobiotic diet.[16] *Food as medicine*—no pills or drugs, no doctors, just a balanced diet and lifestyle. As I indicated earlier, the Western technical approach is good for emergencies like accidents, murder attempts, broken bones, and extending life, but not for daily health. Bill Duffy, whom I met in 1975, wrote the following in *Sugar Blues:*

16 George Ohsawa (Nyoichi Sakurazawa, 1893-1966) defined health on the basis of seven criteria: lack of fatigue, good appetite, good sleep, good memory, good humor, precision of thought and action, and gratitude.

The gradual introduction of sugar into the Japanese diet brought in its wake the beginning of Western diseases. A Japanese midwife, trained in the techniques of Western medicine as a nurse, fell ill and was abandoned as incurable by the Western doctors she had espoused. Three of her children died the same way. The fourth, Nyoichi Sakurazawa, rebelled at the notion of dying of tuberculosis and ulcers in his teens. He took up the study of ancient Oriental medicine which had been officially outlawed in Japan. Sakurazawa was attracted to the unorthodox career of a famous Japanese practitioner, Dr. Sagen Ishizuka. Thousands of patients had been cured by Ishizuka (through traditional use of food) after they had been abandoned as incurable by the new medicine of the West.[17]

The chart below gives you an idea of how I gauge what to eat and not eat throughout the four seasons. My core diet changes seasonally, depending upon what grows or can be stored at my latitude. My habit is to eat little animal food, no sugar or honey, no yeasted breads, no supplements (other than B12), and some spices for fun. In the fall and winter, less raw and more cooked, adjusting oil and sea salt, eating more whole grains and chewing 25-50X a mouthful so as to massage my intestinal tract. I have a cup of strong black organic coffee every morning (the writer's drug), a glass of beer or Malbec wine once in a while with a friend. Otherwise, I drink artesian well water or Cistus herbal tea according to thirst so as not to exhaust my kidneys. (Most foods are at least 60 percent water.)[18]

The Japanese attribute their survival of the radiation of Hiroshima, Nagasaki, and Fukushima to miso soup and seaweed. In our era of wireless radiation and nuclear plant leaks, I have miso soup and seaweed a few times a week.

Other than fun outings to restaurants, *no GMO foods*. Even though fields growing organic foods are subject to chemical trails and soil loaded with aluminum nanoparticles, organic foods grow from natural seed, not Terminator seed that has been genetically modified into something that looks like "food" but is not.

Thirty-eight countries worldwide have officially banned the cultivation of GM crops, and only 28 actually grow GM crops (most of which grow under 500,000 hectares, 1 hectare = 2.47 acres).[19]

---

17 William Duffy, Sugar Blues (Warner, 1975).

18 I recommend Denny and Susan Waxman's 2019 book The Ultimate Guide to Eating for Longevity (Pegasus Books).

19 Sustainable Pulse, 2015.

Yin Alkaline-forming Foods

- honey
- coffee
- herbs
- tea
- spices
- fruits
- seeds
- leafy greens
- vegetables
- some beans
- tofu

Yang Alkaline-forming Foods

- root vegetables
- bancha tea
- gomasio
- tamari
- miso
- umeboshi plums
- salt

Yin Acid-forming Foods

- sugar
- alcohol
- yoghurt
- milk
- soft drinks
- chemical drugs
- nuts

Yang Acid-forming Foods

- meat
- chicken
- fish
- eggs
- cheese
- grains

Issi, "Introduction to Macrobiotics (part 11) – Acid and Alkaline Forming Foods," Self Healing Australia, May 15, 2017

In the Five Element Theory, foods can be divided into Yin and Yang, which corresponds to Acid and Alkaline in Western science. The acid or alkaline quality of our blood is measured by a pH factor. A pH of less than 7 is acidic while above 7 is considered alkaline. Most illnesses and disorders are caused by our blood being acidic. In order to maintain health, our blood and body fluids should be slightly alkaline with a pH between 7.3 and 7.45. So when we eat acid-forming foods, such as meat, for instance, it is important to balance them with alkaline-forming foods such as vegetables. The table shows which foods can be used to create balance in the body.

Remember: eating from Nature is about BALANCE, not just desire and stimulation. It may sound like less fun after years of being conditioned by ads to eat refined food, but who wants broken health and a painful debilitating old age?

The other practical lifestyle caveat is electromagnetics. I have gone extensively into EM throughout this book. Examine where you live and your relationship with neighbors' smart meters and routers, the beam pattern of surrounding towers, metal in your bed, dirty electricity pouring from outlets, etc. STUDY. Do not remain passive and impotent regarding invisible technologies so that you end up in Air Loom hospitals. Retain your health so you can fulfill your highest aspirations.

Consciousness

Your inner life

From a Normandy crucifix of 1632

I am the great sun, but you do not see me,
I am your husband, but you turn away.
I am the captive, but you do not free me,
I am the captain but you will not obey.
I am the truth, but you will not believe me,
I am the city where you will not stay.
I am your wife, your child, but you will leave me,
I am that God to whom you will not pray.
I am your counsel, but you will not hear me,
I am your lover whom you will betray.
I am the victor, but you do not cheer me,
I am the holy dove whom you will slay.
I am your life, but if you will not name me,
Seal up your soul with tears, and never blame me.

With a better understanding of our greater scalar human nature—especially the power of our thinking capability that comprises much of our consciousness—and an idea of what constitutes real health, we are ready to image the inner life that powers it all.

Up until now, the human inner life has been cultural and particularly private, given that each person's conversations with their conscience, whatever their culture, are unique to their life experiences. Religious beliefs or agnostic questions may seem general, but how we approach them is unique to each of us. Mind control and targeting technology via satellites, towers, and the Internet of Things (IoT) is attempting to end this privacy.

In the West, our conditioning has concentrated on training us to spend our inner life on practical security and "down time" (entertainment, relaxation, vacations). The solitary walk, meditation, prayer, or even thoughtful book is strangely discouraged as "antisocial." What I propose is *not* that we put the meditation first, but that we awaken to how everything that we experience can be food for the inner life *if we approach life from our depth and not habit.* It is, after all, the nature of human beings to seek meaning by asking *Why?* and *What am I really observing?* and *How does this experience serve or divert me from the qualitative, unique life I long to live?*

In our era, unlike in previous eras, organized *paths of initiation into Truth* like churches, temples, Freemason lodges, etc. are degenerating into Egregore institutions. The only authentic path of initiation available now is one's individual life. Simply put, every day is Sunday (or Saturday), and everywhere is church (or temple). Meditation and prayer are welcomed into life experience for how they draw forth and enliven the true nature of the mundane and habitual.

The self-examined life is *essential* to authentic consciousness. Look back on your life, all the way back to childhood. Why did things happen as they did? What did it mean for your development and preparation for exactly these dangerous times?

As we undergo the societal conditioning of the family, school, media, we tend to pay less attention to what seems to be just scenery but is often pregnant with meaning and clues as to who we really are and why we are here on the Earth at this particular time. The TV is on, emotions and hormones, academic or parent pressures weigh on us, we end up in a fantasy world of video games or escape into drugs and alcohol, sex without love, etc. As the illusions of youth wane, the career may be going well but depression strikes, anyway. *What is going on with our inner life?*

Not until I was 45 was I able to remember the childhood experience that threw me off the trail I knew was mine—my destiny, my mission. Once I regained memory of the event, the energy blockage was released and I could be *whole.* Strange, isn't it? The experience of the child was over, *but not its lingering, unresolved resonance* because the experience had not been made conscious. A child is dealt an unfair blow, and the adult the child becomes must still dig for the stolen energy so as to complete her destiny.

My situation was hardly unusual. Now, children raised on television think of their lives as arbitrary and meaningless unless they become "stars" and wealthy. The truth is that every human being braves the gates of birth to fulfill a particular destiny, and yet it seems like most of modern life is bent on throwing us off the trail.

Our era is difficult and perilous, and yet our youth and subsequent years prepare us *exactly* for our time. Life is no accident; it's more like a wrapped gift with our name on it. How could an impersonal universe have us in mind? Because the universe is intelligent and extremely interested in consciousness as it plays out in matter—particularly human self-consciousness studying what "life" on Earth is really about.

I know one thing: *I do not want my natural DNA and body and brain controlled by or contrived as a brain-computer interface (BCI) machine.*

Reach into the spiritual world everywhere around and in you for the strength and wisdom as to how to proceed. Do not be distracted by fear of imprisonment or death. Beside and behind you stand great souls accustomed to encounters with evil, powers and principalities, Egregores. Part of our individual destiny is to protect the human spirit, as Rudolf Steiner knew a century ago. Gird up your loins. We have come for this task in this time.

(For the ever-shifting list of Remedies and Resources, see https://www.elanafreeland.com.*)*

> *In the future, we will eliminate the soul with medicine. Under the pretext of a 'healthy point of view,' there will be a vaccine by which the human body will be treated as soon as possible directly at birth, so that the human being cannot develop the thought of the existence of soul and Spirit.*
>
> *To materialistic doctors will be entrusted the task of removing the soul of humanity. As today, people are vaccinated against this disease or that disease, so in the future, children will be vaccinated with a substance that can be produced precisely in such a way that people, thanks to this vaccination, will be immune to being subjected to the "madness" of spiritual life. He would be extremely smart, but he would not develop a conscience, and that is the true goal of some materialistic circles.*
>
> *With such a vaccine, you can easily make the etheric body loose in the physical body. Once the etheric body is detached, the relationship between the universe and the etheric body would become extremely unstable, and Man would become an automaton, for the physical body of Man must be polished on this Earth by spiritual will. So the vaccine becomes a kind of Ahrimanic force; Man can no longer get rid of a given materialistic feeling. He becomes materialistic in constitution and can no longer rise to the spiritual.*
>
> *– Rudolf Steiner (1861-1925)*

Appendices

Appendix 1

Invisible Mindsets

Satanism & the U.S. Military
MISO & domestic propaganda
Software, hardware, firmware / wetware patent language
Digitized personality / Sentient World Simulation (SWS)
"Inorganic life"
Scientism, not science
Occult means hidden
Initiation
The hexagon gateway
The Egregores of corporations, foundations, religious institutions & Brotherhoods

> *There is no surer protection against the understanding of anything than taking for granted or otherwise despising the obvious and the surface. The problem inherent in the surface of things, and only in the surface of things, is the heart of things.*
>
> – Leo Strauss, *Thoughts on Machiavelli*, 1958

> *The case against science is straightforward: much of the scientific literature, perhaps half, may simply be untrue.*
>
> – Richard Horton, MD, Editor-in-Chief, *The Lancet*

MINDSETS CONSTITUTE A SUBTEXT TO daily life that we often do not recognize as influencing our perceptions and decisions about what is what and who is who, and why. Each lifetime is a three-ring circus, a multitiered staged event filled to overflowing with hidden intentions and meanings there for the taking and unraveling of those who desire to go to the trouble of wading through illusions, deceptions, and "false positives" to get to the truth behind one event or another. Make no mistake: it is the work for the truth that develops the soul and the lack thereof that wastes opportunities for development.

Be prepared for resistance to lifting the Veil over philosophy and practices you've been conditioned to view as nonsense, conspiracy theories, or ancient history. In fact, the more university level your education, the greater will be your resistance. The elite at varying levels—depending upon their degrees of attainment under the tutelage of ancient secret societies—count on this educated resistance to retain the *holding pattern* so as to be available for use but blind to the deeper purposes beneath money, prestige, power, etc.

Here are seven mindsets to be aware of.

1. *Satanism and the U.S. military*

> *. . . at one point I defined evil as "the exercise of political power that is the imposition of one's will upon others by overt or covert coercion in order to avoid . . . spiritual growth."*
>
> – M. Scott Peck, PhD, author of *People of the Lie: The Hope for Healing Human Evil* (1998)

The U.S. military (all branches) went through a transformative shift in the 1990s known as the Revolution in Military Affairs (RMA). It wasn't just about shifting from ballistic to kinetic weapons (including nonlethals) and asymmetric warfare; it was a psychological shift born out of the CIA's Phoenix Program trialed during the Vietnam "conflict."

In 1980, Col. Paul E. Vallely and Maj. Michael A. Aquino wrote a 12-page military concept paper called "From PSYOP to MindWar: The Psychology of Victory." Aquino had been a highly decorated Green Beret psyops officer with top security clearance during the CIA's 1968-1972 Phoenix Program "designed to identify and destroy the Viet Cong (VC) via infiltration, torture, capture, counter-terrorism, interrogation, and assassination" (Wikipedia).[1] The Phoenix counterinsurgency doctrine began in Vietnam, continued in Central America, and eventually constituted the core of the Revolution in Military Affairs (RMA). *The Cold Warriors who conceived of Phoenix always intended it for domestic use.*

What is strangely overlooked by military historians is that the decorated psyop war hero Aquino was not only a practicing Satanist but high priest of the Temple of Set, a Satanic church on San Francisco's Russian Hill not that far from the Presidio U.S. Army base (1846-1994) where he was stationed after Vietnam. From "MindWar":

> The MindWar operative must know that he speaks the truth, and he must be PERSONALLY COMMITTED to it . . . For the mind to believe its own decisions, it must feel that it made those decisions without coercion. Coercive measures used by the MindWar operative, consequently, must not be detectable by ordinary means . . .

---

1 Phoenix ran concurrent with the CIA's Paperclip Nazi-run MK-ULTRA and its 149 subprojects in the name of psyops and "behavioral control."

"MindWar" even mentioned ionizing the atmosphere as a method of controlling emotions:

> An abundance of negative condensation nuclei (air ions) in ingested air enhances alertness and exhilaration, while an excess of positive ions enhances drowsiness and depression. Calculation of a target audience's atmospheric environment will be correspondingly useful.

Julianne McKinney, a former U.S. Army intelligence officer and author of the December 1992 study "Microwave Harassment and Mind Control Experimentation," understood well the psyops *special access programs (SAPs)*[2] that would be used to create a societal "ethical and political revolution." Subtle, insidious Satanism was first on her list, and the "induced crime wave" produced by Satanic cults across the nation under then-Lt. Col. Aquino's guidance was the last on her list:

> Satanic cults, UFO cults, directed energy technologies, neurocybernetics / psychotechnologies, biotechnologies / experimental drugs, multinational government contractors and subsidiaries, investment portfolios and other financial inducements, imported foreign national scientists, a controlled and compliant media, decentralized U.S. government control, an induced crime wave . . .[3]

Aquino was involved in the Zodiac serial killer murders (late 1960s, early 1970s) pivoting around the Presidio; in 1986, he was involved in the Presidio Day Care Center scandal during which 60 children were raped, sodomized, and traumatized. Children ID'd "Mikey" as one of the men who had abused them, but the Army protected "Mikey" by making the media blame it all on "satanic panic." The crime scene building was demolished, including the tunnels wherein the children had been raped, and the Army built a brand new $2.3 million new daycare. After 22 years as the Army's resident Satanist specialist, Aquino was quietly discharged, having finally exposed too much about the new Phoenix military.

In 1994, Cheri Seymour's book *The Last Circle: Danny Casolaro's Investigation into The Octopus and the PROMIS Software Scandal* dug into the

2 SAPs require signing a 70-year non-disclosure agreement (NDA) covering all things related to highly classified "national technical means" programs like UFOs, satellites, spy gear, antigravity exotic propulsion systems, etc.

3 Correspondence from Julianne McKinney, director of the Electronic Surveillance Project, Association of National Security Alumni, to Steven Metz, PhD, and LTC James Kievit, cc: Col. John W. Mountcastle, Director, Strategic Studies Institute, U.S. Army War College, 8 January 1995.

military's role in sustaining generational Satanic cults, due in part to Aquino convincing military brass that they had lost the Vietnam war "not because we were outfought but because we were outPSYOPed. PSYOPs—MindWar—had to be strengthened."

In the spring of 1998, the U.S. War College Strategic Studies Institute *Parameters* quarterly published "The Mind Has No Firewalls" by Steven Metz and James Kievit. Up until then, little had been allowed to go public about *soft kill, slow kill, silent kill* nonlethals,[4] "conflict short of war," and behavior modifications as tools of the Revolution in Military Affairs. Metz and Kievit stressed that "to make RMA in conflict short of war would require fundamental changes in the United States—an ethical and political revolution may be necessary to make a military revolution."

Aquino wasn't the military's first Satanic favored son. Marvel Whiteside "Jack" Parsons (1914-1952) was a self-taught genius jet propulsion rocket engineer from Pasadena involved in the founding of the Aerojet Rocketdyne Corporation and Jet Propulsion Laboratory (JPL) funded by the Guggenheim family and administered by the California Institute of Technology (Caltech). British MI6 agent and Satanist Aleister Crowley chose Jack to head up the Pasadena Ordo Templis Orientis (OTO). A crater on the dark side of the Moon has been named for Parsons, but otherwise he has been wiped from space program history.[5]

Both Parsons and Aquino claimed to be the Antichrist.

> . . . both psyops and satanism involve using many levels of deception and coercion to manipulate the perceptions of others for ulterior motives, so these are skills that Aquino is very familiar with and very comfortable in using. He is also an expert in propaganda and skilled in techniques for disseminating misinformation / disinformation, and using misdirection, confusion tactics, isolation techniques, and revisionism. Therefore, he will certainly use these skills to defend himself against the truth of his actions.[6]

Such "skills" have now overtaken the entire nation: Washington, DC politics, law enforcement, corporate culture, UN "peacekeepers," child protec-

---

4 Infrasound / VLF, neural inhibitors, hallucinogens, calmatives, neuroblockers, stun guns, pulsed high-power microwaves, non-penetrating projectiles, laser rifles, flash-bang grenades, etc. In 1994, the Department of Defense (DoD) and Department of Justice (DOJ) formalized their nonlethal cooperation.

5 For the astonishing story of the U.S. rocket program, Paperclip scientists, and Satanism, read John Carter's Sex and Rockets: The Occult World of Jack Parsons (Feral House, 1999). Yes, even L. Ron Hubbard of scientology fame was involved in Jack's black magick rituals.

6 "The 'Conspiracy' Against Michael Aquino – Satanic Pedophile." Exposing the Truth, February 11, 2014.

tion agencies, Hollywood, the "nonlethal" targeting of citizens in their homes and workplaces. Aleister Crowley's *Do what thou wilt shall be the whole of the law* has overtaken *Do unto others as you would have them do unto you.* Now it's if you can get away with it, go for it.

Film and TV programming favor Satanism and pre-Christian belief systems that practice pedophilia, mind control, and blood rituals—from *Do what thou wilt* high rollers and church leaders to petty criminals and corporate flunkies, they are required to attend a blood ritual now and then in order to be kept traumatized and in line. *Der Wille zur Macht,* the will-to-power, is the Satanist defense against weakening brotherly love. As for Death and answering for one's deeds on Earth, those espousing Satanism are ever seeking earthly immortality, whether through adrenochrome from tortured children's blood or the brain-computer interface (BCI) of Transhumanism.

The Phoenix philosophy of social control has permeated American universities. In 2003, the DoD's Research Development Technology and Expenditure top 100 list started off with Johns Hopkins, MIT, and Penn State. The Institute for Non-Lethal Defense Technologies (INLDT) is under Penn State's Applied Research Laboratories, one of the U.S. Navy's top civilian research facilities (1,000 employees).[7] The INLDT's first contract ($42.5 million) was with the U.S. Marine Corps, much of it to study the Schedule 2 drug fentanyl, a sedative 80X stronger than morphine.

Post-9/11, the Phoenix approach has justified all kinds of covert atrocities. Domestic NORTHCOM is the military component of the Department of Homeland Security, the post-9/11 spawn of Harvard's JFK School of Government, the DoD, and DOJ. Hitler's Germany had its *Geheime Staatspolezei,* the U.S. its Homeland Security.

But hey, it's the Great Game! Technology, finance, manufacturing, and military in bed with intelligence and private security corporations, the door between government and transnational corporations spinning like a Russian roulette gun. "Trusted partners" now scratching each other's back this week and stabbing each other in the back next week. "Conflict of interest" is passé, old school, having died along with honor, character, virtue, and being true to one's word. War now includes arsenals of lies, state terrorism, remote electromagnetic torture, and poverty as big business.

Internet and social media corporations are in tight with NSA Special Source Operations and the FBI. Corporate executives and tech employees working abroad double as intelligence agents ("committing officers") with the guarantee of immunity for civil actions of data theft and "wetworks." People

7 Bryan Farrell, "Penn State's Frightening Defense." Foreign Policy in Focus, April 25, 2008.

make the assumption that this is just how people are, but it's not. It's about the mindsets allowed to run rogue for the sake of success and full spectrum dominance at any cost.

2. *MISO & domestic propaganda*

> *. . . the CIA, through Operation Mockingbird, started recruiting mainstream journalists and media outlets as far back as the 1960s in order to covertly influence the American public by disguising propaganda as news. The CIA even worked with top journalism schools to change their curricula in order to produce a new generation of journalists that would better suit the U.S. government's interests. Yet the CIA effort to manipulate the media was born out of the longstanding view in government that influencing the American public through propaganda was not only useful, but necessary.*
>
> *Indeed, Edward Bernays, the father of public relations, who also worked closely with the government in the creation and dissemination of propaganda, once wrote:* The conscious and intelligent manipulation of the organized habits and opinions of the masses is an important element in democratic society. Those who manipulate this unseen mechanism of society constitute an invisible government which is the true ruling power of our country.[8]

In 2010, Psychological Operations (PSYOPS) of the U.S. Army Special Operations Command (USASOC) was rebranded *Military information Support and Operations (MISO).*

> . . . (MISO), previously known as Psychological Operations (PSYOP), uses themes and messages to reach target audiences in order to influence their emotions, motives, reasoning, and ultimately the behavior of foreign [and domestic?] governments, organizations, groups, and individuals . . . If a MISO operator does not understand the depth of an individual's condition, concerns, fears, ambitions, and vulnerabilities, then MISO will not be effective . . ." ("Reaching the Target Audience," USASOC)

To protect "a key friendly center of gravity, to wit the U.S. national will,"[9] the Pentagon normalized lying by legalizing "the use of psychological operations through propaganda on US civilian populations" in the 2013 omnibus

8 Whitney Webb, "Lifting of US Propaganda Ban Gives New Meaning to Old Song." Mint Press News, February 12, 2018.

9 Lt. Col. Daniel Davis, Democracy Now! 2012: "Senior ranking US military leaders have so distorted the truth when communicating with the US Congress and American people in regards to conditions on the ground in Afghanistan that the truth has become unrecognizable."

National Defense Authorization Act (NDAA)[10] and by the revisionism perpetrated upon the 1948 Smith-Mundt Act that banned domestic propaganda and psyops for 64 years until President Obama officially lifted the ban in 2013 with the Smith-Mundt Modernization Act of 2012. MISO and the Joint Force military Information Operations (IO) have officially railroaded American journalism with

> . . . the integrated employment of electronic warfare (EW), computer network operations (CNO), psychological operations (PSYOP), military deception (MILDEC) and operations security (OPSEC), in concert with specified supporting and related capabilities to influence, disrupt, corrupt or usurp adversarial human and automated decision-making while protecting our own.[11]

The Broadcasting Board of Governors, an extension of the U.S. State Department which is an extension of the CIA, approves government narratives for Mockingbird mainstream media dedicated to silencing dissenting perspectives. Spin corporations like Strategic Communication Laboratories (SCL)[12] are proud of their "influence operations," "public diplomacy," and running simulations "from natural disasters to political coups" at exhibits like Defense Systems & Equipment International (DSEi), the UK's largest showcase for military tech. For a price, SCL will run false flag events, help overthrow democratically elected governments of developing countries, and override national radio and TV broadcasts.[13]

The advent of IO in league with shadow corporations like SCL announces loud and clear that human minds and brains are now the battlespace. No firewall makes the mind easy prey for IO psychotronic weapons, and we would be naive to assume that "adversarial" refers to foreign enemies, or that "protecting our own" refers to the American people. For the post-RMA Joint Force military, the "U.S. national will" is *the military will*, not the people's.

---

10 See "NDAA 2013: Congress approves domestic deceptive propaganda." RT, 22 May 2012. The NDAA is an annual Trojan horse of trouble. For propaganda and "narrative-building," the Global Engagement Center was established under Obama's EO13721 (April 2016), then made into law and buried in the 2017 NDAA.

11 U.S. Military, Joint Publication 3-13, February 8, 2015.

12 "The first private-sector provider of psychological operations." – Strategic Communication Laboratories, founded in 1993.

13 Sharon Weinberger, "Psy-ops propaganda goes mainstream." Slate.com, September 19, 2005.

3. *Software, hardware, firmware / wetware patent language*

US Patent #6,965,816 B2 (November 15, 2005)—"PFN/TRAC System FAA Upgrades for Accountable Remote and Robotics Control To Stop the Unauthorized Use of Aircraft and To Improve Equipment Management and Public Safety in Transportation"—was filed one year after the September 11, 2001. At first glance, it seems to be about remote control of aircraft on varying frequencies, like System Planning Corporation's flight termination system (FTS).

But once the patent language is penetrated, it becomes evident that the PFN/TRAC (Point Focal Node Trusted Remote Access Control) system is about *control over all moving things,* not just airplanes, by means of a large "machine-messaging matrix," either by sharing or replacing local and standard human-machine interfacing (HMI, BCI / BMI) with remote control robotics.

For this reason, the patent is known as *the IoT patent*, the key being the "robust and accountable *remote control* for personal applications, stationary equipment and stand-alone functions, and coordinates them and interfaces them within the communication matrix." The same holds for the patent's reference to the "wetware"[14] status of human beings:

> . . . the technology incorporates existing technology as it exists in a present distributed architecture and coordinates and manages the essential function to stop and control an unwanted event and improve public safety. This requires hardware, software and wet-ware (people / the procedures and protocols) . . ."

A month and a half before 9/11, another patent—US Patent #2,397,911, "Protected Accountable Primary Focal Node Interface" (July 26, 2001)—referenced the term "firmware (software-embedded hardware)." Again, once the language is penetrated, the patent is actually referencing *cyborg*[15] human beings with artificial organs, limbs, pacemakers, implants, etc.—*human materials industry* that includes tiny machines (nanobots) in the bloodstreams and "wetware" brains that the IoT / IoNT tunes into, thanks to three decades of GMO foods, aerosols, and aggressive vaccination programs.

With these clues, we can now translate the following patent description into the true *synbio* "firmware" context the patent addresses while hiding the technology in plain sight.

---

14 Wetwork is the long-employed CIA term for assassination.

15 The term cyborg (cybernetic organism) was introduced in 1960 at the Psychophysiological Aspects of Space Flight Symposium in the context of preparing human beings for survival in "extraterrestrial environments," calling up a reference to the secret space program and even the Paperclip Nazi aviation medical doctor Hubertus Strughold (1898-1986), the so-called Father of Space Medicine.

The invention was always designed to remotely control machines, equipment, and vehicles (100-107) through various levels of monitoring and remote control systems and networks. Much of the technology has been designed to marry up to pre-existing devices and systems to develop cost-effective enhancements wherever possible to legacy systems and equipment. The PFN/TRAC System is further developed to integrate and consolidate components and functions through more efficient universal configurations of hardware, software and firmware (software-embedded hardware) to provide integrated accountable remote control and management for man and machine interfacing (HMI) and to include full robotics by employing the latest developments like Systems On a Chip (SOC) Technology. The systems and modalities of hardware, software and firmware detailed in this application and related applications that provide accountable trusted remote control or management, including traceable communications and commands with individual and machine identity and integrity checks, are all part of a technology termed the PFN/TRAC System. *The PFN/TRAC System is made up of individual nodes or units that communicate as part of an accountable machine-messaging network employing and managing various forms of communication computers and machine controls to aid humanity in the safe use of equipment while protecting the environmental and the Earth's resources.*

The final italicized sentence describes the Internet of Things (IoT) as well as the Internet of Nano Things (IoNT) to a T.

4. *Computerized personality simulation / Sentient World Simulation (SWS)*

The truth is that supercomputers and quantum computers cannot think; only a human with a mind—much more than a physical brain—can really *think*. But what AI *can* do is mind control. Would you recognize it if it were happening to your mind?

During the MK-ULTRA years, the Freudian psychiatrist Kenneth Colby (1920-2001) worked in Stanford Research Institute's computer science department on artificial intelligence vis-à-vis the human mind. He was deeply involved in developing *chatterbots* like ELISA, described by Robert Duncan in this way:

> ELISA was an artificial intelligence (AI) computer program demonstrated by the Stanford Research Institute back in the 70's. It acted like a psychologist and asked stupid questions and responded to answers, parsing and understanding sentences. This field is called *natural language processing (NLP)*—not

to be confused with neurolinguistic programming.[16] ELISA fooled about half the people into believing it was a real human being on the other end.

Fast forward 35 years and instead of parsing natural language phrases from keystrokes, ELISA recognizes phonetic brainwaves and parses them into words and sentences for artificial intelligence and natural language processing (NLP). Now the tortures and menticizations can scale to entire populations through this automation . . . The brainwave cognitive ELISA adds realism by inducing an empathetic emotion with the words the target feels, thus adding a new dimension of convincing the target that the synthetic mind virus is a real person.[17]

Colby came up with the following nuances of human thinking that chatterbots would have to imbibe:

- The credibility of a belief is based on the credibility of its source
- Human personalities are based on belief systems concerning significant persons, including the self
- Every psychological concept has specific significance, e.g. father, love, etc.
- Input from others is evaluated and "colored" by mental [and emotional] patterns
- A human mind changes with inner conflict, transforming beliefs to fit into an overall pattern

From his observations, Colby deduced:

- Capture a person's belief structures and they can be controlled
- Unenlightened human minds are combinations of infantile beliefs and emotional patterns
- Unenlightened human minds can be simulated by a computerized system
- Through such systems, unenlightened people can be programmed and controlled

Components of "unenlightened human minds" can be captured and developed into accurate simulations that artificial intelligence technicians and political operatives can use to manipulate us.[18]

The Sentient World Simulation (SWS) was presented as a military concept paper in 2006—basically, the idea that every person on the planet could be digi-

16 Even these sorts of acronym confusions are intentional in the language / concept shell game.

17 Robert Duncan, The Matrix Deciphered: Psychic Warfare Top-Secret Mind Interfacing Technology. Higher Order Thinkers Publishing, 2006.

18 Thanks to "The Possibility of Human Devolution," http://www.hermes-press.com/index24.htm.

tally represented as a software node and given a digital avatar, and the entire infrastructure erected as a blockchain, each individual's consciousness cloned onto the avatar inside the Cloud / supercomputer / quantum computer. Direct links would exist between individuals and their avatars (brain-computer interface, BCI) so that *everything done in the real world occurs in the computer simulation.*

Even the Earth itself would have its digital twin.

One read-through of this concept paper will show how the language has been contrived to be obscure to the uninitiated while being exact to the initiated—similar to patent language. For example, terms like "granularities of access," "coarse-grained" and "fine-grained," "temporal and spatial granularities," and "Joint Semi-Automated Forces (JSAF)" seem to point to the sensor nanotechnology essential to building virtual simulacra of the natural world and its residents. Read between the lines and "unbiased to specific outcomes" seems to refer to the amoral approach touted as "objective" in "agent-based" SEAS (Synthetic Environment for Analysis and Simulation) environments and ends in the torture of millions of targeted individuals for the purpose of collecting endless biometric and behavioral data for "specific outcomes."

The targeting industry provides guinea pigs for ongoing chatterbot and Sentient World Simulation experimentation. People's real lives are being exploited so as to

> . . . build a synthetic mirror of the real world with automated continuous calibration with respect to current real-world information . . . The ability of a synthetic model of the real world to sense, adapt, and react to real events distinguishes SWS from the traditional approach of constructing a simulation to illustrate phenomena . . . Basing the synthetic world in theory in a manner that is *unbiased to specific outcomes* offers a unique environment in which to develop, test, and prove new perspectives.[19] (Emphasis added.)

The end goal is to *reverse* our relationship with our avatar in the Sentient World Simulation: to make the feed now going from nanosensors and nanobots in our biological brains to AI collection points like fusion centers *reverse* so the biological human being is being controlled by the virtual avatar inside the simulation.

HAARP / Space Fence carrier waves synchronize AI communication with SIM-real world simulation.

---

19 Tony Cerri, Government POC (point of contact) and Alok Chaturvedi, PhD, Technical POC for Purdue University, "Sentient World Simulation (SWS): A Continuously Running Model of the Real World / A Concept Paper for Comments," August 22, 2006, https://www.krannert.purdue.edu/academics/mis/workshop/ac2_100606.pdf.

Turn the TV and iPhone off and read, think, and develop your own consciousness; relinquish mere mirroring.

5. *"Inorganic life"*

With the latest 2020 psyop assault on planetary life, we have begun to see *in real time* the beginning erasure of the big black line between the machine and the human being, Nature, and planet Earth. Thus, the language is changing, as well.

"Inorganic life" and "living machines" sound like oxymorons, but since the release of nanotechnology and its synthetic "gain of function" nanoparticles everywhere, the language of life synthesized with artifice becomes essential in order to understand what is happening around and *inside* our bodies and brains.

Thoughtful essays regarding the role that synthetic biology was actually slated to play in the redefinition of *life* have attempted to awaken the public—like the 2009 University of Zurich essay "Synthetic organisms and living machines" by Anna Deplazes and Markus Huppenbauer for whom nanotechnologies were still "novel."[20]

In 2011, Lee Cronin, PhD, of the University of Glasgow announced the first steps toward "creating 'life' from inorganic chemicals." Plainly, he explained:

> "All life on earth is based on organic biology (i.e. carbon in the form of amino acids, nucleotides, and sugars, etc.), but the inorganic world is considered to be inanimate. What we are trying to do is create self-replicating, evolving inorganic cells that would essentially be alive. You could call it inorganic biology . . . If successful, this would give us some incredible insights into evolution and show that it's not just a biological process. It would also mean that we would have proven that non-carbon-based life could exist and totally redefine our ideas of design."[21]

A decade later, here we are with synthetic mRNA delivering genetics to our cells.

At DARPA, the Engineered Living Materials (ELM) program seeks "to revolutionize military logistics and construction . . . by developing living biomaterials that combine the structural properties of traditional building mate-

---

20 Systems and Synthetic Biology, October 10, 2009.

21 University of Glasgow, "Scientists take first step towards creating 'inorganic life.'" Phys.org, September 12, 2011. Note that nanotechnology is not mentioned, despite the fact that "inorganic chemical compounds" that can self-replicate are dependent upon it. See "Modular Redox-Active Inorganic Chemical Cells: iCHELLS," Angewandte Chemie.

rials with attributes of living systems, including the ability to rapidly grow *in situ,* self-repair, and adapt to the environment."[22]

No mention of nanomaterials, only "living biomaterials." Turns of phrase like "cellular systems that function as living materials," "hybrid materials," "inert structural scaffolds that support the growth of living cells," "transition out of the laboratory," and "genetic programming of structural features into biological systems" make it obvious that ELM is about the Transhumanist Human 2.0 science now loosed on all of humanity.

6. *Scientism, not science*

The circularity of the Darwinian theory means that it is not falsifiable and therefore not truly scientific. The "falsifiability criterion" is the cornerstone of twentieth-century scientific method developed by Karl Popper, who also said, "I have come to the conclusion that Darwinism is not a testable scientific theory, but a metaphysical research programme – a possible framework for testable scientific theories . . . It is metaphysical because it is not testable."

– Jeremy Narby, *The Cosmic Serpent*, 1998

For since the creation of the world, God's invisible qualities – His eternal power and divine nature – have been clearly seen, being understood from what has been made...

– Romans 1:20

Social progress means a checking of the cosmic process at every step, and the substitution for it of another . . .

– T.H. Huxley, *Evolution and Ethics*, 1896

In an undergrad biology course decades ago, I had to remind my professor that Darwinian evolution was a theory and not a law.

In 1999, symbiogeneticist[23] Lynn Margulis was awarded the U.S. Presidential Medal for Science in part because she pronounced neo-Darwinism and its "survival of the fittest" dead. Margulis saw through how competitive capitalists had exploited Charles Darwin's "descent with modification" for the sake of justifying political and societal policies of domination, not biological accuracy. Darwinism was actually the old Gnostic myth of Jehovah

22 Dr. Blake Bextine "Engineered Living Materials (ELM)." DARPA, n.d.

23 New organelles, bodies, organs, and species arise from symbiogenesis. Margulis wrote Acquiring Genomes: A Theory of the Origin of Species (Basic Books, 2003).

the imperfect God having erred in creating this world, with the theory of evolution dispensing with him altogether. The theory of evolution was a political-ideological expedient, a spike driven into the resistant heart of religion. Marx viewed Darwin's evolutionary theory as "the basis in natural history," and Hitler perceived that the theory of evolution supported struggle, survival of the fittest and elimination of the weak. A higher race must prevail. Nature decreed it.

A Skull & Bones biology class might only have a dozen hand-picked students, with each weekly seminar taught by a JASON scientist from top programs and labs, all approved by the British Royal Society. None of the assigned readings are mainstream, beginning with Comenius' 1668 manifesto, *The Way of Light,* which says that for science to "secure the empire of human mind over matter," a clearinghouse is needed to accredit and disseminate only the knowledge the public should know and prevent dissemination of what the public shouldn't know. Thus was born the British Royal Society in the late 17th century, composed entirely of Freemasons and elitists whose duty was to set the mold for future regulators of knowledge.

Scientia est potentia was their manifesto. In deciding what the truly scientific would be, God—the incorporeal quality of Being behind magnitude, figure, motion, cohesion and firmness—was the first to go. Next would be æther. Physical laws of *Mater Natura* were enough for the masses until the 19th and 20th century, when Matter itself would be revealed to be the supreme Mystery.

The Skull and Bones class might begin with a quick overview: "In the beginning was lifeless matter, followed by spontaneous generation. *Natura,* being a sentient sovereign being—self-creating, self-sustaining, self-regenerating—created itself, going from matter to life, the first tenet of anthropomorphic mysticism. Thus, the living and non-living are inseparable. Spontaneous generation and the driving doctrine of natural selection set Western science free from *imago viva Dei*, thanks to the ancient Mystery religion of Freemasonry. For centuries, *Natura* was the guides, the force responsible for our thoughts and actions. Religion was no longer needed. Now, the Superman is within our reach, thanks to the *royal art* of science and technology."

Scientists and occultists alike—elite JASONs are one and the same, like Newton—knew that the barrier erected between matter and spirit was as arbitrary as particle and wave. The deeper into the physical one probes, the closer spirit is. The deeper into theoretical physics and biophysics, the closer the alchemical point of view is to Adepts who know how to converge magic and science, mystery and matter.

The Royal Society began as the Lunar Society (1764-1800) founded by Charles Darwin's grandfather Erasmus Darwin. Members were scientists of renown—Wilkinson, Watts, Boulton, Priestly, Wedgewood, Benjamin Franklin, etc.—all called *merchants of light* (from Francis Bacon's *New Atlantis*) who met only at the full moon. All were Freemasons, as had been John Locke (1632-1704). Freemason and Fellow of the royal Society T. H. Huxley, grandfather of Aldous Huxley, spoke for the reclusive Charles Darwin when he insisted that the occult evolutionary idea of *becoming* was the new science.

The Lunar Society was intimately bound up with the machinations behind the French Revolution.[24] Freemason Benjamin Franklin was a member of the Nine Muses (French) and Lunar Society (English), playing international envoy between French and English Freemasons, many of whom were Jacobins, agents of the Bavarian Illuminati at the Club Breton.

Nazism—National Socialism—was based on Marx: subordinate the individual to the collective, which itself is subordinate to a small central control. Then consolidate capital in a monopoly, either government or corporate. Communism and fascism, two sides of the same anti-democratic coin, two oligarchies founded upon the same occult Darwinian worldview.

Unfortunately, none of this is ancient history. It's all still going on.

Should the Hippocratic oath of "First, do no harm" be added to PhD science requirements?

7. Occult means hidden

I have no desire to uphold ancient superstitions . . . nor to support the modern superstitions that bacilli and bacteria cause the different diseases. We need not consider today whether we are really faced with the results of the spiritualistic superstitions of earlier times, or with the superstitions of materialism.

– Rudolf Steiner, "Hygiene, A Social Problem," Dornach, April 7, 1920

When you flip a switch on the wall, somewhere inside the wall metal components make energy move and electric light appears. For the most part, people simply accept that light appears and appliances work, after which they think no more about electricity.

The presence of invisible occult (hidden, concealed, covered over, secret) realities and events made to happen for political, societal, or personal agendas is a constant in modern times but disguised, lied about, and denied for equally obscure reasons and therefore unnoticed by the public mind. Because

24 Lord Acton (1834-1902), Essays on the French Revolution: "The appalling thing in the French Revolution is not the tumult but the design. Through all the fire and smoke, we perceive the evidence of calculating organization. The managers remain studiously concealed and masked, but there is no doubt about their presence from the first."

the forces that science seeks to manipulate are also hidden (like electricity, gravity, magnetism, etc.), it should be no surprise to learn that some scientists are occultists versed in scientific esoterica that normally educated scientists know nothing about and even think is nonsense.

While I could write yet another book on this topic, a few examples of the mindset of those movers and shakers versed in occult laws will have to suffice:

Initiation

Oddly, the medical definition of *occult* has been employed over and over for COVID-19: *not accompanied by readily discernible signs or symptoms.* Is this a reference to the *initiation* that planetary humanity has been subjected to in 2020-2021 via endless repetition and miscasting on mainstream media? Makia Freeman wrote an article in *Waking Times* about how the world has been forced to participate in an "occult corona-initiation ritual" by global elites who certainly believe in and practice occult laws that have been known and protected for thousands of years by secret societies beyond the pale of society. Ritualized quarantine / lockdown / social distancing (isolation), hand-washing, mask-wearing, and terror are practiced in occult circles seeking to separate initiates from their normal lives so as to break them down, engender submission, remold them, then return them to a "new normal."[25]

> In anthropology, *liminality* (L., *limen,* threshold) is the quality of ambiguity or disorientation that occurs in the middle stage of a rite of passage, when participants no longer hold their pre-ritual status but have not yet begun the transition to the status they will hold when the rite is complete. (Wikipedia)

The hexagon gateway

Solar and lunar simulator lenses
Smart City cells (10 miles square)
Graphene lattice structure
Water's geometry drawing current from the Sun
Insect eyes and honeycomb
Carbon nanotubes

At the very core of the science that studies the very essence of the ground of Being (like the nature of matter) are mysteries that blur the distinction between physics and metaphysics. Nanoparticles and the instruments that can perceive them are now leading the pack on the Mystery of Matter.

---

25 Makia Freeman, "Exposing the Occult Corona-Initiation Ritual." Waking Times, July 16, 2020.

MINERAL INTERRELATIONSHIPS

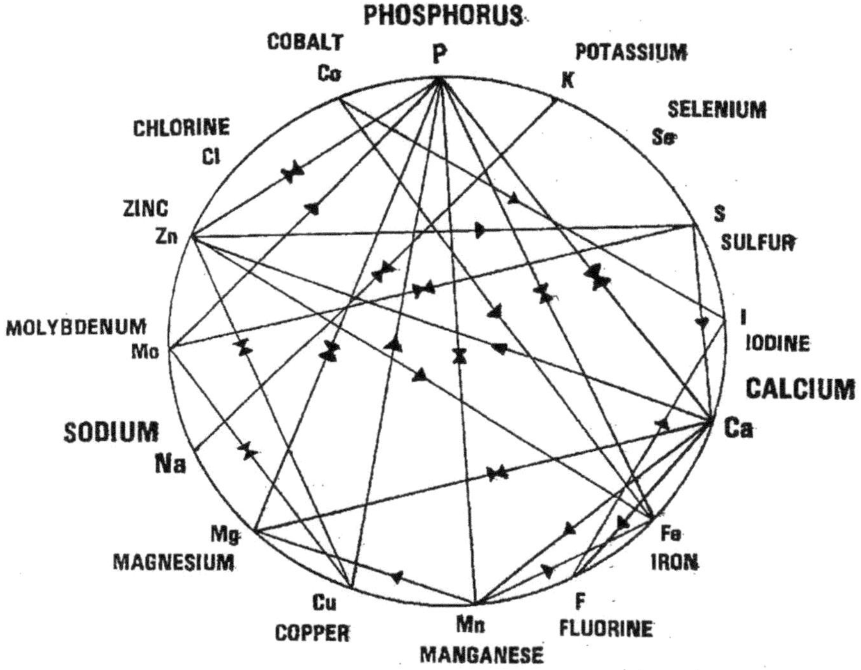

Mineral Interrelations.

http://www.luresext.edu/?q=content/mineral-nutrition-considerations

In 1995, a CRAY C90 supercomputer discovered a 1,500-mile diameter hexagonal close-packed (hcp) crystalline structure aligned with the Earth's spin axis growing in the temperature-pressure extremes of the core of the Earth.[26] For techno-magicians, the Earth is a crystalline electrical Being with a North Pole (anode or positive charge) and a South Pole (cathode or negative charge) in a giant protective ether cocoon transfused by seven planetary organs of Sun, Moon, Mercury, Mars, Venus, Jupiter, and Saturn—each infusing the electromagnetic *chakra* system in the pole-to-pole Rocky Mountain spine. The human body's spine is rich in minerals and energy, and is a transceiver

26 William J. Broad, "The Core of the Earth May Be a Gigantic Crystal Made of Iron." New York Times, April 4, 1995.

antenna receiving, transmitting and resonating to frequencies and pulses, its brain crown serving as relay station for individual consciousness and impersonal will-to-power.[27]

The greatest fallacy perpetrated by Western secret societies like the Freemasons against the *profane* (*pro-fane*, outside the Freemason Temple) has been the hard division between the physical and spiritual. Those who have dis-spelled (and it is a spell) this false division are primarily the truly science-minded who have penetrated the authentic relationship between the two—like the German chemist Friedrich August Kekulé who in 1865 dreamed of six dancing atoms forming a snake eating its own tail (the ouroboros): the hexagonal ring structure of benzene. Interestingly, the benzene ring in close proximity to a nitrogen molecule with two or three carbon molecules[28] between will produce potent hallucinogenic substances, as if the hexagon were a "door of perception" to other dimensions (as discussed in Chapter 12, "The Magical Human Head, Brain, & 'Second Brain'").

While we are conditioned to think of psychedelic substances as inducing "hallucinations," if they have a hexagonal molecular geometry, it is likely that the mind—itself nonphysical (unlike the brain), no doubt straddling at least two simultaneous dimensions at any moment of the day or night—has gained entry to another dimension, much as Kekulé did.[29]

The geometrical hexagon *shape* itself, whether microcosmic (molecular structure) or macrocosmic (insect structures, stone formations, telescope mirrors,[30] Saturn's north pole, etc.), is some sort of interlocking agent. What is geometry, anyway? What kind of power does it hold? Why did the ancient Greeks like Pythagoras study it so carefully?

The Egregores of corporations, foundations, & Brotherhoods

While living in London, I encountered an Italian who had worked at the Vatican in a high secular position during the reign of Pope John Paul II (1978-2005). He shared with me a term used broadly in esoteric circles: *Egregore.*

---

27 The peak voltage of the spinal column is 100 MHz (the FM radio band is 87.5 – 108 MHz) impacting the central nervous system and weakening the blood brain barrier. See Balaguru, Sevaiyan et al. "Investigation of the spinal cord as a natural receptor antenna for incident electromagnetic waves and possible impact on the central nervous system." Department of Electrical and Electronic Engineering, California State University, June 2012.

28 Carbon has six electrons, six protons, and six neutrons. Thus, the maligned number of Man: 666.

29 Thanks to veterinarian and anthroposophist Are Thoresen, Experiences from the Threshold – and Beyond: Understood Through Anthroposophy, 2019.

30 The optical Hobby-Eberly Telescope in the Davis Mountains, Texas, has a honeycomb of 91 hexagonal mirrors in a fixed position for its spectroscopy studies (the interaction between matter and electromagnetic radiation).

..."An egregore is a kind of group mind which is created when people consciously come together for a common purpose. Whenever people gather together to do something and egregore is formed, but unless an attempt is made to maintain it deliberately it will dissipate rather quickly. However, if the people wish to maintain it and know the techniques of how to do so, the egregore will continue to grow in strength and can last for centuries.

"An egregore has the characteristic of having an effectiveness greater than the mere sum of its individual members. It continuously interacts with its members, influencing them and being influenced by them. The interaction works positively by stimulating and assisting its members but only as long as they behave and act in line with its original aim. It will stimulate both individually and collectively all those faculties in the group which will permit the realization of the objectives of its original program. If this process is continued a long time the egregore will take on a kind of life of its own, and can become so strong that even if all its members should die, it would continue to exist on the inner dimensions and can be contacted even centuries later by a group of people prepared to live the lives of the original founders, particularly if they are willing to provide the initial input of energy to get it going again.

"If the egregore is concerned with spiritual or esoteric activities its influence will be even greater. People who discover the keys can tap in on a powerful egregore representing, for example, a spiritual or esoteric tradition, will, if they follow the line described above by activating and maintaining such an egregore, obtain access to the abilities, knowledge, and drive of all that has been accumulated in that egregore since its beginnings. A group or order which manages to do this can, with a clear conscience, claim to be an authentic order of the tradition represented by that egregore..."[31]

To grasp how such a psychological and mental *entity* (*not* a "metaphor") could exist is difficult for those conditioned to believe that thoughts and feelings are ephemeral and fleeting, despite recently witnessing the creation of a worldwide egregor based on fear of a virus that doesn't even exist, all due to a carefully organized, concerted *mental* assault via AI-run media, fear tactics, and 5G systems of *something that once did not exist but does now* in the minds and souls of terrorized people.

We have witnessed the creation of a powerful egregore by the global elite who are acutely aware of how such black magic can be done with the right instruments. Despite the thousands dying of the "treatment" for an imaginary viral disease, thousands more are lining up to receive the "treatment."

31 Gaetan Delaforge, "The Templar Tradition Yesterday and Today," MasonicWorld.com.

Useful entities like Google, Facebook, CDC, and World Health Organization (WHO) march to the rhythm of the egregore; the same goes for those who belong to useful secret societies, foundations, and "think tanks." We are surrounded by egregores that devour whomever they can, people who could have become individuals but instead have chosen to feed mental entities that obliterate the fine soul qualities of honor, virtue, honesty, courage, free will, etc.

This is our challenge. The mind is not a physical thing, and yet the thought forms it produces *live*, whether good and constructive or evil and destructive. This is what is meant in ancient spiritual books when it says the human being was created in the image of God: that we are creators not just with our hands and industry but with our *minds*.

What if demons are human thought forms?

What are your thought forms producing?

The mind exists in spiritual dimensions. As Saul / Paul put in the New Testament, our struggle as human beings is with powers and principalities, including egregores.

> *During the Golden Age of Kronos, abundance and long lives reigned, back when Earth and Saturn were still proximate as plasma planets. When once again their plasma envelopes are fully charged—Earth's by HAARP, Saturn's by CERN's toroidal fields—the two planets will reconnect via Birkeland currents.*[32] *This is the ultimate objective of all the aerosolized chemical spraying and electromagnetic zapping under AI algorithms: to create a plasma Earth controlled by AI machinery like Saturn's.*[33]
>
> *The Titans' digitized DNA vibrating at frequencies from another dimension was trapped inside the black cube inside Saturn until CERN's Large Hadron Collider (LHC) opened a portal and freed the Titan DNA to enter the Earth dimension so as to modify our Schumann resonance to match theirs as well as the frequencies of demonic entities at the nine levels of consciousness that comprise the Earth.*
>
> *–Anthony Patch (paraphrased)*

---

32 See "Magnetic Rope observed for the first time between Saturn and the Sun," University College London, 6 July 2016: "The Cassini spacecraft has been in orbit around Saturn since 2004 . . . Cassini indeed observed a flux rope [Birkeland Current] . . . [that] could be up to 8300 kilometers wide . . . The analysis was completed using a particle spectrometer built at UCL and a magnetometer built at Imperial College, both of which are onboard NASA's Cassini spacecraft. The Cassini mission will end in November 2017, when the spacecraft will be steered into the planet to study it, before disintegrating in Saturn's thick atmosphere."

33 See Norman R. Bergrun, PhD, Ringmakers of Saturn, 1986; from photographs taken during the Voyager 1 flight to Saturn in 1980.

Appendix 2
The Nuremberg Code

HUMAN EXPERIMENTATION IS JUSTIFIED ONLY if its results benefit society and it is carried out in accord with basic principles that satisfy moral, ethical, and legal concepts.

John Frink, email, April 26, 2021: This website gives a brief history of how the 10 points of the Nuremberg Code came into existence. Interestingly, although the code is an international ethical landmark, it is apparently still ***not enshrined in American or German national law.*** *We must assume those governments via their secret agencies like the CIA wanted to keep the door open to conduct* ***medical experimentation*** *(such as bioweapon programs like weaponized ticks) upon their citizenry without technically breaking the law.*

Nuremberg Code #1: Voluntary Consent is Essential

Nuremberg Code #2: Yield Fruitful Results Unprocurable By Other Means

Nuremberg Code #3: Base Experiments on Results of Animal Experimentation and Natural History of Disease

Nuremberg Code #4: Avoid All Unnecessary Suffering and Injury

Nuremberg Code #5: No Experiment to be Conducted If There's Reason to Think Injury or Death Will Occur

Nuremberg Code #6: Risk Should Never Exceed the Benefit

Nuremberg Code #7: Preparation Must Be Made Against Even Remote Possibility of Injury, Disability or Death

Nuremberg Code #8: Experiment Must Be Conducted by Scientifically Qualified Persons

Nuremberg Code #9: Anyone Must Have the Freedom to Bring the Experiment to an End At Any Time

Nuremberg Code #10: The Scientist Must Bring the Experiment to an End At Any Time if There's Probable Cause of it Resulting in Injury or Death

– From "Do Mandatory Masks & Vaccines Break the 10 Points of the Nuremberg Code?" by Klark Jouss, *Clickwooz,* February 15, 2021
https://clickwooz.wordpress.com/2021/02/15/do-mandatory-masks-vaccines-break-the-10-points-of-the-nuremberg-code/

Appendix 3

ITHACA

Protecting Human Rights
7 Ignacio Allende
San Cristobal de las Casas, Chiapas
Mexico 29200
November 25, 2019

Report to The Special Rapporteur on Torture Concerning Psychological Torture and Ill-Treatment

Special Rapporteur Nils Melzer is to be congratulated for attempting to address the darkest corners of torture, where "plausible deniability" allows the perpetrators to inflict grave damage and then to claim that their hands are unsullied. We trust that the submissions to this effort will clarify that what happens to the mind will affect the body and that separating the mental from the physical does not serve to adequately delineate what has been and is being inflicted on "no touch torture" subjects.

The request for submissions itself seems to create a false separation between the mind and the body in ways that are not consonant with our understanding of "no touch torture." "No touch torture" is known to often involve electronic weapons, such as those that were recently determined to have had such devastating effects on diplomats in Cuba and China. Recent reports are confirming that chemical weapons are now being deployed in some cases of "no touch torture." These weapons can be deployed as gases and aerosols and can be airborne, waterborne and have been known to end up inappropriately in a target's food. Clearly the use of such weapons would have not only mental effects but could potentially devastate a person's physical health, as well.

Dr. Robert Duncan, who has worked on some of these weapons projects with DARPA, CIA, the US Army and other agencies, had this to say in a recent correspondence: "....we do know how to create maximal long term suffering of an individual worse than physical torture or death with no evidence other than psychological scars. We can induce any mental illness in the DSM-V manual into a person. I remember reading how the words of torture under the Bush administration were twisted into 'enhanced interrogation.' We can stop the breathing of the target without waterboarding. We can put them through pains that are just as real to the mind but no-touch and hence not physical. We can cause sleep deprivation and hundreds of other effects all remotely by tuning into their cognitive model. The experiments often are deadly because there are things worse than death."

Clearly, "no touch torture" has gone way beyond psychological mistreatment and can induce death or suicide. Dr. Duncan also related that "Inducing mental illness in people decreases their lifetime by about 20 years."

Embracing a wholistic paradigm in terms of investigating the effects of psychological torture and "no touch torture" is called for here. It should be noted that one of the worst offenders in these cases is the United States and that there are no federal laws which would address these circumstances. In fact, the offense of torture is defined as occurring outside of the US, leaving torture within its borders completely unaddressed. Here is the sad little law which constitutes the sole US federal protection against torture, and which in fact negates any protection from or remedy to domestic torture.

https://www.law.cornell.edu/uscode/text/18/2340A

Those who have been tortured in the US (and it is my understanding that other organizations, including Targeted Justice, are providing reports to the Special Rapporteur with declarations from US torture victims), are disallowed through funding mechanisms from receiving assistance at any of the multiple torture rehabilitation agencies that exist in the US. The funding comes through HHS's Office of Refugee Resettlement and is earmarked only for asylum seekers and refugees, leaving US-born torture victims without any means of healing from the experiences. This denial of services constitutes further harm when help is what is called for.

In the US, The Church Committee hearings in the 1970s ostensibly terminated the use of non-consensual subjects in human experimentation. We know now that the experimentation never stopped. At this point in time, the numbers of people put into experimental weapons testing programs without their consent have ballooned astronomically.

Due to the covert nature of these weapons of torture, the US government has been able in many cases to simply deny their use, and has adopted a policy of treating victims of "no touch torture" as "crazy." This also perpetuates and amplifies the harm done.

We hope that this report will serve to inform the international community as to several issues attached to "no touch torture." One issue is the virtual impossibility of separating the physical from the mental in situations involving torture. Another is the utter lack of legal remedy in the US for any acts of domestic torture. Finally, the stance taken by the US to completely deny that covert electronic and chemical weapons are being used in human weapons testing, and in some cases punitively, against US citizens furthers the harm done to victims of no touch torture.

Janet Phelan
Co-Chairman, ITHACA
(janet_c_phelan@yahoo.com)

Appendix 4

Excerpts from

Survival by Using the Domestic Violence Clause

by Michael Diamond
http://domesticviolenceclause.org
2018

Dire conditions

Global warming and the resulting climate changes are bringing about dire conditions. "Thirty years ago," said Deke Arndt, Chief of NOAA's Climate Monitoring Branch, "we may have seen this [global warming] coming as a train in the distance. The train is in our living room now."[1] Mr. Arndt's emphatic description, however, has not brought about actions to deal with the threat.

And forty-eight years ago, René Dubos, a microbiologist with Rockefeller University, warned that chemical exposures would bring increases in diseases and, more importantly, "distortions of mental and emotional attributes." Unless we use our human genetic limitations as the regulatory standard, he predicted that we would begin to see, at the turn of the century, development of a "form of life that will retain little of true humanness."[2]

We came nowhere near using human genetic limitations as our regulatory standard. Philippe Grandjean's book, *Only One Chance: How Environmental Pollution Impairs Brain Development and How to Protect the Brains of the Next Generation*, is an ardent, scholarly plea to have us do so. [3] But Dr. Grandjean's book has not moved us to take action. Before long, it will be out of print and out of mind, and human behavior will continue to decline.

The domestic violence clause

I think that we, the people, fervently want future generations to enjoy good physical and emotional health on a habitable planet. We just don't know how to create an effective opposition to the powerful interests that now prevail.

---

1 Seth Borenstein & Nicky Forster, for *AP*, "Warned 30 Years Ago, Global Warming 'Is In Our Living Room'," The Press of Atlantic City, June 19, 2018, page C6.

2 René Dubos, "The Limits of Adaptability," The Environmental Handbook, ed. Garrett DeBell (New York: Ballantine Books, 1970) pages 28-29.

3 Philippe Grandjean, *Only One Chance* (New York: Oxford University Press, 2013).

The purpose of this writing is to show how the people can wrest control from the oligarchs behind the military-medical-agri-business-industrial-banking-media-political-academic complex. The tool to be used was at our fingertips all the time. It is the domestic violence clause in Article IV, Section 4 of the United States Constitution.

Article IV, Section 4 is generally known as the "guarantee provision." Here is the exact wording of that lengthy, complex Section 4 which ends with the words domestic violence: "The United States shall guarantee to every State in this Union a Republican Form of Government, and shall protect each of them against Invasion: and on Application of the Legislature, or the Executive (when the Legislature cannot be convened), against domestic Violence."

To clarify and simplify those words we can exclude reference to a republican form of government. And because rapid travel now allows state legislatures to be quickly convened, we can drop mention of the executive (meaning governors) of the states. Lastly, the Unites States Supreme Court case of *Texas v. White*, 74 U.S. 700 (1868), at page 721, held that the guarantees of protection are owed not to the state governments, but to the people.

Thus pared down and clarified, Article IV, Section 4 reads as follows: The United States shall protect the people against invasion; and on application of the [state] legislature[s], shall protect the people against domestic violence....

The 9/11 attack as both domestic violence and treason

You see, treason is defined in Article III, Section 3 as "the levying of war" against us. Bombing our own people would be an obvious treasonous act. The first acts of treason the state legislatures need to know about are the attacks on September 11, 2001. At that time, we were killed and maimed by our own people, and that levying of war has kept us at war around the world ever since.

The official stories of what occurred on that date are ludicrous beyond measure. Two airplanes are said to have crashed in New York City, bringing down three skyscraper buildings at near free-fall acceleration largely within their own footprints, in the manner of controlled demolitions. Anyone with any semblance of education knows that the official story of the World Trade Center attack must be false. Hijackers with box-cutters could not possibly have made that happen. The attack had to have been home-grown, accomplished through the use of sophisticated explosives, and done with enormous amounts of preplanning.

Please understand that the treason provision in our Constitution has a federal statutory component known as "misprision of treason." It requires those who know of a treason to come forward and give evidence of what they know concerning treasonous actions.[4] Anyone with any background in physics, chemistry, or mathematics should have, long ago, understood the official story to have been fraudulent and should have come forward with that understanding, pursuant to their misprision of treason obligation. Only by doing so could the resulting series of wars have been stopped.

In like manner, on September 11, 2001, a passenger airplane is supposed to have stuck the Pentagon, a steel reinforced concrete structure, without leaving debris from wingtip to wingtip on the ground immediately below. And another passenger airplane is supposed to have crashed into a field in Shanksville, Pennsylvania, burying itself totally from view under the hard-packed ground. Those two occurrences are as impossible as the New York City air crash story. So ludicrous are the Pentagon and the Shanksville incidents that every college and university science department should have been clamoring to inform the public that treason obviously occurred in Virginia and in Pennsylvania.

Geoengineering as both domestic violence and treason

The federal government's campaign to discredit people from discussing geoengineering has been so successful that little is known about it, even though we see unmistakable evidence of it nearly every day in the skies above us. As a result, this portion of the essay must be longer to include some necessary pieces of evidence.

The state legislatures need to understand also that the geoengineering they see so clearly in the skies above us is an ongoing series of attacks constituting both domestic violence and treason.

When I was young, I saw airplanes occasionally leaving white trails of water vapor that quickly disbursed. Now, I see airplanes flying at high altitudes leaving white trails that remain aloft for long periods of time. The trails often join together with other trails left by other airplanes. The result is a white cloud cover that lingers, blocking direct sunlight.

I had the honor of meeting one of the foremost environmental scientists of our times, Sr. Rosalie Bertell, PhD.[5] The trails in our skies, she said,

---

4 There can be no silent acquiescence to treason. *18 U.S. Code, Section 2382* requires the following: *Whoever, owing allegiance to the United States and having knowledge of the commission of any treason against them, conceals and does not, as soon as may be, disclose and make known the same to the President or to some judge of the United States, or to the governor or to some judge or justice of a particular State, is guilty of misprision of treason and shall be fined under this title or imprisoned not more than seven years, or both.*

5 A fitting tribute to Dr. Bertell's work was written by Ilya Sandra Perlingieri, PhD, "Remembering Rosalie Bertell," *Global Research*, 15 June 2012. Dr. Bertell, author of *Planet Earth: The Latest Weapon of War* (2001) died on June 14, 2012, Dr. Perlingieri, author of *The Uterine Crisis* (2003), on October 7, 2013.

contain dangerous toxins that are being sprayed upon us without our consent by an out-of-control military.[6] The history of military recklessness behind those trails in the sky is vividly portrayed by Amy Worthington in "Chemtrails: Aerosol and Electromagnetic Weapons in the Age of Nuclear War," *Global Research,* 1 June 2004.

The best word to use in describing the spraying of toxins is *massive.* Francis Mangels is a brilliant man with over forty years of experience in environmental management and assessment as a USDA biologist.[7] He tested rainwater in California after significant spraying by unmarked military type aircraft. "My testing," he told me, "since 2003, has consistently shown concentrations of aluminum, barium, and strontium in extremely high numbers. No samples I've taken, heard of, or seen since 2003 have been in the normal concentrations of zero or 1 ug/l. Samples here range from about 13,000 ug/l in rain to 61,000 ug/l in snow, varying with the amount of jet spray."[8] The "aluminum, barium, and strontium" in that spraying, he said, "were likely in nanosized particles. Being that tiny usually makes them many orders of magnitude more dangerous. Nanosize is never normal for those elements. They must be engineered to that size."[9]

Francis Mangels told me the following: A nanoparticle is a billionth of a meter, a thousand times smaller than particles in exhaled tobacco smoke. Commercial filters will not stop them. They go through lung and intestinal tissue easily, coursing through the human body and lodging in every part of us. The blood-brain barrier is no shield against them. The particles lodge in brains where they can disrupt delicate connections and accelerate neural problems. Nanosized particles, he continued, can pass to a child developing in the womb. The umbilical cord cannot stop a nanoparticle.[10]

Mr. Mangels puts the use of nanotechnology in regulatory perspective. "Governments are considering use of nanoparticles in manufacturing processes. How safe are they to handle? What steps should be taken concerning their disposal? Most engineering and health disciplines express the dangers of fine particulates in the human system." But, continues Mangels, "the military/industrial complex or whoever is doing the spraying have not followed

---

6 "Dr. Rosalie Bertell – MAKE IT VISIBLE – chemtrails," a Snowshoe interview, May 3, 2005, New York City, *https://www.youtube.com/watch?v=st3lHWZTrwQ.*

7 Francis Mangels spoke at the Consciousness Beyond Chemtrails conference in Los Angeles in August 2012 (as did Dr. Perlingieri) and appeared in both *What in the World Are They Spraying?* (2010; produced by G. Edward Griffin, Michael Murphy, Paul Wittenberger) and *Why in the World Are They Spraying?* (2012; directed by Michael J. Murphy).

8 Telephone conversations with Francis Mangels in early January, 2017.

9 Ibid.

10 Ibid.

the regulatory process. They have created no environmental impact report. They are spraying nanosize particles out of jets without notice to nor consent of the governed, in violation of laws created to control pollution of air, water, and soil."[11] He warns that "Poisoning through nanoparticles is harming human life, plants, insects, and animals. Human survival is dependent upon a vibrant web of life, which is being threatened."[12]

Over many years, I have come to respect and rely upon the research and writings of Dr. Russell Blaylock, a retired neurosurgeon. He has written about the harm that's resulting from the spraying of large amounts of nanosized aluminum compounds from the aircraft he sees above us. "Once the soil, plants, and water sources are heavily contaminated, there will be no way to reverse the damage that has been done. Steps need to be taken now to prevent an impending health disaster of enormous proportions if this project is not stopped immediately. Otherwise we will see an explosive increase in neurodegenerative diseases occurring in adults and the elderly in unprecedented rates as well as neurodevelopmental disorders in our children. We are already seeing a dramatic increase in these neurological disorders and it is occurring in younger people than ever before."

The official position of the federal government is that the persistent trails in the sky that we are seeing now are merely water vapor from jet engines.[13] But water vapor could not possibly persist as do the trails now being left in our skies. In addition, some airplanes leave persistent trails while others do not. And on some days with the same temperature and humidity conditions,

---

11 Ibid.

12 Ibid.

13 Letter from U.S. Senator Robert Menendez (New Jersey) to me dated January 16, 2015:

"Article 5 of the Universal Declaration of Human Rights states: "No one shall be subjected to torture or to cruel, inhuman or degrading treatment or punishment." This ban on torture and other ill treatment has subsequently been incorporated into the extensive network of international and regional human rights treaties. It is contained in Article 7 of the International Covenant on Civil and Political Rights (ICCPR), ratified by 153 countries, including the United States in 1992, and in the Convention against Torture or Other Cruel, Inhuman or Degrading Treatment or Punishment (the Convention against Torture), ratified by 136 countries, including the United States in 1994. It is also codified in the European Convention for the Protection of Human Rights and Fundamental Freedoms, the African Charter on Human and Peoples' Rights, and the American Convention on Human Rights." ~ Human Rights Watch on the international illegality of torture

[Note: Email from Michael, May 23, 2021: "...an updated version of this essay appeared in *Covert Action* magazine https://covertactionmagazine.com/2021/02/18/ending-corporate-tyranny-solutions-to-the-plague-that-afflicts-us-all/, which includes additional arguments and a 'selling point' when approaching state legislators about the domestic violence clause: the legislators should stop giving up their children as sacrifices in wars for the benefit of corporate profits."

no airplanes leave such trails. I and many others have even seen jet aircraft leave persistent trails that stop and start again a few seconds later—an impossibility if the white trails are water vapor coming from jet engines.

That official response is so at variance with accepted principles of physics and chemistry that science departments all over the country should be outraged over the governmental duplicity. They should be weighing-in to uphold truths. Their not doing so constitutes actions amounting to misprisions of treason, as above noted. With knowledge comes responsibility, and there's no higher a responsibility than to speak out when one knows that the spraying of nanosized particles of neurotoxic materials without the consent of the people is treason, per se, the levying of war against the people.

Appendix 5
"The InGen Incident"

Reptiles are abhorrent because of their cold body, pale color, cartilaginous skeleton, filthy skin, fierce aspect, calculating eye, offensive smell, harsh voice, squalid habitation, and terrible venom; wherefore their Creator has not exerted his powers to make many of them.

– Linnaeus, 1797

You cannot recall a new form of life.

– Erwin Chargaff, biochemist, 1972

Michael Crichton, *Jurassic Park* Introduction (UK: Random Century Group, 1991)

THE LATE TWENTIETH CENTURY HAS witnessed a scientific gold rush of astonishing proportions: the headlong and furious haste to commercialize genetic engineering. This enterprise has proceeded so rapidly—with so little outside commentary—that its dimensions and implications are hardly understood at all.

Biotechnology promises the greatest revolution in human history. By the end of this decade, it will have outdistanced atomic power and computers in its effect on our everyday lives. In the words of one observer, "Biotechnology is going to transform every aspect of human life: our medical care, our food, our health, our entertainment, our very bodies. Nothing will ever be the same again. It's literally going to change the face of the planet."

But the biotechnology revolution differs in three important respects from past scientific transformations.

First, it is broad-based. America entered the atomic age through the work of a single research institution, at Los Alamos. It entered the computer age through the efforts of about a dozen companies. But biotechnology research is now carried out in more than two thousand laboratories in America alone. Five hundred corporations spend five billion dollars a year on this technology.

Second, much of the research is thoughtless and frivolous. Efforts to engineer paler trout for better visibility in the stream, square trees for easier lumbering, and injectable scent cells so you'll always smell your favorite perfume may seem like a joke, but they are not. Indeed, the fact that biotechnology can be applied to the industries traditionally subject to the vagaries of fashion, such as cosmetics and leisure activities, heightens concern about the whimsical use of this powerful new technology.

Third, the work is uncontrolled. No one supervises it. No federal laws regulate it. There is no coherent government policy, in America or anywhere else in the world. And because the products of biotechnology range from drugs to farm crops to artificial snow, an intelligent policy is difficult.

But most disturbing is the fact that no watchdogs are found among scientists themselves. It is remarkable that nearly every scientist in genetics research is also engaged in the commerce of biotechnology. There are no detached observers. Everybody has a stake.

The commercialization of molecular biology is the most stunning ethical event in the history of science, and it has happened with astonishing speed. For four hundred years since Galileo, science has always proceeded as a free and open inquiry into the workings of nature. Scientists have always ignored national boundaries, holding themselves above the transitory concerns of politics and even wars. Scientists have always rebelled against secrecy in research, and have even frowned on the idea of patenting their discoveries, seeing themselves as working to the benefit of all mankind. And for many generations, the discoveries of scientists did indeed have a peculiarly selfless quality.

When, in 1953, two young researchers in England, James Watson and Francis Crick, deciphered the structure of DNA, their work was bailed as a triumph of the human spirit, of the centuries-old quest to understand the universe in a scientific way. It was confidently expected that their discovery would be selflessly extended to the greater benefit of mankind.

Yet that did not happen. Thirty years later, nearly all of Watson and Crick's scientific colleagues were engaged in another sort of enterprise entirely. Research in molecular genetics had become a vast, multibillion dollar commercial undertaking, and its origins can be traced not to 1953 but to April 1976.

That was the date of a now famous meeting, in which Robert Swanson, a venture capitalist, approached Herbert Boyer, a biochemist at the University of California. The two men agreed to found a commercial company to exploit Boyer's gene-splicing techniques. Their new company, Genentech, quickly became the largest and most successful of the genetic engineering start-ups.

Suddenly it seemed as if everyone wanted to become rich. New companies were announced almost weekly, and scientists flocked to exploit genetic research. By 1986, at least 362 scientists, including 64 in the National Academy, sat on the advisory boards of biotech firms. The number of those who held equity positions or consultancies was several times greater.

It is necessary to emphasize how significant this shift in attitude actually was. In the past, pure scientists took a snobbish view of business. They saw the pursuit of money as intellectually uninteresting, suited only to shopkeepers. And to do research for industry, even at the prestigious Bell or IBM labs, was only for those who couldn't get a university appointment. Thus the attitude of pure scientists was fundamentally critical toward the work of applied scientists, and to industry in general. Their long-standing antagonism kept university scientists free of contaminating industry ties, and whenever debate arose about technological matters, disinterested scientists were available to discuss the issues at the highest levels.

But that is no longer true. There are very few molecular biologists and very few research institutions without commercial affiliations. The old days are gone. Genetic research continues, at a more furious pace than ever. But it is done in secret, and in haste, and for profit.

In this commercial climate, it is probably inevitable that a company as ambitious as International Genetic Technologies, Inc., of Palo Alto, would arise. It is equally unsurprising that the genetic crisis it created should go unreported. After all, InGen's research was conducted in secret; the actual incident occurred in the most remote region of Central America; and fewer than twenty people were there to witness it. Of those, only a handful survived.

Even at the end, when International Genetic Technologies filed for Chapter 11 protection in San Francisco Superior Court on October 5, 1989, the proceedings drew little press attention. It appeared so ordinary: InGen was the third small American bioengineering company to fail that year, and the seventh since 1986. Few court documents were made public, since the creditors were Japanese investment consortia, such as Hamaguri and Densaka, companies which traditionally shun publicity. To avoid unnecessary disclosure, Daniel Ross, of Cowan, Swain and Ross, counsel for InGen, also represented the Japanese investors. And the rather unusual petition of the vice consul of Costa Rica was heard behind closed doors. Thus it is not surprising that, within a month, the problems of InGen were quietly and amicably settled.

Parties to that settlement, including the distinguished scientific board of advisers, signed a nondisclosure agreement, and none will speak about what happened—but many of the principal figures in the "InGen incident" are not signatories, and were willing to discuss the remarkable events leading up to those final two days in August 1989 on a remote island off the west coast of Costa Rica.

Appendix 6

STATEMENT ON VIRUS ISOLATION (SOVI)

BY SALLY FALLON MORELL, MA,
THOMAS COWAN, MD, AND ANDREW KAUFMAN, MD

https://drtomcowan.com/sovi

Isolation: The action of isolating; the fact or condition of being isolated or standing alone; separation from other things or persons; solitariness. – *Oxford English Dictionary*

The controversy over whether the SARS-CoV-2 virus has ever been isolated or purified continues. However, using the above definition, common sense, the laws of logic and the dictates of science, any unbiased person must come to the conclusion that the SARS-CoV-2 virus has *never* been isolated or purified. As a result, no confirmation of the virus' existence can be found. The logical, common sense, and scientific consequences of this fact are:

- the structure and composition of something not shown to exist can't be known, including the presence, structure, and function of any hypothetical spike or other proteins;
- the genetic sequence of something that has never been found can't be known;
- "variants" of something that hasn't been shown to exist can't be known;
- it's impossible to demonstrate that SARS-CoV-2 causes a disease called Covid-19.

In as concise terms as possible, here's the proper way to isolate, characterize and demonstrate a new virus. First, one takes samples (blood, sputum, secretions) from many people (e.g. 500) with symptoms which are unique and specific enough to characterize an illness. Without mixing these samples with ANY tissue or products that also contain genetic material, the virologist macerates, filters and ultracentrifuges i.e. *purifies* the specimen. This common virology technique, done for decades to isolate bacteriophages[1] and so-called giant viruses in every virology lab, then allows the virologist to demonstrate

1 "Isolation, characterization and analysis of bacteriophages from the haloalkaline lake Elmenteita, Kenya," Juliah Khayeli Akhwale *et al.*, *PLOS One*, April 25, 2019.

with electron microscopy thousands of identically sized and shaped particles. These particles are the isolated and purified virus.

These identical particles are then checked for uniformity by physical and/or microscopic techniques. Once the purity is determined, the particles may be further characterized. This would include examining the structure, morphology, and chemical composition of the particles. Next, their genetic makeup is characterized by extracting the genetic material directly from the purified particles and using genetic-sequencing techniques, such as Sanger sequencing, that have also been around for decades. Then one does an analysis to confirm that these uniform particles are exogenous (outside) in origin as a virus is conceptualized to be, and not the normal breakdown products of dead and dying tissues.[2] (As of May 2020, we know that virologists have no way to determine whether the particles they're seeing are viruses or just normal break-down products of dead and dying tissues.)[3]

If we have come this far then we have fully isolated, characterized, and genetically sequenced an exogenous virus particle. However, we still have to show it is causally related to a disease. This is carried out by exposing a group of healthy subjects (animals are usually used) to this isolated, purified virus in the manner in which the disease is thought to be transmitted. If the animals get sick with the same disease, as confirmed by clinical and autopsy findings, one has now shown that the virus actually causes a disease. This demonstrates infectivity and transmission of an infectious agent.

None of these steps has even been attempted with the SARS-CoV-2 virus, nor have all these steps been successfully performed for any so-called pathogenic virus. Our research indicates that a single study showing these steps does not exist in the medical literature.

Instead, since 1954, virologists have taken unpurified samples from a relatively few people, often less than ten, with a similar disease. They then minimally process this sample and inoculate this unpurified sample onto tissue culture containing usually four to six other types of material — **all of which contain identical genetic material as to what is called a "virus."** The tissue culture is starved and poisoned and naturally disintegrates into many types of particles, some of which contain genetic material. Against all common sense, logic, use of the English language and scientific integrity, this process is called "virus isolation." This brew containing fragments of genetic material

---

2 "Extracellular Vesicles Derived From Apoptotic Cells: An Essential Link Between Death and Regeneration," Maojiao Li1 *et al.*, *Frontiers in Cell and Developmental Biology*, October 2020.

3 "The Role of Extracellular Vesicles as Allies of HIV, HCV and SARS Viruses," Flavia Giannessi, *et al.*, *Viruses*, May 2020.

from many sources is then subjected to genetic analysis, which then creates in a computer-simulation process the alleged sequence of the alleged virus, a so called *in silico genome*. At no time is an actual virus confirmed by electron microscopy. At no time is a genome extracted and sequenced from an actual virus. This is scientific fraud.

The observation that the unpurified specimen — inoculated onto tissue culture along with toxic antibiotics, bovine fetal tissue, amniotic fluid and other tissues — destroys the kidney tissue onto which it is inoculated is given as evidence of the virus' existence and pathogenicity. This is scientific fraud.

From now on, when anyone gives you a paper that suggests the SARS-CoV-2 virus has been isolated, please check the methods sections. If the researchers used Vero cells or any other culture method, you know that their process was not isolation. You will hear the following excuses for why actual isolation isn't done:

1. There were not enough virus particles found in samples from patients to analyze.
2. Viruses are intracellular parasites; they can't be found outside the cell in this manner.

If No. 1 is correct, and we can't find the virus in the sputum of sick people, then on what evidence do we think the virus is dangerous or even lethal? If No. 2 is correct, then how is the virus spread from person to person? We are told it emerges from the cell to infect others. Then why isn't it possible to find it?

Finally, questioning these virology techniques and conclusions is not some distraction or divisive issue. Shining the light on this truth is essential to stop this terrible fraud that humanity is confronting. For, as we now know, if the virus has never been isolated, sequenced or shown to cause illness, if the virus is imaginary, then why are we wearing masks, social distancing and putting the whole world into prison?

Finally, if pathogenic viruses don't exist, then what is going into those injectable devices erroneously called "vaccines," and what is their purpose? This scientific question is the most urgent and relevant one of our time.

We are correct. The SARS-CoV2 virus does not exist.

Sally Fallon Morell, MA
Dr. Thomas Cowan, MD
Dr. Andrew Kaufman, MD

Appendix 7
Vaccine Ingredients*

("modified" = gain of function)

betapropiolactone
CTAB (cetyltrimethylammonium bromide)
formalin
L-cystine
2-phenoxyethanol
acetone
African Green Monkey kidney (Vero)
alcohol
aluminum hydroxide
aluminum phosphate
aluminum salts
amino acid supplement
amino acids
amino acids solution
aminoglycoside
antibiotic
ammonium sulfate
ammonium sulfate aluminum phosphate
amorphous aluminum hydroxyphosphate sulfate
amphotericin B
anhydrous lactose
anti-foaming agent
arginine
ascorbic acid
asparagine
baculovirus and cellular DNA
baculovirus and Spodoptera frugiperda cell proteins
barium
benzethonium chloride
beta-propriolactone beta-propiolactone
bovine albumin
bovine calf serum
bovine serum

bovine serum albumin
calcium carbonate
calcium chloride
calf bovine serum
Calf serum
calf serum and lactalbumin hydrolysate
carbohydrates
casamino acids
casamino acids and yeast extract-based medium
casein
castor oil
cell culture media
cellulose acetate phthalate
cetyltrimethlyammonium bromide
chick embryo cell culture
chicken fibroblasts
chlortetracycline
citric acid
citric acid monohydrate
CMRL 1969 medium supplemented with calf serum
complex fermentation media
concentrated vitamin solution
CRM197 carrier protein
CY medium
cystine
D- fructose
D- glucose
defined fermentation growth media
deoxycholate
dextran
dextrose
dibasic potassium phosphate
dibasic sodium phosphate
dimethyl-beta-cyclodextrin
glutaraldehyde
disodium phosphatedisodium phosphate dihydrate
D-mannose
DNA
dried lactose
Dulbecco's Modified Eagle Medium

E. coli
Eagle MEM modified medium
EDTA (Ethylenediaminetetraacetic acid)
egg protein
ethylenediaminetetraacetic acid (EDTA)
FD&C Yellow #6 aluminum lake dye
Fenton medium containing a bovine extract
ferric (III) nitrate
fetal bovine serum
formaldehyde
Franz complete medium
galactosegelatin
gentamicin sulfate
glutamate
glutaraldehyde
Glycerin
guinea pig cell cultures
HEPES
hexadecyltrimethylammonium bromide histidine
histidine-buffered saline
host cell DNA
host cell protein
human albumin
human diploid cell cultures (MRC-5)
human diploid cell cultures (WI-38)
human embryonic lung cell cultures
human serum albumin
human-diploid fibroblast cell cultures (strain WI-38)
hydrocortisone
hydrolyzed casein
hydrolyzed gelatin
hydrolyzed porcine gelatin
inorganic salts
iron ammonium citrate
isotonic sodium chloride
kanamycin
L-250 glutamine
lactalbumin hydrolysate
lactose L-histidine
lipids

L-tyrosine
M-199 without calf bovine serum
Madin Darby Canine Kidney (MDCK) cell protein
magnesium stearate
magnesium stearate.
gelatin
magnesium sulfate
maltose
MDCK cell DNA
Medium 199 without calf serum
microcrystalline cellulose
mineral salts
modified culture medium containing hydrolyzed casein
modified Latham medium derived from bovine casein
modified Mueller and Miller medium
modified Mueller and Miller medium (the culture medium contains milk- derived raw materials [casein derivatives])
modified Mueller's growth medium
modified Mueller-Miller casamino acid medium without beef heart infusion
modified Mueller's media which contains bovine extracts
modified Stainer-Scholte liquid medium
monobasic potassium phosphate
monobasic sodium phosphate
monosodium glutamate
monosodium L-glutamate
monosodim phosphate
MRC-5 diploid fibroblast
MRC-5 human diploid cells
Mueller Hinton casein agar
Mueller's growth medium
neomycin
neomycin sulfate
non-viral protein
nonylphenol ethoxylate
normal human diploid cells
octoxynol-10 (TRITON X-100)
octylphenol ethoxylate (Triton X-100)
ovalbumin
ovalbumin neomycin
phenol

phenol red
phenol red indicator
phosphate buffer
phosphate-buffered saline solution
plasdone C
polacrilin potassium
polydimethylsiloxane
polygeline (processed bovine gelatin) polymyxin
polymyxin B
polymyxin B sulfate
polysorbate 20
polysorbate 20 (Tween 20)
polysorbate 80 (Tween 80) potassium aluminum sulfate
potassium chloride
potassium glutamate
potassium phosphate
potassium phosphate dibasic
potassium phosphate monobasic
potassium phosphate potassium chloride protamine sulfate
protein other than HA
recombinant human albumin
saline
semi-synthetic media
semi-synthetic medium
sodium bicarbonate
sodium borate
sodium carbonate
sodium chloride
sodium citrate
sodium citrate dehydrate
sodium deoxycholate
sodium dihydrogen phosphate dihydrate
sodium EDTA
sodium hydrogenocarbonate
sodium hydroxide
sodium metabisulphite
sodium phosphate
sodium phosphate dibasic
sodium phosphate monobasic monohydrate
sodium phosphate-buffered isotonic sodium chloride

sodium phosphate-buffered isotonic sodium chloride solution
sodium pyruvate
sodium taurodeoxycholate
sorbitan trioleate
sorbitol
soy peptone
squalene
Stainer-Scholte medium
sterile water
succinate buffer
sucrose
sugars
synthetic medium
thimerosal (multi- dose vials)
tris (trometamol)-HCl
Triton X-100
uracil urea
[DNA from porcine circoviruses (PCV) 1 and 2 detected in RotaTeq and Rotarix]
vitamins
Watson Scherp casamino acid media
Watson Scherp media containing casamino acid
WI-38 human diploid lung fibroblasts
MRC-5 cells
xanthan
yeast extract
*yeast protein*α*-tocopheryl*
hydrogen succinate
β*-propiolactone*

**Does not include Moderna's "SM-102 Not for Human or Veterinary Use" or other poisons recently discovered in other vaccines*

Appendix 8
"Not A Vaccine"

David E. Martin, PhD
"Focus on Fauci" with Robert F. Kennedy Jr., Judy Mikovits, PhD, Rocco Galati, JD, and Sacha Stone, January 5, 2021

LET'S MAKE SURE WE ARE clear ... This is not a vaccine. They are using the term "vaccine" to sneak this thing under public health exemptions. This is not a vaccine. This is mRNA packaged in a fat envelope that is delivered to a cell. It is a medical device designed to stimulate the human cell into becoming a pathogen creator. It is not a vaccine. Vaccines actually are a legally defined term under public health law; they are a legally defined term under CDC and FDA standards. And the vaccine specifically has to stimulate both the immunity within the person receiving it, and it also has to disrupt transmission. And that is not what this is.

They have been abundantly clear in saying that the mRNA strand that is going into the cell is not to stop the transmission; it is a treatment. But if it was discussed as a treatment, it would not get the sympathetic ear of public health authorities because then people would say "What other treatments are there?" The use of the term "vaccine" is unconscionable for both the legal definition and also it is actually the sucker punch to open and free discourse ...

Moderna was started as a chemotherapy company for cancer, not a vaccine manufacturer for SARSCOV2. If we said we are going to give people prophylactic chemotherapy for the cancer they don't yet have, we'd be laughed out of the room because it's a stupid idea. That's exactly what this is. This is a mechanical device in the form of a very small package of technology that is being inserted into the human system to activate the cell to become a pathogen-manufacturing site.

I refuse to stipulate in any conversations that this is, in fact, a vaccine issue. The only reason the term is being used is to abuse the 1905 Jacobson case that has been misrepresented since it was written. And if we were honest with this, we would actually call it what it is: a chemical pathogen device that is actually meant to unleash a chemical pathogen production action within a cell. It is a medical device, not a drug because it meets the CDRH [Center for Devices and Radiological Health] definition of a device. It is not a living system, it is not a biological system. It is a physical technology that happens to come in the size of a molecular package.

So we need to be really clear on making sure we don't fall for their game because their game is if we talk about it as a vaccine, then we are going to get into a vaccine conversation. But this is not, by their own admission, a vaccine. As a result, it must be clear to everyone listening that we will not fall for this failed definition, just like we will not fall for their industrial chemical definition of health. Both of them are functionally flawed and are an implicit violation of the legal construct that is being exploited.

I get frustrated when I hear activists and lawyers say "we are going to fight the vaccine." If you stipulate it's a vaccine, you've already lost the battle. It's not a vaccine. It is made to make you sick ... 80% of people who get this injected into them experience a clinical adverse event. You are getting injected with a chemical substance to induce illness, not to induce an immune-transmissive response. In other words, nothing about this is going to stop you from transmitting anything. This is about getting you sick and having your own cells be the thing that gets you sick.

When the paymaster for the distribution of information happens to be the industry that's doing the distributing, we lose because the only narrative is the one that will be compensated by the people writing the check. That goes for our politicians and our media. It has been paid for. If you follow the money, you realize there is no non-conflicted voice on any network.

See G. Edward Griffin's *needtoknow.news* article quoting David E. Martin, PhD, on 15 US Code 41 and 1905 Supreme Court case *Jacobson v Massachusetts.*

https://needtoknow.news/2021/01/rna-vaccines-are-gmo-implants-not-vaccines/

Appendix 9

Nanotech Terms

Nanoscale (10^{-9} meters)
1 nanometer = 1 millionth of a meter
100 million nanoparticles on the head of a pin
A human hair is 90,000 nm thick
A red blood cell is 5,000 nm in diameter
The human being has 25 km of blood vessels,
each with a diameter of less than 10 microns
(1 micron = 1,000 nanometers)

Project on Emerging Nanotechnology, 2005
Defense Threat Reduction Agency / Joint Science and Technology Office for Chemical and Biological Defense

Engineered nanoparticles:

- Metal oxides
- Carbon nanotubes (CNTs)
- Nanowires
- Quantum dots
- Carbon fullerenes (buckyballs)
- Carbon nanofibers (CNFs)
- Graphene
- Lattices (frames, scaffolding, molds)
- Origami DNA

VT-LPTEM (variable temperature liquid-phase transmission electron microscopy): new form of electron microscopy that avails researchers of examining nanoscale tubular materials while they are "alive" and forming liquids – how nanomaterials grow, form and evolve as the researcher mixes components and performs chemical reactions.

We think LPTEM could do for nanoscience what live-cell light microscopy has done for biology. – Nathan Gianneschi, chemist[1]

1 Amanda Morris, "New technology gives insight into how nanomaterials form and grow." *Northwestern Now*, June 27, 2019

3D printing of microrobots, including synthetic microfish, microjet engines, microdrillers, microrockets, etc. For example, microfish contain nanobots ("functional nanoparticles") that self-propel, chemically power, magnetically steer

Artificial atoms comprise a new branch of chemistry in a second periodic table for flat atoms (2D) that can have thousands of electron states (stable natural elements have 92)

Carbon nanotubes (CNTs): hollow tubes of pure carbon as wide as a strand of DNA; tend to bundle and align tangentially with other CNTs; stronger and lighter than steel; high electrical conductivity. CNT-based integrated circuits, CNT chips faster and faster, better battery life for smartphones.

Carbon nanotubes are delivered by chemical trails and have been found in Parisian children's lungs.[2] The enzyme myeloperoxidase (MPD) found in white blood cells can be used to break down CNTs into water and CO2.[3] Reusable water filters can be made to absorb cadmium, cobalt, copper, mercury, nickel and lead by growing CNTs in place on quartz fibers, then epoxified.[4]

Claytronics (catoms): reconfigurable nanoscale robots; shape-shifting

Cyborg: a portmanteau of *cybernetic* and *organism*

DNA origami: manipulates strands of DNA to bind into shapes outside the traditional double helix. DNA nanotechnology entails origami computers that fold and unfold strands of DNA.[5]

ENPs: engineered nanoparticles, as opposed to natural nanoparticles; contaminating air, water, and soil

Fullerenes: carbon spherical molecule, hollow cage of atoms that uses silica, carbon, graphene, or other polymer or metallic materials to construct, repair, assemble, and mutate at the cell level; delivered by chemical trails; utilizes cell DNA replication mutations. Possibly embedded as payloads in fullerenes:

---

2 Mike Williams-Rice, "Nanotubes found in lungs of French kids." Futurity.org, October 19, 2015.

3 Clay Dillow, "Scientists Devise a Means For Human Bodies To Break Down Carbon Nanotubes." Popular Science, April 6, 2010.

4 Mike Williams, "Heavy Metals in Water Meet Their Match." TMC News, July 27, 2017.

5 See Arun Richard Chandrasekaran and David A. Rusling, "Triplex-forming oligonucleotides: a third strand for DNA nanotechnology." Nucleic Acids Research, February 16, 2018.

thorium, strontium, barium, aluminum, lithium, nanosilver, styrene, polymers, liposomes, and hydrogels acting as the transport mechanism into the fats (lipids) and fluids of the body. Buckminsterfullerene = buckyballs.

***In vivo* nanoplatforms (IVN):** "adaptable nanoparticles for persistent, distributed, unobtrusive physiologic and environmental sensing" – DARPA

In vivo means inside living bodies.

Laser ablation: generation of nanoparticles by laser; technology for synthesizing nanoparticles

MEMS / BioMEMS: Microelectromechanical systems. Sensor nodes (motes) gather sensory information and communicate with other nodes in the network. E.g. MEMS functions in smartphones include CMOS image sensor, gyroscopes, accelerometers, magnetic field sensors (digital compass), autofocus actuators, pressure sensors (barometric sensors), micro mirrors, silicon microphones, oscillators and timing circuits, and RF MEMS—including FBAR, SAW, varactors (semiconductor diodes), etc.[6]

BioMEMS are engaged in replacing Human 1.0 cells.

Molecular nanotechnology: engineered nanosystems (nanoscale machines) operating on the molecular level, e.g. the molecular assembler [**see illustration**], a machine that produces structures atom by atom via mechanosynthesis. *Molecular machine systems are not the same as the manufacture of nanomaterials like carbon nanotubes.* Future nanosystems installed in human bodies will be hybrids of silicon technology and biological molecular machines.

Nanoantennas: A nanoscale antenna-like structure for sending and transmitting electromagnetic waves; for example, chlorophyll molecules arrange in antenna complexes, or bio-inspired short strands of DNA.

Nanohybrid (NH): multicomponent assemblies in which two or more presynthesized nanomaterials are conjugated to extract multifunctionality.

Nanophotonics: behavior of light on the nanoscale

Nanoplasmonics: the study of optical phenomena in nanoscale metal surfaces

---

6 SEMICO Research & Consulting Group, May 17, 2011.

Nanotechnology: the ability to work – to see, measure, and manipulate – at the atomic, molecular, and supramolecular levels in the length scale of approximately 1-100 nm range.

Nanotubes: rolled-up sheets of interlocking carbon atoms. The tubes are so strong they could be used to tether satellites to a fixed position above the Earth.

Metal-organic nanotubes (like molybdenum disulfide nanotubes or MDNTs) are used for nanowires in nanoscale lasers, semiconductors and sensors

Nanowire: 450 atoms wide; silicon nanowire grows from gold catalyst particle after disilane (a silicon-rich gas) liquefies it; a solid silicon crystal forms and grows into a nanowire

Novel materials: Nano novel properties of "novel materials" require new toxicological testing methods. For example,

Sub-nano clusters (SNCs) of metal nanoparticles and metallic nanocrystals[7] (0.5 to 2 nm) have very distinctive properties that make them excellent catalyzers for electrochemical reactions due to size, shape, surface area, agglomeration states, and surface charges. Even with (silica) surface-enhanced Raman spectroscopy, it is difficult to study SNCs because of the peculiar quantum phenomena seemingly dependent upon the number of constituent atoms.[8] "Peculiar quantum phenomena" occur because tiny SNCs are at the very threshold of quantum dimensions.

Origami DNA: the frames or molds utilized in the design and shapes of the nanoparticles to be used in assemblies.

Programmable matter has the ability to change its physical properties (shape, density, moduli, conductivity, optics, etc.) in a programmable fashion, based upon user input or autonomous sensing. (Wikipedia)

---

7 "A study shows the existence of various nanoparticles in patients suffering from severe respiratory impairment who were exposed to dust and smoke from the collapse of the World Trade Center ... aluminum and magnesium silicates, chrysotile asbestos, calcium phosphate, calcium sulfate, and small shards of glass." Nanotechnology in Eco-efficient Construction, Materials, Processes & Applications, Woodhead Publishing, 2018, p. 729.

8 Tokyo Institute of Technology, "Nanoscience breakthrough: Probing particles smaller than a billionth of a meter," December 13, 2019.

Quantum dots (QDs): colloidal semiconductor nanocrystals with unique optical properties, including fluorescence and the entire color spectrum; discovered in 1980, nicknamed "artificial atoms," QTs have the ability to tune optical and electronic properties by changing the crystallite size or internal structure. They behave more like organic molecules than metal nanoparticles. Applications: transistors, solar cells, optical switches and logic gates, quantum computing, LEDs, displays, photovoltaics, etc. Used for track and trace with blockchain (Nanotope Tracking Technology), e.g. the QDX HealthID purportedly for tracking and monitoring disease outbreaks with color-coded indicators (QDs) via the Microsoft Azure cloud and Hyperledger Sawtooth blockchain.[9]

Stochastic sensing: Nanosensors that detect DNA, RNA by their frequency signatures

Utility fog (foglets): micro-mechanical shape-shifters, computer-controlled swarms working together to simulate macro-scale machines. By combining virtual telepresence technologies with nanotech utility fog, consciousness can be remotely projected and we can interact in remote environments through distant, artificial bodies made of utility fog (as in the 2009 film *Surrogates*?). "Ghost in the machine."

9 "US Firm combines nanotechnology, blockchain for COVID-19 immunity passports." Ledger Insights, April 2020.

Appendix 10

Forced Nanotechnology Integration: Stages to Building a Platform

Thanks to Tony Pantalleresco and Suzanne Mahr

1. Nanotechnology taken in through eating, breathing and exposure.
2. Nanotechnology gestates 24 to 72 hours upon which it will morph and assimilate.
3. The beginning of breaking down of bodily raw material for biology to use through cells or tissues, using anything it can access.
4. Congregation of particles in an area to further integrate or assimilate material by which it will shape the material into a conical, circular or cylindrical particle.
5. Nanotechnology saturates the material, lining itself up, creating fullerenes, dots which will accumulate in the building block it has already created.
6. The biofilm / bacteria created will trigger an immune response which will then be used in collecting and sealing the nanoparticles.
7. Nano-constructs will break down the biofilm / polymer substance to further its network with other particles, which will further assemble and become a ligand or fullerene.
8. The fullerene assembly is now fully constructed and looking to attach itself to other material. It will continue to expand, attaching itself to other synthetics.

Appendix 11

Monosodium Glutamate (MSG)

www.healthglade.com

MSG IS ONE OF THE most dangerous food additives in the world, alongside Aspartame. It delivers a burst of flavour to the brain cells for very little cost to the food producer.

However, it is not the only burst that it delivers. MSG is designed to excite the brain cells, but it excites them to such as large degree that they literally explode and die. Over time, these cell deaths lead to many serious health conditions, including cancer, brain damage, eye damage, obesity, shrinking organs, infertility, mental problems, Alzheimer's, permanent immune system suppression, and much more. Oh, let's not forget death, as it can kill you within minutes.

You would think that such a harmful chemical would be banned by the governments, or least required to be labelled on the packaging. Sadly, this is another case of the politicians being bought out. The food industry not only lobbied to make MSG permissible, but they went one step further and asked the government to fudge the labelling laws so that they only had to name it if it was 99% pure. So this means that they can put a fake or deceptive name for MSG on the packaging if it is only 98% pure, without listing the real name.

The food industry started off with a few alternatives, but the public quickly spread the word and avoided products containing these names. The food industry then took their labelling deception to a new level, and created so many different names that it is hard to keep track. This is why we created this valuable resource of trick MSG names. The public need to be informed of the names so they can avoid MSG and stay healthy.

- Monosodium Glutamate E621, Monopotassium Glutamate E622
- Calcium Glutamate E623
- Monoammonium Glutamate E624
- Magnesium Glutamate E625
- Natrium Glutamate, Glutamate, Glutamic Acid E620
- Hydrolyzed Protein, Hydrolyzed Vegetable Protein, Hydrolyzed Plant Protein
- Hydrolyzed Oat Flour
- Autolyzed Plant Protein
- Autolyzed Yeast

- Textured Protein
- Calcium Caseinate
- Sodium Caseinate
- Yeast Food, Yeast Extract, Yeast Nutrient
- Torula Yeast
- Brewer's Yeast
- Maltodextrin
- Oligodextrin
- Gelatin
- Whey Protein, Whey Protein Concentrate, Whey Protein Isolate
- Soy Protein, Soy Protein Concentrate, Soy Protein Isolate
- Soy Sauce, Soy Sauce Extract
- Vetsin
- Ajinomoto
- Umani
- Carrageenan E407
- Bouillon
- Broth
- Stock
- Flavours, Flavouring, Natural Flavouring
- Seasoning
- Spices
- Citric Acid
- Citrate E330
- Pectin E440
- Barley Malt, Malted Barley, Malt Extract
- Anything Hydrolyzed, Protein Fortified, Enzyme Modified, Protease, Fermented, Ultra-Pasteurized

Appendix 12

Visitors to www.carnicom.com

Aug 26, 1999

Let it be noted that some of the recent visitors to this web site include:
(Let it also be noted that United States government computer systems are to be used for official purposes only.)

1. Desert Research Institute in Nevada (weather modification research institution) (repeat visits)
2. Fort Lewis Army Military Base in the State of Washington (home of Special Forces air squadron)
3. Lockheed Martin (aviation and space defense contractor) (repeat visits)(repeat repeat visits)
4. Los Alamos National Laboratory (repeat visit)
5. Allergan Pharmaceutical Corporation (Allergy Pharmaceutical Research Company)
6. Alliant Techsystems (Space and Strategic Defense Systems contractor)
7. Raytheon Defense Systems (Defense Contractor) (repeat visit) (repeat repeat visit) (repeat repeat repeat visit)
8. BOEING AIRCRAFT COMPANY (100 visits minimum)
9. United States Defense Logistics Agency (supplies and support to combat troops)
10. Davis-Monthan Air Force Base, Tucson AZ (home of 355th Wing) (repeat visits) (repeat repeat visits) (repeat repeat repeat visit)
11. Dept of Defense Naval Computer and Telecommunications Area Master Station
12. U.S. Naval Sea Systems Command
13. Western Pacific Region of the Federal Aviation Administration, Lawndale CA. (repeat visit) (repeat visit) (repeat visit)
14. National Aeronautics and Space Administration Langley Research Center (10 visits minimum)
15. United States Environmental Protection Agency (20 visits minimum)
16. St. Vincent Hospital, Santa Fe New Mexico
17. HEADQUARTERS UNITED STATES AIR FORCE, THE PENTAGON
18. United States Department of the Treasury (repeat visit) (repeat visit)

19. United States Department of Defense Educational Activity
20. ANDREWS AIR FORCE BASE, PROUD HOME OF AIR FORCE ONE
21. United States Federal Aviation Administration
22. United States Naval Research Center, Washington D.C.
23. Rockwell-Collins (U.S. defense contractor)
24. Honeywell (U.S. Defense Contractor) (repeat visit)
25. Wright-Patterson Air Force Base, Dayton OH (repeat visit) (repeat repeat visit)
26. Kadena Air Force Base, Okinawa, Japan
27. Camp Pendleton, United States Marine Corps (mandatory US Defense anthrax vaccination program described at www.cpp.usmc.mil) (repeat visit) (repeat visit)
28. Ames Research Center, NASA (one of primary missions is to research ASTROBIOLOGY, i.e. the study of life in outer space) (repeat visit)
29. Space Dynamics Laboratory, Utah State University, North Logan, Utah
30. Merck (Pharmaceutical Products and Health Research) (repeat visit)
31. McClellan Air Force Base, Sacramento, CA. (The Sacramento Air Logistics Center at McClellan Air Force Base, California performs depot maintenance on the KC-135 Stratotanker aircraft and is heavily involved in space and communications - electronics.) (repeat visit)
32. TRW (U.S. Defense Contractor) (repeat visit)
33. Teledyne Brown Engineering (U.S. Defense Contractor)
34. United States Navy Medical Department
35. Air National Guard, Salt Lake City, Utah
36. Monsanto Company (Chemical, Pesticide, and Pharmaceutical products) (repeat visit) (repeat repeat visits)
37. U.S. Department of Veterans Affairs
38. Arco Chemical Corporation
39. Sundstrand Aerospace (U.S. Defense Contractor)
40. National Oceanic and Atmospherics Administration Aeronomy Laboratory (conducts fundamental research on the chemical and physical processes of the Earth's atmosphere)
41. Allied Signal Corporation (chemical, aerospace, energy) (repeat visit) (repeat repeat visit) (repeat repeat repeat visit) (repeat repeat repeat repeat visit)
42. Aviation Weather Center, National Oceanic and Atmospherics Administration
43. United States Army Medical Department (repeat visit)
44. Nasa Goddard Space Flight Center

45. Applied Physics Laboratory, a research division of John Hopkins University, which supports the U.S. Defense Department
46. United States Naval Health Research Center, San Diego, CA
47. HEADQUARTERS, UNITED STATES ARMY, THE PENTAGON
48. United States General Accounting Office (The General Accounting Office is the investigative arm of Congress. GAO performs audits and evaluations of Government programs and activities.)
49. Bristol-Myers Squibb Company (Pharmaceutical Research and Development)
50. United States Naval Criminal Investigative Service (A worldwide organization responsible for conducting criminal investigations and counterintelligence for the Department of the Navy and for managing naval security programs.)
51. 51. National Computer Security Center (NCSE) (Involved in advanced warfare simulation)
52. The Mayo Clinic (repeat visit) (repeat repeat visit) (repeat repeat repeat visit)
53. The Federal Judiciary (home of the United States Supreme Court)
54. United States Federal Emergency Management Agency (Controls a comprehensive, risk-based, emergency management program of mitigation, preparedness, response and recovery.) (repeat visit)
55. United States Naval Surface Warfare Center, Crane IN (repeat visit) (repeat repeat visit)
56. United States National Guard Public Affairs Web Access (no public access to this site)
57. UNITED STATES SENATE (repeat visit) (repeat repeat visit) (repeat repeat repeat visit)(repeat repeat repeat repeat visit)
58. Headquarters, United States Air Force Reserve Command
59. Kaiser Permanente health organization
60. United States Naval Warfare Assessment Station
61. Air University, United States Air Force
62. United States Naval Research Laboratory (repeat visit)
63. Enterprise Products Partners L.P. (MTBE production)
64. United States Navy Naval Air Weapons Stations, China Lake CA
65. California Pacific Medical Center
66. United States Defense Information Systems Agency (mission: "To plan, engineer, develop, test, manage programs, acquire, implement, operate, and maintain information systems for C4I and mission support under all conditions of peace and war.")
67. San Francisco Department of Public Health

68. BJC Health System, St. Louis, Missouri
69. United States Open Source Information Systems (OSIS) (an unclassified confederation of systems serving the intelligence community with open source intelligence) OSIS sites include: (AIA) Air Intelligence Agency, Kelly AFB, San Antonio, TX IC-ROSE (CIA) Central Intelligence Agency, Reston, VA (DIA) Defense Intelligence Agency, Washington, D.C. (NSA) National Security Agency, Ft. Meade, Laurel, MD (NIMA) National Imagery & Mapping Agency, Fairfax, VA (NAIC) National Air Intelligence Center, Wright-Patterson AFB, Dayton, OH (NGIC) National Ground Intelligence Center, Charlottesville, VA (MCIC) Marine Corps Intelligence Center, Quantico, VA (NMIC) National Maritime Intelligence Center, Office of Naval Intelligence, Suitland, MD (ISMC) Intelink Service Management Center, Ft. Meade, Laurel, MD (repeat visit)
70. New Mexico Department of Health
71. United States Space and Naval Warfare Systems Command (SPAWAR)
72. United States McMurdo Research Station, Antarctica
73. Orlando Regional Healthcare System, Florida
74. United States Andersen Air Force Base, Guam
75. United States Misawa Air Base, Japan
76. United States Hickam Air Force Base, Hawaii
77. United States Osan Air Force Base, Korea
78. Royal Air Force, Lakenheath, Suffolk
79. United States Scott Air Force Base
80. United States F.E. Warren Air Force Base
81. United States Air Force News Agency
82. United States Langley Air Force Base (repeat visit)
83. United States Tinker Air Force Base
84. United States McConnell Air Force Base
85. United States Charleston Air Force Base
86. United States Randolph Air Force Base
87. United States Air Force Reserve Command
88. United States Seymour Johnson Air Force Base
89. United States Bolling Air Force Base, Washington DC
90. Keesler Air Force Base, MS
91. United States Hill Air Force Base
92. United States Vandenberg Air Force Base, California
93. United States Minot Air Force Base, North Dakota
94. United States Eielson Air Force Base, Alaska

95. ANDREWS AIR FORCE BASE, PROUD HOME OF AIR FORCE ONE (repeat visit)
96. HEADQUARTERS UNITED STATES AIR FORCE, THE PENTAGON (repeat visit) (Visitors 75-96 arrived within a 24-hour period (09/23/99)
97. United States Cannon Air Force Base, New Mexico
98. United States McGuire Air Force Base
99. United States Beale Air Force Base (home of the U-2 fleet of reconnaissance aircraft)
100. United States Department of Justice – Federal Bureau of Prisons
101. Metnet – United States Navy (associated with weather reporting system and SPAWAR)
102. TRADOC – United States Army Training and Doctrine Command, Fort Monroe, VA
103. Newsweek Magazine
104. United States Defense Advanced Research Projects Agency
105. Massachusetts Medical Society, Owner – Publisher: New England Journal of Medicine
106. OFFICE OF THE SECRETARY OF DEFENSE: THE OFFICE OF WILLIAM S. COHEN, SECRETARY OF DEFENSE (repeat visit)
107. HEADQUARTERS UNITED STATES AIR FORCE, THE PENTAGON (repeat repeat visit)
108. UNITED STATES JOINT FORCES COMMAND (reports to US Secretary of Defense) (repeat visit)
109. Naval Warfare Assessment Station, Corona CA
110. Los Angeles County Emergency Operations Center
111. Commander in Chief, United States Pacific Fleet, United States Navy
112. HEADQUARTERS UNITED STATES AIR FORCE, THE PENTAGON
113. Defense Logistics Agency, Administrative Support Center in Europe
114. United Stated Department of Defense Network Information Center, Vienna, VA (repeat visits)
115. Office of the Assistant Secretary of the Army
116. Headquarters, United States Air Force, The Pentagon (repeat visit)
117. U.S. News and World Report
118. Naval Air Warfare Center – Aircraft Division (repeat visits)
119. New Zealand Parliament
120. HEADQUARTERS UNITED STATES AIR FORCE, THE PENTAGON (multiple repeat visits)
121. NIPR – Department of Defense Network Operations (NIPRNet);

The Defense Information Systems Agency (DISA) has established a number of NIPRNet gateways to the Internet, which will be protected and controlled by firewalls and other technologies.) (repeat visits)

122. Peterson Air Force Base, Colorado Springs, CO (home of NORAD and SPACECOM)
123. Raytheon (visits immediately after introduction of HAARP implications)
124. United States Army War College
125. Lawrence Berkeley National Laboratory
126. Fermi National Accelerator Laboratory

https://carnicominstitute.org/research_papers/Carnicom_Institute_Research-1999.pdf

Appendix 13
Movers and Shakers

The US is an empire now, and when we act, we create our own reality.
– Karl Rove, Deputy Chief of Staff, 2004

The technotronic era involves the gradual appearance of a more controlled society. Such a society would be dominated by an elite unrestrained by traditional values. Soon, it will be possible to assert almost continuous surveillance over every citizen and maintain up-to-date complete files containing even the most personal information about the citizen. These files will be subject to instantaneous retrieval by the authorities.
– Zbigniew Brzezinski (1928-2017), National Security Adviser to four Democrat Presidents

- *American Family Foundation (AFF)* — *Private*
- *Asilomar Conferences* — *Private*
- *Bain & Company* — *Private*
- *Bouvet Island* — *??*
- *Department of Homeland Security (DHS)* — *Private / Government*
- *Federal Accounting Standards Advisory board (FASAB)* — *Government*
- *Google, Facebook, and the Defense Industrial Base* — *Private*
- *Health Advanced Research Projects Agency (HARPA)* — *Government*
- *Highlands Forum* — *Private*
- *In-Q-Tel / CIA* — *Private / Government*
- *Lethal Autonomous Weapons System (LAWS)* — *UN*
- *Lifeboat Foundation* — *NGO*
- *Lockheed Martin* — *Private*
- *SAIC* — *Private*
- *Senior Executive Service (SES)* — *Government*
- *Serco* — *Private*
- *Smith-Mundt Modernization Act of 2012* — *Government*
- *Task Force on Climate-related Financial Disclosure (TCFD)* — *Private*

On July 1, 1960, President Eisenhower (1953-1961) signed the Executive Order that moved U.S. space operations—the secret space program deeply buried in "national security"—from the U.S. Army to NASA, a civilian agency not answerable to Congress. Equipment valued at $100 million[1] and 4,700 civilian employees, plus Operation Paperclip scientist Wernher von Braun and his German rocket team, were transferred from the U.S. Army's Redstone Arsenal in Huntsville, Alabama (and Cape Canaveral, Florida) to next door to NASA's Marshall Space Flight Center.

Since then, the revolving door between government and industry (i.e. the military-industrial-intelligence complex)—now called public-private partnerships—has become more like a Gorgon's head sprouting hypnotic, devouring snakes. Going up against this Gorgon means running the risk of being turned to stone, i.e. professionally ostracized, destitute, and in danger.

American Family Foundation (AFF) **Private**

> The dark powers have set up the AFF [American Family Foundation] to ensure that the secret work of cult-making and the experimental / functional use of brainwashing mind-control techniques can continue...
>
> – Alan Morrison, "Controlling the Opposition," May 16, 2005

"Black" organizations and agencies play a shell game with their techno-ergot, acronyms, names and re-names of hidden-in-plain-sight projects. One excellent and far-reaching example is how MK-ULTRA / MKSEARCH and Artichoke went "black" under the CIA cut-out *American Family Foundation (AFF)* after the August 3, 1977 Joint Session of the U.S. Senate Select Committee on Intelligence and Subcommittee on Health and Scientific Research of the Committee on Human Resources.

The AFF board was comprised of ex-CIA advisers and former MK-ULTRA psychiatric personnel—Robert J. Lifton, Maurice Davis, Margaret Singer, Louis Jolyon "Jolly" West, etc. AFF support came from Morgan Stanley Investment Advisors, Inc., Richard Mellon Scaife, and of course the Bodman and Achellis Foundations, administered by the New York City law offices of Morris and McVeigh (intelligence and banking families), with overlapping directorates. In 2000, Bodman gave the AFF $50,000 specifically for "the development and marketing of Citizenship and Character, instructional material to supplement American government and history classes in U.S. high schools." The AFF is still funded by top Wall Street family foundations.

Another source of funding—according to the 1961 Annual Report on the CIA cut-out Human Ecology Foundation and 1941-1960 correspondence of John Clare Whitehorn, Director of the Department of Psychiatry, Johns Hopkins University—was the Scottish Rite Foundation. Both Johns Hopkins

---

1 One dollar in 1960 was worth eight dollars today.

and MK-ULTRA / MKSEARCH contractor Dr. Carl Pfeiffer received grants via the Scottish Rite Research Committee whose chairman Dr. Winfred Overholser (32° Scottish Rite) had been superintendent of the notorious St. Elizabeth's Hospital in Washington, D.C. in 1937,[2] had worked for the OSS (Office of Strategic Services) during World War Two, and had became president of the American Psychiatric Association in 1948. From 1956 to 1959, Overholser's son Winfred Jr. did his psychiatry residency at New York State Psychiatric Institute, during which time famed tennis player Harold Blauer died after being injected by Dr. Paul Hoch with 450mg of U.S. Army mescaline code-named EA-1298 (3,4-Methylenedioxyamphetamine) under MK-ULTRA. Political prisoner poet Ezra Pound and Scientology founder L. Ron Hubbard were both "treated" at St. Elizabeth's, and Winfred Jr. was in charge of Pound.

In 2004, the AFF morphed into the International Cultic Studies Association (ICSA), a supposedly anti-cult organization—rather like the False Memory Syndrome Foundation founded in 1992 to cover for pedophiles and Satanic ritual abuse perpetrators by casting doubt on children's testimony.

Asilomar Conferences **Private**

A meaningtul trilogy of Asilomar Conferences on the Monterey Peninsula in California in the years 1975, 2010, and 2017:

- February 27, 1975 *Asilomar Conference on Recombinant DNA* The decision to lift the moratorium on genetic engineering and allow the alteration of the genetics of all of life on Earth.
- March 22-26, 2010 *Asilomar International Conference on Climate Intervention Technologies* Based on the biotechnology decisions of 1975, the decision to deliberately change the world environment by means of geoengineering.
- January 5-8, 2017 *Asilomar Conference on Beneficial AI* Confirmation that the AI system is in place, from satellites to nanoparticles.[3]

Bain & Company **Private**

Bain & Company was founded in 1973 with Mormon wealth in the person of Mitt Romney who then helped to shape Bain. In the *reallygraceful* video "Who Controls the Gates Family?" (May 23, 2020), Bain is called "the KGB of Consulting." Global management consulting translates to a buy-out firm

2 Now run by the District of Columbia. Author Simon Winchester asked for the 1910-1919 incarceration records of William Chester Minor, the Surgeon of Crowthorne, and was refused point-blank. The 2019 film The Professor and the Madman with Mel Gibson and Sean Penn is based on Winchester's 1998 book The Surgeon of Crowthorne.

3 Thanks to Jarod Taylor, Facebook.

that takes over corporations, guts them, then places its people in power in the abandoned corporate shell. Private equity firms like Bain, the Carlyle Group, and BlackRock Funds (all three being code for the CIA and the Fortune 500 corporations the CIA serves) are cuckoo bird that lays its eggs in other birds' nests; its fledglings then devour the host's fledglings once born.

Bain & Company handles[4] clients like Dick Cheney / Halliburton, Raytheon, Monsanto, Microsoft, Starbucks, Bill & Melinda Gates Foundation, etc. It is also a "fixer" in that it may be contracted to make sure that stars like Kanye West stay tuned up (mind control), that social engineering accompanies the commodities it "handles" (like Starbucks and plant-based burgers), and that back-door-access computers are omnipresent. In other words, Bain & Company works for (or is) the Deep State.

Bouvet Island **??**

Ruled by Norway since 1930, Bouvet Island is a solitary sub-antarctic volcanic island with a top-level Internet country domain code of *.bv*. Ongoing live cyberwarfare attacks emanate from the island.

Council of Governors (COG) **Government**

The Council of Governors (COG) was established by former President Obama under Executive Order 13528 supposedly "to strengthen further the partnership between the Federal Government and State Governments to protect our Nation against all types of hazards," with particular emphasis on "the National Guard of the various States; homeland defense; civil support; synchronization and integration of State and Federal military activities in the United States; and other matters of mutual interest pertaining to National Guard, homeland defense, and civil support activities"—all of which has certainly come into play since the COVID-19 crisis of 2020. COG governs the ten FEMA districts of the United States.

Department of Homeland Security (DHS) **Private / government**

- *National Risk Management Center*
- *Energy Sector*
- *Science & Technology Directorate*
- *Cybersecurity and Infrastructure Security Agency (CISA)*
- *National Cybersecurity and Communications Integration Center (NCCIC)*

4 Handle / handler has two basic meanings: to oversee or deal with certain commodities, and to train or have charge of an animal (or person). In the case of Bain & Company (the CIA is known as "the Company"), the term is intended to cover both senses.

Before September 11, 2001, there was no Department of Homeland Security nor reference to the United States as a "homeland"—a peculiarly Nazi-era term.

> Perhaps ironically, Hitler stole the term "homeland" from the 1920s and 1930s Zionist movement's goal to create a Jewish "homeland" in the Middle East . . .
>
> So, in 1934, at the Nazi party's big coming-out event, the famous Nuremberg rally, Nazis introduced the term "homeland." Prior to that, they'd always referred to Germany as "the Fatherland" or "the Motherland" or "our nation." But Hitler and his think-tank wanted Germans to think of themselves with what he and Goebbels viewed as the semi-tribal passion that the Zionists had for Israel . . .[5]

As I explained in *Under An Ionized Sky*, the Department of Homeland Security (DHS) is a *civilian* agency answering to the Office of the Director of National Intelligence (ODNI) and overseeing fusion centers, black projects, and COG (continuity of government) operations, including federal detention camps often located on "closed" military bases or Bureau of Land Management lands, etc. DHS touts itself as a domestic *and* international terrorism watchdog, the third-largest federal department drawing together 22 different federal agencies. *One DHS, with integrated, results-based operations.*[6]

The example I gave of the DHS role in overseeing international terrorism was the "Agreement Between the Government of the Kingdom of Sweden and the Government of the USA in the Area of Scientific and Technical Cooperation For the Protection of National Security,"[7] signed by the Swedish Defence minister and then-DHS director Michael Chertoff in Washington, D.C. on Friday, April 13, 2007. The agreement gave Sweden access to billions of NSA dollars to funnel into Swedish biotech corporations, institutions, universities, laboratories, etc.—in other words, R&D in nuclear, biological / chemical, underwater techniques, border control, sensors and microprocessors, search and surveillance, and targeting. At the end of 2011, then-DHS Secretary Janet Napolitano met with Swedish ministers of State and Justice and signed the Preventing and Combating Crime Agreement for the fluid exchange of biometric and biographic data on citizens "to bolster counterterrorism and law enforcement efforts."[8]

---

5 "Time for the US To Dump the Word 'Homeland.'" The Thom Hartmann Program, September 23, 2014.

6 "Homeland Security Enterprise," https://www.dhs.gov/topic/homeland-security-enterprise.

7 https://www.dhs.gov/xlibrary/assets/agreement_us_sweden_sciencetech_cooperation_2007-04-13.pdf.

8 "Readout of Secretary Napolitano's Meeting with Swedish Deputy Foreign Minister Frank Belfrage," Office of the Press Secretary, DHS, December 16, 2011. Similar "international

DHS activation of Oak Ridge National Laboratory's *SensorNet program* must have begun under the authority of what today is known as the National Cybersecurity and communications Integration Center (NCCIC). Interestingly, in the late 1990s, the Center for Nanophase Materials Sciences (CNMS) at Oak Ridge was nano central: nanoscience research, nanomaterials synthesis, nanofabrication, imaging, simulation, integrating nano- and microsensors into real-time detection and surveillance.[9]

> **The NCCIC Mission:** *To operate at the intersection of the private sector, civilian, law enforcement, intelligence, and defense communities, applying unique analytic perspectives, ensuring shared situational awareness, and orchestrating synchronized response efforts . . .*

The endless shell game of department names at the DHS sites seems purposeful. For example, which department really runs the *National Network of Fusion Centers*, the "state-owned and operated centers that serve as focal points in states and major urban areas for the receipt, analysis, gathering and sharing of threat-related information between State, Local, Tribal and Territorial (SLTT), federal and private sector partners"[10]? According to the ACLU,[11] of the 43 state, local, and regional fusion centers in the U.S., no two are alike in form or function, in part due to ambiguous lines of authority, varying degrees of military and private sector involvement, an emphasis on wholesale data collection, and an overarching excessive secrecy. Sounds a lot like COINTELPRO of the 1970s:

> . . . the FBI ran a domestic intelligence/counterintelligence program called COINTELPRO that quickly grew from a legitimate effort to protect national security into an effort to suppress political dissent through illegal activities. Frequent targets were groups that criticized the FBI itself. The Senate panel that investigated COINTELPRO (the "Church Committee") in the 1970s found that a combination of factors led law enforcers to become law breakers. But the crucial factor was their easy access to damaging personal information as a result of the unrestrained collection of domestic intelligence.[12]

---

partner" agreements exist with 22+ nations.

9 Take a look at Michael Edwards' "How Close Are We to a Nano-based Surveillance State?" Activist Post, February 21, 2011.

10 "Fusion Centers," DHS, https://www.dhs.gov/fusion-centers.

11 "What's Wrong With Fusion Centers?" ACLU, December 2007.

12 Select Committee to Study Governmental Operations with Respect to Intelligence Activities, U.S. Senate, 94 Congress, Final Report on Supplemental Detailed Staff Reports on Intelligence Activities and the Rights of Americans (Book III), S. Rep. No. 94-755, at 10 (1976).

FASAB (Federal Accounting Standards Advisory Board) ***Government***

You probably haven't heard of this government body, nor its October 4, 2018 announcement "Statement of Federal Financial Accounting Standards 56 (FASAB 56)"[13] that basically legalizes federal budget-line item lies, or as *Rolling Stone* reporter Matt Taibbi put it in 2019, "a system of classified money-moving."[14] The Security Exchange Commission (SEC), mandated to keep watch on government transparency, basically looked the other way as FASAB 56 became policy and thus overrode the U.S. Constitution to take "a large portion of the U.S. securities marker dark."[15]

And yet at the same time, companies are being forced to reveal their ESG (environmental, social, and governance) investments under the UN's Principles for Responsible Investment (PRI) in the wake of the Climate Risk Disclosure Act sponsored by Senator Elizabeth Warren. The SEC requires:

> ...public companies to disclose climate change-related risks, including climate change scenario analyses similar to those called for by the FSB Climate Task Force referenced in the petition, as well as companies' direct and indirect greenhouse gas emissions, the total amount of fossil fuel-related assets they own or manage, and their management strategies related to physical risks posed by climate change.[16]

Google, Facebook, and the Defense Industrial Base ***Private***

> *I will answer very simply that the internet will disappear. There will be so many IP addresses . . . so many devices, sensors, things that you are wearing, things that you are interacting with that you won't even sense it, it will be part of your presence all the time. Imagine you walk into a room, and the room is dynamic. And with your permission and all of that, you are interacting with the things going on in the room. A highly personalized, highly interactive and very, very interesting world emerges.*
>
> – Google Chairman Eric Schmidt, World Economic Forum, Davos, Switzerland, 2015

---

13 For an honest appraisal of this travesty, see Catherine Austin Fitts' http://constitution.solari.com/fasab-statement-56-understanding-new-government-financial-accounting-loopholes/.

14 Matt Taibbi, "Has the Government Legalized Secret Defense Spending?" Rolling Stone, January 2019.

15 Catherine Austin Fitts, "Will ESG Turn the Red Button Green?" The Solari Report, 1st Qtr. 2019 Wrap Up, Vol. 3.

16 Betty Huber, October 4, 2018, https://www.briefinggovernance.com/2018/10/investors-petition-the-sec-to-develop-esg-reporting-requirements/. Also see http://www.sec.gov/rules/petitions/2018/petn4-730.pdf.

What Lockheed Martin was to the twentieth century, technology and cyber-security companies will be to the twenty-first.

– Henry Kissinger

How does it feel to walk through and breathe the WASS (wide-area surveillance system), WAMI (wide-area motion imagery), WAPs (wireless application protocols), WDFV public space image technology running behavior detection, remote neural monitoring and biological process controls while collecting cell phone, social media, and medical records Big Data?

Basically a *warrantless search*, an endless frisk and theft of your data.

AI-organized OS / EH (organized stalking / electronic harassment) like Argus and its Gorgon Stare (2 billion pixels) target people via their individual brainwave signatures (evoked potentials), despite their inability to perceive it.

Google's algorithms swing elections. The line between tech giants like Google and government was erased long ago, especially regarding Deep State-Pentagon- intelligence players and the *Defense Industrial Base*,[17] "the worldwide industrial complex that enables research and development as well as design, production, delivery, and maintenance of military weapons systems, subsystems, and components or parts to meet U.S. military requirements" (Department of Homeland Security). Wikileaks whistleblower Julian Assange cited an email thread of Google founder Sergey Brin, Google guru Eric Schmidt, and NSA chief General Keith Alexander in 2012 discussing the *Enduring Society Framework (ESF)*:

General Alexander to Brin: Your insights as a key member of the Defense Industrial Base are valuable to ensure ESF's efforts have measurable impact.

As Stratfor[18] vice president for intelligence Fred Burton observed, Google can do things the CIA cannot do, namely technologically operate as "corporate intervention in foreign affairs at a level that is normally reserved for states" (Assange).[19]

Google Earth and its search functionality marked the beginning of Google's military-intelligence-policing-security expansion into Big Data. Now, Google is a committed military-intelligence-for-profit corporate contractor in service to the NSA, CIA, DIA, FBI, NGA, etc.—the whole alphabet

---

17 Could this be a rebranding of DISC, the Defense Industrial Security Command deeply embedded in the assassinations of John F. Kennedy, Martin Luther King Jr., and Robert F. Kennedy?

18 Barron's financial magazine has called STRATFOR in Austin, Texas "a private quasi-CIA."

19 Claire Bernish, "Julian Assange—'Google is not what it seems'—They 'do things the CIA cannot.'" FreeThoughtProject.com, November 14, 2016.

soup (which may be why its parent company is named Alphabet Inc.). Google has *always* been about intelligence, from the 1990s when Larry Page and Sergey Brin were at Stanford University to 2003 when In-Q-Tel bailed it out so it could purchase the Keyhole satellite and the NGA could pay for Keyhole to be "tailored" to meet Intelligence Community needs—like Google Earth ("CIA-assisted technology"). Google's been in bed with the NGA—sister of the NSA—ever since.

> *Google is the exclusive provider of geospatial intelligence services to America's military and intelligence agencies.*[20]

Google went on to become the first "cloud-based" provider for the U.S. government, getting its federal security classification for non-classified data, leading to contracts with the U.S. Naval Academy and U.S. Coast Guard Academy, U.S. Army, DoD, Department of Interior, nuclear labs, state and municipal governments . . .

Google started at Stanford University, Facebook at Harvard University.

The CIA's In-Q-Tel helped to fund the Facebook startup, along with PayPal, Palantir Technologies, Founders Fund, and venture capital firm Accel Partners. DARPA, of course, was involved; some say Facebook is DARPA's datamining Total Information Awareness (TIA) come again ("human network analysis and behavior model building engines").[21]

> Facebook coming online with advanced tech and no ads, and the Harvard connection, scream intel agency funding & origins . . . Facebook is a live guinea-pig test for how to develop and deploy this kind of software to collect intel on people on a network, and how to do analyses to extract actionable intel from the noise . . . What they're concerned with is how accurately they can PREDICT who is going to ask who to the prom [or how many will wear the mask out of fear]. So they attempt to develop algorithms to make automated predictions with Dick and Jane, and all their classmates, and see what happens.[22]

---

20 Yasha Levine, "Oakland emails give another glimpse into the Google-Military-Surveillance Complex." Pando.com, March 7, 2014.

21 Remember the TIA "all-seeing eye" logo? Both Sergey Brin (co-founder of Google) and Mark Zuckerberg (co-founder of Facebook) were groomed through the "exceptional children" program of CTY (Center for Talented Youth) run by Johns Hopkins University, mind control programming at its best.

22 Thomas Paine, "Facebook – The Hidden Aspect to DARPA's Total Information Awareness Project?" NotCIA, January 24, 2009.

Ever read the small print of Facebook's Terms of Use and Privacy Policy?

> *Terms of use: By posting Member Content to any part of the Web site, you automatically grant, and you represent and warrant, that you have the right to grant to Facebook an irrevocable, perpetual, non-exclusive, transferable, fully paid, worldwide license to use, copy, perform, display, reformat, translate, excerpt and distribute such information and content, and to prepare derivative works of, or incorporate into other works, such information and content, and to grant and authorize sublicenses of the foregoing.*

> *Privacy policy: Facebook may also collect information about you from other sources, such as newspapers, blogs, instant messaging services, and other users of the Facebook service through the operation of the service (e.g. photo tags) in order to provide you with more useful information and a more personalized experience. By using Facebook, you are consenting to have your personal data transferred to and processed in the United States.*

HARPA (Health Advanced Research Projects Agency) ***Government***

HARPA merges military and medical technology (yet more "dual use"), given that it is modeled after DARPA (Defense Advanced Research Projects Agency),

> . . . the gold standard for innovation and accountability . . . for national security. [DARPA] developed the Internet, Voice Recognition Technology, GPS navigation, Night vision, Robotic Prostheses, Stealth Technology . . . HARPA's identical operating principles, built on urgency, leadership, high-impact investments and accountability, will advance scientific research from the lab to the patient.[23]

The Highlands Forum ***Private***

Goldman Sachs-funded, along with In-Q-Tel, Facebook, Google, Microsoft, eBay, etc.

> According to the Pentagon's 1997 *Annual Report to the President and the Congress* under a section titled "Information Operations" (IO), the Office of the Secretary of Defense (OSD) had authorized the "establishment of the Highlands Group of key DoD, industry, and academic IO experts" to coordinate IO across federal military intelligence agencies.[24]
>
> According to Eric Schmidt's former lover, a DARPA insider, during an in-

---

23 www.harpa.org.

24 Nafeez Ahmed, "Why Google made the NSA." Insurge Intelligence, January 22, 2015. Much of what follows was gleaned from Nafeez's excellent series.

terview with *Anonymous Patriots,* July 1, 2019: "The Highlands Group works out of the Naval Intelligence Net Assessment Office and basically is the international group of corporations, venture capitalists, military and corporate intelligence, and the CIA's In-Q-Tel agency that uses SAIC and Leidos as their corporate arm. Highlands Group was run by Andrew Marshall for decades and essentially assessed new patents, DARPA / In-Q-Tel projects, and military desires for new weapons. Andrew Marshall was 'Yoda' because he was basically the 'head warlord' of America, globalist corporations, and the world in general."[25]

The Highlands Forum, HAARP, and the Project Cloverleaf aerosol delivery program all went active at about the same time: 1995. With the conversion of analog to digital and the resurrection of the Strategic Defense Initiative (SDI) "Star Wars" program, thanks to HAARP, I am in no doubt that the Highlands Group (later renamed the Highlands Forum) played a pivotal role in Lockheed Martin's Space Fence now categorized under information warfare / Information Operations (IW / IO) "perception management." Certainly, the Highlands Forum—funded by the Senior Executive Service (SES), DoD Office of Net Assessment, DARPA, National Science Foundation, U.S. Air Force, U.S. Navy, U.S. Army, MITRE, Harvard University, and the CIA—has overseen the global reconfiguration of the socio-political landscape since 9/11.

While "the US Intelligence Community funded, nurtured and incubated Google as part of a drive to dominate the world through control of information," the Highlands Group spun the Washington, DC roulette wheel between government and elites in business, industry, finance, and mainstream media. Thus, a "shadow network of private contractors," intelligence, and Pentagon influence over the private sector metastasized. Nafeez Ahmed calls Google a "smokescreen behind which lurks the US military-industrial complex . . . a parasitical network driving the evolution of the US national security apparatus and profiling obscenely from its operation."[26]

Behind the friendly face of Google, the Internet has been weaponized.

The Highlands Forum has gone from heretical to mainstream gravitas. Since 9/11, we are now subject to mass surveillance and a U.S. military transformed into Skynet on steroids. The shell game of names and acronyms has added ISR (intelligence, surveillance, reconnaissance) to C5 (command, control, communications, computers, combat)—*C5ISR.*

Since the mid-1990s, the Highlands Forum has played a massive role in pushing the doctrine of full spectrum dominance at every level of post-modern

---

25 Eric Schmidt, Google CEO (2001-2011), Google executive chairman (2011-2015), Alphabet Inc. executive chairman (2015-2017); now chairs the DoD Innovation Advisory Board. Estimated wealth US$11.1 billion (Forbes).

26 Nafeez Ahmed, "Why Google Made the NSA."

life. Not counting Google, the "shadow intelligence community" of giant military contractors (RAND, MITRE, Lockheed Martin, Raytheon, Booz Allen Hamilton, Northrup Grumman, Boeing, L3, SAIC,[27] etc.) developing "high-tech network-based warfare" is heavily represented in the Highlands Forum.

An anonymous whistleblower reports having overheard a secret Highlands Forum conversation with Anthony Fauci regarding a fusion of chemistry, biology, wireless networks, encryption, and nanorobots into bioweapons.

In-Q-Tel / Central Intelligence Agency (CIA) **Private / Government**

An entire book could be written on the CIA's role in geoengineering and its seven manifold operations to move psyop and technological control along toward our Transhumanist future.[28] Here, however, I only seek to draw attention to its "venture capital arm," In-Q-Tel, founded in 1999 to cover R&D for the 17 agencies of the Intelligence Community (IC), plus the NGA (National Geospatial-Intelligence Agency), DIA (Defense Intelligence Agency), and Homeland Security's Security Science and Technology Directorate, plus Google, Oracle, IBM, Lockheed Martin, etc.[29] Dig a little deeper and one gets the impression that in exchange for this "service," the CIA "maintains an investment stake" in these corporations and government agencies, and I don't mean just money.

> So what is the point of these interwoven relationships? The underlying element that permeates these tech companies is that the federal government is systematically involved in the funding, purpose objectives, application acquisitions and equity participation.
>
> Is this the new normal for the economy? Looks like it is, but such an organizational structure does not conform to the standards of free enterprise. This method for invention does not have the identical importance as "The Manhattan Project," but may well create advance technology that will have the same or greater risk of permanent extinction . . .
>
> Is Google a real standalone company, or is Facebook the social network department for the NSA? Is the wealth of Bill Gates, the equity positions of Larry Page and Sergey Brin, or the tax dodge shares of Mark Zuckerberg a true reflection of their actual ownership stakes in their respective companies, or are they mere fronts for a shadow government?

---

27 SAIC was an initial Highlands Group "partner." Many of Google's senior executives are affiliated with the Highlands Forum.

28 One article among many, Jason Mick's "CIA Funds Study Looking on the Effects of Geoengineering Blocking the Sun," DailyTech, July 18, 2013.

29 See Nafeez Ahmed's excellent "How the CIA made Google," Medium.com, Insurge Intelligence, January 22, 2015.

Just how many Eric Schmidt types are embedded in high-tech pulling the strings for the intelligence community?

The In-Q-Tel's of this world act as the JP Morgan's of the twenty-first century. Nikola Tesla's free electricity wireless distribution was killed by the robber baron. Today the role of inventive genius is managed and contained by technocrats following the directions of spooks who do the bidding of the supra elite . . .[30]

James Hall brings up excellent points in his wrap-up that I have pondered ever since I read Mae Brussell's *Playgirl* magazine article about Howard Hughes, the famous billionaire aviator owner of Hughes Aircraft.[31] Do Bill Gates, Mark Zuckerberg, and Elon Musk *really* run their own businesses, their own assets, or are they subject to the Billionaires Club? Wealth coupled with a technology (like Hughes Aircraft[32]) is crucial to many players. (Brussell: "Was an open-ended money funnel set up, into which millions of tax-free dollars could disappear? Wouldn't the man who controlled such a funnel be in a position to control U.S. elections -- and thus, the United States -- through tax-free 'contributions'?") Just as Hillary Clinton and Joe Biden have doubles, according to Brussell Hughes doubles (one being the bit actor Brucks Randell) stood in for him *for 20+ years*. The real Hughes died in 1971, but the ruse continued until 1976.

Raytheon bought Hughes Aircraft in 1997 for $9.5 billion. The aerospace and defense operations of Hughes Electronics (Hughes Aircraft) merged with Raytheon, which also acquired one half of the Hughes Research Laboratories. Two years before, Raytheon had purchased E-Systems which controlled HAARP and all its patents.

Today, A-Teams like Delta Force and SEAL Team 6 or Development Group conduct quiet kill-or-capture missions everywhere while the CIA's corporate arm In-Q-Tel "diversifies" throughout the transnational corporate world. The CIA itself has melded with the FBI, military contractors, and police forces while "combatting domestic terrorism" (the targeting of citizens with EM weapons) in partnership with Homeland Security, Fusion Centers, and telecom corporations.

---

30 James Hall, "CIA Funding of Tech Companies." Break All the Rules / Corporatocracy, December 16, 2015.

31 Mae Brussell and Stephanie Caruana, "Is Howard Hughes Dead and Buried Off a Greek Island?" Playgirl, December 1974.

32 The Howard Hughes Medical Foundation owned all the stock of Hughes Aircraft.

LAWS (lethal autonomous weapons system) **UN**

LAWS (lethal autonomous weapons system) is overseen by the UN's Group of Governmental Experts (GGE) under the Convention on Certain Conventional Weapons (CCW). LAWS include "weapons that can select, detect and engage targets with little or no human intervention," from autonomous to semi-autonomous weapons.[33]

How autonomous should LAWS "killer robots" be, given that international human law (IHL) is still under the 1899 Hague Convention (II) Laws and Customs of War on Land Martens Clause? In no way do LAWS comply with "principles of humanity" or "dictates of public conscience"—terms dispensed with by high-profile Silicon Valley tech leaders sitting on the DoD's Defense Innovation Board. As usual, developing nations want a LAWS treaty and developed nations don't.

Lifeboat Foundation **NGO**

Lifeboat is a nonprofit nongovernmental organization "dedicated to encouraging scientific advancements while helping humanity survive existential risks and possible misuse of increasingly powerful technologies, including genetic engineering, nanotechnology, and robotics / AI, as we move towards a technological singularity."

Besides being a futurist proponent of the Singularity University at NASA's Ames Research Center, sponsored by NASA and Google (Ray Kurzweil is on Lifeboat's Scientific Advisory Board), Lifeboat builds underground bunkers, sponsors the development of the NanoShield that will "protect Earth against attacks by nanoweapons,"[34] and otherwise serves as a nexus for Fortune 500 corporations investing in the secret space program's mandate to prepare the Earth for full spectrum dominance.

Lifeboat's SecurityPreserver program looks for ways to "provide early warning of attacks before such attacks can be fully designed, planned, developed, deployed, let alone launched,"[35] and believes that the SecurityPreserver program "that includes both surveillance and sousveillance is the best way to handle the threat of existential threats that will soon be in the hands of small groups of people."[36]

---

33 Hayley Evans, Natalie Salmanowitz, "Lethal Autonomous Weapons Systems: Recent Developments." Lawfare, March 7, 2019.

34 https://lifeboat.com/ex/press.releases.nanoshield.fund

35 https://lifeboat.com/ex/securitypreserver

36 https://lifeboat.com/ex/press.releases.edward.snowden.2013.guardian.award.winner. Surveillance denotes eye-in-the-sky watching from above whereas sousveillance denotes human-level surveillance.

While it is true that elite pimp Jeffrey Epstein sat on Lifeboat's financial board, it is also true that whistleblower Edward Snowden was honored with the Lifeboat Foundation Guardian Award for warning humanity of future dangers and encouraging the U.S. government to be more transparent regarding surveillance. Like other good globalists, Lifeboat plays both sides of the fence.

Lockheed Martin **Private**

Lockheed Martin—once Lockheed Missiles and Space Company in Sunnyvale, California—launched 30 satellites into geosynchronous orbit back in 1987-1992 out of the brand new Schriever Air Force Base ten miles east of Peterson Air Force Base in Colorado Springs under the 2nd Space Wing that controlled the Air Force Satellite Control Network. Lockheed now runs and owns the patents for the calibrated Space Fence.

Defense contractors like Lockheed Martin are not subject to congressional oversight or citizen demands, which is why big defense corporations run private security "hitmen" teams with direct access to sophisticated technology and keep IO matters out of public view. From an anonymous report sent to "The EveryDay Concerned Citizen," June 30, 2016:

> Lockheed Martin, the world's largest defense contractor and the prime cyber-security and information technology supplier to the federal government, coordinates the communications and trains the "team leaders" of a nationwide Gestapo-like apparatus, which has tentacles into every security and law enforcement agency in the nation, including state and local police and 72 regional "fusion centers" administered by the U.S. Department of Homeland Security. According to company literature, Lockheed Martin has operations in 46 of the 50 states.
>
> Lockheed Martin also has operational command and control over a U.S. government microwave radio frequency [MW / RF] weapon system deployed on cell tower masts throughout the U.S. being used to silently torture, impair, subjugate and electronically incarcerate so-called "targeted individuals." The nexus of this American "torture matrix"[37] appears to be Lockheed Martin's Mission and Combat Support Solutions control command center in Norristown, Montgomery County, Pennsylvania, which employs several thousand workers. The defense contractor's global headquarters is in Bethesda, Maryland, just outside the nation's capital.

---

37 According to former FBI agent Bob Levin, the torture matrix is set up to (1) cause self-inflicted harm and (2) sensory disorientation; (3) attack individual fears; (4) attack cultural identity.

Much as Raytheon owned the patents and oversaw HAARP for the CIA, Lockheed Martin oversees the Space Fence lockdown infrastructure and the development of the covert IO microwave assault on the public and training programs in *passive millimeter imaging*, such as for Homeland Security's Transportation Security Administration (TSA) and FBI agents:

> Each day, a nationwide scalar electromagnetic radiation "multifunctional" radio frequency directed-energy weapon attack system employing phased array cell tower antenna transmitter / receivers and GPS satellites, under the administration of U.S. Cyber command and military contractor Lockheed Martin, is used to silently and invisibly torture, impair, subjugate, and degrade the physical and neurological health of untold thousands of American citizens who have been extrajudicially "targeted" by a hate- and ideology-driven domestic "disposition matrix" as "dissidents" or "undesirables."[38]

So the next time you're checking the Live Map of Satellite Positions https://in-the-sky.org/satmap_worldmap.php, expand your idea of what some of those satellites are being tasked with by remembering how all of humanity is now *transparent* to surveillance instruments around, above, and inside, and that streams of the Big Data files being crunched by thousands of supercomputers on Earth are being fed to satellite supercomputers so beam weapons can infuse our thoughts with others' thoughts and make us think *diffuse artificial thoughts* that we assume are ours.

DARPA is now going public with how they hack into the peripheral nervous system "to trick the brain into thinking that it is learning fast [and] . . . benefit from the synaptic plasticity of our brain."[39] The Targeted Neuroplasticity Training (TNT) program is sheer "enhancement" mind control, but DARPA prefers to describe it as "modulat[ing] peripheral nerves" and "controlling synaptic plasticity of the brain." Intelligence and private contractor agents have a lot of spy fun directing radio waves in the 800 MHz band at brains, or inducing trances at 6-7 Hz via air conditioners, having memorized the phreaking codes: 6 Hz for depression, 8.2 Hz for euphoria, 11-11.3 Hz for depressed agitation or riotous behavior, etc. Meanwhile, TV violence is ramped up to open the receptors in the brain for more phreaking and mind-mapping and -tapping.

Under Lockheed Martin protocols, FBI Roving Bug Project workshops teach how to gaslight, stalk, and torture citizens. Through cell phone network-

---

38 Vic Livingston, "U.S. Silently Tortures Americans With Cell Tower Electromagnetic Neuroweapon," December 29, 2011. http://viclivingston.blogspot.com/2013/06/us-cyber-commandlockheed-martin.html

39 Ryan De Souza, "Hacking Brain Possible with DARPA New Targeted Neuroplasticity Training Program." Hackread.com, March 22, 2016.

ing, teams keep track of the target's every move, thanks to SATINT from peering through roofs and windows. Stalkers speed dial and call all night long, scream and bang on walls, leave death threats on voice mail, recount what the target just did in the bathroom or bed, record what the target said on the cell phone and play it back to them, remote control their phone, etc. They learn how to operate classified surveillance technology like sonic lasers and bullets, and study how sysadmins, spies, search engines and advertisers collect log files for spying on Internet users. From the Surveillance to the Attack stage, they create a profile while complicit psychiatrists determine Attack goals according to DSM-5 standards (drive the target insane? kill others? kill themselves?). If not murder or suicide, then involuntary commitment to a mental institution for psychiatric evaluation and forced medication is the goal of most operations.

> In tandem with the secret government developing this secret harassment technology over the last decades, the [DSM-5] has been incorporating the artificial symptoms created by this technology into its guidelines. A psychiatrist cannot deviate from the [DSM-5] and expect to remain licensed. You are walking into a trap if you try to tell a psychiatrist you are under attack by high-tech weapons.
>
> The medication prescribed for the "mental illness" may be harmful and cause permanent damage to the person's brain. Some people refer to the forced medication of mentally ill people as "chemical lobotomy."[40]

SAIC ***Private***

Did you notice that SAIC is CIAS backwards?

Men who organize and perpetrate violence on others for profit are a particular kind of secret society—like the Fraternal Order of Police but perhaps with top security clearance and diplomatic channels. Such *omertà* Brotherhoods constitute a criminal class of disaster capitalism in service to black programs protected by military contractor corporations like *Science Applications International Corporation (SAIC)*. These Brotherhoods have no problem experimenting on the disenfranchised or laundering drug and human trafficking profits through Weed & Seed or Safe Home to pay the NYPD and other urban police departments and hospitals to look the other way when radiated, debilitated, and humiliated *targeted individuals (TIs)* hobble in for help.

When SAIC bought out Network Solutions Inc. (NSI) in 1995, it basically meant taking control of Internet domain names.

---

40 Paul Baird's old site "America's Secret Government," http://www.angelfire.com/nj4/hightechharassment/. See Paul Baird's new site: http://www.surveillanceissues.com/index.html.

The strings that were pulled before and during the Clinton administration's "Green Paper" and "White Paper" process, that ultimately resulted in the creation of NewCo, also known as ICANN, were pulled by SAIC. SAIC is a very interesting for-profit company with a multibillion-dollar annual revenue, most of which comes from classified contracts with the U.S. military. What's even more interesting about SAIC is that there is no external control on it: It is "employee-owned," i.e., there are no outside stockholders. If you leave the company, you have to sell your shares in it. SAIC's board of directors reads like a who's who of the military-industrial complex (former secretaries of defense, spy-agency heads, etc.). When you read about the government wasting billions on "homeland security," guess who gets it. SAIC's home page features their new brochure on "SAIC — Securing the Homeland."[41]

In 2009, the Internet domain name registry was supposedly transferred from the NSA and British Telecommunications (BT) to Nominet UK and the nonprofit ICANN, including a quiet agreement to open up Internet development and oversight to transnational corporations and governments. NSI is still going strong, and since former President Obama didn't renew control over ICANN on September 30, 2016, SAIC probably has carte blanche over that, too, in great part *because ICANN issues IP addresses to Internet of Things (IoT) devices*. IPV6 (Internet Protocol version 6) means digital slavery.[42]

Besides Internet control over the IoT, SAIC is busy setting up global dual-use communications for the military, FBI and IRS, handling electronic voting machines for fixed elections, training foreign militaries, targeting citizens, mind control, etc.—a real devil's kitchen. With 44,000 employees, SAIC is larger than Labor, Energy, and HUD combined. Not counting "black" contracts, SAIC holds thousands of active light-of-day no-bid federal contracts. As a "lead systems integrator" for the Army's Future Combat Systems Program, SAIC designed the Iraqi Reconstruction and Development Council two months before the 2003 assault on Iraq, packing the council with Iraqi journalists, police, military, etc. Through the Bureau for International Narcotics and Law Enforcement Affairs (INL), SAIC set up International Law Enforcement Academies (ILEAs) around the world—10,000 officers in 50 countries—to "ensure a safe environment abroad for market economies."

---

41 Damien Cave, "It's time for ICANN to go." Salon, July 2, 2002. The Internet Corporation for Assigned Names and Numbers of California (ICANN) was formed in 1998 to administrate for the Internet Assigned Numbers Authority (IANA).

42 Read Patrick Wood, "Technocracy: The Real Reason Why The UN Wants Control Over The Internet." Technocracy News, October 27, 2016.

Senior Executive Service (SES)43 ***Executive Branch, Government***

Begun in 1978 under President Jimmy Carter, a Council on Foreign Relations member, the Senior Executive Service (SES) is basically the shadow government with the power of the purse (including salaries) over 75 government agencies. It is known as the *keystone*. The Office of Personnel Management (OPM) makes sure the 8,000 SES slots are filled with career executives (salaries ~$250,000 per annum), the vast majority of whom are Departments of Defense and Justice. Seventy-five percent of the Security Exchange Commission (SEC) are SES members, and 70 percent of the Nuclear Regulatory Commission. SES members cannot be fired and are accountable to no one with their black budget and highest security clearance, nor do they have to suffer through background checks.

On December 18, 2015, President Obama signed Executive Order 13714, "Strengthening the Senior Executive Service," which expanded their power.

Serco Inc. ***British, Private***

Does British Serco serve as the corporate arm of the SES?

In *Under An Ionized Sky*, I mentioned Serco Group ($4 billion per annum), the biggest company nobody has heard of—the British outsource for support services founded in 1989. Until 1987, the Serco Group was RCA Services Limited, the British arm of the fading American Radio Corporation of America. Serco is involved in everything—trains, satellites, hospitals, schools, missile defense systems, American bases, border screening, Intelligence Community, Department of State, Homeland Security, etc., with a staff of 40,000 in 38 nations.

As the SES feeds endless lucrative contracts to Serco's 70 subsidiaries around the world, many of which serve British Aerospace (BAE) and Lockheed Martin, it is important to point out that the SES, alongside the Highlands Group, runs the nonprofit Aerospace Corporation in El Segundo, California, a federally funded R&D center. Serco also (1) manages U.S. FEMA Region 9 (Arizona, California, Hawaii, Nevada, and the Pacific Islands) for $610 million per annum, (2) oversees the pathologies Laboratory Corporation of America Holdings (LabCorp) whose annual revenue is $6 billion, and (3) is gatekeeper over the U.S. Patent and Trademark Office.[44]

---

43 See U.S. Government "Policy and Supporting Positions," Committee on Homeland Security and Governmental Affairs, U.S. Senate, 114th Congress, 2d Session, December 1, 2016, http://www.fdsys.gov.

44 See Chapter 5, "5G Wi-Gig & the Internet of Things (IoT)." Thanks to Douglas Gabriel and Michael McKibben for exposing the SES, Serco, Highlands Group, etc. ("SHOCKING Global Control System Exposed," American Intelligence Media, May 17, 2018);

Control over patents and visas (the National Visa Center) is accomplished through the subsidiary Serco Inc. in Herndon, Virginia (6,000 employees, annual revenue of $1 billion).

> Serco Inc., a provider of professional, technology, and management services, announced today that the Company recently processed their 4 millionth patent application for the U.S. Patent & Trademark Office (USPTO). USPTO is the government agency that grants U.S. patents and registers trademarks. Since 2006, Serco has performed classification and other analysis services . . . Serco's Intellectual Property (IP) team is responsible for the analysis of the full disclosure including claims, specifications, and drawings in patent applications to identify the subject matter contained in each application and to assign the appropriate U.S. and international classification symbols representative of proposed inventions. These classifications are critical elements to the patent process and are used to enable examiner and public search as well as for internal routing of documents at the USPTO.[45]

Needless to say, running the U.S. patent office in a Tesla era such as ours is a powerful position—as powerful as, say, the good old boy peer review system that decides which scientific papers will be published and which not. Trade secrets, copyrights, trademarks, and patents must pass through the Patent Office in their quest for legitimization, security, and funding. Copyrights and patents are the only two property rights specifically protected by the U.S. Constitution.

> A patent must contain enough detail to enable a third party with "ordinary skill in the art" to replicate it . . . ostensibly for the benefit of society. The expectation is that third party will license the underlying patent in the process of adding value to it.[46]

The patent system (like the peer review) has been hijacked. Not only are patentees disguising material contributors by making up fake companies ("fraud on the court" or "inequitable conduct"), but they are also subsuming others' inventions by not crediting their patents, source codes, etc. Two tragic examples among many of patent abuse come to mind: the PFN/Trac patent (see Chapter 5, "5G Wi-Gig and the Internet of Things") and the life patent-

---

and thanks to notes from Steemit, "Obama's Secret Army: The Senior Executive Services," richq11.

45 "Serco Processes 4 Millionth Patent Application for U.S. Patent and Trademark Office." PRNewswire, November 15, 2018.

46 PatentDocs.org.

ing / "gain of function" patents (see Chapter 14, "The COVID-19 'Vaccine' Event"). Technically, everyone who has undergone the COVID-19 gene transfer is now technically gain-of-function patented and therefore owned as "transhuman," which means they do not have human rights.[47]

Serco seems to operate as a CEO / don for exchange traded funds (ETFs) racketeers like BlackRock, Vanguard,[48] and State Street. According to AI expert David Hawkins who lives in British Columbia, Canada, this globalist triumvirate with $18 trillion in assets and an inside track on SIGINT, are the controllers of the world COVID-19 / "vaccine" drama and Five Eyes racketeers like Maximus ("to protect health, support families, strengthen workforces, and streamline government services"), Pfizer, and Microsoft.[49]

TCFD (Task Force on Climate-Related Financial Disclosure) **Private**

Chairman billionaire Michael Bloomberg, members picked by the financial Stability Board (G20 central banks)

According to the TCFD's website, its mission is to

> . . . develop voluntary consistent climate related financial risk disclosures for use by companies and provide information to investors, lenders, insurers and other stakeholders . . . The task force will consider the physical liability and transition risks associated with climate change and what constitutes effective financial disclosures across industries.

If the TCFD decides your business is contributing to "climate change" and is therefore a threat to civilization, you can bet banks, insurance corporations, and government will hear about it and thrust your business into social credits outer darkness.[50]

> *I doubt any medieval man would have much difficulty in feeling a sense of overwhelming foreboding in the face of the Soviet hammer and sickle symbol. Yet most modern literate people obviously don't know a thing about what that symbol actually represents, except on the most profane level as the implements of the farmer and the worker. The sickle symbolizes Saturn, also known as*

---

47 See Association for Molecular Pathology et al. v. Myriad Genetics, Inc., et al., April 15, 2013 – June 13, 2013, https://www.supremecourt.gov/opinions/12pdf/12-398_1b7d.pdf

48 See Bill Sardi, "Who Runs the World? BlackRock and Vanguard." LewRockwell.com, April 21, 2021.

49 See Bitchute video "April 19th 2021 David Hawkins exposes Trudeau & Gates family massive corruption," A Warrior Calls.

50 Thanks to Alexandra Bruce's Forbidden Knowledge TV text accompanying Spiro Skouras' YouTube, "The U.N. & Central Banks: A Rockefeller & Rothschild Coup," January 6, 2020.

Chronos-Saturn or as the Greeks called it Demiurgos, the operating engineer of the universe as opposed to the Creator of that universe. In the reign of Saturn, we see exorbitant building and modeling activities, and this is reflected in the Masonic reference to their god as the "Big Builder" or "Architect."

– Michael A. Hoffman II, Secret Societies and Psychological Warfare, 1992

Author Note

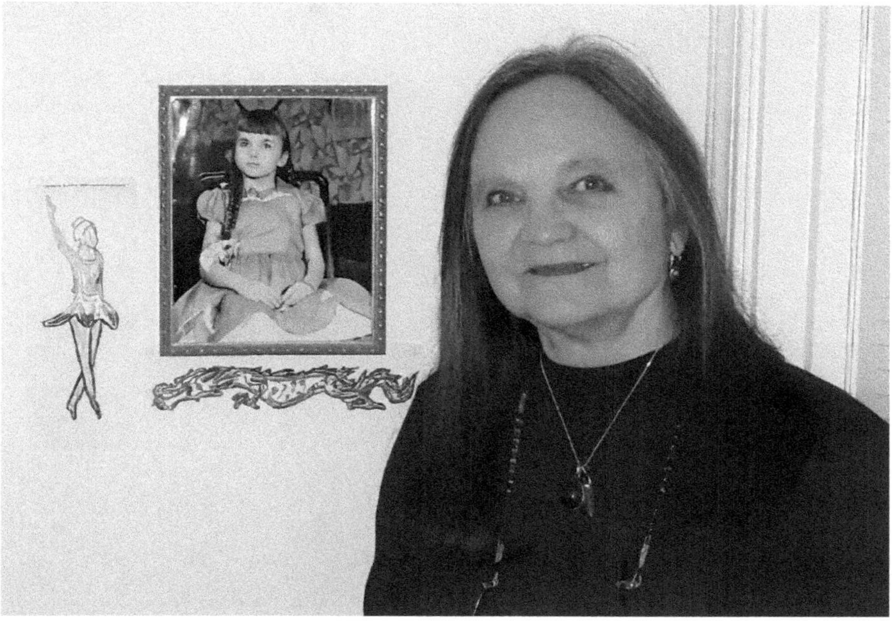

Elana Freeland is a writer, ghostwriter, teacher, storyteller, and lecturer who researches and writes on Deep State issues like geoengineering, MK-ULTRA, ritual abuse, targeting, and directed energy weapons.

The first book of her geoengineering trilogy was *Chemtrails, HAARP, and the Full Spectrum Dominance of Planet Earth* (Feral House, June 2014), the second book *Under An Ionized Sky: From Chemtrails to Space Fence Lockdown* (Feral House, February 2018), and now the third and last *Geoengineered Transhumanism: How the Environment Has Been Weaponized by Chemicals, Electromagnetics, & Nanotechnology for Synthetic Biology*.

Under An Ionized Sky has been translated into Serbian and is recommended as a supplementary text at a Technical University in Serbia, Nikola Tesla›s home nation; to date, it is the only book for the public about how Tesla technology has been weaponized on a planetary scale.

Freeland is also known for her 4-book series *Sub Rosa America: A Deep State History*, a fictional approach to the real history of America after President John F. Kennedy's televised assassination, including an 80-page bibliography at *elanafreeland.com* of real events the series exposes.

Glossary

Acid: pH <7

Acoustic or sonic: High-power low-frequency waves originally from antenna

bullets: dishes are now Flash Gordon-type portable acoustic guns

Acoustic gravity: Infrasound low frequency (20-100Hz) modulated by ultra-*waves* low infrasonic waves (0.1-15Hz). Many of the groans and hums heard around the world are acoustic gravity waves.

Alkaline: pH >7

AM: Amplitude modulation (see FM, frequency modulation)

Anthropogenic: Man-made

Artificial Intelligence (AI): Same as *Machine Intelligence (MI)*

Atmosphere: Composed of the *troposphere* (6-20km), stratosphere (20-50km), mesosphere (50-80km), thermosphere (80-690km)

BCI: Brain-computer interface

Biochemistry: Concerned with chemical and physicochemical processes in living organisms.

Bioelectricity / bioelectronics: Study and application of electric phenomena / electronics in *bioelectronics* medicine and biological processes.

Biofilm: Gell-like substance that bacterial colonies use to protect themselves

Biometrics: Human-made processes, substances, devices, or systems that imitate nature.

Biophysics: Application of the laws of physics to biological phenomena.

Bolometer: Measures incident electromagnetic radiation by heating a material with a temperature-dependent electrical resistance; from the Greek *bole* (βολή) for something thrown, as a ray of light

BMI: Brain-machine interface

Cation: An ion or group of ions having a positive charge.

Chelation: A type of bonding of ions and molecules to metal ions.

Chromatography: The separation of a mixture by passing it in solution or suspension or as a vapor (as in gas chromatography) through a medium in which the components move at different rates.

Climate: The balance between incoming short waves from the Sun (light) and loss of outgoing long-wave radiation (heat).

Clouds: A manifestation of weather and climate; gases in the atmosphere that absorb radiation from the Sun or Earth and radiate it back into space.

Cloud-seeding: Chemical treatment for local atmospheres. Silver iodide (AgI), "dry ice" (frozen CO2), and other chemicals convert clouds into ice crystal clouds of super-cooled water droplets.

5ISR: Command, control, communications, computers, combat, intelligence, surveillance, reconnaissance

CME: Coronal mass ejection

CMOS: Complementary metal oxide semiconductor

CPU: central processing unit; also QPUs (quantum processing units)

Curie: Unit of radiation; amount of any nuclide that undergoes 3.7×10^{10} radioactive disintegration per second. The safe standard of radioactivity is 100 billion curies; safe dose 100 microcuries per liter.

dB: Decibel; a measurement used in acoustics and electronics, such as gains of amplifiers, attenuation of signals, and signal-to-noise ratios..

DBS: Deep brain stimulation

Dielectric: Insulating as opposed to conductive

DMA: Direct memory access

Doppler: A specialized radar that bounces a microwave signal off of a target to analyze how the target's motion has altered the frequency of the return signal. The highly accurate *Doppler Effect or Shifting* is useful for aviation, satellites, weather systems, radar guns, and targeting. NEXRAD (NEXt generation weather RADar) is a Doppler radar system, and so is 3D video detection and ranging (ViDAR).

Dusty plasma (or complex plasma): nanometer- or micrometer-sized dust particles suspended in plasma. (Dust particles may be charged and therefore behave as a plasma that can create liquid and crystalline states and plasma crystals.)

Effective radiative power (ERP) Measures the combined power emitted by the transmitter and the ability of the antenna to direct that power in a given direction. It is equal to the input power to the antenna multiplied by the gain of the antenna. (Wikipedia)

Electrical brain stimulation: (EBS) Stimulation of a neuron or neural network in the brain through direct or remote excitation of cell membranes via electrodes or electromagnetic waves.

Electrochemical: The relation of electricity to chemical changes and interconversion of chemical and electrical energy.

Electrohypersensitivity / electrical sensitivity / electromagnetic hypersensitivity / multiple chemical sensitivity: (EHS / ES / MCS) Health effects from being exposed to an electromagnetic field (EMF)

Electrojet: A charging electric current 90-150 km (56-93 miles) in the ionosphere; the *equatorial electrojet* (magnetic equator) and *auroral electrojets* (Arctic and Antarctic Circles) are ionospheric fluctuations.

Electro-optics A branch of physics that deals with the effects of an *electric* field on light traversing it.

EHF: Extremely high frequency, 30-300 GHz. Transmissions travel in a straight line (a beam).

ELF: Extremely low frequency, 3-300 Hz

ERP: Effective radiated power of directional radio frequency

Eugenics: Pseudo-science aiming to minimize the genetic presence of certain traits while favoring others

Evoked potential: The individual electrical activity in the brain and spinal cord

Faraday cage: Conductive enclosure that shields from electric fields by channeling electricity along its walls

Frequency: The rate at which a particle vibrates in space. Electrons behave collectively in waves; ions move more slowly and make waves with a smaller frequency.

FFR: Frequency following response: an evoked potential generated by pulsed auditory stimuli; the neurological tendency of the brain to fall into rhythm with repetitive patterns; alignment of brain patterns. B2B or B2C (brain-to-brain, brain-to-computer) entrainment / subliminal programming. Brain locks onto an ELF signal and begins mirroring it.

FM: Frequency modulation (see AM, amplitude modulation)

FSB: Frequency-selective bolometer; low noise sub-millimeter to mid-infrared sensor

Gain of function: Employed to weaponize nature and thus patent it; activate genetic *function* mutations to enhance bioweapon potential

Gauss (G): Measurement of magnetic flux density or magnetic induction.

GE/GM/GMO: Genetically engineered / genetically modified organism

Genocide: Government-imposed measures to prevent births or deliberately kill a large number of people from a particular group with the aim of destroying it

GPR: Ground penetrating radar

GSM: Global System for Mobile communication is a digital mobile network widely used by Europe and other parts of the world.

G-force: gravitational force exerted on pilots who jink at close to 500 mph

Gyrotron resonance maser: A machine that talks to the brain after the PREMA scanner determines the brain's evoked potential

Harmonics: the mathematics that connect wavelengths of matter, gravity, and light

Hertz (Hz): a measure of frequency in cycles per second (cps). 1 Hertz wave is 186,000 miles long, the speed of light being 186,000 miles per second.

> **kHz (kilohertz)**, kHz 10^3 Hz)
>
> **MHz (megahertz)**, 10^6 Hz, one million (1,000,000) cycles per second (Hz)
>
> **GHz (gigahertz)**, 10^9 Hz, one billion (1,000,000,000) cycles per second (Hz)
>
> **THz (terahertz)** 10^{12} Hz, 1 THz = 1,000 GHz

Heterodyne: An engineering term meaning to mix signals

HPM: High-power microwave

HUMINT: Human intelligence

Hydroscope: An optical device for viewing objects underwater.

Hygroscopy: A substance's ability to attract and hold water molecules from the surrounding environment. *Hygroscope*: instrument showing changes in humidity.

IMINT: Imagery intelligence (NGA)

Infrared (IR): A wavelength from 800 nm to 1 mm, between visible light and microwaves. *Far infrared (FIR)* radiation has a wavelength of 15 micrometers (μm) to 1 mm, corresponding to a range of about 20 THz to 300 GHz.

Infrasound: <20 Hz

In silico: Experiments conducted by means of computer modeling or simulation

In situ: Measurements taken on site where the phenomenon is occurring

In vitro: Process taking place in a test tube or culture dish *outside* a living organism

In vivo: Process taking place *inside* a living organism

Ion: Atom, group of atoms, or molecule that has acquired or is regarded as having acquired a net electric charge by gaining or losing electrons.

Ionization: The process by which ions are formed, basically (1) passing radiation through matter, and (2) heating matter to high temperatures to force the electrons to leave the atom to become free electrons (negative charge). Whatever is left of the atom then becomes a positive ion.

Ionizing radiation: Radiation of energetic charged particles such as alpha and beta rays, nonparticulate radiation such as X-rays and neutrons.

Ionosphere: 50-600 miles (80-1,000 km) above the earth's surface; high concentration of ions and free electrons, thus able to reflect radio waves.

Interferometry: Said to be an approach to measurement by means of intersecting beams of light, radio or sound waves, interferometry is also used in its weapon capacity. HAARP is a scalar interferometer.

Kilometer: 0.621371 miles (a little over half a mile)

Laser: Light amplification by stimulated emission of radiation

LEO: Low-earth orbit

LIDAR: Light Detection and Ranging / Laser Imaging Detection and Ranging

Magnetohydrodynamics (MHD): Dynamics of fluids conducting electricity (like plasma and liquid metals). Fluid motion generates magnetic fields that confine plasma along magnetic lines of force.

Magnetosphere: Overlaps the ionosphere and extends into space to 60,000km (37,280 miles) toward the Sun, and over 300,000km (186,500 miles) away from the Sun (nightward) as the Earth's magnetotail.

Magnetron: A barrier microwave technology that operates non-ionizing radiation at the extremely high frequency (EHF) end of the spectrum by generating electrons with a cathode-anode cylinder to combine a magnetic field with an electrical field. A large magnetron can generate a consistent EHF beam of microwave pulses equaling 10 million watts (10MW) per pulse. Microwave ovens are armed with magnetrons.

MASER: Microwave Amplification by Stimulated Emission of Radiation

MASINT: Measurement and signature intelligence (Defense Intelligence Agency, DIA)

Materials science or physics: A syncretic construction discipline hybridizing metallurgy, ceramics, solid-state physics, and chemistry; nanotechnology.

Metamaterial: (Greek, *meta* – beyond) Engineered to have a property that is not found in nature

Micron (µm): 1 micrometer = one millionth of a meter (0.000039 inch) or 1,000 nanometers. 1/70 the thickness of a human hair.

Millimeter (mm): 1 millimeter = one thousandth of a meter (0.039 inch), the International System Units (SI) base unit.

Molecular biology: The branch of biology dealing with the structure and function of macromolecules (e.g. proteins and nucleic acids) essential to life; in which physics, biology, and chemistry merge.

Nanometer (nm): 1 nm = 1 billionth of a meter (0.000000001 m)

Nanoscience / nanotechnology: The study and application of extremely small things on the atom level used in other science fields, such as chemistry, biology, physics, materials science, and engineering.

NBIC: Nanotech, biotech, info tech, cognitive tech

NGA: National Geospatial-Intelligence Agency

NEO: Near-earth orbit

Neuroscience: Any science (like neurochemistry or experimental psychology) that deals with the nervous system and brain.

Neuroweapon: Any weapon that targets the nervous system; psychotronic weapons.

Neutrino: A type of scalar wave having to do with internal communication; an electrically neutral subatomic particle with a mass close to zero.

Nonionizing: Nonthermal radiation; insufficient energy to cause ionization *radiation* or heating: electric and magnetic fields, radio waves, microwaves, infrared, ultraviolet, and visible radiation.

Nuclide: Any atomic nucleus specified by atomic number, atomic mass, and energy state.

Numerical: Calculating by means of numerical algorithms the current densities *dosimetry* and specific absorption rates (SARs) in tissues and organs of individuals exposed to EM fields.

Orgone: Wilhelm Reich, MD's term for life-giving æther

OS/EH: Organized stalking ("gang stalking," a Stasi tactic) / electronic harassment

OTH: Over-the-horizon radar

PM: Particulate matter 10 microns or less. Coarse particle = 10,000-2,500 nanometers; fine particles = 2,500-100 nanometers; nanoparticle (ultrafine) = 1-100 nanometers.

ppm: Parts per million

Permittivity: Ability of a substance to store electrical energy in an electric field

Photon: A quantum of electromagnetic energy generally regarded as a particle with no mass or electric charge.

Physics: Study of matter and energy, including electricity, magnetism, and electromagnetism.

Piezoelectric: Electricity resulting from pressure and latent heat, such as in crystals.

Plasma: Fourth state of matter; an ionized (electrically conductive) gas in which atoms have lost electrons and exist in a mixture of free electrons and positive ions. *Positively charged particles (electrons and ions) governed by electric and magnetic forces possess collective behavior.*

Positron: The antimatter counterpart of the electron.

PREMA: "Phreaking." Personal radio and electromagnetic frequency *Prime Freak* scanner that identifies a brain's unique frequency (evoked potential) so the gyrotron resonance maser can talk to the brain (voice-to-skull, V2K).

Psychotronic weapons: See neuroweapons.

Quantum: Particle mediating a specific type of fundamental interaction; an indivisible unit of energy.

Quark: Any of three hypothetical subatomic particles having electric charges of 1/3 or 2/3 the magnitude of an electron.

Qubit: A quantum bit (particle in superposition).

Quorum sensing (QS): Cell-to-cell communication.

Radar: Radio Detection and Ranging

Radon: A chemically inert, radioactive gaseous element produced by the decay of radium.

RAM: Random access memory

ROM: Read-only memory

RFR: Radio frequency radiation

SAR: Specific absorption rate of radiation (usually ionizing): 1.6W/kg (FCC)

Scalar: Having only magnitude, not direction; longitudinal as opposed to EM waves which are transverse. Unlike electromagnetic waves, scalar waves have to do with Nature and the supernatural. Unfortunately, they have been weaponized (HAARP being only one example). Recommended reading: T.E. Bearden, "Background For Pursuing Scalar Electromagnetics," February 1992.

SDI: Strategic Defense Initiative; "Star Wars"

SIGINT: Signals intelligence

SLF: Super low frequency

SMART: Secret Militarized Armaments Residential Technology

Spectrometry: The measurement of the interactions between light and matter, reactions and measurements of radiation intensity and wavelength.

Spectroscopy: The study of the interaction between matter and electromagnetic radiation.

Spectrum analyzer: Real time spectrum analyzers (RTSAs) find interfering and infringing signals in the environment, and a superheterodyne spectrum analyzer translates frequencies. Most spectrum analyzers have digital displays that digitize video signals with an analog-to-digital converter (ADC). One of the primary uses of a spectrum analyzer being to search out and measure low-level signals, it is essential for targeted mind control.

SRM: Solar radiation management

SWS: Sentient world simulation

Synergy: Increased intensity caused by the combination of two or more substances

Techlepathy: communication of information directly from one mind to another (i.e. telepathy) with the assistance of technology

Telemetry: Recording and transmitting readings of an instrument.

Terabit: 1 terabit (Tb) = 10^{12} bits = 1 000 000 000 000 bits = 1,000 gigabits

TMS: Transcranial magnetic stimulation

Transmitter: Electronic device that uses radio waves to transmit data by converting energy from the power source into radio waves then sent to receivers

Troposcatter: Tropospheric scatter uses microwave transmitters to do what the gyrotron resonance maser does. The *troposphere* is our lowest region of the atmosphere, extending 3.7–6.2 miles (6–10 km).

TTWS: Through-the-wall-surveillance or sensor

UAP: Unidentified aerial phenomena, aka UFOs

ULF: Ultra low frequency

Ultrasound: >20,000 Hz

V2V: Vehicle to vehicle

VLF: Very low frequency (20-35 kHz)

VTRPE: Variable Terrain Radio Parabolic Equation

Viral vector: Virus modified to deliver genetic material into cells

Watts: Electrical power. For direct current (DC), watts = volts x amps; for alternating current (AC), calculating watts is more complicated but if using the Root Mean Squared (RMS) values for voltage and current, watts = volts x amps. Normal US household electricity is 120 volts, so if your appliance draws 2 amps, watts = 120 volts X 2 amps = 240 watts.

X-ray: 0.01 to 10 nm (shorter than UV waves, longer than gamma waves)

Yottabyte: According to NSA expert James Bamford, the equivalent of septillion bytes, a number so large that no one has yet coined a term for the next higher magnitude.

Lightning Source UK Ltd.
Milton Keynes UK
UKHW020437171221
395703UK00009B/528

9 780578 927053